Nursing Diagnosis Reference Manual

Twelfth Edition

LINDA LEE PHELPS, DNP, RN
Nursing Education
Escondido, California

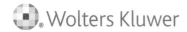 Wolters Kluwer

Philadelphia · Baltimore · New York · London
Buenos Aires · Hong Kong · Sydney · Tokyo

Vice President and Publisher: Julie K. Stegman
Senior Acquisitions Editor: Jonathan Joyce
Director of Nursing Education and Practice Content: Jamie Blum
Manager of Content Editing: Staci Wolfson
Editorial Coordinator: Marisa Solorzano-Taylor
Editorial Assistant: Devika Kishore
Marketing Manager: Sarah Schuessler
Senior Production Project Manager: Sadie Buckallew
Manager, Graphic Arts & Design: Stephen Druding
Manufacturing Coordinator: Margie Orzech
Prepress Vendor: S4Carlisle Publishing Services

Twelfth edition

Credits

Nursing diagnoses, definitions, and characteristics from Herdman, T. H., Kamitsuru, S., & Takáo Lopes, C. (Eds.). *Nursing Diagnoses: Definitions and Classification 2021-2023* (12th ed.). NANDA International, Inc. Copyright © 2021 by NANDA International, ISBN 978-1-68420-454-0 used by arrangement with the Thieme Group, Stuttgart/New York. 3/2022

Suggested NOC labels: Moorhead, S., Swanson, E., Johnson, M., & Maas, M. (Eds.). (2018). *Nursing outcomes classification (NOC): Measurement of health outcomes* (6th ed.). Elsevier.

Suggested NIC labels: Butcher, H. K., Bulechek, G. M., Dochterman, J. M., & Wagner, C. M. (Eds.). (2018). *Nursing interventions classification* (NIC) (7th ed.). Elsevier.

The clinical treatments described and recommended in this publication are based on research and consultation with nursing, medical, and legal authorities. To the best of our knowledge, these procedures reflect currently accepted practice. Nevertheless, they can't be considered absolute and universal recommendations. For individual applications, all recommendations must be considered in light of the patient's clinical condition and, before administration of new or infrequently used drugs, in light of the latest package-insert information. The authors and publisher disclaim any responsibility for any adverse effects resulting from the suggested procedures, from any undetected errors, or from the reader's misunderstanding of the text.

9 8 7 6 5 4 3 2 1

Printed in Mexico

Library of Congress Cataloging-in-Publication Data

ISBN-13: 978-1-9751-9895-4

ISBN-10: 1-9751-9895-6

Cataloging in Publication data available on request from publisher.

This work is provided "as is," and the publisher disclaims any and all warranties, express or implied, including any warranties as to accuracy, comprehensiveness, or currency of the content of this work.

This work is no substitute for individual patient assessment based upon healthcare professionals' examination of each patient and consideration of, among other things, age, weight, gender, current or prior medical conditions, medication history, laboratory data and other factors unique to the patient. The publisher does not provide medical advice or guidance and this work is merely a reference tool. Healthcare professionals, and not the publisher, are solely responsible for the use of this work including all medical judgments and for any resulting diagnosis and treatments.

Given continuous, rapid advances in medical science and health information, independent professional verification of medical diagnoses, indications, appropriate pharmaceutical selections and dosages, and treatment options should be made and healthcare professionals should consult a variety of sources. When prescribing medication, healthcare professionals are advised to consult the product information sheet (the manufacturer's package insert) accompanying each drug to verify, among other things, conditions of use, warnings and side effects and identify any changes in dosage schedule or contraindications, particularly if the medication to be administered is new, infrequently used or has a narrow therapeutic range. To the maximum extent permitted under applicable law, no responsibility is assumed by the publisher for any injury and/or damage to persons or property, as a matter of products liability, negligence law or otherwise, or from any reference to or use by any person of this work.

QUADM0722

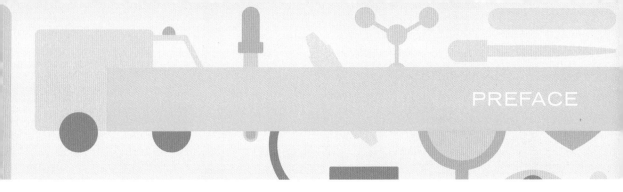

*N*ursing Diagnosis Reference Manual, 12th edition, offers clearly written, authoritative care plans to meet the health care needs of patients throughout the life span. This edition contains monographs for 46 new/revised nursing diagnoses, updated information for 67 nursing diagnoses, and updated definitions and content to meet the 2021 to 2023 NANDA-I standards. An updated feature in this edition highlights interventions that meet the Quality and Safety Education for Nurses (QSEN) criteria for patient-centered care or safe practice. Look for the icons throughout the book: **PCC** Patient-Centered Care; **EBP** Evidence-Based Practice; **S** Safety; **T&C** Teamwork and Collaboration; **QI** Quality Improvement; **I** Informatics.

The nursing process is the foundation for all nursing actions. Each monograph included in *Nursing Diagnosis Reference Manual*, 12th edition, has been constructed utilizing the nursing process. There are 267 comprehensive monographs for NANDA-I-approved nursing diagnoses included in this edition of the book. The monographs were written and reviewed by leading nursing clinicians, educators, and researchers. Each monograph is complete and can be used independently, thereby eliminating the need to search for material in different places.

Nursing Diagnosis Pocket Guide, fourth edition, is a pocket-sized companion to this manual. The pocket guide contains one monograph for each diagnosis and is organized using the NNN Taxonomy of Nursing Practice and the International Classification of Nursing Practice (ICNP) intervention terminology. Both the pocket guide and the reference manual include the linkages between NANDA International and the Nursing Interventions Classification (NIC) and Nursing Outcomes Classification (NOC) labels. You'll find the monographs invaluable in every health care setting you encounter throughout your career.

STUDENT AND INSTRUCTOR RESOURCES

Visit the Point to find additional resources for students and instructors. Available resources include journal articles, case studies, assignments, and more!

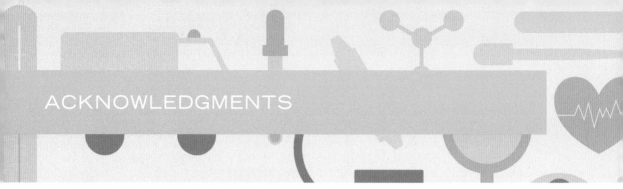

ACKNOWLEDGMENTS

I wish to express my sincere appreciation to everyone who helped make the *Nursing Diagnosis Reference Manual*, 12th edition, possible. I am grateful to Jonathan Joyce and Wolters Kluwer for allowing me to continue my passion for nursing language and teaching.

I dedicate this book to all nurses, students to expert clinicians, who are tirelessly dedicated to providing quality patient care.

—Linda Lee Phelps

CONTENTS

PREFACE   iii

ACKNOWLEDGMENTS   iv

OVERVIEW OF THE NURSING PROCESS   vii

INTRODUCTION   1

A 2

B 44

C 81

D 156

E 199

F 226

G 277

H 293

I 344

K 380

L 385

M 401

N 431

O 450

P 463

R 535

S 575

T 685

U 719

V 733

W 745

APPENDIX A   Selected Nursing Diagnoses by Medical Diagnosis   751

APPENDIX B   Select Nursing Diagnoses by Population Focus   790

APPENDIX C   Organizing Assessment Data   796

INDEX   799

The nursing process provides a framework for independent nursing action, promotes a consistent structure for professional practice, and helps bring focus more precisely on each patient's health care needs. The nursing process is a systematic method for making decisions and implementing care. Steps in the nursing process include:

- assessing the patient's problems;
- forming a diagnostic statement;
- identifying expected outcomes;
- creating a plan to achieve expected outcomes and solve the patient's problems;
- implementing the plan or assigning others to implement it;
- evaluating the plan's effectiveness.

These phases of the nursing process—assessment, nursing diagnosis formation, outcome identification, care planning, implementation, and evaluation—are dynamic, flexible, and frequently overlap. The American Nurses Association (2015) has established these phases to meet professional Standards of Practice.

Becoming familiar with the nursing process has many benefits. It will allow you to apply your knowledge and skills in an organized, goal-oriented manner. It will also enable you to communicate about professional topics with colleagues from all clinical specialties and practice settings. Using the nursing process is essential to documenting nursing's role in the provision of comprehensive, quality patient care.

The recognition of the nursing process is an important development in the struggle for greater professional autonomy. By clearly defining those problems a nurse may treat independently, the nursing process has helped to dispel the notion that the nursing practice is based solely on carrying out the physician's orders.

Nursing remains in a state of professional evolution. Nurse researchers and expert practitioners continue to develop a body of knowledge specific to the field. Nursing literature is gradually providing direction to students and seasoned practitioners for evidence-based practice. A strong foundation in the nursing process will enable you to better assimilate emerging concepts and to incorporate these concepts into your practice. (See Table 1, *Nursing's Approach to Problem Solving*.)

TABLE 1. Nursing's Approach to Problem Solving

Dynamic and flexible, the phases of the nursing process resemble the steps that many other professions rely on to identify and correct problems. Here's how the nursing process phases correspond to the standard problem-solving method.

NURSING PROCESS	PROBLEM-SOLVING METHOD
Assessment	
• Collect and analyze subjective and objective data about the patient's health problem	• Recognize the problem • Learn about the problem by obtaining facts
Diagnosis	
• State the health problem	• State the nature of the problem
Outcome identification	
• Identify expected outcomes	• Establish goals and a time frame for achieving them
Planning	
• Write a care plan that includes the nursing interventions designed to achieve expected outcomes	• Think of and select ways to achieve goals and solve the problem
Implementation	
• Put the care plan into action • Document the actions taken and their results	• Act on ways to solve the problem
Evaluation	
• Critically examine the results achieved • Review and revise the care plan as needed	• Decide if the actions taken have effectively solved the problem

ASSESSMENT

The first and most critical phase in the nursing process—assessment—consists of the patient history, the physical examination, and pertinent diagnostic studies. Nurses also collect information about patient strengths and areas where potential problems exist. The other nursing process phases—nursing diagnosis formation, outcome identification, planning care, implementation, and evaluation—depend on the quality of the assessment data for their effectiveness.

A properly recorded initial assessment provides:

- a way to communicate patient information to other caregivers;
- a method of documenting initial baseline data;
- a foundation on which to build an effective care plan.

Your initial patient assessment begins with the collection of data (patient history, physical examination findings, and diagnostic study data) and ends with a statement of the patient's deficiency in, risk for, or readiness for enhancement of a specific problem that is written as the nursing diagnosis.

Building a Database

The information you collect when taking the patient's history, performing a physical examination, and analyzing test results serves as your assessment database. Your goal is to gather and record information that will be most helpful in assessing your patient. You can't realistically collect—or use—*all* the information that exists about the patient. To limit your database appropriately, ask yourself these questions:

- What data do I want to collect?
- How should I collect the data?
- How should I organize the data to make care planning decisions?

Your answers will help you to be selective in collecting meaningful data during patient assessment.

The well-defined database for a patient may begin with admission signs and symptoms, chief complaint, or medical diagnosis. It may also center on the type of patient care given in a specific setting, such as the intensive care unit (ICU), the emergency department (ED), or an outpatient care center. For example, you wouldn't ask a trauma patient in the ED about a family history of breast cancer nor would you perform a routine breast examination. You would, however, do these types of assessment during a comprehensive health checkup in an outpatient care setting.

If you work in a setting where patients with similar diagnoses are treated, choose your database from information pertinent to this specific patient population. Even when addressing patients with similar diagnoses, complete a thorough assessment to make sure unanticipated problems don't go unnoticed.

Collecting Subjective and Objective Data

The assessment data you collect and analyze fall into two important categories: subjective and objective. The patient's *history*, embodying a *personal perspective* of problems and strengths, provides subjective data. It's your most important assessment data source. Because it's also the most subjective source of patient information, it must be interpreted carefully.

In the *physical examination* of a patient—involving inspection, palpation, percussion, and auscultation (IPPA)—you collect *objective data* about the patient's health status or about the pathologic processes that may be related to illness or injury. In addition to adding to the patient's database, this information helps you interpret the patient's history more accurately by providing a basis for comparison. Use it to validate and amplify the historical data. However, don't allow the physical examination to assume undue importance—formulate your nursing diagnosis by considering all the elements of your assessment, not just the examination.

Laboratory test results are another objective form of assessment data and the third essential element in developing your assessment. Laboratory values will help you interpret—and usually clarify—your history and physical examination findings. The advanced technology used in laboratory tests enables you to assess anatomic, physiologic, and chemical processes that can't be assessed subjectively or by physical examination alone. For example, if the patient complains of fatigue (history) and you observe conjunctival pallor (physical examination), check the patient's hemoglobin level and hematocrit (laboratory data).

Both subjective (history) and objective (physical examination and laboratory test results) data are essential for comprehensive patient assessment. They validate each other and together provide more data than either can provide alone. By considering history, physical examination, and laboratory data in their appropriate relationships to one another, you'll be able to develop a nursing diagnosis on which to formulate an effective care plan.

Taking a Complete Health History

This portion of the assessment consists of the subjective data you collect from the patient. A complete health history provides the following information about a patient:

- Biographical data, including ethnic, cultural, health-seeking, and spiritual factors
- Chief complaint (or concern)

- History of present illness (or current health status)
- Health promotion behaviors, motivation
- Past health history
- Family medical history
- Psychosocial history
- Activities of daily living (ADLs)
- Review of systems

Follow this orderly format in taking the patient's history, but allow for modifications based on the patient's chief complaint or concern. For example, the health history of a patient with a localized allergic reaction will be much shorter than that of a patient who complains vaguely of mental confusion and severe headaches.

If the patient has a chief complaint, use information from the health history to decide whether problems stem from physiologic causes or psychophysiologic maladaptation and how nursing interventions may help. The depth of such a history depends on the patient's cooperation and your skill in asking insightful questions.

A patient may request a complete physical checkup as part of a periodic (perhaps annual) health maintenance routine. Such a patient may not have a chief complaint. Therefore, this patient's health history should be comprehensive with detailed information about lifestyle, self-image, family and other interpersonal relationships, and degree of satisfaction with current health status.

Be sure to record health history data in an organized fashion to ensure the information will be meaningful to everyone involved in the patient's care. Some health care facilities provide patient questionnaires or computerized checklists. (See Box 1, *Using an Assessment Checklist.*)

These forms make history-taking easier, but they aren't always available. Therefore, you must know how to take a comprehensive health history without them. This is easy to do if you develop an orderly and systematic method of interviewing. Ask the history questions in the same order every time. With experience, you'll know which types of questions to ask in specific patient situations.

REVIEW OF SYSTEMS

When interviewing the patient, use this review of systems as a guide.

- *General:* Overall state of health, ability to carry out ADLs, weight changes, fatigue, exercise tolerance, fever, night sweats, repeated infections
- *Skin:* Changes in color, pigmentation, temperature, moisture, or hair distribution; eruptions; pruritus; scaling; bruising; bleeding; dryness; excessive oiliness; growths; moles; scars; rashes; scalp lesions; brittle, soft, or abnormally formed nails; cyanotic nail beds; pressure ulcers
- *Head:* Trauma, lumps, alopecia, headaches
- *Eyes:* Nearsightedness, farsightedness, glaucoma, cataracts, blurred vision, double vision, tearing, burning, itching, photophobia, pain, inflammation, swelling, color blindness, injuries (also ask about use of glasses or contact lenses, date of last eye examination, and past surgery to correct vision problems)
- *Ears:* Deafness, tinnitus, vertigo, discharge, pain, tenderness behind the ears, mastoiditis, otitis or other ear infections, earaches, ear surgery
- *Nose:* Sinusitis, discharge, colds, or coryza more than four times per year; rhinitis; trauma; sneezing; loss of sense of smell; obstruction; breathing problems; epistaxis
- *Mouth and throat:* Changes in color or sores on tongue, dental caries, loss of teeth, toothaches, bleeding gums, lesions, loss of taste, hoarseness, sore throats (streptococcal),

BOX 1. Using an Assessment Checklist

Use an assessment checklist such as this to ensure that you cover all key points during your health history interview. Although the format may vary from one facility to another, all assessment checklist guides include the same key elements.

- *Reason for hospitalization or chief complaint:* As patient sees it
- *Duration of this problem:* As patient recalls it (Has it affected the patient's lifestyle?)
- *Other illnesses and previous experience with hospitalization(s):* Reason, date(s), results, impressions of previous hospitalizations, problems encountered, effect of this hospitalization on education, family, child care, employment, finances
- *Observation of patient's condition:* Level of consciousness, well-nourished, healthy, color, skin turgor, senses, headaches, cough, syncope, nausea, seizures, edema, lumps, bruises or bleeding, inflammation, integrity of skin, pressure areas, temperature, range of motion, unusual sensations, paralysis, odors, discharges, pain
- *Mental and emotional status:* Cooperative, understanding, anxious, language, expectations, feelings about illness, state of consciousness, mood, self-image, reaction to stress, rapport with interviewer and staff, compatibility with roommate
- *Review of systems:* Neurologic; eye, ear, nose, throat (EENT); pulmonary; cardiovascular; gastrointestinal (GI); genitourinary (GU); skin; reproductive; musculoskeletal; and so forth
- *Allergies:* Food, drugs, other allergens, type of reaction
- *Medication:* Dosage, why taken, when taken, last dose, does the patient have it, any others taken occasionally, recently, why, use of over-the-counter drugs or cough preparations, use of alcohol or recreational drugs
- *Prostheses:* Pacemaker, intermittent positive-pressure breathing unit, tracheostomy tube, drainage tubes, feeding tube, catheter, ostomy appliance, breast form, hearing aid, glasses or contact lenses, dentures, false eye, prosthetic limb, cane, brace, walker, does the patient have the device, need anything
- *Hygiene patterns:* Dentures, gums, teeth, bath or shower, when taken
- *Rest and sleep patterns:* Usual times, aids, difficulties
- *Activity status:* Self-care, ambulatory aids, daily exercise
- *Bladder and bowel patterns:* Continence, frequency, nocturia, characteristics of stools and urine, discharge, pain, ostomy, appliances, who cares for these, laxatives, medications
- *Meals and diet:* Feeds self, diet restrictions (therapeutic and cultural or preferential), frequency, snacks, allergies, dislikes, fad diets, usual dietary intake
- *Health practices:* Breast self-examination, physical examination, Papanicolaou test, testicular self-examination, digital rectal examination, smoking, electrocardiogram, annual chest x-ray, practices related to other conditions, such as glaucoma testing, urine testing, weight control
- *Lifestyle:* Parent, family, number of children, residence, occupation, recreation, diversion, interests, financial status, religion, sexuality, education, ethnic background, living environment
- *Typical day profile:* As patient describes it
- *Informant:* From whom did you obtain this information: patient, family, old records, ambulance driver?

tonsillitis, voice changes, dysphagia, date of last dental checkup, use of dentures, bridges, or other dental appliances

■ *Neck:* Pain, stiffness, swelling, limited movement, or injuries

■ *Breasts:* Change in development or lactation pattern, trauma, lumps, pain, discharge from nipples, gynecomastia, changes in contour or in nipples, history of breast cancer (also ask whether the patient knows how to perform breast self-examination)

■ *Cardiovascular:* Palpitations, tachycardia, or other rhythm irregularities; pain in chest; dyspnea on exertion; orthopnea; cyanosis; edema; ascites; intermittent claudication; cold extremities; phlebitis; orthostatic hypotension; hypertension; rheumatic fever (also ask whether an electrocardiogram has been performed recently)

▨ *Respiratory:* Dyspnea, shortness of breath, pain, wheezing, paroxysmal nocturnal dyspnea, orthopnea (number of pillows used), cough, sputum, hemoptysis, night sweats, emphysema, pleurisy, bronchitis, tuberculosis (contacts), pneumonia, asthma, upper respiratory tract infections (also ask about results of chest x-ray and tuberculin skin test)

▨ *Gastrointestinal:* Changes in appetite or weight, dysphagia, nausea, vomiting, heartburn, eructation, flatulence, abdominal pain, colic, hematemesis, jaundice (pain, fever, intensity, duration, color of urine), stools (color, frequency, consistency, odor, use of laxatives), hemorrhoids, rectal bleeding, changes in bowel habits

▨ *Renal and genitourinary:* Color of urine, polyuria, oliguria, nocturia (number of times per night), dysuria, frequency, urgency, problem with stream, dribbling, pyuria, retention, passage of calculi or gravel, sexually transmitted disease (discharge), infections, perineal rashes and irritations, incontinence (stress, functional, total, reflex, urge), protein or sugar ever found in urine

▨ *Reproductive:* Male—lesions, impotence, prostate problems (also ask about use of contraceptives and whether the patient knows how to perform a testicular self-examination); female—irregular bleeding, discharge, pruritus, pain on intercourse, protrusions, dysmenorrhea, vaginal infections (also ask about number of pregnancies; delivery dates; complications; abortions; onset, regularity, and amount of flow during menarche; last normal menses; use of contraceptives; date of menopause; last Papanicolaou test)

▨ *Neurologic:* Headaches, seizures, fainting spells, dizziness, tremors, twitches, aphasia, loss of sensation, weakness, paralysis, numbness, tingling, balance problems

▨ *Psychiatric:* Changes in mood, anxiety, depression, inability to concentrate, phobias, suicidal or homicidal thoughts, hallucinations, delusions

▨ *Musculoskeletal:* Muscle pain, swelling, redness, pain in joints, back problems, injuries (such as fractured bones, pulled tendons), gait problems, weakness, paralysis, deformities, range of motion, contractures

▨ *Hematopoietic:* Anemia (type, degree, treatment, response), bleeding, fatigue, bruising (also ask whether patient is receiving anticoagulant therapy)

▨ *Endocrine and metabolic:* Polyuria, polydipsia, polyphagia, thyroid problem, heat or cold intolerance, excessive sweating, changes in hair distribution and amount, nervousness, swollen neck (goiter), moon face, buffalo hump

ENSURING A THOROUGH HISTORY

When documenting the health history, be sure to record both negative and positive findings, that is, note the absence of symptoms that other history data indicate might be present. For example, if a patient reports abdominal pain and burning, ask about experiencing nausea and vomiting or noticing blood in stools. Record the presence or absence of these symptoms.

Remember that the information you record will be used by others who will be caring for the patient. Recorded information can be used as a legal document in a liability case, a malpractice suit, or an insurance disability claim. With these considerations in mind, record history data thoroughly and precisely. Continue your questioning until you're satisfied that you've recorded sufficient detail. Don't be satisfied with inadequate answers, such as "a lot" or "a little"; such subjective terms must be explained within the patient's context to be meaningful. If taking notes seems to make the patient anxious, explain the importance of keeping a written record. To facilitate accurate recording of the patient's answers, familiarize yourself with standard history data abbreviations.

When you complete the patient's health history, it becomes part of the permanent written record. It will serve as a subjective database with which you and other health care professionals can monitor the patient's progress. Remember that history data must be specific and precise. Avoid generalities. Instead, provide pertinent, concise, detailed information that will help determine the direction and sequence of the physical examination—the next phase in your patient assessment.

Physical Examination

After taking the patient's health history, the next step in the assessment process is the *physical examination*. During this assessment phase, you obtain objective data that usually confirm or rule out suspicions raised during the health history interview.

Use four basic techniques to perform a physical examination: *inspection*, *palpation*, *percussion*, and *auscultation*. These skills require you to use your senses of sight, hearing, touch, and smell to formulate an accurate appraisal of the structures and functions of body systems. Using IPPA skills effectively lessens the chances that you'll overlook something important during the physical examination. In addition, each examination technique collects data that validate and amplify data collected through other IPPA techniques.

Accurate and complete physical assessments depend on two interrelated elements. One is the critical act of sensory perception, by which you receive and perceive external stimuli. The other element is the conceptual, or cognitive, process by which you relate these stimuli to your knowledge base. This two-step process gives meaning to your assessment data.

Develop a system for assessing patients that identifies problem areas in priority order. By performing physical assessments systematically and efficiently instead of in a random or indiscriminate manner, you'll save time and identify priority problems quickly. First, choose an *examination method*. The most commonly used methods for completing a total systematic physical assessment are *head-to-toe* and *major body systems*.

The head-to-toe method is performed by systematically assessing the patient by—as the name suggests—beginning at the head and working toward the toes. Examine all parts of one body region before progressing to the next region to save time and to avoid tiring the patient or yourself. Proceed from left to right within each region so you can make symmetrical comparisons, that is, when examining the head, proceed from the left side of the head to the right side. After completing both sides of one body region, proceed to the next.

The major body systems method of examination involves systematically assessing the patient by examining each body system in priority order or in an established sequence.

Both the head-to-toe and the major body systems methods are systematic and provide a logical, organized framework for collecting physical assessment data. They also provide the same information; therefore, neither is more correct than the other. Choose the method (or a variation of it) that works well for you and is appropriate for your patient population. Follow this routine whenever you assess a patient, and try not to deviate from it.

To decide which method to use, first determine whether the patient's condition is life-threatening. Identifying the *priority* problems of a patient suffering from a life-threatening illness or injury—for example, severe trauma, a heart attack, or gastrointestinal hemorrhage—is essential to preserve the patient's life and function and prevent additional damage.

Next, identify the *patient population* to which the patient belongs and take the common characteristics of that population into account in choosing an examination method. For example, elderly or debilitated patients tire easily; for these patients, you should select a method that requires minimal position changes. You may also defer parts of the examination to avoid tiring the patient.

Try to view the patient as an integrated whole rather than as a collection of parts, regardless of the examination method you use. Remember, the integrity of a body *region* may reflect adequate functioning of many body *systems*, both inside and outside the region in question. For example, the integrity of the chest region may provide important clues about the functioning of the cardiovascular and respiratory systems. Similarly, the integrity of a body *system* may reflect adequate functioning of many body *regions* and of the various systems within these regions.

You may want to plan your physical examination around the patient's *chief complaint* or *concern*. To do this, begin by examining the body system or region that corresponds to the chief complaint. This allows you to identify priority problems promptly and reassures the patient that you're paying attention to his or her chief complaint.

Physical examination findings are crucial to arriving at a nursing diagnosis and ultimately to developing a sound nursing care plan. Record your examination results thoroughly, accurately, and clearly. Although some examiners don't like to use a printed form to record physical assessment findings, preferring to work with a blank paper, others believe that standardized data collection forms can make recording physical examination results easier. These forms simplify comprehensive data collection and documentation by providing a concise format for outlining and recording pertinent information. They also remind you to include all essential assessment data.

When documenting, describe exactly what you've inspected, palpated, percussed, or auscultated. Don't use general terms, such as *normal*, *abnormal*, *good*, or *poor*. Instead, be specific. Include positive and negative findings. Try to document as soon as possible after completing your assessment. Remember that abbreviations aid conciseness. (See Box 2, *Documentation Tips*.)

NURSING DIAGNOSIS

According to NANDA International, the nursing diagnosis is a "clinical judgment concerning a human response to health conditions/life processes, or *susceptibility to that* response, by an individual, family, group, or community" (Herdman et al., 2021, p. 80). The nursing diagnosis must be supported by clinical information obtained during patient assessment. (See Box 3, *Nursing Diagnoses and the Nursing Process*.)

Each nursing diagnosis describes a patient problem that a nurse can legally manage. Becoming familiar with nursing diagnoses will enable you to better understand how nursing

---

BOX 2. Documentation Tips

Remember these rules about documenting your initial assessment:

- Always document your findings as soon as possible after you take the health history and perform the physical examination.
- Complete documentation of your assessment away from the patient's bedside. Jot down only key points while you're with the patient.
- If you're using an assessment form, answer every question. If a question doesn't apply to your patient, write "N/A" or "not applicable" in the space. (Unanswered questions give the appearance that the question was not assessed.)
- Focus your questions on areas that relate to the patient's chief complaint. Record information that has significance and will help you build a care plan.
- If you delegate the job of filling out the first section of the form to another nurse or an ancillary nursing person, remember—you must review the information gathered and validate it if you aren't sure it's correct.
- Always accept accountability for your assessment by signing your name to the areas you've completed.
- Always directly quote the patient or family member who gave you the information if you fear that summarizing will lose some of its meaning.
- Always write or print legibly, in ink.
- Be concise, specific, and exact when you describe your physical findings.
- Always go back to the patient's bedside to clarify or validate information that seems incomplete.

BOX 3. Nursing Diagnoses and the Nursing Process

When first described, the nursing process included only assessment, planning, implementation, and evaluation. However, during the past three decades, several important events have helped to establish diagnosis as a distinct part of the nursing process.

* The American Nurses Association (ANA), in its 1973 publication *Standards of Nursing Practice*, mentioned nursing diagnosis as a separate and definable act performed by the registered nurse. In 1991, the ANA published its revised standards of clinical practice, which continued to list nursing diagnosis as a distinct step of the nursing process.
* Individual states passed nurse practice acts that listed diagnosis as part of the nurse's legal responsibility.
* In 1973, the North American Nursing Diagnosis Association, now NANDA International, began a formal effort to classify nursing diagnoses. NANDA International continues to meet biennially to review proposed new nursing diagnoses and examine applications of nursing diagnoses in clinical practice, education, and research. NANDA International also publishes *Nursing Diagnoses: Definitions and Classification 2021–2023*, a complete list of nursing diagnoses, definitions, and defining characteristics. Currently, members of NANDA-I are working in cooperation with the ANA and the International Council of Nurses to develop an International Classification of Nursing Practice.
* The emergence of the computer-based patient record has underscored the need for a standardized nomenclature for nursing.

practice is distinct from medical practice. Although the identification of problems commonly overlaps in nursing and medicine, the approach to treatment clearly differs. Medicine focuses on curing disease; nursing focuses on holistic care that includes care and comfort. Nurses can independently diagnose and treat the patient's response to illness, certain health problems and risk for health problems, readiness to improve health behaviors, and the need to learn new health information. Nurses comfort, counsel, and care for patients and their families until they're physically, emotionally, and spiritually ready to provide self-care.

Developing Your Diagnosis

The nursing diagnosis expresses your professional judgment of the patient's clinical status, responses to treatment, and nursing care needs. In effect, the nursing diagnosis *defines* the practice of nursing. Translating the patient's history, physical examination, and laboratory data into a nursing diagnosis involves organizing the data into clusters and interpreting what the clusters reveal about the patient's ability to meet basic needs. In addition to identifying the patient's needs in coping with the effects of illness, consider what assistance the patient requires to grow and develop to the fullest extent possible.

Your nursing diagnosis describes the cluster of signs and symptoms indicating an actual or potential health problem that you can identify—and that your care can resolve. Nursing diagnoses that indicate potential health problems can be identified by the words "risk for," which appear in the diagnostic label. There are also nursing diagnoses that focus on prevention of health problems and enhanced wellness.

Creating your nursing diagnosis is a logical extension of collecting assessment data. In your patient assessment, you asked each history question, performed each physical examination technique, and considered each laboratory test result because it provided evidence of how the patient could be helped by your care or because the data could affect nursing care.

To develop the nursing diagnosis, use the assessment data you've collected to develop a problem list. Less formal in structure than a fully developed nursing diagnosis, this list describes the patient's problems or needs. It's easy to generate such a list if you use a conceptual model or an accepted set of criterion norms. Examples of such norms include normal physical and psychological development and Gordon's functional health patterns.

You can identify the patient's problems and needs with simple phrases, such as *poor circulation*, *high fever*, or *poor hydration*. Next, prioritize the problems on the list and then develop the working nursing diagnosis.

Writing a Nursing Diagnosis

Some nurses are confused about how to document a nursing diagnosis because they think the language is too complex. However, by remembering the following basic guidelines, you can ensure that your diagnostic statement is correct:

- Use proper terminology that reflects the patient's *nursing* needs.
- Make your statement concise so it's easily understood by other health care team members.
- Use the most precise words possible.
- Use a problem-and-cause format, stating the problem and its related cause.

Whenever possible, use the terminology recommended by NANDA-I.

NANDA-I diagnostic headings, when combined with suspected etiology and supported by defining characteristics or risk factors (Herdman et al., 2021), provide a clear picture of the patient's needs. Thus, for clarity in charting, start with one of the NANDA-I categories as a heading for the diagnostic statement. The category can reflect an actual or potential problem. Consider this sample diagnosis:

- *Heading*: Impaired physical mobility
- *Etiology*: Related to pain and discomfort following surgery
- *Signs and symptoms* (*these are the defining characteristics or risk factors*): "I can't walk without help." Patient hasn't ambulated since surgery on ____ (give date and time). Range of motion limited to 10 degrees flexion in the right hip. Patient can't walk 3 ft from the bed to the chair without the help of two nurses.
- This format links the patient's problem to the etiology without stating a direct cause-and-effect relationship (which may be hard to prove). Remember to state only the patient's problems and the probable origin. Omit references to possible solutions. (Your solutions will derive from your nursing diagnosis, but they aren't part of it.)

Avoiding Common Errors

One major pitfall in developing a nursing diagnosis is writing one that nursing interventions can't treat. Errors can also occur when nurses take shortcuts in the nursing process, either by omitting or hurrying through assessment or by basing the diagnosis on inaccurate assessment data.

Keep in mind that a nursing diagnosis is a statement of a health problem that a nurse is licensed to treat—a problem for which you'll assume responsibility for therapeutic decisions and accountability for the outcomes. A nursing diagnosis is *not* a

- diagnostic test ("schedule for cardiac angiography")
- piece of equipment ("set up intermittent suction apparatus")
- problem with equipment ("the patient has trouble using a commode")
- nurse's problem with a patient ("Mr. Jones is a difficult patient; he's rude and won't take his medication.")

- nursing goal ("encourage fluids up to 2,000 mL/day")
- nursing need ("I have to get through to the family that they must accept the fact that their father is dying.")
- medical diagnosis ("cervical cancer")
- treatment ("catheterize after each voiding for residual urine")

At first, these distinctions may not be clear. The following examples should help clarify what a nursing diagnosis is:

- Don't state a need instead of a problem.
  - Incorrect: Fluid replacement related to fever
  - Correct: Deficient fluid volume related to fever
- Don't reverse the two parts of the statement.
  - Incorrect: Lack of understanding related to noncompliance with diabetic diet
  - Correct: Noncompliance with diabetic diet related to lack of understanding
- Don't identify an untreatable condition instead of the problem it indicates (which can be treated).
  - Incorrect: Inability to speak related to laryngectomy
  - Correct: Social isolation related to inability to speak because of laryngectomy
- Don't write a legally inadvisable statement.
  - Incorrect: Skin integrity impairment related to improper positioning
  - Correct: Impaired skin integrity related to immobility

- Don't identify as unhealthful a response that would be appropriate, allowed for, or culturally acceptable.
  - Incorrect: Anger related to terminal illness
  - Correct: Ineffective therapeutic regimen management related to anger over terminal illness
- Don't make a tautological statement (one in which both parts of the statement say the same thing).
  - Incorrect: Pain related to alteration in comfort
  - Correct: Acute pain related to post-operative abdominal distention and anxiety
- Don't identify a nursing problem instead of a patient problem.
  - Incorrect: Difficulty suctioning related to thick secretions
  - Correct: Ineffective airway clearance related to thick tracheal secretions

How Nursing and Medical Diagnoses Differ

You assess your patient to obtain data in order to make a nursing diagnosis, just as the physician examines a patient to establish a medical diagnosis. It is important to understand the differences between the two and remember that they sometimes overlap. You perform a complete assessment to identify patient problems that nursing interventions can help resolve; your nursing diagnoses state these problems. (Some problems may be secondary to medical treatment.) If you plan your care of a patient around only the medical aspects of an illness, you'll probably overlook significant problems.

For example, suppose the patient's medical diagnosis is a fractured femur. In your assessment, take a careful history. Include questions to determine whether the patient has adequate financial resources to cope with prolonged disability. To assess the patient's capacity to adjust to the physical restrictions caused by the disability, gather data about his or her previous lifestyle.

Suppose your physical examination of this patient—in addition to uncovering signs and symptoms pertaining to the medical diagnosis—reveals actual or potential skin breakdown secondary to immobility. Your nursing diagnoses, in that case, may include home maintenance management impairment, diversional activity deficit (related to prolonged immobility), and risk for skin integrity impairment.

The care plan you prepare for this patient should include the nursing interventions suggested by your nursing diagnoses as well as the nursing actions necessary to fulfill the patient's medical treatment plan. When integrated into a care plan, the nursing and medical diagnoses describe the complete nursing care the patient needs. See Box 4, *Examples of Medical and Nursing Diagnoses*, for examples of differences between medical and nursing diagnoses.

OUTCOME IDENTIFICATION

During this phase of the nursing process, you will identify expected outcomes for the patient. Derived from the patient's nursing diagnoses, expected outcomes are goals that are measurable, patient focused, realistic, clear, concise, and time limited. These goals may be short- or long term. Short-term goals include those of immediate concern that can be achieved quickly. Long-term goals take more time to achieve and usually involve prevention, patient teaching, and rehabilitation.

In many cases, you can identify expected outcomes by converting the nursing diagnosis into a positive statement. For instance, for the nursing diagnosis "impaired physical mobility related to a fracture of the right hip," the expected outcome might be "The patient will ambulate independently before discharge."

When writing the care plan, state expected outcomes in terms of the patient's behavior— for example, "the patient correctly demonstrates turning, coughing, and deep breathing." Also, identify a target time or date by which the expected outcomes should be accomplished. The expected outcomes will serve as the basis for evaluating your nursing interventions.

If possible, consult with the patient and the patient's family when establishing expected outcomes. As the patient progresses, expected outcomes should be increasingly directed toward planning for discharge and follow-up care.

BOX 4. Examples of Medical and Nursing Diagnoses

Study the following examples here to better understand the difference between medical and nursing diagnoses:

- Frank Smith, age 67, complains of "stubborn, old muscles." He has difficulty walking, as you can see by his shuffling gait. During the interview, Mr. Smith speaks in a monotone and seems very depressed. Physical examination shows a pill-rolling hand tremor. Laboratory tests reveal a decreased dopamine level.
  - *Medical diagnosis:* Parkinson disease
  - *Nursing diagnoses:* Impaired physical mobility related to decreased muscle control; disturbed body image related to physical alterations; deficient knowledge related to lack of information about progressive nature of illness
- For 5 consecutive days, Judy Wilson, age 26, has had sporadic abdominal cramps of increasing intensity. Most recently, the pain has been accompanied by vomiting and a slight fever. Your examination reveals rebound tenderness and muscle guarding.
  - *Medical diagnosis:* Appendicitis
  - *Nursing diagnoses:* Acute pain related to biologic agents; deficient fluid volume related to vomiting
- During an extensive bout with respiratory tract infections, Tom Bradley, age 7, complains of throbbing ear pain. Tom's mother notes his hearing difficulty and his fear of the pain and possible hearing loss. On inspection, his tympanic membrane appears red and bulging.
  - *Medical diagnosis:* Acute suppurative otitis media
  - *Nursing diagnoses:* Acute pain related to swollen tympanic membrane; fear related to progressive hearing loss

Outcome statements should be tailored to your practice setting. For example, in the ICU, you may focus on maintaining hemodynamic stability, whereas in a rehabilitation unit, you would focus on maximizing the patient's independence and preventing complications. (See Box 5, *Understanding NOC.*)

Writing Expected Outcome Statements

Expected outcomes must be stated in measurable terms. Measurable terms describe observable results and provide the criteria for success; they clearly describe the expected result after interventions are implemented. Avoid ambiguous language such as *better*, *improve*, or *decrease* because such terms are difficult to quantify. When writing expected outcomes in your care plan, always start with a specific action verb that focuses on the patient's behavior. By telling your reader how the patient should *look*, *walk*, *eat*, *drink*, *turn*, *cough*, *speak*, or *stand*, for example, you give a clear picture of how to evaluate progress.

Avoid starting expected outcome statements with *allow*, *let*, *enable*, or similar verbs. Such words focus attention on your own and other health care team members' behavior—not on the patient's.

With many documentation formats, you won't need to include the phrase "The patient will …" with each expected outcome statement. You will, however, have to specify which person the goals refer to when family, friends, or others are directly concerned.

Make sure target dates are realistic. Be flexible enough to adjust the date if the patient needs more time to respond to your interventions.

PLANNING

The nursing care plan refers to a written plan of action designed to help you deliver quality patient care. It includes relevant nursing diagnoses, expected outcomes, and nursing interventions. Keep in mind that the care plan usually forms a permanent part of the patient's health record and will be used by other members of the nursing team. The care plan may be integrated into an interdisciplinary plan for the patient. In this instance, clear guidelines should outline the role of each member of the health care team in providing care.

Benefits of a Care Plan

To provide quality care for each patient, you must plan and direct that care. Writing a care plan allows you to document the scientific method used throughout the nursing process. In the care plan, you summarize the patient's problems and needs (as nursing diagnoses) and identify appropriate nursing interventions and expected outcomes. A care plan that's well conceived and properly written helps decrease the risk of incomplete or incorrect care by

BOX 5. Understanding NOC

The Nursing Outcomes Classification (NOC) is a standardized language of patient or client outcomes that was developed by a nursing research team at the University of Iowa. It contains 540 outcomes organized into 34 classes and 7 domains. Each outcome has a definition, list of measurable indicators, and references. The outcomes are research based, and studies are ongoing to evaluate their reliability, validity, and sensitivity. More information about NOC can be found at the Center for Nursing Classification and Clinical Effectiveness (https://nursing.uiowa.edu/cncce/nursing-outcomes-classification-overview).

- *Giving direction:* A written care plan gives direction by showing colleagues the goals you have set for the patient and gives clear instructions for assisting in goal achievement. The care plan also makes clear exactly what to document on the patient's progress notes. For instance, the plan should list what observations to make and how often, what nursing measures to take and how to implement them, and what to teach the patient and the patient's family before discharge.
- *Providing continuity of care:* A written care plan identifies the patient's needs to each caregiver and tells what must be done to meet those needs. With this information, nurses caring for the patient at different times can adjust their routines to meet the patient's care demands. A care plan also provides caregivers with specific instructions on patient care, eliminating the confusion that can exist. If the patient is discharged from your health care facility to another, your care plan can help ease this transition.
- *Establishing communication between you and other nurses who will care for the patient, between you and health care team members in other departments, and between you and the patient:* Soliciting the patient's input as you develop the care plan demonstrates that you value the patient's opinions and feelings. By reviewing the care plan with other health care team members and with other nurses, you can regularly evaluate the patient's response or lack of response to the nursing care and medical regimen.
- *Serving as a key for patient care assignments:* If you're a team leader, you may want to delegate some specific routines or duties described in each nursing intervention—not all of them need your professional attention.

Reviewing the Planning Stages

Formulating the care plan involves three stages:

- *Assigning* priorities to the nursing diagnoses: Any time you develop more than one nursing diagnosis for the patient, you must assign priorities to them and begin your care plan with those having the highest priority. High-priority nursing diagnoses involve the patient's most urgent needs (such as emergency or immediate physical needs). Intermediate priority diagnoses involve nonemergency needs, and low-priority diagnoses involve needs that don't directly relate to the patient's specific illness or prognosis.
- *Selecting* appropriate nursing actions (interventions): Next, you'll select one or more nursing interventions to achieve each of the expected outcomes identified for the patient. For example, if one expected outcome statement reads, "The patient will transfer to chair with assistance," the appropriate nursing interventions include placing the wheelchair facing the foot of the bed and assisting the patient to stand and pivot to the chair. If another expected outcome statement reads, "The patient will express feelings related to recent injury," appropriate interventions might include spending time with the patient each shift, conveying an open and nonjudgmental attitude, and asking open-ended questions.
- *Documenting* the nursing diagnoses, expected outcomes, nursing interventions, and evaluations on the care plan: Reviewing the second part of the nursing diagnosis statement (the part describing etiologic factors) may help guide your choice of nursing interventions. For example, for the nursing diagnosis "Risk for injury related to inadequate blood glucose levels," you would determine the best nursing interventions for maintaining an adequate blood glucose level. Typical interventions for this goal include observing the patient for evidence of hypoglycemia and providing an appropriate diet. Try to think creatively during this step in the nursing process. It's an opportunity to describe exactly what you and your patient would like to have happen and to establish the criteria against which you'll judge further nursing actions.

The planning phase culminates when you write the care plan and document the nursing diagnoses, expected outcomes, nursing interventions, and evaluations for expected outcomes. Write your care plan in concise, specific terms so that other health care team members can follow it. Keep in mind that because the patient's problems and needs will change, you'll have to review your care plan frequently and modify it when necessary.

Elements of the Care Plan

Care planning formats vary from one health care facility to another. For example, you may write your care plan on a form supplied by the hospital or you can use software that's approved by your facility. Nearly all care planning formats include space in which to document the nursing diagnoses, expected outcomes, and nursing interventions. In many health care facilities, you may also document assessment data and discharge planning on the care plan.

No matter which format you use, be sure to sign and date the care plan, even though you may have to make revisions if your nursing interventions don't work. Remember—the patient's care plan becomes part of the permanent record and shouldn't be erased or destroyed. The information must remain intact, enabling you and other health care team members to readily refer to nursing interventions used in the past. (See Box 6, *Guidelines for Writing a Care Plan*.)

Be specific when writing your care plan. By discussing specific problems, expected outcomes, nursing interventions, and evaluations for expected outcomes, you leave no doubt as to what needs to be done by other health care team members. For example, when listing nursing interventions, be sure to include *when* the action should be implemented, who should be involved in each aspect of implementation, and the *frequency*, *quantity*, and *method* to be used. Specify dates and times when appropriate. List target dates for each expected outcome.

BOX 6. Guidelines for Writing a Care Plan

Keeping these tips in mind will help you write an accurate and useful care plan.

- Write your patient's care plan in ink or use the facility's electronic form—it's part of the permanent record.
- Be specific; don't use vague terms or generalities on the care plan.
- Never use abbreviations that may be confused or misinterpreted. In general, it's better to use only established abbreviations and acronyms.
- Take time to review all your assessment data *before* you select an approach for each problem. (*Note:* If you can't complete the initial assessment, immediately note "insufficient database" on your records.)
- Write down a specific expected outcome for each problem you identify and record a target date for its completion.
- Avoid setting an initial goal that's too high to be achieved. For example, the outcome for a newly admitted patient with stroke stating, "Patient will ambulate with assistance," is an unrealistic initial goal because several patient outcomes will need to be achieved before this goal can be addressed.
- Consider the following three phases of patient care when writing nursing interventions: What observations to make and how often, what nursing measures to do and how to do them, and what to teach the patient and family before discharge.
- Make each nursing intervention specific.
- Make sure nursing interventions match the resources and capabilities of the staff. Combine what's necessary to correct or modify the problem with what's reasonably possible in your setting.
- Be creative when you write your patient's care plan; include a drawing or an innovative procedure if either will make your directions more specific.
- Don't overlook any of the patient's problems or concerns. Include them on the care plan so they won't be forgotten.
- Make sure your care plan is implemented correctly.
- Evaluate the results of your care plan and discontinue any nursing diagnoses that have been resolved. Select new approaches, if necessary, for problems that haven't been resolved.

If your nursing interventions have resolved the problem on which you've based the nursing diagnosis, write "discontinued" next to the diagnostic statement on the care plan and list the date you discontinued the interventions. If your nursing interventions haven't resolved the problem by the target date, reevaluate your plan and do one of the following:

■ Extend the target date and continue the intervention until the patient responds as expected.
■ Discontinue the intervention and select a new one that will achieve the expected outcome.

You'll need to update and modify a patient's care plan as problems (or priorities) change and resolve, new assessment information becomes available, and you evaluate the patient's responses to nursing interventions.

IMPLEMENTATION

During this phase, you put your care plan into action. Implementation encompasses all nursing interventions directed toward solving the patient's nursing problems and meeting health care needs. While you coordinate implementation, you also seek help from other caregivers, the patient, and the patient's family. (See Box 7, *Understanding NIC*.)

Implementation requires some (or all) of the following interventions:

■ Assessing and monitoring (e.g., recording vital signs)
■ Therapeutic interventions (e.g., giving medications)
■ Making the patient more comfortable and helping him or her with ADLs
■ Supporting the patient's respiratory and elimination functions
■ Providing skin care
■ Managing the environment (e.g., controlling noise to ensure a good night's sleep)
■ Providing food and fluids
■ Giving emotional support
■ Teaching and counseling
■ Referring the patient to appropriate agencies or services

Incorporate these elements into the implementation stage:

■ *Reassessing:* Although it may be brief or narrowly focused, reassessment should confirm that the planned interventions remain appropriate.
■ *Reviewing and modifying the care plan:* Never static, an appropriate care plan changes with the patient's condition. As necessary, update the assessment, nursing diagnoses, implementation, and evaluation sections. (Entering the new data in a different color of ink alerts other staff members to the revisions.) Date the revisions.
■ *Seeking assistance:* Determine, for example, whether you need help from other staff members or additional information before you can intervene.

BOX 7. Understanding NIC

The Nursing Interventions Classification (NIC) is a research-based clinical tool that standardizes and defines the knowledge base for nursing practice; it was developed by a nursing research team at the University of Iowa. It contains 565 interventions organized into 30 classes and 7 domains. Each intervention has a definition, list of indicators, publication facts line, and references (Butcher et al., 2018). The interventions are research based, and studies are ongoing to evaluate the effectiveness and cost of nursing treatments. More information about NIC can be found at the Center for Nursing Classification and Clinical Effectiveness (https://nursing.uiowa.edu/cncce/nursing-interventions-classification-overview).

Documentation

Implementation isn't complete until you've documented each intervention, the time it occurred, the patient's response, and any other pertinent information. Make sure each entry relates to a nursing diagnosis. Remember that any action not documented may be overlooked during quality assurance monitoring or evaluation of care. Thorough documentation offers a way for you to take rightful credit for your contribution in helping a patient achieve the highest possible level of wellness. After all, nurses use a unique and worthwhile combination of interpersonal, intellectual, and technical skills when providing care. (See Box 8, *Nursing Interventions: Three Types*.)

Evaluation

In this phase of the nursing process, you assess the effectiveness of the care plan by answering such questions as:

- How has the patient progressed in terms of the plan's projected outcomes?
- Does the patient have new needs?
- Does the care plan need to be revised?

Evaluation also helps you determine whether the patient received high-quality care from the nursing staff and the health care facility.

Steps in the Evaluation Process

Include the patient, family members, and other health care professionals in the evaluation. Then follow these steps:

- *Select evaluation criteria:* The care plan projected outcomes—the desired effects of nursing interventions—form the basis for evaluation.
- *Compare the patient's response with the evaluation criteria:* Did the patient respond as expected? If not, the care plan may need revision.
- *Analyze your findings:* If your plan wasn't effective, determine why. You may conclude, for example, that several nursing diagnoses were inaccurate.
- *Modify the care plan:* Make revisions (e.g., change inaccurate nursing diagnoses) and implement the new plan.
- *Reevaluate:* Like all steps in the nursing process, evaluation is ongoing. Continue to assess, plan, implement, and evaluate for as long as you care for the patient.

BOX 8. Nursing Interventions: Three Types

Knowing the three types of nursing interventions will help you document implementation appropriately.
- *Independent interventions.* These interventions fall within the purview of nursing practice and don't require a physician's direction or supervision. Most nursing actions required by the patient's care plan are independent interventions. Examples include patient teaching, health promotion, counseling, and helping the patient with activities of daily living.
- *Dependent interventions.* Based on written or oral instructions from another professional—usually a physician—dependent interventions include administering medication, inserting indwelling urinary catheters, and obtaining specimens for laboratory tests.
- *Interdependent interventions.* Performed in collaboration with other professionals, interdependent interventions include following a protocol and carrying out standing orders.

Questions to Answer

When evaluating and documenting the patient's care, collect information from all available sources—for example, the patient's medical record, family members, other caregivers, and the patient. Include your own observations.

During the evaluation process, ask yourself these questions:

- Has the patient's condition improved, deteriorated, or remained the same?
- Were the nursing diagnoses accurate?
- Have the patient's nursing needs been met?
- Did the patient meet the outcome criteria documented in the care plan?
- Which nursing interventions should I revise or discontinue?
- Why did the patient fail to meet some goals (if applicable)?
- Should I reorder priorities? Revise expected outcomes?

NURSING DIAGNOSES AND CRITICAL PATHWAYS

In a growing number of health care settings—inpatient and outpatient, acute and long-term care—critical pathways are being used to guide the process of care for a patient. Critical pathways describe the course of a specific health-related condition. A critical pathway may be used along with or instead of a nursing care plan, depending on the standards set by the individual health care facility. These tools may also be referred to as clinical pathways, care maps, collaborative care plans, or multidisciplinary action plans. (See Box 9, *Developing a Critical Pathway*.)

The concept of the critical pathway evolved out of the growth of managed care and the development of the case management model in the early 1990s. Pressure from managed care organizations to control costs led to the evolution of case management.

BOX 9. Developing a Critical Pathway

The critical pathway is an interdisciplinary tool that requires the collaborative efforts of all disciplines involved in patient care. The interdisciplinary team must decide on a diagnosis, select a set of achievable outcomes, and agree on a plausible time line for achieving the desired outcomes. Note that when establishing standard practices for treatment of a given condition, it has usually proved difficult for physicians to achieve consensus.

ESTABLISHING A TIMELINE

Time intervals allocated on a critical pathway vary according to the patient's condition and its acuity. For a hip replacement, the time line extends over days; for a cardiac catheterization procedure, time intervals are expressed in hours. In the post-anesthesia period, a critical pathway can be defined in minutes.

Average length of stay is an important concept in developing a critical pathway. If agency data indicate that the average length of stay for an inpatient who has had a modified radical mastectomy with reconstruction is 4 days, then the team begins planning around a 4-day stay.

BUILDING THE PATHWAY

The interdisciplinary team must choose a framework for developing outcomes and interventions. Some agencies build pathways around nursing diagnoses. If interdisciplinary collaboration is strong, an agency may build pathways around general aspects of care, for example, pain, activity, nutrition, assessment, medications, psychosocial status, treatments, teaching, and discharge planning.

In an acute care setting, outcomes and interventions for each aspect of care are determined for each day of an expected length of stay. In long-term care and other community-based settings, progress may be measured in longer intervals.

In case management, one professional—usually a nurse or a social worker—assumes responsibility for coordinating care so that patients move through the health care system in the shortest time and at the lowest cost possible.

Early on, case managers used the nursing process and based their plans on nursing diagnoses. Over time, however, it became evident that a multidisciplinary approach was needed to adequately monitor the length of stay and reduce overall costs. This led to the development of the critical pathway concept.

In critical pathways, a time line is defined for each condition and for the achievement of expected outcomes. By reading the critical pathway, caregivers can determine on any given day where the patient should be in his or her progress toward optimal health.

The critical pathway provides a method for physicians and nurses to standardize and organize care for routine conditions. These pathways also make it easier for case managers to track data needed to

- streamline utilization of material resources and labor
- ensure that patients receive quality care
- improve the coordination of care
- reduce the cost of providing care

The most successful critical pathways have been developed for medical diagnoses with predictable outcomes, such as hip replacement, mastectomy, myocardial infarction, and cardiac catheterization. Critical pathways work best with high-volume, high-risk, high-cost conditions or procedures for which there are predictable outcomes.

Care Planning for Students

Developing a care plan helps the nursing student improve problem-solving technique, learn the nursing process, improve written and verbal communication, and develop organizational skills. More important, it shows how to apply classroom and textbook knowledge to practice.

Because the purpose is to teach the care planning process, the student care plan is longer than the standard plan used in most health care facilities. In a step-by-step manner, student care plans progress from assessment to evaluation. However, some teaching institutions model the student care plan on the plan used by the affiliated health care institution, adding a space for the scientific rationale for each nursing intervention selected.

Writing out all of your planned actions enables you to review planned nursing activities with your clinical instructor. This is an opportunity to consider whether you have complete assessment data to support your diagnoses and interventions and whether you've taken into consideration all the problems that a more experienced nurse is likely to identify. See Box 10, *Care Plans*, for an explanation of each section of a care plan.

The Importance of Nursing Diagnoses

Using a critical pathway can be helpful, especially for nursing students and new graduates. You may be assigned to provide care to a particular patient for only 1 or 2 days. Seeing the entire pathway and examining the outcomes the patient is expected to achieve will help you obtain a broader clinical perspective on care.

Using a critical pathway as a guide for delivering care does not negate the need to formulate and utilize nursing diagnoses. Nursing diagnoses continue to define the primary responsibility of nursing—to diagnose and treat human responses to actual or potential health problems. The full nursing care needs of any patient are unlikely to be documented in a critical pathway. When using a pathway, always keep in mind that the patient may require nursing intervention beyond what's specified in the critical pathway.

BOX 10. Care Plans

All care plans contain the following sections:

* *Diagnostic statement.* Each diagnostic statement includes a NANDA-I-approved diagnosis and, in most cases, a related etiology. This edition of the *Nursing Diagnosis Reference Manual* contains all the diagnoses approved by NANDA-I to date.
* *Definition.* This section offers a brief explanation of the diagnosis.
* *Assessment.* This section suggests parameters to use when collecting data to ensure an accurate diagnosis. Data may include health history, physical findings, psychosocial status, laboratory studies, patient statements, and other subjective and objective information.
* *Defining characteristics.* This section lists clinical findings that confirm the diagnosis. For diagnoses expressing the possibility of a problem, such as "risk for injury," this section is labeled Risk Factors.
* *Expected outcomes.* Here you'll find realistic goals for resolving or ameliorating the patient's health problem, written in measurable behavioral terms. You should select outcomes that are appropriate to the condition of your patient. Outcomes are arranged to flow logically from admission to discharge of the patient. Outcomes identified by NOC research have been added to correlate with the NANDA-I expected outcomes.
* *Interventions and rationales.* This section provides specific activities you carry out to help attain expected outcomes. Each intervention contains a rationale, highlighted in italic type. Rationales receive typographic emphasis because they form the premise for every nursing action. You'll find it helpful to consider rationales before intervening. Understanding the why of your actions can help you see that carrying out repetitive or difficult interventions is an essential element of your nursing practice. More importantly, it can improve critical thinking and help you to avoid mistakes. Interventions from NIC research have been added to correlate with the interventions.
* *Evaluations for expected outcomes.* Here you'll find evaluation criteria for the expected outcomes. These criteria will help you determine whether expected outcomes have been attained or provide support for revising outcomes or interventions to meet changing patient conditions.
* *Documentation.* This section lists critical topics to include in your documentation—for example, patient perceptions, status, and response to treatment as well as nursing observations and interventions. Using the information provided in this section will enable you to write the careful, concise documentation required to meet professional nursing standards.

For example, a patient enters a hospital for a hip replacement and can't communicate verbally because of a recent stroke. The critical pathway wouldn't include measures to assist the patient to disclose personal needs. Therefore, you would develop a nursing care plan around the diagnosis, "Impaired verbal communication related to decreased circulation to the brain."

Even if you practice in a clinical setting that relies on critical pathways to fill documentation requirements, the *Nursing Diagnosis Reference Manual*, 12th edition, will prove to be a valuable resource for identifying and treating each patient's unique nursing needs. Creating a care plan based on carefully selected nursing diagnoses and using it along with a critical pathway will enable you to provide your patients with high-quality collaborative care that includes a strong nursing component.

REFERENCES

American Nurses Association. (2015). *Nursing: Scope and standards* of practice (3rd ed.). Silver Spring, MD: Author.

Butcher, H. K., Bulechek, G. M., Dochterman, J. M., & Wagner, C. M. (Eds.). (2018). *Nursing interventions classification* (NIC) (7th ed.). Elsevier.

Herdman, T. H., Kamitsuru, S., & Takáo Lopes, C. (Eds.). (2021). *Nursing diagnoses: Definitions and classification 2021–2023* (12th ed.). Thieme.

INTRODUCTION

This section includes the alphabetically organized diagnostic labels and associated care plans that identify health problems responsive to independent nursing action. Many focus on meeting the patient's actual physiologic needs. For example, you'll find care plans that will assist you in planning the care of a patient with decreased cardiac output, help an injured patient maintain joint range of motion, and teach an immunosuppressed patient measures to prevent infection. In addition, you'll find plans for warding off potential health problems, such as risk for infection or injury.

Other care plans focus on the psychological and psychosocial problems. For example, if a patient with a chronic illness experiences related emotional difficulties, such diagnostic labels as *hopelessness*, *ineffective role performance*, and *disturbed body image* may help pinpoint the patient's needs. If a patient lacks adequate financial, social, or spiritual resources, appropriate care plans provide instructions for documenting such hardships and interventions for ameliorating them.

Still other care plans focus on more specialized patient problems. For example, you'll find plans for patients undergoing surgery.

In summary, the diagnostic labels and associated care plans covered in this manual encompass the full range of nursing responsibilities. To make full use of this broad database, you'll need to perform a complete and careful nursing assessment. When appropriate, include questions about the patient's cultural background. Ask about self-concept, stressors, daily living habits, and coping mechanisms. Discuss the patient's health goals. How well does the patient understand his or her condition? Will family members or friends take an active role in patient care? Your assessment should also include information derived from your own observations.

Use information gathered during assessment to select an accurate diagnostic statement and an appropriate care plan. That way, you can ensure your patient's comprehensive, individualized, and consistent nursing care.

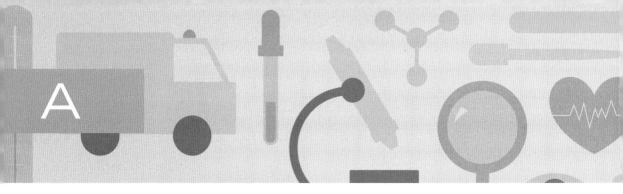

Decreased Activity Tolerance

DEFINITION

Insufficient endurance to complete required or desired daily activities

RELATED FACTORS (R/T)

- Decreased muscle strength
- Depressive symptoms
- Fear of pain
- Imbalance between oxygen supply/demand
- Impaired physical mobility
- Inexperience with an activity
- Insufficient muscle mass
- Malnutrition
- Pain
- Physical deconditioning
- Sedentary lifestyle

ASSOCIATED CONDITIONS

- Neoplasms
- Neurodegenerative diseases
- Respiration disorders
- Traumatic brain injuries
- Vitamin D deficiency

ASSESSMENT

- History of present illness
- History of circulatory disease, respiratory disease, or both
- Patient's perception of tolerance for activity
- Current medications, effectiveness
- Respiratory status, including pulse oximetry; pulmonary function studies; breath sounds; and respiratory rate, depth, and pattern at rest and with activity
- Cardiovascular status, including blood pressure, complete blood count, skin color, hemoglobin level and hematocrit, stress electrocardiogram (ECG) results, and heart rate and rhythm at rest and with activity
- Neurologic status, including orientation, and motor and sensory status
- Musculoskeletal status, including range of motion (ROM) and muscle size, strength, and tone

- Knowledge, including understanding of present condition; perception of need to maintain or restore an activity level consistent with capabilities; and physical, mental, and emotional readiness to learn
- Past experience with prolonged bed rest

DEFINING CHARACTERISTICS

- Abnormal blood pressure response to activity
- Abnormal heart rate response to activity
- Anxious when activity is required
- Electrocardiogram change
- Exertional discomfort
- Exertional dyspnea
- Expresses fatigue
- Generalized weakness

EXPECTED OUTCOMES

- Patient's blood pressure, pulse, and respiratory rates will remain within prescribed limits during activity.
- Patient will perform self-care activities to tolerance level.
- Patient will state desire to increase activity level.
- Patient will state understanding of the need to increase activity level gradually.
- Patient will identify controllable factors that cause fatigue.
- Patient will state a sense of satisfaction with each new level of activity attained.
- Patient will demonstrate skill in conserving energy while carrying out daily activities to tolerance level.
- Patient will explain illness and connect symptoms of activity intolerance with deficit in oxygen supply or use.

Suggested NOC Outcomes

Activity Tolerance; Discharge Readiness; Endurance; Energy Conservation; Psychomotor Energy; Self-Care: Activities of Daily Living (ADLs); Self-Care: Instrumental Activities of Daily Living (IADLs)

INTERVENTIONS AND RATIONALES

- Assess for cause of activity intolerance. *Cause of the intolerance will guide interventions.*
- **PCC** Discuss with patient the need for activity. *Lack of activity causes physical deconditioning and may also have a negative impact on psychological well-being.*
- **PCC** Involve patient in planning and decision-making *to encourage greater compliance with activity plan.*
- **PCC** Identify activities the patient considers desirable and meaningful. *Engaging patient in activities that have personal meaning gives the patient a greater sense of independence and may motivate patient to continue developing tolerance.*
- **EBP** Teach patient exercises for increasing strength and endurance *to improve breathing and promote general physical reconditioning.*
- **PCC** Encourage patient to help plan activity progression, being sure to include activities the patient considers essential. *Participation in planning may encourage patient compliance with the plan.*

EBP ▪ Encourage active exercise:

EBP ▪ Provide a trapeze or other assistive device whenever possible. *Such devices simplify moving and turning for many patients and help them to strengthen upper-body muscles.*

EBP ▪ Teach isometric exercises *to help patient maintain or increase muscle tone and joint mobility.*

EBP ▪ Have patient perform self-care activities and assist with turning and transfer. Begin slowly and increase daily as tolerated. *Performing self-care activities helps patient regain independence and enhances self-esteem.*

▪ Monitor physiologic responses to increased activity level, including respirations, heart rate and rhythm, and blood pressure *to ensure they return to normal within 2 to 5 minutes after stopping exercise.*

PCC ▪ Support and encourage activity to patient's level of tolerance *to help foster patient's independence.*

EBP ▪ Gradually increase activity to meet patient's abilities. *Activity progression builds strength and endurance.*

▪ Instruct and help patient alternate periods of rest and activity. *Providing rest periods prevents fatigue and encourages patient to continue improving activity tolerance.*

EBP ▪ Teach patient how to conserve energy while performing ADLs—for example, sitting in a chair while dressing, wearing lightweight clothing that fastens with Velcro or a few large buttons, and wearing slip-on shoes. *These measures reduce cellular metabolism and oxygen demand.*

▪ Remove barriers that prevent patient from achieving goals that have been established *to minimize factors that may decrease patient's exercise tolerance.*

T&C ▪ Refer patient to physical therapist. *Physical therapist can develop plan to increase activity level and build strength.*

EBP ▪ Turn and reposition patient at least every 2 hours. Establish a turning schedule for the dependent patient. Post schedule at bedside and monitor frequency. *Turning and repositioning prevent skin breakdown, atelectasis, and improve lung expansion.*

S ▪ Maintain proper body alignment *to avoid contractures and to maintain optimal musculoskeletal balance and physiologic function.*

S ▪ Perform active or passive ROM exercises to all extremities every 2 to 4 hours. *These exercises foster muscle strength and tone, maintain joint mobility, and prevent contractures.*

PCC ▪ Provide emotional support and encouragement *to improve patient's self-concept and motivate patient to perform ADLs.*

PCC ▪ Before discharge, formulate a plan with patient and caregivers that will enable the patient either to continue functioning at maximum activity tolerance or to gradually increase tolerance. For example, teach patient and caregivers to monitor patient's pulse during activities, to recognize the need for oxygen (if prescribed), and to use oxygen equipment properly. *Participation in discharge planning encourages patient satisfaction and compliance.*

T&C ▪ Make sure that a case manager or social worker has assessed patient's home and made the appropriate modifications to accommodate patient's level of mobility. *Making adjustments in the home allows patient a greater degree of independence in performing ADLs, thus better conserving energy.*

Suggested NIC Interventions

Activity Therapy; Body Mechanics Promotion; Energy Management; Environmental Management; Exercise Promotion; Exercise Therapy: Ambulation; Exercise Therapy: Balance; Exercise Therapy: Joint Mobility; Exercise Therapy: Muscle Control; Mutual Goal Setting; Oxygen Therapy; Progressive Muscle Relaxation

- Patient states a desire to increase activity level.
- Patient identifies a plan to increase activity level.
- Patient lists factors that cause fatigue.
- Patient's blood pressure and pulse and respiratory rates remain within normal parameters.
- Patient expresses satisfaction with increase in activity level.
- Patient is proficient in conserving energy while performing ADLs.
- Patient verbalizes understanding of the need to maximize activity level.
- Patient performs self-care activities at optimal level within restrictions imposed by illness.
- Patient demonstrates an understanding of the relationship between signs and symptoms of activity intolerance and deficits in oxygen supply or use.

DOCUMENTATION

- Patient's perception of need for activity
- Patient's priorities in performing selected activities
- Patient's description of physical effects of various activities
- Observations of physical findings in response to activity
- Skills demonstrated by patient in conserving energy during activity
- Teaching activities performed with patient or caregivers
- New activities patient was able to perform
- Evaluations for expected outcomes

REFERENCES

Brunjes, D., Kennel, P., & Christian Schulze, P. (2017). Exercise capacity, physical activity, and morbidity. *Heart Failure Reviews, 22*(2), 133–139.

Hammarlund, C. S., Lexell, J., & Brogårdh, C. (2017). Perceived consequences of ageing with late effects of polio and strategies for managing daily life: A qualitative study. *BMC Geriatrics, 17*, 179.

Miranda, N. A., Boris, J. R., Kouvel, K. M., & Stiles, L. (2018). Activity and exercise intolerance after concussion: Identification and management of postural orthostatic tachycardia syndrome. *Journal of Neurologic Physical Therapy, 42*(3), 163–171.

O'Donnell, D. E., Webb, K. A., Langer, D., Elbehairy, A. F., Neder, J. A., & Dudgeon, D. J. (2016). Respiratory factors contributing to exercise intolerance in breast cancer survivors: A case-control study. *Journal of Pain and Symptom Management, 52*(1), 54–63.

Risk for Decreased Activity Tolerance

DEFINITION

Susceptible to experiencing insufficient endurance to complete required or desired daily activities

RISK FACTORS

- Decreased muscle strength
- Depressive symptoms
- Fear of pain
- Imbalance between oxygen supply/demand

- Impaired physical mobility
- Inexperience with an activity
- Insufficient muscle mass
- Malnutrition
- Pain
- Physical deconditioning
- Sedentary lifestyle

ASSOCIATED CONDITIONS

- Neoplasms
- Neurodegenerative diseases
- Respiration disorders
- Traumatic brain injuries
- Vitamin D deficiency

ASSESSMENT

- History of present illness
- Past experience with immobility or prescribed bed rest
- Pain
- Environmental factors, including safety hazards
- History of chronic illnesses (cardiopulmonary, cardiovascular, musculoskeletal, and neuromuscular)
- Sensory deficits, including hearing, vision, and tactile
- Psychosocial status, including cognitive and mental status, mood, affect, behavior, family support, and coping style
- Economic status
- Medication history, including use of prescription and over-the-counter medications
- Cardiovascular status, including blood pressure, heart rate, and rhythm at rest and with activity, complete blood count, skin temperature and color, edema, and chest pain or discomfort
- Respiratory status, pulse oximetry, auscultation of breath sounds, pain or discomfort associated with respiration, and rate, rhythm, depth, and pattern of respirations at rest and with activity
- Neurologic status, including level of consciousness; orientation; and mental, sensory, and motor status
- Musculoskeletal status, including range of motion (ROM), muscle size, strength, and tone, and functional mobility as follows:
  0 = completely independent
  1 = requires use of equipment or device
  2 = requires help, supervision, or teaching from another person
  3 = requires help from another person and equipment or device
  4 = dependent; doesn't participate in activity

EXPECTED OUTCOMES

- Patient will maintain muscle strength and joint ROM.
- Patient will carry out isometric exercise regimen.
- Patient will communicate understanding of the rationale for maintaining activity level.
- Patient will avoid risk factors that may lead to activity intolerance.

- Patient will perform self-care activities to tolerance level.
- Patient will seek help in performing activities of daily living (ADLs), as needed.
- Patient will demonstrate willingness to perform activities needed to follow prescribed care plan.
- Patient will verbalize acceptance of decreased activity level.
- Patient will experience less discomfort when ambulating, transferring, or performing other activities.
- Patient's blood pressure, pulse, and respiratory rate will remain within prescribed range during periods of activity (specify).

Suggested NOC Outcomes

Activity Tolerance; Endurance; Energy Conservation; Self-Care: Activities of Daily Living (ADLs); Self-Care: Instrumental Activities of Daily Living (IADLs)

INTERVENTIONS AND RATIONALES

- Assess patient's level of functioning using the functional mobility scale *to determine patient's capabilities.*
- **EBP** Monitor the patient's medication regimen regularly *to identify drugs that may cause gait, posture, or ambulatory problems.*
- **EBP** Explain rationale for maintaining or improving activity level. Discuss factors that increase risk of activity intolerance. *Education helps patient avoid activity intolerance.*
- **PCC** Encourage patient to become involved in planning care and making decisions related to treatment. *Participation in planning enhances patient compliance and self-esteem.*
- **PCC** Help the patient identify activities that are personally meaningful and develop a realistic plan to incorporate meaningful activities into the daily routine *to heighten satisfaction with energy expenditure.*
- Establish realistic goals for improving the patient's activity level, taking into account the patient's physical limitations and energy level *to help improve the patient's quality of life. Keep in mind that in some older patients with chronic conditions, even minimal improvements in activity level are noteworthy.*
- Encourage the patient to take part in exercise and social activities as tolerated *to increase stamina and decrease social isolation.*
- **EBP** Establish progressive goals to increase ambulation, for example:
  Older patients may tire easily; therefore, the activity level should be increased gradually.
  - **EBP** Ambulate 20 ft (6.1 m) three times/day for 1 week
  - **EBP** Ambulate 40 ft (12.2 m) three times/day for 1 week
  - **EBP** Ambulate 60 ft (18.3 m) three times/day for 1 week
- **S** Demonstrate the use of assistive devices, such as a cane or walker, shopping cart on wheels, or trapeze, *to teach methods of conserving energy and maintaining independence.*
- **S** Position patient to maintain proper body alignment. Use assistive devices as needed *to maintain joint function and prevent musculoskeletal deformities.*
- **S** Turn and position patient at least every 2 hours. Establish turning schedule for the dependent patient. Post at bedside and monitor frequency. *Turning helps prevent skin breakdown by relieving pressure and reduces the risk of atelectasis and pneumonia.*
- **S** Assess patient's physiologic response to increased activity (blood pressure, respirations, heart rate, and rhythm). *Monitoring vital signs helps assess tolerance for increased exertion and activity.*

`T&C` ▪ Communicate patient's level of functioning to all staff. *Communication among staff members ensures continuity of care and enables patient to preserve identified level of independence.*

`S` ▪ Unless contraindicated, perform ROM exercises every 2 to 4 hours. Progress from passive to active, according to patient tolerance. *ROM exercises prevent joint contractures and muscular atrophy.*

`S` ▪ Perform periodic health assessments and monitor for complaints of weakness or fatigue *to assess whether acute illness or exacerbation of chronic condition is causing activity intolerance.*

▪ Teach patient how to perform isometric exercises *to maintain and improve muscle tone and joint mobility.*

`S` ▪ Teach patient symptoms of overexertion, such as dizziness, chest pain, and dyspnea, *to help patient take responsibility for monitoring activity level.*

▪ Encourage patient to carry out ADLs. Provide emotional support and offer positive feedback when patient displays initiative. *Offering emotional support enhances patient's self-esteem and motivation.*

▪ Assist patient in carrying out self-care activities, turning, and transfer. Increase patient's participation in self-care, as tolerated, *to foster independence and improve mobility.*

`S` ▪ Modify the environment *to maximize independent activity.* For example, place the bed on the first floor of the home with easy access to the bathroom, and instruct the patient to obtain and use energy-saving devices, such as an elevated toilet seat, trapeze bar on the bed, and a chair with arms and a seat that raises the patient to standing position, *to promote independence.*

▪ Teach patient, family members, or other caregiver methods to maximize patient's participation in self-care. *Informed caregivers can encourage patient to become more independent.*

`T&C` ▪ Coordinate the activities of the interdisciplinary team when developing an activity regimen for the patient. For example, the physician can prescribe treatment for the medical condition, a physical therapist can design an exercise program, a dietitian can devise a nutrition plan, and a social worker can locate community resources, such as Meals on Wheels or home health care services. *All of these measures address the patient's physical and psychosocial needs.*

`T&C` ▪ Refer the patient to a home health care agency for follow-up care. Encourage the patient to interview and select home health care personnel *to foster the patient's sense of independence.*

Suggested NIC Interventions

Energy Management; Exercise Promotion: Strength Training; Exercise Therapy: Joint Mobility; Home Maintenance Assistance; Hope Instillation; Nutrition Management; Self-Care Assistance; Teaching: Prescribed Activity/Exercise; Body Mechanics Promotion

EVALUATIONS FOR EXPECTED OUTCOMES

▪ Functional mobility scale indicates that muscle strength and joint ROM remain stable.

▪ Patient demonstrates isometric exercises.

▪ Patient explains rationale for maintaining activity level.

▪ Patient states at least five risk factors for activity intolerance.

▪ Patient performs self-care activities in preparation for discharge.

▪ Patient doesn't exhibit evidence of cardiovascular or respiratory complications during or after activity.

DOCUMENTATION

- Patient's expressions of motivation to maintain maximum activity level within restrictions imposed by illness
- Activities performed by patient
- Teaching instructions provided to patient and family member or other caregivers
- Patient's physiologic response to increased activity
- Evaluations for expected outcomes

REFERENCES

Brunjes, D., Kennel, P., & Christian Schulze, P. (2017). Exercise capacity, physical activity, and morbidity. *Heart Failure Reviews, 22*(2), 133–139.

Elbehairy, A. F., Ciavaglia, C. E., Webb, K. A., Guenette, J. A., Jensen, D., Mourad, S. M., ... O'Donnell, D. E. (2015). Pulmonary gas exchange abnormalities in mild chronic obstructive pulmonary disease. Implications for dyspnea and exercise intolerance. *American Journal of Respiratory and Critical Care Medicine, 191*(12), 1384–1394.

Fox, M. T., Sidani, S., Brooks, D., & McCague, H. (2018). Perceived acceptability and preferences for low-intensity early activity interventions of older hospitalized medical patients exposed to bed rest: A cross sectional study. *BMC Geriatrics, 18*, 53.

Liu, S., Marcinek, D., Liu, S. Z., & Marcinek, D. J. (2017). Skeletal muscle bioenergetics in aging and heart failure. *Heart Failure Reviews, 22*(2), 167–178.

Ineffective Activity Planning

DEFINITION

Inability to prepare for a set of actions fixed in time and under certain conditions

RELATED FACTORS (R/T)

- Flight behavior when faced with proposed solution
- Hedonism
- Insufficient information processing ability
- Insufficient social support
- Pattern of procrastination
- Unrealistic perception of events
- Unrealistic perception of personal abilities

ASSESSMENT

- Patient's perception of problem, coping mechanisms, problem-solving ability, decision-making competencies
- Neurologic status, including level of consciousness; orientation; and mental, sensory, and motor status
- Cultural status, including affiliation with racial, ethnic, or religious groups

DEFINING CHARACTERISTICS

- Absence of pain
- Excessive anxiety about a task to be undertaken
- Fear about a task to be undertaken
- Insufficient organizational skills
- Insufficient resources

- Pattern of failure
- Pattern of procrastination
- Unmet goals for chosen activity
- Worried about a task to be undertaken

EXPECTED OUTCOMES

- Patient will demonstrate improved self-confidence to accomplish tasks.
- Patient will demonstrate improved concentration in task planning and execution.
- Patient will minimize procrastination.
- Patient will articulate personal goals for activity planning and completion.
- Patient will verbalize diminished fear and anxiety concerning task planning and execution.

Suggested NOC Outcomes

Cognition; Cognition Orientation; Concentration; Decision-Making; Information Processing; Memory

INTERVENTIONS AND RATIONALES

PCC
- Assess patient's concerns related to activity planning and execution *to be able to suggest strategies to overcome challenges.*
- Model effective techniques for planning and executing activities. *Patients who are challenged by planning and executing activities often find it helpful to observe practical approaches instead of solely hearing theoretical information.*
- Teach behavior management strategies *to help patient minimize fears of failure.*
- Praise successes in any steps of planning or executing activities. *Positive reinforcement enhances self-confidence.*

T&C
- Refer or collaborate with physical and/or occupational therapists in managing the patient's activity. *Colleagues in related disciplines bring valuable additional perspectives to complex clinical situations.*

Suggested NIC Interventions

Anxiety Reduction; Behavior Management; Calming Technique; Memory Training; Planning Assistance; Sequence Guidance

EVALUATIONS FOR EXPECTED OUTCOMES

- Patient demonstrated improved self-confidence and concentration with task accomplishment.
- Patient was able to minimize procrastination.
- Patient stated personal goals for activity planning and execution.
- Patient verbalized diminished fear and anxiety concerning task planning and execution.

DOCUMENTATION

- Patient's statements of improved self-confidence in task accomplishment
- Patient's stated goals for activity planning and execution
- Evaluations for expected outcomes

REFERENCES

Barz, M., Lange, D., Parschau, L., Lonsdale, C., Knoll, N., & Schwarzer, R. (2016). Self-efficacy, planning, and preparatory behaviours as joint predictors of physical activity: A conditional process analysis. *Psychology & Health, 31*(1), 65–78.

Blouin, H. E. C., & Pychyl, T. A. (2017). A mental imagery intervention to increase future self-continuity and reduce procrastination. *Applied Psychology: An International Review, 66*(2), 326–352.

Hassan, N. (2017). "Putting music on": Everyday leisure activities, choice-making and person-centred planning in a supported living scheme. *British Journal of Learning Disabilities, 45*(1), 73–80.

Kroese, F. M., & de Ridder, D. T. D. (2016). Health behaviour procrastination: A novel reasoned route towards self-regulatory failure. *Health Psychology Review, 10*(3), 313–325.

Risk for Ineffective Activity Planning

DEFINITION

Susceptible to an inability to prepare for a set of actions fixed in time and under certain conditions, which may compromise health

RISK FACTORS

- Flight behavior when faced with proposed solution
- Hedonism
- Insufficient information processing ability
- Insufficient social support
- Pattern of procrastination
- Unrealistic perception of events
- Unrealistic perception of personal abilities

ASSESSMENT

- Patient's perception of problem, coping mechanisms, problem-solving ability, decision-making competencies
- Neurologic status, including level of consciousness; orientation; and mental, sensory, and motor status
- Cultural status, including affiliation with racial, ethnic, or religious groups

EXPECTED OUTCOMES

- Patient will express an interest in activity planning.
- Patient will minimize procrastination.
- Patient will set attainable realistic goals for activity planning and completion.
- Patient will demonstrate ability to make decisions and resolve problems.

Suggested NOC Outcomes

Information Processing; Decision-Making; Concentration; Motivation

INTERVENTIONS AND RATIONALES

- Assess patient's support system. *Family involvement can help patient feel more in control.*

PCC ▥ Assess patient's feelings related to decision-making and activity planning *to help identify underlying fears.*

PCC ▥ Listen to patient's concerns *to validate his or her feelings and your willingness to help.*

▥ Assist the patient to set simple, achievable short-term goals *to promote feeling of achievement.*

S ▥ Educate patient regarding recognition of early symptoms of anxiety related to decision-making. *This will keep anxiety from escalating.*

EBP ▥ Explore possible behavior management strategies *that will minimize fears of failure.*

▥ Provide positive reinforcement for independent behaviors. *This will promote confidence and feeling of achievement.*

EBP ▥ Explore the use of alternative methods to minimize concerns regarding activity planning, for example, therapeutic breathing techniques or temporary avoidance technique, *which will allow the buildup of confidence before taking action.*

T&C ▥ Provide community resources for follow-up support *to ensure continuation of care.*

T&C ▥ Refer to behavioral specialist as needed *to provide care for more complex issues.*

Suggested NIC Interventions

Anxiety Reduction; Behavior Management; Behavior Modification

EVALUATIONS FOR EXPECTED OUTCOMES

▥ Patient plans activities.

▥ Patient minimizes procrastination.

▥ Patient has reasonable goals.

▥ Patient has decision-making skills.

DOCUMENTATION

▥ Patient's expressions of concern about lack of activity planning

▥ Observations of physiologic and behavioral manifestations of lack of activity

▥ Interventions performed to promote activity planning

▥ Patient's response to interventions

▥ Evaluations for expected outcomes

REFERENCES

Barz, M., Lange, D., Parschau, L., Lonsdale, C., Knoll, N., & Schwarzer, R. (2016). Self-efficacy, planning, and preparatory behaviours as joint predictors of physical activity: A conditional process analysis. *Psychology & Health, 31*(1), 65–78.

Blouin, H. E. C., & Pychyl, T. A. (2017). A mental imagery intervention to increase future self-continuity and reduce procrastination. *Applied Psychology: An International Review, 66*(2), 326–352.

Hassan, N. (2017). "Putting music on": Everyday leisure activities, choice-making and person-centred planning in a supported living scheme. *British Journal of Learning Disabilities, 45*(1), 73–80.

Kroese, F. M., & de Ridder, D. T. D. (2016). Health behaviour procrastination: A novel reasoned route towards self-regulatory failure. *Health Psychology Review, 10*(3), 313–325.

Acute Substance Withdrawal Syndrome

DEFINITION

Serious, multifactorial sequelae following abrupt cessation of an addictive compound

RISK FACTORS

▪ Developed dependence to alcohol or other addictive substance
▪ Heavy use of an addictive substance over time
▪ Malnutrition
▪ Sudden cessation of an addictive substance

ASSOCIATED CONDITIONS

▪ Comorbid mental disorder
▪ Comorbid serious physical illness

ASSESSMENT

▪ History of patient use of ethyl alcohol (ETOH), recreational drugs, or other addictive compounds
▪ Symptoms of withdrawal which may include nausea and vomiting, anxiety, insomnia, perspiration, muscle cramps, and diarrhea
▪ Mental status changes including disorientation, confusion, and hallucinations
▪ Seizures
▪ Vital signs including resting pulse rate
▪ Restless behavior
▪ Neurologic assessment with pupil size and reaction
▪ Presence of tremors
▪ Excessive yawning
▪ Hot or cold flashes
▪ Teary eyes
▪ Runny nose
▪ Perceptual distortions
▪ Nutritional status, including dietary intake, appetite, current weight, and change from normal weight

DEFINING CHARACTERISTICS

▪ Acute confusion
▪ Anxiety
▪ Disturbed sleep pattern
▪ Nausea
▪ Risk for electrolyte imbalance
▪ Risk for injury

EXPECTED OUTCOMES

▪ Patient will remain free from harm.
▪ Patient will not experience seizure activity.
▪ Patient will comply with treatment regimen.
▪ Patient will develop effective coping behaviors.
▪ Patient will have decreased anxiety.
▪ Patient will experience undisturbed sleep.
▪ Patient will have balanced electrolytes.
▪ Patient will consume _____ calories per day.

Suggested NOC Outcomes

Alcohol Abuse Cessation Behavior; Anxiety Level; Anxiety Self-Control; Drug Abuse Cessation Behavior; Electrolyte Balance; Nutritional Status: Nutrient Intake; Substance Addiction Consequences; Substance Withdrawal Severity

INTERVENTIONS AND RATIONALES

PCC ▪ Perform thorough nursing history and head-to-toe assessment and document *to establish baseline of patient's condition for future comparison and to ensure continuity and consistency of care among nursing staff.*

S ▪ Monitor and record level of consciousness (LOC), temperature, heart rate and rhythm, and blood pressure at least every 4 hours, or more often if necessary, *to detect deterioration from possible hypoxia or decreased cardiac output.*

S ▪ Report complaints of anxiety, confusion, dizziness, or syncope promptly; *these may indicate neurological decline.*

PCC ▪ Assess sleeping patterns. *Rest reduces symptoms of anxiety and fosters patient coping.*

PCC ▪ Include patient in plan of action *to promote self-care.*

S ▪ Have a staff member stay at patient's bedside if necessary *to protect patient from harm during episodes of confusion.*

EBP ▪ Limit noise and environmental stimulation *to prevent patient from becoming overstimulated.*

S ▪ Use appropriate safety measures *to protect patient from injury.* Avoid physical restraints *to prevent agitating patient.*

PCC ▪ Provide positive feedback when patient assumes responsibility for own behavior *to reinforce effective coping behaviors.*

PCC ▪ Convey attitude of acceptance, separating individual from unacceptable behavior. *Promotes feelings of dignity and self-worth.*

PCC ▪ Provide nonjudgmental care. Monitor for changes in behavior (restlessness, increased tension). *Agitation can lead to compromised patient safety.*

PCC ▪ Assist patient to assess current life situation and impact of substance use. *Allows patient to see the relationship between substance use and physical problems.*

PCC ▪ Assess patient's support system. *Family involvement can help patient feel more in control.*

T&C ▪ Encourage patient to attend recovery support and therapy groups regularly. *Attendance fosters healing relationships and maintenance of a long-term substance-free existence.*

T&C ▪ Refer the patient to a mental health specialist and/or social worker for follow-up treatment after hospitalization. *Continuing therapy is usually necessary to assist the patient in coping with health care status.*

Suggested NIC Interventions

Anxiety Reduction; Behavior Modification; Electrolyte Monitoring; Seizure Management; Self-Esteem Enhancement; Substance Use Treatment; Substance Use Treatment: Alcohol Withdrawal; Substance Use Treatment: Drug Withdrawal

EVALUATIONS FOR EXPECTED OUTCOMES

▪ Patient doesn't exhibit self-harming behaviors.

- Patient maintains neurologic, cardiovascular, respiratory, GI, nutritional, genitourinary, musculoskeletal, and integumentary functioning.
- Patient does not experience seizure activity.
- Patient complies with treatment regimen and plan of care.
- Patient doesn't exhibit altered LOC, mental status, sensory ability, or motor ability.
- Patient develops healthy effective coping strategies.
- Patient's anxiety level remains at a manageable level.
- Patient experiences undisturbed sleep.
- Patient electrolyte levels remain within normal limits.
- Patient consumes _____ calories per day.

DOCUMENTATION

- Patient's vital signs
- Patient's concerns or perceptions of circumstances; willingness to accept and participate in treatment
- Assessment of body systems at risk for deterioration
- Observations of patient's behaviors
- Interventions to provide preventive or supportive care and prescribed treatment
- Treatment given to patient and patient's understanding and demonstrated ability to carry out instructions
- Patient's response to nursing interventions
- Evaluations for expected outcomes

REFERENCES

Grover, S., Kate, N., Sharma, A., Mattoo, S. K., Basu, D., Chakrabarti, S., … Avasthi, A. (2016). Symptom profile of alcohol withdrawal delirium: Factor analysis of Delirium Rating Scale-Revised-98 version. *American Journal of Drug and Alcohol Abuse, 42*(2), 196–202.

Heron, N. (2018). Opioid use disorder in critical care: Recognizing, managing, and advocating for our patients. *Canadian Journal of Critical Care Nursing, 29*(2), 38–39.

Lee, K. Y., & Park, J. Y. (2018). Pediatric nurses' knowledge and attitude on iatrogenic narcotic analgesic withdrawal symptoms management. *Journal of Korean Critical Care Nursing, 11*(3), 107.

Stockmann, T., Odegbaro, D., Timimi, S., & Moncrieff, J. (2018). SSRI and SNRI withdrawal symptoms reported on an internet forum. *International Journal of Risk & Safety in Medicine, 29*(3/4), 175–180.

Risk for Acute Substance Withdrawal Syndrome

DEFINITION

Susceptible to serious, multifactorial sequelae following abrupt cessation of an addictive compound, which may compromise health

RISK FACTORS

- Developed dependence to alcohol or other addictive substance
- Heavy use of an addictive substance over time
- Malnutrition
- Sudden cessation of an addictive substance

ASSOCIATED CONDITIONS

- Comorbid mental disorder
- Comorbid serious physical illness

ASSESSMENT

- History of patient use of ethyl alcohol (ETOH), recreational drugs, or other addictive compounds
- Symptoms of withdrawal, which may include nausea and vomiting, anxiety, insomnia, perspiration, muscle cramps, and diarrhea
- Mental status changes including disorientation, confusion, and hallucinations
- Vital signs including resting pulse rate
- Restless behavior
- Nutritional status, including dietary intake, appetite, current weight, and change from normal weight

EXPECTED OUTCOMES

- Patient will remain free from harm.
- Patient will not experience withdrawal symptom complications.
- Patient will comply with treatment regimen.
- Patient will consume _____ calories per day.

Suggested NOC Outcomes

Alcohol Abuse Cessation Behavior; Anxiety Level; Anxiety Self-Control; Drug Abuse Cessation Behavior; Substance Addiction Consequences; Substance Withdrawal Severity

INTERVENTIONS AND RATIONALES

- **S** Perform thorough nursing history and head-to-toe assessment and document *to establish baseline of patient's condition for future comparison and to ensure continuity and consistency of care among nursing staff.*
- **S** Monitor and record level of consciousness (LOC), temperature, heart rate and rhythm, and blood pressure at least every 4 hours, or more often if necessary, *to detect deterioration from possible hypoxia or decreased cardiac output.*
- **S** Report complaints of anxiety, confusion, dizziness, or syncope promptly; *these may indicate neurological decline.*
- **PCC** Include patient in plan of action *to promote self-care.*
- **S** Use appropriate safety measures *to protect patient from injury.* Avoid physical restraints *to prevent agitating patient.*
- **PCC** Provide positive feedback when patient assumes responsibility for own behavior *to reinforce effective coping behaviors.*
- **PCC** Convey attitude of acceptance, separating individual from unacceptable behavior. *Promotes feelings of dignity and self-worth.*
- **PCC** Provide nonjudgmental care. Monitor for changes in behavior (restlessness, increased tension). *Agitation can lead to compromised patient safety.*
- **PCC** Assist patient in assessing current life situation and impact of substance use. *Allows patient to see the relationship between substance use and physical problems.*
- **PCC** Assess patient's support system. *Family involvement can help patient feel more in control.*
- **T&C** Encourage patient to attend support and therapy groups regularly. *Attendance fosters healing relationships and maintenance of a long-term substance-free existence.*
- **T&C** Refer the patient to a mental health specialist and/or social worker for follow-up treatment after hospitalization. *Continuing therapy is usually necessary to assist the patient to cope with health care status.*

Suggested NIC Interventions

Anxiety Reduction; Behavior Modification; Self-Esteem Enhancement; Substance Use Treatment; Substance Use Treatment: Alcohol Withdrawal; Substance Use Treatment: Drug Withdrawal

EVALUATIONS FOR EXPECTED OUTCOMES

- Patient maintains neurologic, cardiovascular, respiratory, gastrointestinal (GI), nutritional, genitourinary, musculoskeletal, and integumentary functioning.
- Patient does not sustain any injuries.
- Patient complies with treatment regimen and plan of care.
- Patient doesn't exhibit altered LOC, mental status, sensory ability, or motor ability.
- Patient develops healthy effective coping strategies.

DOCUMENTATION

- Patient's vital signs
- Patient's concerns or perceptions of circumstances; willingness to accept and participate in treatment
- Assessment of body systems at risk for deterioration
- Observations of patient's behaviors
- Interventions to provide preventive or supportive care and prescribed treatment
- Treatment given to patient and patient's understanding and demonstrated ability to carry out instructions
- Patient's response to nursing interventions
- Evaluations for expected outcomes

REFERENCES

Larney, S., Zador, D., Sindicich, N., & Dolan, K. (2017). A qualitative study of reasons for seeking and ceasing opioid substitution treatment in prisons in New South Wales, Australia. *Drug and Alcohol Review, 36*(3), 305–310.

Tewell, R., Edgerton, L., & Kyle, E. (2018). Establishment of a pharmacist-led service for patients at high risk for opioid overdose. *American Journal of Health-System Pharmacy, 75*(6), 376–383.

Traynor, K. (2018). Medical treatment is key in battling opioid crisis. *American Journal of Health-System Pharmacy, 75*(5), 254–256.

Vogel, L. (2018). Acute care model of addiction treatment not enough for substance abuse. *CMAJ: Canadian Medical Association Journal, 190*(42), E1268–E1269.

Risk for Adverse Reaction to Iodinated Contrast Media

DEFINITION

Susceptible to noxious or unintended reaction associated with the use of iodinated contrast media that can occur within seven days after contrast agent injection, which may compromise health

RISK FACTORS

- Dehydration
- Generalized weakness

- Chronic illness
- Concurrent use of pharmaceutical agents
- Contrast media precipitates adverse event
- Fragile vein
- Unconsciousness

- History of experience with illness, hospitalization, and surgery
- Health history, including accidents, exposure to pollutants, falls, hyperthermia, hypothermia, poisoning, sensory or perceptual changes (auditory, gustatory, kinesthetic, olfactory, tactile, and visual), and trauma
- Allergies
- Mental status, including cognitive and emotional function, problems with concentration, memory, orientation, mood, and behavior
- Risk factors
- History of previous adverse effect from iodinated contrast media
- History of allergies
- Extremes of age
- Dehydration
- Concurrent use of medications (e.g., beta-blockers, interleukin-2, metformin, nephrotoxic medications)
- Fragile veins
- Underlying disease (e.g., heart disease, pulmonary disease, blood dyscrasias, endocrine disease, renal disease, pheochromocytoma, autoimmune disease)
- General debilitation

- Patient will not experience an adverse reaction to iodinated contrast media.
- Patient will recognize personal risk factors for adverse reaction.
- Patient will ask questions if new information requires clarification.

Suggested NOC Outcomes

Risk Control; Risk Detection; Knowledge: Treatment Procedure; Immune Hypersensitivity Response; Allergy Response

- **S** Assess for any previous adverse reaction to contrast media.
- **S** Identify preexisting disease states and current medications history that may trigger reaction to iodinated contrast media. *This is essential for the safe administration of contrast media and prevention of adverse effects.*
- **S** Assess for history of asthma, food allergies, or other allergies, *which may increase likelihood of an adverse reaction.* Assess for presence of other medical conditions including heart failure and renal insufficiency, *which may increase risk of adverse reaction.*
- **EBP** Consider prehydration with normal saline solution *to decrease risk of renal damage.*

EBP ▪ Withhold metformin before any administration of contrast media, and resume after 48 hours once renal function has been evaluated. *This will reduce any medication-associated renal tissue damage due to contrast media.*

EBP ▪ Premedication with corticosteroids or antihistamines may be indicated *to reduce incidence of reaction in patients with known risk factors.*

PCC ▪ Educate patient regarding risk factors associated with adverse reaction to iodinated contrast media. *Knowledge of risk factors is essential in preventing adverse reaction and possible organ damage.*

S ▪ Ensure patient is aware of personal risk factors to share with future providers. *This will promote continued safe administration of iodinated contrast media.*

PCC ▪ Encourage patient to share concerns about procedures requiring use of iodinated contrast media *to reduce anxiety.*

T&C ▪ Collaborate with other members of the health care team regarding presence of risk factors associated with adverse reaction to iodinated contrast media. *This will allow for modifications in the preparation for the procedure and prevent complications.*

Suggested NIC Interventions

Risk Identification; Teaching: Individual

EVALUATIONS FOR EXPECTED OUTCOMES

▪ Patient has no reaction to iodinated contrast media.
▪ Patient recognizes possibility of adverse reaction to iodinated contrast media.
▪ Patient asks questions regarding the preparation for the procedure.

DOCUMENTATION

▪ Patient's expressions of concern about adverse reaction and symptoms of previous episodes
▪ Observations of physiologic and behavioral manifestations of adverse reaction
▪ Interventions performed to allay adverse reaction
▪ Patient's response to interventions
▪ Evaluations for expected outcomes

REFERENCES

Cantais, A., Hammouda, Z., Mory, O., Patural, H., Stephan, J.-L., Gulyaeva, L., & Darmon, M. (2016). Incidence of contrast-induced acute kidney injury in a pediatric setting: A cohort study. *Pediatric Nephrology, 31*(8), 1355–1362.

Ehrmann, S., Quartin, A., Hobbs, B., Robert-Edan, V., Cely, C., Bell, C., ... Ng, C. S. (2017). Contrast-associated acute kidney injury in the critically ill: Systematic review and Bayesian meta-analysis. *Intensive Care Medicine, 43*(6), 785–794.

Matthews, E. (2018). Acute kidney injury and iodinated contrast media. *Radiologic Technology, 89*(5), 467CT–477CT.

Patschan, D., Buschmann, I., & Ritter, O. (2018). Contrast-induced nephropathy: Update on the use of crystalloids and pharmacological measures. *International Journal of Nephrology, 2018*, 1–8.

Ineffective Airway Clearance

DEFINITION

Reduced ability to clear secretions or obstructions from the respiratory tract to maintain a clear airway

RELATED FACTORS (R/T)

- Dehydration
- Excessive mucus
- Exposure to harmful substance
- Fear of pain
- Foreign body in airway
- Inattentive to second-hand smoke
- Mucus plug
- Retained secretions
- Smoking

ASSOCIATED CONDITIONS

- Airway spasm
- Allergic airway
- Asthma
- Chronic obstructive pulmonary disease
- Congenital heart disease
- Critical illness
- Exudate in the alveoli
- General anesthesia
- Hyperplasia of the bronchial walls
- Neuromuscular diseases
- Respiratory tract infection

ASSESSMENT

- History of present illness
- Patient's ability to clear airway
- Knowledge of physical condition
- Neurologic status, including level of consciousness, orientation, and sensory and motor status
- Respiratory status, including symmetry of chest expansion; use of accessory muscles; cough (productive or nonproductive); respiratory rate, depth, and pattern; sputum characteristics; palpation for fremitus; percussion of lung fields; auscultation for breath sounds; pulse oximetry; chest x-ray; arterial blood gas (ABG) values; and hemoglobin level and hematocrit; pulmonary function studies
- Psychosocial status, including interest, motivation, and knowledge

DEFINING CHARACTERISTICS

- Absence of cough
- Adventitious breath sounds
- Altered respiratory rhythm

- Altered thoracic percussion
- Altered thoraco-vocal fremitus
- Bradypnea
- Cyanosis
- Difficulty verbalizing
- Diminished breath sounds
- Excessive sputum
- Hypoxemia
- Ineffective cough
- Ineffective sputum elimination
- Nasal flaring
- Orthopnea
- Psychomotor agitation
- Subcostal retraction
- Tachypnea
- Uses accessory muscles to breathe

EXPECTED OUTCOMES

- Airway will remain patent.
- Adventitious breath sounds (crackles, rhonchi, wheezes, or stridor) will be absent.
- Chest x-ray will show no abnormality.
- Oxygen level will be in normal range.
- Patient will breathe deeply and cough to remove secretions.
- Patient will expectorate sputum.
- Patient will demonstrate controlled coughing techniques.
- Ventilation will be adequate.
- Patient will demonstrate skill in conserving energy while attempting to clear airway.
- Patient will state understanding of changes needed to diminish oxygen demands.

Suggested NOC Outcomes

Anxiety Level; Anxiety Self-Control; Aspiration Prevention; Respiratory Status: Airway Patency; Respiratory Status: Ventilation

INTERVENTIONS AND RATIONALES

- **S** Assess respiratory status at least every 4 hours or according to established standards. *Obstruction in the airway leads to atelectasis, pneumonia, or respiratory failure.*
- **EBP** Turn patient every 2 hours. Always position for maximal aeration of lung fields and mobilization of secretions. *This prevents pooling and stasis of respiratory secretions.*
- Mobilize patient to full capabilities *to facilitate chest expansion and ventilation.*
- **S** Avoid placing patient in supine position for extended periods. Encourage lateral, sitting, prone, and upright positions as much as possible *to enhance lung expansion and ventilation.*
- **EBP** When helping patient cough and deep breathe, use whatever position best ensures cooperation and minimizes energy expenditure, such as raising the head of the bed or sitting on side of bed. *Such positions promote chest expansion and ventilation of basilar lung fields.*
- Suction, as ordered, to stimulate cough and clear airways. Be alert for progression of airway compromise. Maintaining a patent airway will *prevent respiratory distress.*

▥ Perform postural drainage, percussion, and vibration to facilitate secretion movement. Monitor sputum, noting amount, odor, and consistency. *Sputum amount and consistency are indicators of hydration status and effectiveness of therapy. Foul-smelling sputum may indicate respiratory infection.*

PCC ▥ Teach patient an easily performed cough technique *to clear airway without fatigue.*

▥ Provide adequate humidification *to loosen secretions.*

▥ Encourage adequate water intake (3 to 4 L/day) *to ensure optimal hydration and loosening of secretions, unless contraindicated.*

▥ Encourage sputum expectoration *to remove pathogens and prevent spread of infection.* Provide tissues and paper bags for hygienic disposal *to prevent spread of infection.*

▥ Give expectorants, bronchodilators, and other drugs, as ordered, and monitor effectiveness. *These measures enhance clearance of secretions from airways.*

▥ Provide bronchodilator treatments before chest physical therapy *to optimize results of the treatment.*

S ▥ Administer oxygen, as ordered, *to promote oxygenation of cells throughout the body.*

S ▥ Monitor ABG values and hemoglobin levels *to assess oxygenation and ventilatory status.* Report deviations from baseline levels; oxygen saturation should be higher than 90%.

▥ If conservative measures fail to maintain partial pressure of arterial oxygen (PaO_2) within an acceptable range, prepare for endotracheal intubation, as ordered, *to maintain artificial airway and optimize PaO_2 level.*

PCC ▥ Assess patient's learning needs and provide appropriate information *to help prevent recurrence of obstruction and promote change in daily activities to reduce oxygen demands.*

Suggested NIC Interventions

Airway Management; Aspiration Precautions; Cough Enhancement; Infection Protection; Oxygen Therapy; Positioning; Respiratory Monitoring; Ventilation Assistance

EVALUATIONS FOR EXPECTED OUTCOMES

▥ Patient's airway remains clear and allows for adequate ventilation.
▥ Auscultation of patient's lung fields reveals no adventitious breath sounds.
▥ Patient's chest x-ray is normal.
▥ Patient's oxygen level remains within normal range.
▥ Patient coughs and deep breathes to expectorate secretions.
▥ Patient expectorates sputum.
▥ Patient performs controlled coughing techniques.
▥ Patient doesn't experience dyspnea or change in respiratory pattern.
▥ Patient performs energy conservation techniques.
▥ Patient demonstrates understanding of changes needed to diminish oxygen demands.

DOCUMENTATION

▥ Patient's perceptions of ability to cough
▥ Observations of physical findings
▥ Effectiveness of medications
▥ Patient's attempts to clear airway
▥ Maneuvers performed to clear airway
▥ Evaluations for expected outcomes

REFERENCES

Dilektaşlı, A. G., & Önen, Z. P. (2018). Essentials in the comprehensive management of chronic respiratory diseases: Airway clearance and vaccination. *Turkish Thoracic Journal, 19*(3), 101–102.

Lee, L., Hill, A., & Patman, S. (2017). A survey of clinicians regarding respiratory physiotherapy intervention for intubated and mechanically ventilated patients with community-acquired pneumonia. What is current practice in Australian ICUs? *Journal of Evaluation in Clinical Practice, 23*(4), 812–820.

Reychler, G., Debier, E., Contal, O., & Audag, N. (2018). Intrapulmonary percussive ventilation as an airway clearance technique in subjects with chronic obstructive airway diseases. *Respiratory Care, 63*(5), 620–631.

Spors, D., & Sawyer, C. (2018). Connected solutions for pediatric airway clearance: Airway clearance therapy adherence for adults can be complicated by a variety of factors, but pediatric patients face additional barriers to proper management simply due to their age. *RT: The Journal for Respiratory Care Practitioners, 31*(1), 22–24.

Risk for Allergy Reaction

DEFINITION

Susceptible to an exaggerated immune response or reaction to substances, which may compromise health

RISK FACTORS

- Exposure to allergen
- Exposure to environmental allergen
- Exposure to toxic chemical

ASSESSMENT

- History of reactions to allergens in the environment, medications, chemicals
- Physical symptoms: eyes, ears, nose, throat, breathing, skin
- History of when symptoms occur
- Environmental factors: air systems, dust, carpet, pets
- Knowledge level, including patient's current understanding of physical condition and physical, mental, and emotional readiness to learn

EXPECTED OUTCOMES

- Patient will not experience an adverse reaction to allergen.
- Patient will recognize personal risk factors for allergic reaction.
- Patient will express awareness of personal allergy.
- Patient will ask questions if new information requires clarification.

Suggested NOC Outcomes

Risk Control; Risk Detection; Knowledge: Medication; Knowledge: Diet; Immune Hypersensitivity Response; Allergy Response: Localized

INTERVENTIONS AND RATIONALES

PCC ■ Determine whether patient has had any previous allergic reaction to substances and explore related details of the reaction. *Thorough history will provide a more effective prevention plan.*

EBP ▪ Suggest that patient keep a diary noting when symptoms occur. *This will help in the development of a risk reduction plan.*

▪ Assess for presence of any other conditions that may indicate an altered immune response, for example, multiple food intolerances, sensitivity to flowers or perfumes. *This will help to identify those at risk and promote early interventions for risk reduction.*

PCC ▪ Remove any known allergens from patient environment if possible *to reduce risk of reaction in patient.*

▪ Assist with any allergy testing and any prescribed treatment interventions such as long-term prophylaxis *and reinforce treatment plan as needed.*

S ▪ Review signs and symptoms of allergic reaction and emergency interventions *to ensure rapid response to critical situations.*

S ▪ Instruct patient and family to inform health care providers of allergy to medications, and consider wearing a warning bracelet *to further protect patient from unnecessary harm.*

PCC ▪ Assist patient with modifying environment *to minimize exposure to allergens.*

S ▪ For food allergens: Encourage patient to read all food labels *to minimize exposure.* Suggest development of a food allergen card to use when dining out. *This will help chefs prepare a safe meal.*

EBP ▪ For airborne allergens: Encourage frequent washing of bed linens and using vacuum with special filter *to minimize exposure.*

T&C ▪ Refer patient to primary provider to discuss possible need for emergency medication, for example, EpiPen. *This will ensure immediate treatment for severe allergic reaction.*

Suggested NIC Interventions

Allergy Management; Risk Identification; Teaching: Individual

EVALUATIONS FOR EXPECTED OUTCOMES

▪ Patient has no episodes of reaction to allergens.
▪ Patient recognizes possibility of adverse reaction allergen and the response needed.
▪ Patient asks questions regarding the use of EpiPen or other measures to reduce allergic response.

DOCUMENTATION

▪ Patient's expressions of concern about adverse reaction and symptoms of previous episodes of allergic reactions
▪ Observations of physiologic and behavioral manifestations of adverse reaction to allergens
▪ Interventions performed to allay adverse reaction
▪ Patient's response to interventions
▪ Evaluations for expected outcomes

REFERENCES

Böhm, R., Proksch, E., Schwarz, T., & Cascorbi, I. (2018). Drug hypersensitivity: Diagnosis, genetics, and prevention. *Deutsches Aerzteblatt International, 115*(29/30), 501–512.

Caltekin, İ., Akyol, P. Y., Topal, F. E., Karagöz, A., & Ünlüer, E. E. (2017). Contrast-induced nephropathy and allergic reaction in patients who were given intravenous contrast material in emergency department. *Journal of Emergencies, Trauma and Shock, 10*(1), 48–49.

Chang, K.-L., & Guarderas, J. C. (2018). Allergy testing: Common questions and answers. *American Family Physician, 98*(1), 34–39.

Lyons, S. A., van Dijk, A. M., Knulst, A. C., Alquati, E., Le, T.-M., & van Os-Medendorp, H. (2018). Dietary interventions in pollen-related food allergy. *Nutrients, 10*(10), 1520.

Ring, J., Klimek, L., & Worm, M. (2018). Adrenaline in the acute treatment of anaphylaxis. *Deutsches Aerzteblatt International, 115*(31/32), 528–534.

Anxiety

DEFINITION

An emotional response to a diffuse threat in which the individual anticipates nonspecific impending danger, catastrophe, or misfortune

RELATED FACTORS (R/T)

- Conflict about life goals
- Interpersonal transmission
- Pain
- Stressors
- Substance misuse
- Unfamiliar situation
- Unmet needs
- Value conflict

ASSOCIATED CONDITIONS

- Mental disorders

ASSESSMENT

- Current health status
- History of stress-related signs or symptoms
- History of panic symptoms (choking feeling in throat, hyperventilation, light-headedness, dizziness, and other physical signs and symptoms of anxiety)
- Sociologic status, including support systems, hobbies, interests, work history, family makeup, family roles (evidence of harmony or disharmony), family coping mechanisms, evidence of reinforcement of problem by family, and lifestyle (how this reinforces irrational fears)
- Medication history, including response, effectiveness, and adverse effects
- Cultural influences
- Physiologic status
- Patient's perception of problem, onset of problem, recent stressors, life changes, and other precipitants
- Mental status, including orientation to time, place, and person; insight regarding current situation; judgment; abstract thinking; general information; mood; affect; recent and remote memory; thought processes; and thought content
- Coping and problem-solving ability
- Ability to perform activities of daily living
- Sleep habits
- Dietary and nutritional status
- Available support systems, including family members, friends, clergy, and health care agencies

Behavioral/Emotional

- Crying
- Decreased productivity
- Expresses anguish
- Expresses anxiety about life event changes
- Expresses distress
- Expresses insecurity
- Expresses intense dread
- Helplessness
- Hypervigilance
- Increased wariness
- Insomnia
- Irritable mood
- Nervousness
- Psychomotor agitation
- Reduced eye contact
- Scanning behavior
- Self-focused

Affective

- Anguish
- Apprehensiveness
- Distress
- Fear
- Feeling of inadequacy
- Helplessness
- Increase in wariness
- Irritability
- Nervousness
- Overexcitement
- Rattled
- Regretful
- Self-focused
- Uncertainty

Physiologic

- Altered respiratory pattern
- Anorexia
- Brisk reflexes
- Chest tightness
- Cold extremities
- Diarrhea
- Dry mouth
- Expresses abdominal pain
- Expresses feeling faint
- Expresses muscle weakness
- Expresses tension
- Facial flushing

- Increased blood pressure
- Increased heart rate
- Increased sweating
- Nausea
- Pupil dilation
- Quivering voice
- Reports altered sleep-wake cycle
- Reports heart palpitations
- Reports tingling in extremities
- Superficial vasoconstriction
- Tremors
- Urinary frequency
- Urinary hesitancy
- Urinary urgency

Sympathetic

- Alteration in respiratory pattern
- Anorexia
- Brisk reflexes
- Cardiovascular excitation
- Diarrhea
- Dry mouth
- Facial flushing
- Heart palpitations
- Increase in blood pressure
- Increase in heart rate
- Increase in respiratory rate
- Pupil dilation
- Superficial vasoconstriction
- Twitching
- Weakness

Parasympathetic

- Abdominal pain
- Alteration in sleep pattern
- Decreased blood pressure
- Decrease in heart rate
- Diarrhea
- Faintness
- Fatigue
- Nausea
- Tingling in extremities
- Urinary frequency
- Urinary hesitancy
- Urinary urgency

Cognitive

- Altered attention
- Confusion

- Decreased perceptual field
- Expresses forgetfulness
- Expresses preoccupation
- Reports blocking of thoughts
- Rumination

EXPECTED OUTCOMES

- Patient will experience reduced anxiety by identifying precipitating situations.
- Patient will identify current stressors.
- Patient will set limits and compromises on behavior when ready.
- Patient will develop effective coping behaviors.
- Patient will maintain autonomy and independence without disabling fears or use of phobic behavior.
- Patient will identify factors that elicit anxious behaviors.
- Patient will discuss activities that decrease anxious behaviors.
- Patient will make use of available emotional support.
- Patient will show fewer signs of anxiety.
- Patient will practice progressive relaxation techniques a specified number of times per day.
- Patient will cope with current medical situation without demonstrating severe signs of anxiety.

Suggested NOC Outcomes

Aggression Self-Control; Anxiety Level; Anxiety Self-Control; Concentration; Coping; Hyperactivity Level; Impulse Self-Control; Psychosocial Adjustment: Life Change; Social Interaction Skills; Stress Level; Symptom Control

INTERVENTIONS AND RATIONALES

- **PCC** — Spend 10 minutes with patient twice per shift. Convey a willingness to listen. Offer understanding and empathy; for example, "I know you're frightened. I'll stay with you." *Specific amount of uninterrupted, non–care-related time spent with anxious patient builds trust and reduces tension. Active listening helps patient ventilate feelings.*
- **PCC** — Give patient clear, concise explanations of anything that's about to occur. Avoid information overload; an anxious patient can't assimilate many details. *Anxiety may impair patient's cognitive abilities.*
- **PCC** — Listen attentively; allow patient to express feelings verbally. *This may allow patient to identify anxious behaviors and discover the source of anxiety.*
- Make no demands on patient. *An anxious patient may respond to excessive demands with hostility and abuse.*
- **PCC** — Attend to patient's comfort needs to increase trust and reduce anxiety.
- Identify and reduce as many environmental stressors (including people) as possible. *Anxiety commonly results from lack of trust in the environment.*
- **PCC** — Have patient state what kinds of activities promote feelings of comfort and encourage patient to perform them. *This gives patient a sense of control.*
- **PCC** — Remain with patient during severe anxiety. *Anxiety is usually related to fear of being left alone.*

`PCC` ▪ Include patient in decisions related to care, when feasible. *Anxious patient may mistrust own abilities; involvement in decision-making may reduce anxious behaviors.*

`PCC` ▪ Support family members in coping with patient's anxious behavior. *Involving family members in the process of reassurance and explanation allays patient's anxiety as well as their own.*

▪ Identify your feelings toward the patient *to keep your feelings from interfering with treatment.*

`PCC` ▪ Accept patient as is. *Forcing patient to change before patient is ready causes panic.*

`EBP` ▪ Explore factors that precipitate phobic reactions and anxiety. *This is important for understanding patient's behavioral dynamics.*

`S` ▪ Reassure patient about being safe. *Patient may perceive being at risk, which may increase patient's level of anxiety.*

`EBP` ▪ Support patient with desensitization techniques *to help overcome patient's problem.*

`PCC` ▪ Give patient a chance to ventilate own feelings. *This reduces patient's tendency to suppress or repress bottled-up feelings, which may continue to affect behavior even though patient may be unaware of them.*

`PCC` ▪ Allow extra visiting periods with family if this seems to allay patient's anxiety. *This allows anxious patient and family to support each other according to their abilities and at their own pace.*

▪ Help patient set limits and compromises on behavior when ready and allow patient to be afraid. *Fear is a feeling, neither right nor wrong.*

`EBP` ▪ Teach patient relaxation techniques to be performed at least every 4 hours, such as guided imagery, progressive muscle relaxation, and meditation. *These measures restore psychological and physical equilibrium by decreasing autonomic response to anxiety.*

`EBP` ▪ Give patient facts about fear and anxiety and their consequences *to reduce anxiety and encourage patient to help manage problem.*

▪ Encourage patient not to run away when afraid *to help patient learn that fear can be faced and managed.*

`PCC` ▪ Help patient develop own techniques for dealing with fears *to establish alternatives to escape or avoidance behaviors.*

`EBP` ▪ Offer relaxing types of music to patient for quiet listening periods. *Listening to relaxing music may provide distraction and have a calming effect on patient.*

`T&C` ▪ Refer patient to community or professional mental health resources to provide ongoing mental health assistance. *Encouraging the use of community resources reinforces the notion that anxiety reduction is a long-term process.*

Suggested NIC Interventions

Active Listening; Anger Control Assistance; Anticipatory Guidance; Anxiety Reduction; Behavior Modification: Social Skills; Calming Technique; Coping Enhancement; Meditation Facilitation; Impulse Control Training; Presence; Progressive Muscle Relaxation; Simple Guided Imagery; Simple Relaxation Therapy; Spiritual Support; Support Group

EVALUATIONS FOR EXPECTED OUTCOMES

▪ Patient identifies precipitating situations and demonstrates fewer physical symptoms of anxiety, improved concentration, and reduced preoccupation with fears.

▪ Patient describes at least two situations that increase anxious behaviors.

▪ Patient states at least two ways to eliminate or minimize anxious behaviors.

- Patient identifies causes of anxiety.
- Patient communicates with nurse or family members to gain reassurance, information, or emotional support.
- Patient participates in desensitization therapy and learns to better manage stress, health, and responsibilities.
- Patient makes decisions, shows greater independence, and decreases behaviors that limit spontaneous activity.
- Patient demonstrates progressive relaxation exercises and practices them a specified number of times per day.
- Patient reports ability to cope with current situation without experiencing severe anxiety.

DOCUMENTATION

- Patient's statement of anxiety and feelings of relief
- Statements about observable signs of patient's anxiety
- Interventions to reduce patient's anxiety
- Effectiveness of nursing interventions that can be observed
- Evaluations for expected outcomes

REFERENCES

Day, P. (2018). Treatment of anxiety in elderly housebound patients. *Journal of Community Nursing,* *32*(2), 52–55.
Edraki, M., Rambod, M., & Molazem, Z. (2018). The effect of coping skills training on depression, anxiety, stress, and self-efficacy in adolescents with diabetes: A randomized controlled trial. *International Journal of Community Based Nursing and Midwifery,* 6(4), 324–333.
Melin, E. O., Svensson, R., & Thulesius, H. O. (2018). Psychoeducation against depression, anxiety, alexithymia and fibromyalgia: A pilot study in primary care for patients on sick leave. *Scandinavian Journal of Primary Health Care,* 36(2), 123–133.
Özakgül, A. A., & Aştı, T. A. (2018). The effect of training provided to the relatives of stroke patients on the life quality, anxiety and depressive symptom levels of patients and their relatives. *Journal of Neurological and Neurosurgical Nursing,* 7(2), 56–63.

Risk for Aspiration

DEFINITION

Susceptible to entry of gastrointestinal secretions, oropharyngeal secretions, solids, or fluids to the tracheobronchial passages, which may compromise health

RISK FACTORS

- Barrier to elevating upper body
- Decreased gastrointestinal motility
- Difficulty swallowing
- Enteral nutrition tube displacement
- Inadequate knowledge of modifiable factors
- Increased gastric residue
- Ineffective airway clearance

ASSOCIATED CONDITIONS

- Chronic obstructive pulmonary disease
- Critical illness

- Decreased level of consciousness
- Delayed gastric emptying
- Depressed gag reflex
- Enteral nutrition
- Facial surgery
- Facial trauma
- Head and neck neoplasms
- Incompetent lower esophageal sphincter
- Increased intragastric pressure
- Jaw fixation techniques
- Medical devices
- Neck surgery
- Neck trauma
- Neurological diseases
- Oral surgical procedures
- Oral trauma
- Pharmaceutical preparations
- Pneumonia
- Stroke
- Treatment regimen

ASSESSMENT

- Patient's ability to cough
- Neurologic status, including level of consciousness (LOC), orientation, and mental status
- Gastrointestinal (GI) status, including gag and swallow reflexes, inspection of abdomen, abdominal girth, auscultation of bowel sounds, palpation for masses and tenderness, percussion of abdomen, and medications
- Nutritional status, including continuous and intermittent tube feeding
- Respiratory status, including skin color, rate and depth of respiration, cough (productive or nonproductive), auscultation of breath sounds, palpation for fremitus, sputum characteristics (color, consistency, amount, and odor), arterial blood gas values, and chest x-ray
- Vital signs
- Laboratory studies, such as white blood cell (WBC) count and sputum culture

EXPECTED OUTCOMES

- Patient's temperature and WBC count will remain normal.
- No pathogens will appear in sputum cultures.
- Respiratory secretions will be clear and odorless.
- Auscultation will reveal no adventitious breath sounds.
- Respiratory rate will remain within normal limits.
- Auscultation will reveal normal bowel sounds.
- Patient and caregiver will apply measures to prevent aspiration.

Suggested NOC Outcomes

Aspiration Prevention; Mechanical Ventilation Response: Adult; Respiratory Status: Airway Patency; Respiratory Status: Ventilation; Risk Control; Swallowing Status

S ▪ Assess respiratory status at least every 4 hours *for signs of possible aspiration (increased respiratory rate, cough, sputum production, or diminished breath sounds), which should be treated as early as possible.*

S ▪ Monitor and record neurologic status *to detect altered LOC, which could affect ability to swallow food or saliva.*

S ▪ Monitor and record vital signs *to detect signs of aspiration or impaired gas exchange due to aspiration.*

S ▪ Keep suction equipment available at all times, especially when feeding the patient, *to ensure ability to keep airway clear.*

S ▪ Assess patient for gag and swallow reflexes. *Decreased gag or swallow reflex may cause aspiration.*

▪ Encourage patient to cough and expectorate sputum *to mobilize secretions.* Provide tissues and paper bags for hygienic sputum disposal *to prevent spreading infection.*

S ▪ Hold infant with head elevated during feeding and position in an infant seat after feeding. *Such positioning uses gravity to prevent regurgitation of stomach contents and promotes lung expansion.*

▪ Auscultate for bowel sounds every shift and report changes. *Delayed gastric emptying and elevated intragastric pressure may promote regurgitation of stomach contents.*

▪ If patient is receiving tube feedings:

   ▪ Assess cuff inflation for patient with artificial airway and adjust appropriately *to protect lower airways from oropharyngeal secretions.*

S   ▪ Add food coloring to tube feeding if patient has altered state of consciousness, diminished gag reflex, or history of aspiration *to help monitor gastric secretions for aspiration.*

   ▪ Begin regimen with a small, diluted amount, as tolerated and ordered, *to allow adjustment to formula osmolality and avoid nausea, vomiting, and diarrhea.*

S   ▪ Elevate head of bed during and after feedings unless contraindicated *to prevent aspiration.*

   ▪ Check for residual tube feeding every shift and record amount. If more than 50 mL remains, withhold feeding *to prevent vomiting and aspiration. Report findings to physician.*

   ▪ Place tube properly before feeding or giving medication *to protect airway.*

S   ▪ Stop feeding immediately if aspiration is suspected; then apply suction as needed and turn patient on side *to avoid further aspiration.*

PCC ▪ Assess need for antiemetic drug *to reduce nausea and vomiting.* Administer, if ordered, and monitor for effectiveness.

S ▪ Review test results *to identify signs of infection*; report abnormalities.

PCC ▪ Explain treatment to patient and caregivers *to encourage compliance.*

Suggested NIC Interventions

Airway Suctioning; Artificial Airway Management; Aspiration Precautions; Enteral Tube Feeding; Positioning; Vomiting Management

▪ Patient's temperature and WBC count remain within normal parameters.

▪ No pathogens appear in patient's cultures.

▪ Patient's respiratory secretions remain clear and odorless.

- Auscultation of lungs reveals no adventitious breath sounds.
- Auscultation of abdomen reveals normal bowel sounds.
- Patient and caregiver discuss measures necessary to prevent aspiration.

DOCUMENTATION

- Verification of tube placement
- Residuals of tube feedings
- Vomiting or aspiration
- Breath sounds
- Patient's indication of situations that may lead to aspiration
- Observations of physical findings
- Interventions performed to prevent aspiration
- Evaluations for expected outcomes

REFERENCES

Miller, S. (2017). Assessment of airway defenses in the neurologically impaired patient. *MEDSURG Nursing, 26*(2), 113–118.
Prevention of Aspiration in Adults. (2017). *Critical Care Nurse, 37*(3), 88.
Sakai, K., Hirano, H., Watanabe, Y., Tohara, H., Sato, E., Sato, K., & Katakura, A. (2016). An examination of factors related to aspiration and silent aspiration in older adults requiring long-term care in rural Japan. *Journal of Oral Rehabilitation, 43*(2), 103–110.
Takenoshita, S., Kondo, K., Okazaki, K., Hirao, A., Takayama, K., Hirayama, K., … Terada, S. (2017). Tube feeding decreases pneumonia rate in patients with severe dementia: Comparison between pre- and post-intervention. *BMC Geriatrics, 17*, 267.
Yagi, N., Nagami, S., Lin, M., Yabe, T., Itoda, M., Imai, T., & Oku, Y. (2017). A noninvasive swallowing measurement system using a combination of respiratory flow, swallowing sound, and laryngeal motion. *Medical & Biological Engineering & Computing, 55*(6), 1001–1017.

Risk for Impaired Attachment

DEFINITION

Susceptible to disruption of the interactive process between parent or significant other and child that fosters the development of a protective and nurturing reciprocal relationship

RISK FACTORS

- Anxiety
- Child's illness prevents effective initiation of parental contact
- Disorganized infant behavior
- Inability of parent to meet personal needs
- Insufficient privacy
- Parental conflict resulting from disorganized infant behavior
- Parent–child separation
- Physical barrier
- Substance misuse

ASSESSMENT

- Family status, including marital status, composition of family, ages of family members, ability of family to meet physical and emotional needs of its members, evidence of abuse, and health history

- Parental status, including level of education, knowledge of normal growth and development, stability of relationship, and available support systems
- Parents' psychological statuses, including energy level, motivation, recent life changes, psychiatric history, maternal history of drug abuse, and alcohol or antidepressant use by either partner
- Child's neurologic status, including muscle tone and reflexes; infant lethargy, irritability, seizures, or tremors; and Brazelton Neonatal Behavioral Assessment, Dubowitz Gestational Age Assessment, and Bayley Scales of Infant Development
- Child's sensory status, including vision or hearing loss, visual and auditory-evoked potentials, and audiometric tests
- Sleep pattern, including infant's usual hours of sleep

EXPECTED OUTCOMES

- Parents will initiate positive interaction with child.
- Parents will hold and talk to child.
- Parents will express confidence in ability to respond to child's needs.
- Parents will respond appropriately to child.
- Parents will express positive feelings about child.
- Parents will express confidence in their ability to care for child.
- Parents will recognize when they need assistance.
- Child will respond positively to parents, show interest in their faces, and become calm when soothed by them.

Suggested NOC Outcomes

Parenting Performance; Role Performance

INTERVENTIONS AND RATIONALES

EBP - Perform ongoing assessment of parent and child interaction *to evaluate whether parent–child attachment is proceeding normally.*
- Speak positively about child in parents' presence *to encourage parents to develop positive view of child.*

PCC - Maintain eye contact with child while providing care, talk to child, and touch appropriately *to demonstrate healthy interactions with child.*
- Help parents learn to understand behavioral cues from child. For example, child may become fussy when ready for a nap or may pull ear if there is an earache. *Developing better understanding of child's behavior will decrease parents' frustration and help them care more effectively for child.*

PCC - Provide parents and child with privacy *to promote attachment.*

EBP - Assess parents' knowledge of child care and development *to develop an appropriate teaching plan.*

EBP - Teach parents to provide physical care for child *to increase their sense of competence and self-confidence.*
- Encourage parents to make eye contact with child, caress and talk to child in soothing tone, call by name, and make positive remarks *to foster a healthy parent–child attachment and to help ensure child's well-being.*

PCC ▪ Observe parents; note whether their responses to child are appropriate. Compliment them when they exhibit successful parenting skills *to increase their confidence.*

PCC ▪ Discuss life changes precipitated by birth *to help parents express their frustrations and feelings about role changes.* Topics may include altered finances, changes in living space, care-taking arrangements, and new roles and responsibilities for parents and siblings.

PCC ▪ Provide parents with sources of ongoing support and care *to ensure adequate follow-up.*

PCC ▪ Assess the home environment. Discuss adaptations parents need to make. *Adaptations in home environment may be needed to help parents properly care for their child.*

Suggested NIC Interventions

Abuse Protection Support: Child; Coping Enhancement; Developmental Enhancement: Child; Parenting Promotion

EVALUATIONS FOR EXPECTED OUTCOMES

▪ Parents initiate positive interactions with child.
▪ Parents make eye contact with child, caress and talk to child, and call by name.
▪ Parents express confidence in their ability to meet child's needs.
▪ Parents respond appropriately to child's behavioral cues, provide stimulation when child is alert and ready, don't overstimulate child, and recognize when child needs to nap.
▪ Parents express positive feelings about child.
▪ Parents express confidence in ability to care for child at home.
▪ Parents recognize when they need assistance and make plans to contact appropriate resources.
▪ Child responds positively to parents, shows interest in their faces, and becomes calm when soothed by them.

DOCUMENTATION

▪ Description of parent and child interactions
▪ Nursing interventions to promote attachment
▪ Parents' response to nursing interventions
▪ Child's response to modifications in parents' behavior
▪ Evaluations for expected outcomes

REFERENCES

Aslan, E., Erturk, S., Demir, H., & Aksoy, O. (2017). Fathers' attachment status to their infants. *International Journal of Caring Sciences, 10*(3), 1410–1418.

Branjerdporn, G., Meredith, P., Strong, J., & Garcia, J. (2017). Associations between maternal-foetal attachment and infant developmental outcomes: A systematic review. *Maternal and Child Health Journal, 21*(3), 540–553.

Cadman, T., Belsky, J., & Pasco Fearon, R. M. (2018). The brief attachment scale (BAS-16): A short measure of infant attachment. *Child: Care, Health and Development, 44*(5), 766–775.

Shoghi, M., Sohrabi, S., & Rasouli, M. (2018). The effects of massage by mothers on mother-infant attachment. *Alternative Therapies in Health and Medicine, 24*(3), 34–39.

Autonomic Dysreflexia

DEFINITION

Life-threatening, uninhibited sympathetic response of nervous system to a noxious stimulus after a spinal cord injury at the 7th thoracic vertebra (T7) or above

RELATED FACTORS (R/T)

Gastrointestinal Stimuli

- Constipation
- Difficult passage of feces
- Digital stimulation
- Enemas
- Fecal impaction
- Suppositories

Integumentary Stimuli

- Cutaneous stimulation
- Skin irritation

Musculoskeletal–Neurological Stimuli

- Irritating stimuli below level of injury
- Painful stimuli below level of injury
- Pressure over bony prominence
- Pressure over genitalia
- Range-of-motion exercises
- Spasm

Regulatory–Situational Stimuli

- Constrictive clothing
- Environmental temperature fluctuations
- Positioning

Reproductive–Urological Stimuli

- Bladder distention
- Bladder spasm
- Instrumentation
- Sexual intercourse

Other

- Insufficient caregiver knowledge of disease process
- Insufficient knowledge of disease process

ASSOCIATED CONDITIONS

- Bowel distention
- Cystitis
- Deep vein thrombosis

- Detrusor sphincter dyssynergia
- Epididymitis
- Esophageal reflux disease
- Fracture
- Gallstones
- Gastric ulcer
- Gastrointestinal system pathology
- Hemorrhoids
- Heterotopic bone
- Labor and delivery
- Ovarian cyst
- Pharmaceutical agent
- Pregnancy
- Pulmonary emboli
- Renal calculi
- Substance withdrawal
- Sunburn
- Surgical procedure
- Urethritis
- Urinary catheterization
- Urinary tract infection
- Wound

ASSESSMENT

- History of spinal cord trauma, including level of injury or lesion, and previous episodes of dysreflexia
- Patient's description of symptoms, including headache, nasal congestion, blurred vision, chest pain, diaphoresis and flushing above level of lesion, chilling, paresthesia, cutis anserina ("goose flesh") above level of lesion, metallic taste, and nausea
- Neurologic status, including level of consciousness, orientation, pupillary response, sensory status, and motor status
- Cardiovascular status, including blood pressure, heart rate and rhythm, and skin temperature and color
- Genitourinary status, including urine output, palpation of bladder, signs of urinary tract infection (UTI), and examination of urinary assistive devices such as catheter
- Gastrointestinal (GI) status, including nausea and vomiting, usual bowel elimination pattern, last bowel movement, inspection of abdomen, auscultation of bowel sounds, palpation for masses, and percussion for areas of dullness
- Environmental conditions, including changes in temperature (e.g., cold draft) and objects putting pressure on skin

DEFINING CHARACTERISTICS

- Blurred vision
- Bradycardia
- Chest pain
- Chilling
- Conjunctival congestion
- Diaphoresis above the injury
- Diffuse pain in different areas of the head

- Horner syndrome
- Metallic taste in mouth
- Nasal congestion
- Pallor below injury
- Paresthesia
- Paroxysmal hypertension
- Pilomotor reflex
- Red blotches on skin above the injury
- Tachycardia

EXPECTED OUTCOMES

- Cause of dysreflexia will be identified and corrected.
- Patient will experience cardiovascular stability as evidenced by ____ systolic range, ____ diastolic range, and _____ heart rate range.
- Patient will avoid bladder distention and UTI.
- Patient will have no fecal impaction.
- Patient's environment will have no noxious stimuli.
- Patient will state relief from symptoms of dysreflexia.
- Patient will have few, if any, complications.
- Patient's bladder elimination pattern will remain normal.
- Patient's bowel elimination pattern will remain normal.
- Patient, family members, or caregiver will demonstrate knowledge and understanding of dysreflexia and will describe care measures.
- Patient will experience few or no dysreflexic episodes.

Suggested NOC Outcomes

Knowledge: Disease Process; Neurologic Status; Neurologic Status: Autonomic; Sensory Function Status; Vital Signs Status

INTERVENTIONS AND RATIONALES

- **S** Assess for signs of dysreflexia (especially severe hypertension) *to detect condition so that prompt treatment may be initiated.*
- Place patient in sitting position or elevate head of bed *to aid venous drainage from brain, lower intracranial pressure, and temporarily reduce blood pressure.*
- Ascertain and correct probable cause of dysreflexia:
    - Check for bladder distention and patency of catheter. If necessary, irrigate catheter with small amount of solution or insert a new catheter immediately. *A blocked urinary catheter can trigger dysreflexia.*
    - Check for fecal mass in rectum. Apply dibucaine ointment (Nupercainal) or another product, as ordered, to anus and 2.5 cm into rectum 10 to 15 minutes before removing impaction. *Failure to use ointment may aggravate autonomic response.*
    - Check environment for cold drafts and objects putting pressure on patient's skin, *which could act as dysreflexia stimuli.*
    - Send urine for culture if no other cause becomes apparent *to detect possible UTI.*
- If hypertension persists despite other measures, administer ganglionic blocking agent, vasodilator, or other medication as ordered. *Drugs may be required if hypertension persists or if noxious stimuli can't be removed.*

S ▪ Take vital signs frequently *to monitor effectiveness of prescribed medications.*

EBP ▪ Instruct patient, family members, or caregiver about dysreflexia, including its causes, signs and symptoms, and care measures *to prepare them to handle possible emergencies related to condition.* Suggest patient carry an autonomic dysreflexia emergency card such as the one from www.sci-info-pages.com *to provide information quickly for responders unfamiliar with autonomic dysreflexia.*

PCC ▪ Implement and maintain bowel and bladder elimination programs *to avoid stimuli that could trigger dysreflexia.*

Suggested NIC Interventions

Airway Management; Bowel Management; Dysreflexia Management; Fluid Management; Neurologic Monitoring; Surveillance; Temperature Management; Vital Signs Monitoring

EVALUATIONS FOR EXPECTED OUTCOMES

▪ Cause of dysreflexia is identified and corrected.

▪ Patient experiences cardiovascular stability as evidenced by ___ systolic range, _____ diastolic range, and ___ heart rate range.

▪ Palpation doesn't reveal a distended bladder or signs of UTI.

▪ Patient's bowel elimination program is successfully implemented and maintained. Fecal impaction is absent.

▪ Patient's environment remains free from noxious stimuli.

▪ Patient expresses relief from signs and symptoms of dysreflexia.

▪ Patient doesn't experience complications of dysreflexia, including contractures, venous stasis, thrombus formation, skin breakdown, and hypostatic pneumonia.

▪ Patient's bladder elimination program is successfully implemented and maintained, urinary catheter is patent and without kinking or blockage, and urine output remains within specified volume.

▪ Patient's bowel elimination pattern remains normal.

▪ Patient, family members, or caregiver expresses understanding of causes, signs and symptoms, and treatment of autonomic dysreflexia, and demonstrates measures to implement if dysreflexia occurs.

▪ Because of successful maintenance of bladder and bowel elimination programs, preventive skin care measures, and patient and family teaching, patient experiences few or no dysreflexic episodes.

DOCUMENTATION

▪ Objective assessment of dysreflexic episode

▪ Patient's description of dysreflexic episode

▪ Interventions to identify and eliminate causes of dysreflexia and patient's response to these

▪ Instructions given to patient, family, and caregiver

▪ Patient's expressions of understanding and demonstrated ability to prevent or manage dysreflexic episode

▪ Implementation, alteration, or continuation of bladder and bowel programs

▪ Evaluations for expected outcomes

REFERENCES

Koyuncu, E., & Ersoz, M. (2017). Monitoring development of autonomic dysreflexia during urodynamic investigation in patients with spinal cord injury. *Journal of Spinal Cord Medicine, 40*(2), 170–174.

Lee, E. S., & Joo, M. C. (2017). Prevalence of autonomic dysreflexia in patients with spinal cord injury above T6. *BioMed Research International, 2017*, 1–6.

Solinsky, R., Kirshblum, S. C., & Burns, S. P. (2018). Exploring detailed characteristics of autonomic dysreflexia. *Journal of Spinal Cord Medicine, 41*(5), 549–555.

Squair, J. W., Phillips, A. A., Harmon, M., & Krassioukov, A. V. (2016). Emergency management of autonomic dysreflexia with neurologic complications. *CMAJ: Canadian Medical Association Journal, 188*(15), 1100–1103.

Risk for Autonomic Dysreflexia

DEFINITION

Susceptible to life-threatening, uninhibited response of the sympathetic nervous system post-spinal shock, in an individual with spinal cord injury or lesion at the 6th thoracic vertebra (T6) or above (has been demonstrated in patients with injuries at the 7th thoracic vertebra [T7] and the 8th thoracic vertebra [T8]), which may compromise health

RISK FACTORS

Gastrointestinal Stimuli

- Bowel distention
- Constipation
- Difficult passage of feces
- Digital stimulation
- Enemas
- Fecal impaction
- Suppositories

Integumentary Stimuli

- Cutaneous stimulation
- Skin irritation
- Sunburn
- Wound

Musculoskeletal–Neurological Stimuli

- Irritating stimuli below level of injury
- Painful stimuli below level of injury
- Pressure over bony prominence
- Pressure over genitalia
- Range of motion
- Spasm

Regulatory–Situational Stimuli

- Constrictive clothing
- Environmental temperature fluctuations
- Positioning

Reproductive–Urological Stimuli

▥ Bladder distention
▥ Bladder spasm
▥ Instrumentation
▥ Sexual intercourse

Other

▥ Insufficient caregiver knowledge of disease process
▥ Insufficient knowledge of disease process

ASSOCIATED CONDITIONS

▥ Bowel distention
▥ Cystitis
▥ Deep vein thrombosis
▥ Detrusor sphincter dyssynergia
▥ Epididymitis
▥ Esophageal reflux disease
▥ Fracture
▥ Gallstones
▥ Gastric ulcer
▥ Gastrointestinal system pathology
▥ Hemorrhoids
▥ Heterotopic bone
▥ Labor and delivery period
▥ Ovarian cyst
▥ Pharmaceutical agent
▥ Pregnancy
▥ Pulmonary emboli
▥ Renal calculi
▥ Substance withdrawal
▥ Sunburn
▥ Surgical procedure
▥ Urethritis
▥ Urinary catheterization
▥ Urinary tract infection
▥ Wound

ASSESSMENT

▥ History of spinal cord trauma or spinal cord tumor, including level of injury or lesion, and previous episodes of dysreflexia
▥ Neurologic status, including level of consciousness, orientation, pupillary response, sensory status, and motor status
▥ Cardiovascular status, including blood pressure, heart rate and rhythm, and skin temperature and color
▥ Genitourinary status, including urine output, palpation of bladder, signs of urinary tract infection (UTI), and urinary assistive devices such as catheter
▥ Gastrointestinal (GI) status, including nausea and vomiting, usual bowel pattern, bowel habits, last bowel movement, inspection of abdomen, auscultation of bowel sounds, palpation for masses and tenderness, and percussion for areas of tympany and dullness

- Environmental conditions, including changes in temperature (e.g., cold drafts) and objects putting pressure on skin

EXPECTED OUTCOMES

- Risk factors for dysreflexia will be identified and reduced.
- Patient will avoid bladder distention.
- Patient won't experience UTI.
- Patient will maintain normal urinary and bowel elimination patterns.
- Patient will be free from fecal impaction.
- Patient's environment will be free from noxious stimuli that may cause dysreflexia.
- Patient, family members, or caregiver will express understanding of causes of dysreflexia.
- Patient, family members, or caregiver will demonstrate understanding of measures to prevent dysreflexia.

Suggested NOC Outcomes

Neurologic Status: Autonomic; Symptom Severity; Vital Signs Status

INTERVENTIONS AND RATIONALES

S - Assess for risk factors of dysreflexia, such as constipation, fecal impaction, distended bladder, and presence of noxious stimuli. *Identifying risk factors can prevent or minimize dysreflexic episodes.*
- Monitor and record intake and output accurately *to ensure adequate fluid replacement, thereby helping to prevent constipation.*
S - Check for bladder distention and patency of catheter. *A blocked catheter can trigger dysreflexia.*
S - Check for abdominal distention and assess bowel sounds. Monitor and record characteristics and frequency of stools. *Fecal impaction may lead to dysreflexia.*
S - Monitor vital signs frequently *to ensure effectiveness of preventive measures.* Severe hypertension may indicate dysreflexia.
- Encourage fluid intake of 3 L daily, unless contraindicated. *Adequate fluid intake helps maintain patency of catheter and aids bowel elimination.*
- Administer laxative, enema, or suppositories, as prescribed, *to promote elimination of solids and gases from GI tract.* Monitor effectiveness.
T&C - Consult with dietitian about increasing fiber and bulk in diet to maximum prescribed by physician *to improve intestinal muscle tone and promote comfortable elimination.*
PCC - Implement and maintain bowel and bladder programs *to avoid stimuli that could trigger dysreflexia.*
EBP - Instruct patient, family members, or caregiver about risk factors, signs and symptoms, and care measures for dysreflexia *to help prevent a possible dysreflexic episode and help patient respond appropriately should dysreflexia occur.* Suggest patient carry an autonomic dysreflexia emergency card such as the one from www.sci-info-pages.com *to provide information quickly for responders unfamiliar with autonomic dysreflexia.*

Suggested NIC Interventions

Dysreflexia Management; Neurologic Monitoring; Vital Signs Monitoring

EVALUATIONS FOR EXPECTED OUTCOMES

- Risk factors for dysreflexia are identified and reduced.
- Patient avoids bladder distention.
- Patient doesn't experience UTI.
- Patient maintains normal urinary and bowel elimination patterns.
- Patient remains free from fecal impaction.
- Patient's environment is free from noxious stimuli that may cause dysreflexia.
- Patient, family members, or caregiver expresses understanding of causes of dysreflexia.
- Patient, family members, or caregiver demonstrates understanding of measures to prevent dysreflexia.

DOCUMENTATION

- Presence of risk factors for dysreflexia
- Interventions to minimize risk of dysreflexia and patient's response
- Patient's, family members', or caregiver's expressions of concern about risk of dysreflexia
- Instructions given to patient, family members, or caregiver regarding prevention of dysreflexic episodes
- Implementation or alteration of bowel and bladder program
- Evaluations for expected outcomes

REFERENCES

Davidson, R., & Phillips, A. (2017). Cardiovascular physiology and responses to sexual activity in individuals living with spinal cord injury. *Topics in Spinal Cord Injury Rehabilitation, 23*(1), 11–19.

Lee, E. S., & Joo, M. C. (2017). Prevalence of autonomic dysreflexia in patients with spinal cord injury above T6. *BioMed Research International, 2017,* 1–6.

Walter, M., Knüpfer, S. C., Cragg, J. J., Leitner, L., Schneider, M. P., Mehnert, U., ... Kessler, T. M. (2018). Prediction of autonomic dysreflexia during urodynamics: A prospective cohort study. *BMC Medicine, 16*(1), 53.

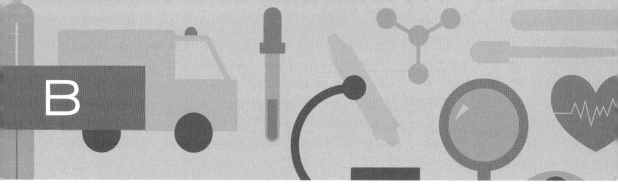

Disorganized Infant Behavior

Disintegration of the physiological and neurobehavioral systems of functioning

- Caregiver cue misreading
- Environmental overstimulation
- Feeding intolerance
- Inadequate physical environment
- Infant malnutrition
- Insufficient caregiver knowledge of behavioral cues
- Insufficient containment within environment
- Insufficient environmental sensory stimulation
- Pain
- Sensory deprivation
- Sensory overstimulation

- Congenital disorder
- Genetic disorder
- Infant illness
- Immature neurological functioning
- Impaired infant motor functioning
- Invasive procedure
- Infant oral impairment

- Cardiovascular status, including heart rate and rhythm
- Respiratory status, including oxygen saturation and respirations
- Gastrointestinal (GI) status, including feeding pattern, food tolerance, defecation pattern, ability to maintain adequate weight, and abdominal bloating and distention
- Neurologic status, including muscle tone, neonatal reflexes, excessive crying, lethargy, irritability, seizures, tremors, and assessments such as Brazelton Neonatal Behavioral Assessment Scale and Dubowitz Gestational Age Assessment
- Sensory status, including responsiveness to visual, tactile, and auditory stimuli and experience with pain
- Parental status, including knowledge of normal growth and development

- Sleep status, including sleep patterns and usual hours of sleep
- Parents' psychological status, including energy level, motivation, self-image, competence, recent life changes, experience with children, and eye contact and interaction with infant

DEFINING CHARACTERISTICS

Attention–Interaction System

- Impaired response to sensory stimuli

Motor System

- Alteration in primitive reflexes
- Exaggerated startle response
- Fidgeting
- Finger splaying
- Fisting
- Hands to face
- Hyperextension of extremities
- Impaired motor tone
- Tremor
- Twitching
- Uncoordinated movements

Physiological

- Abnormal skin color
- Arrhythmia
- Bradycardia
- Feeding intolerance
- Oxygen desaturation
- Tachycardia
- Time-out signals

Regulatory Problems

- Inability to inhibit startle reflex
- Irritability

State-Organization System

- Active-awake
- Diffuse alpha electroencephalogram (EEG) activity with eyes closed
- Irritable crying
- Quiet-awake
- State oscillation

EXPECTED OUTCOMES

- Parents will learn to identify and understand infant's behavioral cues.
- Parents will identify their own emotional responses to infant's behavior.
- Parents will identify means to help infant overcome behavioral disturbance.
- Parents will identify ways to improve their ability to cope with infant's responses.

▓ Infant will begin to show appropriate signs of maturation.

▓ Parents will express positive feelings about their ability to care for infant.

▓ Parents will identify resources for help with infant.

Suggested NOC Outcomes

Knowledge: Infant Care; Neurological Status; Preterm Infant Organization; Sleep

INTERVENTIONS AND RATIONALES

EBP ▓ Educate parents about infant maturation developmental process, emphasizing that parental participation is crucial *to help parents understand the importance of nurturing the infant.*

EBP ▓ Discuss with parents how their actions can help modify some of their infant's behavior. However, make it clear that infant maturation isn't completely within their control. *This explanation may help decrease the parents' feelings of incompetence.*

PCC ▓ Educate parents that infants give behavioral cues to indicate needs. Discuss appropriate ways to respond to behavioral cues—for example, providing stimulation that doesn't overwhelm the infant, stopping stimulation when the infant gives behavioral cues (such as yawning, looking away, or becoming agitated), and finding methods to calm the infant if the infant becomes agitated (such as swaddling, gentle rocking, and quiet vocalizations). Assist parents in identifying and coping with their responses to the infant's behavioral disturbance *to help them recognize and adjust their response patterns. When the infant doesn't respond positively to them, the parents may feel inadequate or become frustrated. Explain to parents that these reactions are normal.*

PCC ▓ Assist parents in exploring ways to cope with stress imposed by the infant's behavior *to help them develop better coping skills.*

PCC ▓ Praise the parents when they demonstrate appropriate methods of interacting with the infant *to provide positive reinforcement.*

T&C ▓ Provide the parents with information on sources of support and special infant services *to help them cope with their infant's long-term needs.*

Suggested NIC Interventions

Environmental Management; Neurologic Monitoring; Newborn Care; Parent Education: Infant; Positioning; Sleep Enhancement

EVALUATIONS FOR EXPECTED OUTCOMES

▓ Parents state their understanding of infant's behavioral cues.

▓ Parents discuss appropriate ways of responding to infant's behavior and exhibit decreased frustration with infant's behavior.

▓ Parents identify ways to help infant overcome behavioral disturbance by recognizing infant's needs and responding appropriately.

▓ Parents report improved ability to cope with stress of caring for infant.

▓ Infant begins to show appropriate signs of maturation, such as longer periods of sleep; shorter periods of crying; longer periods of being awake and alert; smoother transitions between behavioral states; and positive responses to parents' interventions.

▓ Parents express positive feelings about their ability to care for infant.

▓ Parents identify resources for help with infant.

DOCUMENTATION

- Assessment of factors that may enhance or retard infant behavioral development
- Parents' expressed feelings about caring for infant
- Nursing interventions and infant's response to them
- Evaluations for expected outcomes

REFERENCES

Nyström, P., Bölte, S., & Falck-Ytter, T. (2017). Responding to other people's direct gaze: Alterations in gaze behavior in infants at risk for autism occur on very short timescales. *Journal of Autism and Developmental Disorders, 47*(11), 3498–3509.

Santos, A. M. G., Viera, C. S., Bertolini, G. R. F., Osaku, E. F., de Macedo Costa, C. R. L., & Grebinski, A. T. K. G. (2017). Physiological and behavioural effects of preterm infant positioning in a neonatal intensive care unit. *British Journal of Midwifery, 25*(10), 647–654.

Wagner, N., Mills-Koonce, W., Propper, C., Willoughby, M., Rehder, P., Moore, G., ... Cox, M. J. (2016). Associations between infant behaviors during the face-to-face still-face paradigm and oppositional defiant and callous-unemotional behaviors in early childhood. *Journal of Abnormal Child Psychology, 44*(8), 1439–1453.

Readiness for Enhanced Organized Infant Behavior

DEFINITION

An integrated pattern of modulation of the physiological and neurobehavioral systems of functioning, which can be strengthened

ASSESSMENT

- Cardiovascular status, including heart rate and rhythm
- Respiratory status, including oxygen saturation and respirations
- Gastrointestinal status, including feeding and defecation patterns, food tolerance, ability to maintain adequate weight, and abdominal distention and bloating
- Neurologic status, including excessive crying, poor sleep patterns, lethargy, irritability, seizures, tremors, muscle tone, neonate reflexes, and assessments such as Brazelton Neonatal Behavioral Assessment Scale and Dubowitz Gestational Age Assessment
- Sensory status, including responsiveness to visual, tactile, and auditory stimuli and experience with pain
- Sleep status, including usual hours of sleep
- Parental status, including knowledge of normal growth and development
- Parents' psychological status, including energy level, motivation, experience with children, eye contact and interaction with infant, and Home Observation Measurement of the Environment results

DEFINING CHARACTERISTICS

- Parent expresses desire to enhance cue recognition
- Parent expresses desire to enhance environmental conditions
- Parent expresses desire to enhance recognition of infant's self-regulatory behaviors

EXPECTED OUTCOMES

- Parents will express understanding of their role in infant's behavioral development.
- Parents will express confidence in their ability to interpret infant's behavioral cues.

- Parents will identify means to promote infant's behavioral development.
- Parents will express positive feelings about their ability to care for infant.
- Parents will identify resources for help with infant.

Suggested NOC Outcomes

Child Development: 2 Months; Knowledge: Infant Care; Neurological Status; Sleep

INTERVENTIONS AND RATIONALES

EBP ▪ Educate parents about infant maturation developmental process. Include that infants exhibit three behavioral states: sleeping, crying, and being awake and alert. Also explain that infants provide behavioral cues that indicate their needs. *Education will help parents understand the importance of nurturing the infant and prepare them to respond to the infant's behavioral cues.*

EBP ▪ Discuss with parents how their actions can help promote infant development. Make it clear, however, that infant maturation isn't completely within their control. *This explanation may decrease feelings of anxiety and incompetence and help prevent unrealistic expectations.*

▪ Demonstrate appropriate ways of interacting with the infant, such as moderate stimulation, gentle rocking, and quiet vocalizations, *to help parents identify most effective methods of interacting with their child.*

PCC ▪ Assist parents in interpreting behavioral cues from their infant *to foster healthy parent–child interaction.* For example, help them recognize when infant is awake and alert, and point out to them that this is a good time to provide stimulation.

EBP ▪ Assist parents in identifying ways they can promote infant's development, such as providing stimulation by shaking a rattle in front of the infant, talking to infant in a gentle voice, and looking at infant when feeding, *to encourage practices that promote infant's development. Sensory experiences promote cognitive development.*

PCC ▪ Assist parents in exploring ways to cope with stress caused by infant's behavior *to increase their coping skills.*

PCC ▪ Praise parents for their attempts to enhance their interaction with infant *to provide positive reinforcement.*

T&C ▪ Provide parents with information on sources of support and special infant services *to encourage them to continue to foster their infant's development.*

Suggested NIC Interventions

Attachment Promotion; Developmental Care; Family Integrity Promotion: Childbearing Family; Infant Care; Sleep Enhancement

EVALUATIONS FOR EXPECTED OUTCOMES

- Parents express understanding of their role in infant's behavioral development.
- Parents express confidence in their ability to recognize infant's behavioral cues.
- Parents identify activities that foster positive responses from infant and provide appropriate sensory and tactile stimulation.
- Parents express positive feelings about their ability to care for infant.
- Parents identify resources for help with infant.

DOCUMENTATION

- Assessment of factors that may enhance infant's behavioral development
- Parents' expressed feelings about caring for their infant
- Nursing interventions and infant's response to them
- Evaluations for expected outcomes

REFERENCES

Kristensen, I. H., & Kronborg, H. (2018). What are the effects of supporting early parenting by enhancing parents' understanding of the infant? Study protocol for a cluster-randomized community-based trial of the Newborn Behavioral Observation (NBO) method. *BMC Public Health, 18*(832), 1–9. doi:10.1186/s12889-018-5747-4

Smarius, L., Strieder, T., Loomans, E., Doreleijers, T., Vrijkotte, T., Gemke, R., & Eijsden, M. (2017). Excessive infant crying doubles the risk of mood and behavioral problems at age 5: Evidence for mediation by maternal characteristics. *European Child & Adolescent Psychiatry, 26*(3), 293–302.

Vallotton, C. D., Decker, K. B., Kwon, A., Wang, W., & Chang, T. (2017). Quantity and quality of gestural input: Caregivers' sensitivity predicts caregiver-infant bidirectional communication through gestures. *Infancy, 22*(1), 56–77.

Risk for Disorganized Infant Behavior

DEFINITION

Susceptible to disintegration in the pattern of modulation of the physiological and neurobehavioral systems of functioning, which may compromise health

RISK FACTORS

- Caregiver cue misreading
- Environmental overstimulation
- Feeding intolerance
- Inadequate physical environment
- Infant malnutrition
- Insufficient caregiver knowledge of behavioral cues
- Insufficient containment within environment
- Insufficient environmental sensory stimulation
- Pain
- Sensory deprivation
- Sensory overstimulation

ASSOCIATED CONDITIONS

- Congenital disorder
- Genetic disorder
- Infant illness
- Immature neurological functioning
- Impaired infant motor functioning
- Invasive procedure
- Infant oral impairment

ASSESSMENT

- Cardiovascular status, including heart rate and rhythm
- Respiratory status, including oxygen saturation and respirations

- Gastrointestinal status, including feeding and defecation patterns, food tolerance, ability to maintain adequate weight, and abdominal bloating and distention
- Neurologic status, including muscle tone, neonate reflexes, excessive crying, lethargy, irritability, seizures, tremors, and assessments such as Brazelton Neonatal Behavioral Assessment Scale and Dubowitz Gestational Age Assessment
- Sensory status, including infant's responsiveness to visual, tactile, and auditory stimuli and experience with pain
- Sleep status, including sleep pattern and usual hours of sleep
- Parental status, including knowledge of normal growth and development
- Parents' psychological status, including energy level, motivation, experience with children, and eye contact and interaction with infant

EXPECTED OUTCOMES

- Parents will identify factors that place the infant at risk for behavioral disturbance.
- Parents will identify potential signs of behavioral disturbance in infant.
- Parents will identify appropriate ways to interact with infant.
- Parents will identify their reactions to infant (including ways of coping with occasional frustration and anger).
- Parents will express positive feelings about their ability to care for infant.
- Parents will identify resources for help with infant.

Suggested NIC Interventions

Child Development: 2 Months; Knowledge: Infant Care; Knowledge: Parenting; Preterm Infant Organization

INTERVENTIONS AND RATIONALES

EBP ▪ Educate parents about infant maturation developmental process, emphasizing that parental participation is crucial *to help them understand the importance of nurturing the infant.*

EBP ▪ Discuss with parents how their actions can help modify some of their infant's behavior. However, make it clear that infant maturation isn't completely within their control. *This explanation may decrease the parents' feelings of incompetence.*

EBP ▪ Educate parents about certain risk factors that may interfere with the infant's ability to achieve optimal development. These risk factors include overstimulation, lack of stimulation, lack of physical contact, and painful medical procedures. *Educating the parents will help them understand their role in interpreting the infant's behavioral cues and providing appropriate stimulation.*

PCC ▪ Assist parents in identifying the potential signs of a behavioral disturbance in infant: inappropriate responses to stimuli, such as the failure to respond to human contact or tendency to become agitated with human contact; physiologic regulatory problems, such as a breathing disturbance in a premature infant; and apparent inability to interact with the environment. *Education will help parents recognize if infant has a problem in behavioral development.*

- Demonstrate appropriate ways of interacting with infant *to help parents identify and interpret infant's behavioral cues and respond appropriately.* For example, help them recognize when infant is awake and alert, and help them understand when infant needs more stimulation, such as being spoken to or held.

PCC ▪ Assist parents in exploring ways to cope with the stress imposed by infant's behavior *to increase their coping skills*. Help parents identify their emotional responses to infant's behavior *to help them recognize and adjust their response patterns*. Explain that it's normal for parents to experience feelings of inadequacy, frustration, or anger if infant doesn't respond positively to them.

PCC ▪ Praise parents when they demonstrate appropriate methods of interacting with infant *to provide positive reinforcement*.

T&C ▪ Provide parents with information on sources of support and special infant services *to help them cope with infant's long-term needs*.

Suggested NOC Outcomes

Infant Care; Newborn Monitoring; Parent Education: Infant; Positioning; Surveillance

EVALUATIONS FOR EXPECTED OUTCOMES

- Parents identify risk factors for behavioral disturbance.
- Parents identify potential signs of behavioral disturbance in infant.
- Parents identify actions that promote their infant's development.
- Parents report improvement in their ability to cope with the stress of raising an infant.
- Parents express positive feelings about their ability to care for infant.
- Parents identify resources for help with infant.

DOCUMENTATION

- Assessment of factors that could disturb infant's behavioral development
- Parents' expression of feelings about caring for infant
- Nursing interventions and infant's response to them
- Evaluations for expected outcomes

REFERENCES

Alakortes, J., Kovaniemi, S., Carter, A., Bloigu, R., Moilanen, I., & Ebeling, H. (2017). Do child healthcare professionals and parents recognize social-emotional and behavioral problems in 1-year-old infants? *European Child & Adolescent Psychiatry, 26*(4), 481–495.

Smaling, H., Huijbregts, S., Heijden, K., Hay, D., Goozen, S., Swaab, H., … van Goozen, S. H. M. (2017). Prenatal reflective functioning and development of aggression in infancy: The roles of maternal intrusiveness and sensitivity. *Journal of Abnormal Child Psychology, 45*(2), 237–248.

Smarius, L., Strieder, T., Loomans, E., Doreleijers, T., Vrijkotte, T., Gemke, R., & Eijsden, M. (2017). Excessive infant crying doubles the risk of mood and behavioral problems at age 5: Evidence for mediation by maternal characteristics. *European Child & Adolescent Psychiatry, 26*(3), 293–302.

Risk for Bleeding

DEFINITION

Susceptible to a decrease in blood volume, which may compromise health

RISK FACTORS

- Insufficient knowledge of bleeding precautions

- Aneurysm
- Circumcision
- Disseminated intravascular coagulopathy
- Gastrointestinal condition
- Impaired liver function
- Inherent coagulopathy
- Postpartum complication
- Pregnancy complication
- Trauma
- Treatment regimen

- Cardiovascular status, including blood pressure, cardiac output, patient and family history of cardiovascular disease, peripheral pulses, and smoking history
- Nutritional status, including dietary patterns, laboratory tests, and serum protein level
- Neurologic status, including level of consciousness (LOC), mental status, motor function, and sensory pattern
- Reproductive status, including number of pregnancies and complications of pregnancy
- Respiratory status, including breath sounds, respiratory rate, and pattern
- Presence of health condition that may interfere with bleeding, such as coagulopathies
- Gastrointestinal (GI) status, including nausea and vomiting, bowel habits, stool characteristics, history of GI problems, disease, or surgery; bowel sounds
- Laboratory studies, including complete blood count (CBC), liver profile, serum electrolyte levels, platelet count, and blood coagulation studies

- Patient will receive adequate screening/monitoring to alert clinicians of existing risk factors for bleeding.
- Patient will receive appropriate follow-through and evidence-based interventions by clinicians to protect the patient from a bleeding episode.
- Patient will receive appropriate clinician staffing and surveillance for a rapid response to rescue client before bleeding occurs (i.e., avoid a failure to rescue occurrence).
- Patient heart rate, rhythm, blood pressure, and tissue perfusion will remain within expected ranges during episodes of risk.
- Patient will exhibit coping mechanism and functional behavior during episodes of risk.
- Patient and clinicians will identify and avoid risk situations with the potential for trauma injury and falls in the environment.
- Patient will perform self-care activities and functions.
- Patient will experience no bleeding episodes.

Suggested NOC Outcomes

Maternal Status: Antepartum; Maternal Status: Postpartum; Blood Coagulation; Treatment-Related Side Effects: Surgery, Circumcision, Medications, Administration of Blood Products; Circulation Status; Tissue Perfusion: Vital Organs and Cellular; Wound Healing; Blood Loss Severity; Trauma

INTERVENTIONS AND RATIONALES

S ▪ Interview/screen each individual for risk factors for bleeding; *some individuals know their risks for bleeding, others do not, and clinical tests and evaluation by expert clinicians allow for preventive or corrective intervention measures.*

S ▪ Anticipate conditions and episodes of care that may precipitate bleeding. *The clinicians in high-risk areas (trauma, emergency departments, ante/intra/postpartum, surgery) must be prepared and be aware of patient conditions and changes that could precede a bleeding event.*

PCC ▪ Monitor physiologic responses (vital signs, O_2 level, LOC [behavior]) for values that remain in expected or normal ranges; *early bleeding compensatory mechanisms alter respirations, pulse, and blood pressure, and subtle changes can be detected by a perceptive clinician.*

▪ Monitor for frank bleeding and for occult bleeding in urine and feces through assessment of wounds, dressings, and eliminated body fluids either by visual inspection or with the aid of easy chemical testing (guaiac hemoccult).

PCC ▪ Correlate interview findings, risk factors, and current episode of care and patient condition *to determine the imminent level of risk for bleeding.*

▪ Perform vital signs and basic physical assessments according to evidence-based protocols for the in-hospital patient who is at risk for bleeding *until it is assured the patient is no longer at risk for bleeding.*

▪ Obtain clinical laboratory tests (hemoglobin, hematocrit, CBC, thrombin time [TT], prothrombin time [PT], activated partial thromboplastin time [APTT], others) and point-of-care tests (guaiac, urine dip test, gastroccult) *to monitor for trend changes in values that would indicate a risk for bleeding or that a bleeding episode is in process.*

▪ Examine surgical and wound dressings; *drainage tubes and collection canisters to measure the amount of bleeding and seepage the patient experiences and compare this with the expected blood loss for similar conditions.*

EBP ▪ Teach about intended effects of medications (heparin, enoxaparin, warfarin, clopidogrel, aspirin) that increase the risk for bleeding or prolong clotting. *This enables the patient to avoid situations that could cause bleeding (shaving, sports, vigorous tooth brushing) and to observe self for bleeding.*

EBP ▪ Teach about unintended or adverse effects of medications (corticosteroids, aspirin, nonsteroidal anti-inflammatory drugs [NSAIDs]) that increase the risk for bleeding or prolong clotting. *This enables the patient to avoid situations that could cause bleeding (shaving, sports, vigorous tooth brushing) and to observe self for bleeding.*

EBP ▪ Teach patient gentle alternatives in activities of daily living (ADLs) *to avoid trivial trauma that may cause injury and bleeding.*

EBP ▪ Teach patient about inherent conditions (thrombocytopenia, hemophilia) and devise an approach to lifestyle *that protects patient from injury and yet is satisfying and has a positive quality of life.*

EBP ▪ Teach patient patterns of risk management and promotion of a lifestyle that focuses on health promotion and injury avoidance because this will diminish the possibility of injury. *Having the knowledge to participate safely will increase independence and enhance self-esteem.*

PCC ▪ Provide care that protects the individual with a risk for bleeding from injury *to prevent bleeding.*

EBP ▪ Implement evidence-based interventions that reverse or remove the risk for bleeding or the bleeding condition. *These interventions will prevent patient from bleeding or will stabilize patient's physiologic condition and assist in recovery.*

PCC ▪ Provide emotional support to patient who is experiencing an episode of bleeding and also physiologic compensatory responses such as anxiety, fear, and a sense of dread. *This support provides assurance and is calming.*

PCC ▪ Support patient in participating in decisions about the treatment regimen that places the patient at risk for bleeding. *This active participation encourages greater understanding of the rationale and compliance by the patient with the treatment regimen (for medications, see earlier).*

T&C ▪ Refer patient at risk for bleeding secondary to treatment goals (i.e., warfarin, international normalized ratio [INR] level) to a case manager or advanced practice nurse *for clinical monitoring and reinforcement of teaching and lifestyle adjustments.*

S ▪ Manage and monitor the recovery progress of patient who experienced a bleeding episode *because patient may be weak and at safety risk for falls or injury.*

T&C ▪ Refer to a case manager the patient with inherent conditions that require long-term monitoring and management *so that patient can maintain independence safely.*

Suggested NIC Interventions

Hemodynamic Regulation; Intravenous (IV) Therapy; Circulatory Care; Hypovolemic Management; Vital Signs Monitoring; Fluid Management; Laboratory Data Interpretation; Shock Management

EVALUATIONS FOR EXPECTED OUTCOMES

▪ Patient receives careful monitoring of existing risk factors.
▪ Patient receives appropriate intervention to protect from bleeding episodes.
▪ Patient's vital signs remain in the ranges expected during risk for bleeding period.
▪ Patient exhibits adequate coping mechanisms.
▪ Patient is able to articulate an understanding of ways to avoid risk situations.
▪ Patient experiences no incidence of active bleeding.

DOCUMENTATION

▪ Recording of assessments for bleeding
▪ Lab values and vital signs
▪ Signs of any active bleeding episodes
▪ Intake and output
▪ Patient's concern about the risk for bleeding
▪ Patient's understanding of practical ways in which to avoid risk

REFERENCES

Butler, E., Møller, M. H., Cook, O., Granholm, A., Penketh, J., Rygård, S. L., ... Perner, A. (2018). Corticosteroids and risk of gastrointestinal bleeding in critically ill adults: Protocol for a systematic review. *Acta Anaesthesiologica Scandinavica, 62*(9), 1321–1326.

Carlin, N., Asslo, F., Sison, R., Shaaban, H., Baddoura, W., Manji, F., & Depasquale, J. (2017). Dual antiplatelet therapy and the severity risk of lower intestinal bleeding. *Journal of Emergencies, Trauma & Shock, 10*(3), 98–102.

Li, J., Han, B., Li, H., Deng, H., Méndez-Sánchez, N., Guo, X., & Qi, X. (2018). Association of coagulopathy with the risk of bleeding after invasive procedures in liver cirrhosis. *Saudi Journal of Gastroenterology, 24*(4), 220–227.

Zhang, C., Huang, C., Kong, X., Liu, G., Li, N., Liu, J., ... Wang, J. (2018). A randomized double-blind placebo-controlled trial to evaluate prophylactic effect of traditional Chinese medicine supplementing qi and hemostasis formula on gastrointestinal bleeding after percutaneous coronary intervention in patients at high risks. *Evidence-Based Complementary and Alternative Medicine, 2018*, 1–13. doi:10.1155/2018/3852196

Risk for Unstable Blood Glucose Level

DEFINITION

Susceptible to variation in serum levels of blood glucose from the normal range, which may compromise health

RISK FACTORS

- Excessive stress
- Excessive weight gain
- Excessive weight loss
- Inadequate adherence to treatment regimen
- Inadequate blood glucose self-monitoring
- Inadequate diabetes self-management
- Inadequate dietary intake
- Inadequate knowledge of disease management
- Inadequate knowledge of modifiable factors
- Ineffective medication self-management
- Sedentary lifestyle

ASSOCIATED CONDITIONS

- Cardiogenic shock
- Diabetes mellitus
- Infections
- Pancreatic diseases
- Pharmaceutical preparations
- Polycystic ovary syndrome
- Preeclampsia
- Pregnancy-induced hypertension
- Surgical procedures

ASSESSMENT

- Health status, educational level, cultural status, requests for information; demonstrated understanding of material
- Integumentary status, color, elasticity, hygiene, lesions, moisture, sensation, complete blood cell count, hemoglobin/hematocrit, serum albumin, blood coagulation studies, serum electrolytes, mobility status, urinary or bowel incontinence
- Nutritional status, including dietary patterns, laboratory tests, and serum protein level
- Neurologic status, including level of consciousness, mental status, motor function, and sensory pattern
- Behavioral status, understanding of health problem and treatment plan, past history with health care providers, participation in health care planning and decision-making; recognition and realization of potential growth, health, and autonomy
- Gastrointestinal (GI) status, including nausea and vomiting; bowel habits; stool characteristics; history of GI problems, disease, or surgery; and bowel sounds
- Laboratory studies, including serum albumin and glucose

EXPECTED OUTCOMES

- Patient will be free from symptoms of hypoglycemia/hyperglycemia.
- Patient will have serum glucose values in the prescribed desired range.
- Patient will verbalize understanding of how to control blood glucose level.

Suggested NOC Outcomes

Blood Glucose Level; Diabetes Self-Management; Knowledge: Diabetes Management, Weight Control

INTERVENTIONS AND RATIONALES

- **S** Assess patient for symptoms of low serum glucose level and maintain a patent airway if indicated. *A low serum glucose may not be detected in some patients until moderate to severe central nervous system impairment occurs, which can lead to a compromised airway and cardiac arrest.*
- **EBP** Assess for the underlying cause of changes in glucose (e.g., inadequate dietary intake; illness such as nausea, vomiting, or diarrhea; too much insulin) *to help patient prevent future episodes and adapt treatment strategies and lifestyle changes.*
- **S** Monitor or instruct patient to monitor glucose levels with a glucometer at regular intervals *to identify and respond early to fluctuations in glucose levels that occur outside normal parameters.*
- **PCC** Assess family understanding of prescribed treatment regimen. *The family plays an important role in supporting the patient.*
- **PCC** Assess patient's knowledge of hypoglycemia/hyperglycemia *to ensure adequate management and prevent future episodes.*
- **S** Monitor for signs and symptoms of hyperglycemia (polyuria, polydipsia, polyphagia, lethargy, malaise, blurred vision, and headache). *Early detection ensures prompt intervention and management.*
- **EBP** Assess for the underlying cause of elevated serum glucose level, including inadequate dietary intake, illness, and poor medication management, *to prevent future episodes and develop treatment strategies such as changes in lifestyle.*
- **S** Perform immediate finger stick with a glucometer *to determine glucose level, which will guide treatment strategies.* Administer insulin as prescribed *to treat elevated blood glucose levels.*
- **S** Provide patient with glucose tablets or gel if he or she is conscious and has ability to swallow. Administer intravenous (IV) glucose if patient is unconscious or cannot swallow. *Immediate treatment in the form of oral or IV glucose must be administered to reverse the low serum glucose level. If patient becomes nauseated, turn patient on side to prevent aspiration.*
- **S** Protect patient from injuries, such as falls. *Symptoms of low serum glucose place patient at risk for injury, especially when driving and performing other potentially dangerous activities.*
- **EBP** Evaluate serum electrolyte levels. Administer potassium, as prescribed. *With elevated blood glucose levels, potassium and sodium levels may be low, normal, or high, depending on the amount of water loss. Consider performing serum testing for HgbA$_{1c}$ (glycosylated hemoglobin A$_{1c}$ level) to evaluate average blood glucose levels over a period of approximately 2 to 3 months and to assess the adherence and effectiveness of the treatment regimen.*
- **EBP** Teach patient and family self-management of hypoglycemia and hyperglycemia including glucose monitoring at regular intervals *to treat abnormal glucose levels early* and

medication management, nutritional intake, exercise, and regular follow-up visits with the physician *to ensure adequate understanding and management of the treatment regimen to prevent future hyperglycemic events. Patient and family teaching may include referrals to a diabetic educator, diabetic education classes, and a dietitian.*

T&C ▦ Consult physician if signs and symptoms persist. *Changes in prescribed medications may be needed, such as with oral hypoglycemic agents or insulin dosing.* Call for emergency medical services if patient is unstable outside the hospital.

Suggested NIC Interventions

Bedside Laboratory Testing; Health Education; Health Screening; Nutritional Counseling; Teaching: Disease Process; Teaching: Prescribed Medications

EVALUATIONS FOR EXPECTED OUTCOMES

▦ Patient has no episodes of hypoglycemia or hyperglycemia.
▦ Patient has glucose readings within prescribed range.
▦ Patient verbalizes glucose management plan.

DOCUMENTATION

▦ Patient's expressions of concern about symptoms of previous episodes of hypoglycemia or hyperglycemia
▦ Observations of physiologic and behavioral manifestations of poor glucose control
▦ Interventions performed to allay symptoms of hypoglycemia or hyperglycemia
▦ Patient's response to interventions
▦ Evaluations for expected outcomes

REFERENCES

Linden, K., Berg, M., Adolfsson, A., & Sparud-Lundin, C. (2018). Well-being, diabetes management and breastfeeding in mothers with type 1 diabetes—An explorative analysis. *Sexual & Reproductive HealthCare, 15*, 77–82.

McClinchy, J. (2018). Dietary management of older people with diabetes. *British Journal of Community Nursing, 23*(5), 248–251.

Salci, M. A., Meirelles, B. H. S., & da Silva, D. M. V. G. (2017). Prevention of chronic complications of diabetes mellitus according to complexity. *Revista Brasileira de Enfermagem, 70*(5), 996–1003.

Saliva test could improve diabetes control and treatment. (2018). *MLO: Medical Laboratory Observer, 50*(9), 40

Risk for Unstable Blood Pressure

DEFINITION

Susceptible to fluctuating forces of blood flowing through arterial vessels, which may compromise health

RISK FACTORS

▦ Inconsistency with medication regimen
▦ Orthostasis

ASSOCIATED CONDITIONS

- Adverse effects of cocaine
- Adverse effects of nonsteroidal anti-inflammatory drugs (NSAIDs)
- Adverse effects of steroids
- Cardiac dysrhythmia
- Cushing syndrome
- Electrolyte imbalance
- Fluid retention
- Fluid shifts
- Hormonal change
- Hyperosmolar solutions
- Hyperparathyroidism
- Hyperthyroidism
- Hypothyroidism
- Increased intracranial pressure
- Rapid absorption and distribution of antiarrhythmia agent
- Rapid absorption and distribution of diuretic agent
- Rapid absorption and distribution of vasodilator agents
- Sympathetic responses
- Use of antidepressant agents

ASSESSMENT

- History of present illness
- History of circulatory disease
- History of drug abuse
- History of steroid use
- Cardiovascular status including blood pressure, heart rate and rhythm, skin color, temperature, and peripheral pulses
- Current medications, effectiveness
- History of medication compliance
- Medical history including family history, history of cardiovascular disease, and medication history
- Patient knowledge of current medications

EXPECTED OUTCOMES

- Patient will remain hemodynamically stable.
- Patient's blood pressure will be maintained within normal limits.
- Patient will verbalize modifiable risk factors for high blood pressure.
- Patient will identify reportable symptoms of low blood pressure.
- Patient will take medications as directed.

Suggested NOC Outcomes

Cardiac Pump Effectiveness; Cardiopulmonary Status; Knowledge: Cardiac Disease Management; Knowledge: Hypertension Management; Self-Management: Cardiac Disease; Self-Management: Hypertension; Tissue Perfusion: Cardiac

INTERVENTIONS AND RATIONALES

S ▪ Assess hemodynamic status, including blood pressure, heart rate, oxygen saturation, and respiratory rate for any abnormalities *that may be early indicators of high or low blood pressure.*

▪ Assist with preparation and completion of diagnostic tests and postprocedural care. *Safe completion of diagnostic tests will result in improved patient outcomes.*

EBP ▪ Treat episodes of high or low blood pressure promptly. *Perfusion is decreased if blood pressure is not within normal limits.*

EBP ▪ Provide patient with information regarding modifiable risk factors. *Knowledge of risk factors will contribute to informed decisions about lifestyle changes.*

PCC ▪ Encourage patient and family to share concerns regarding outcomes of tests *to reduce anxiety.*

T&C ▪ Collaborate with other members of the health care team to ensure that all underlying medical conditions are being managed effectively. *This will minimize the possibility of high and low blood pressure complications.*

Suggested NIC Interventions

Cardiac Care; Cardiac Care: Acute; Cardiac Risk Management; Health Education; Hemodynamic Regulation; Medication Administration; Medication Management; Medication Monitoring; Vital Signs Monitoring

EVALUATIONS FOR EXPECTED OUTCOMES

▪ Patient remains hemodynamically stable.
▪ Patient's blood pressure is maintained within normal limits.
▪ Patient verbalizes modifiable risk factors for high blood pressure.
▪ Patient identifies and reports symptoms of low blood pressure.
▪ Patient complies with medication regimen as directed.

DOCUMENTATION

▪ Hemodynamic status including vital signs and physical assessment findings
▪ Patient's report of any symptoms related to high or low blood pressure
▪ Patient's understanding of risk reduction interventions
▪ Evaluation of expected outcomes

REFERENCES

Jones, D. W. (2018). Blood pressure management: Beyond the guidelines. *Hypertension, 71*(6), 969–971.
Perry, H., Thilaganathan, B., Khalil, A., & Sheehan, E. (2018). Home blood-pressure monitoring in a hypertensive pregnant population. *Ultrasound in Obstetrics & Gynecology, 51*(4), 524–530.
Schwartz, C. L., Seyed-Safi, A., Haque, S., Bray, E. P., Greenfield, S., Hobbs, F. D. R., ... Mcmanus, R. J. (2018). Do patients actually do what we ask: Patient fidelity and persistence to the targets and self-management for the control of blood pressure in stroke and at risk groups blood pressure self-management intervention. *Journal of Hypertension, 36*(8), 1753–1761.
Weber, M. A., Chapple, C. R., Gratzke, C., Herschorn, S., Robinson, D., Frankel, J. M., ... White, W. B. (2018). A strategy utilizing ambulatory monitoring and home and clinic blood pressure measurements to optimize the safety evaluation of noncardiovascular drugs with potential for hemodynamic effects: A report from the SYNERGY trial. *Blood Pressure Monitoring, 23*(3), 153–163.

Disturbed Body Image

DEFINITION

Negative mental picture of one's physical self

RELATED FACTORS (R/T)

- Body consciousness
- Cognitive dysfunction
- Conflict between spiritual beliefs and treatment regimen
- Conflict between values and cultural norms
- Distrust of body function
- Fear of disease recurrence
- Low self-efficacy
- Low self-esteem
- Obesity
- Residual limb pain
- Unrealistic perception of treatment outcome
- Unrealistic self-expectations

ASSOCIATED CONDITIONS

- Binge-eating disorder
- Chronic pain
- Fibromyalgia
- Human immunodeficiency virus infections
- Impaired psychosocial functioning
- Mental disorders
- Surgical procedures
- Treatment regimen
- Wounds and injuries

ASSESSMENT

- Age
- Gender
- Marital status
- Physiologic changes
- Behavioral changes
- Appetite
- Health history, including eating disorders; dieting; physical, emotional, or sexual abuse; and episodes of emesis and self-induced emesis
- Exercise pattern, including type and duration
- Patient's and family's perception of patient's present health problem
- Patient's usual pattern of coping with stress
- Patient's role in family
- Patient's past experiences with health problems
- Sleep pattern
- Hobbies and interests
- Occupational history

- Use of diuretics and laxatives
- Medication use, either prescription or over-the-counter
- Ethnic background and cultural perceptions

DEFINING CHARACTERISTICS

- Altered proprioception
- Altered social involvement
- Avoids looking at one's body
- Avoids touching one's body
- Consistently compares oneself with others
- Depressive symptoms
- Expresses concerns about sexuality
- Expresses fear of reaction by others
- Expresses preoccupation with change
- Expresses preoccupation with missing body part
- Focused on past appearance
- Focused on past function
- Focused on past strength
- Frequently weighs self
- Hides body part
- Monitors changes in one's body
- Names body part
- Names missing body part
- Neglects nonfunctioning body part
- Nonverbal response to body changes
- Nonverbal response to perceived body changes
- Overexposes body part
- Perceptions that reflect an altered view of appearance
- Refuses to acknowledge change
- Reports feeling one has failed in life
- Social anxiety
- Uses impersonal pronouns to describe body part
- Uses impersonal pronouns to describe missing body part

EXPECTED OUTCOMES

- Patient will acknowledge change in body image.
- Patient will participate in decision-making about his or her care (specify).
- Patient will comply with prescribed treatment.
- Patient will communicate feelings about change in body image.
- Patient will express positive feelings about self.
- Patient will demonstrate increased flexibility and willingness to consider lifestyle changes.
- Patient will talk with someone who has experienced the same problem.
- Patient will demonstrate ability to practice two new coping behaviors.

Suggested NOC Outcomes

Adaptation to Physical Disability; Body Image; Coping; Grief Resolution; Adaptive Psychosocial Adjustment: Life Change; Self-Esteem

INTERVENTIONS AND RATIONALES

PCC ▓ While assisting with self-care measures, involve patient in discussions that will provide further insights into patient's coping patterns and self-esteem. *Patient's usual coping patterns and self-perception provide baseline data for assessing potential threat of current situation.*

PCC ▓ Accept patient's perception of self. *The nurse's acceptance validates patient's self-perception and provides reassurance of successfully overcoming crisis.*

PCC ▓ Assess patient's readiness for decision-making; then involve patient in making choices and decisions related to care and treatment. *This gives patient a sense of control over environment.*

PCC ▓ Convey a positive, caring attitude and take steps to ensure continuity of care throughout treatment *to ensure safety and foster a trusting therapeutic relationship.*

PCC ▓ Encourage patient to express feelings about physical changes. *Active listening conveys a caring and accepting attitude.*

EBP ▓ Provide information on appropriate self-care activities, such as:
  ▓ maintaining a proper diet
  ▓ bathing
  ▓ using skin lotions
  ▓ exercising appropriately to maintain muscle mass, bone strength, and cardiorespiratory health
Providing accurate self-care information helps the patient establish realistic goals.

PCC ▓ Encourage patient to participate actively in performing care. *This gives patient a sense of independence and increases self-esteem.*

PCC ▓ Give patient opportunities to voice feelings. *This helps patient ventilate doubts and resolve concerns.*

PCC ▓ Assist in identifying positive aspects of patient's appearance *to improve self-esteem by correcting distorted perceptions about body image.*

PCC ▓ Encourage patient to consider new grooming styles or to seek advice from a barber or cosmetologist on "updating" hair and makeup styles. *Attractive, tasteful grooming may help the older patient achieve a sense of control over the aging process.*

PCC ▓ Provide positive reinforcement to patient's efforts to adapt *to increase probability that healthy adaptation will continue.*

T&C ▓ Arrange for patient to interact with others who have similar problems. *A support group allows patient to share mutual support and caring with others who can fully understand. This kind of support will help the patient to respond in social situations without undue embarrassment.*

T&C ▓ Refer patient to a mental health professional for further counseling. *Referral is indicated when patient is adapting poorly to situation.*

PCC ▓ Assist patient to identify appropriate coping strategies. Discuss previously effective strategies *to help patient substitute them for maladaptive ones.*

T&C ▓ Encourage participation in support groups *to provide a forum for expressing feelings and obtaining support from individuals who can understand their concerns.*

PCC ▓ Encourage family members to express feelings and concerns about changes in the patient's body appearance or function. Provide accurate information and answer questions thoroughly. *Encouraging open discussion enables you to provide emotional support and may help ease family members' anxiety.*

PCC ▓ Have patient provide feedback about coping behaviors that seem to work. Reinforce the practice of these behaviors. *This allows you to evaluate patient's adaptive abilities.* Positive feedback reinforces adaptability and encourages similar behaviors in future.

Suggested NIC Interventions

Active Listening; Anticipatory Guidance; Body Image Enhancement; Coping Enhancement; Counseling; Grief Work Facilitation; Presence; Self-Care Assistance; Spiritual Support; Support System Enhancement

EVALUATIONS FOR EXPECTED OUTCOMES

- Patient acknowledges change in body image.
- Patient complies with prescribed treatment regimen.
- Patient takes an active role in planning aspects of care (specify).
- Patient expresses emotions associated with change in body image.
- Patient expresses positive feelings about self.
- Patient participates in discussions with support group composed of individuals with a similar change in body image (specify).
- Patient's hair appears clean and well-groomed.
- Patient uses at least two healthy coping skills to deal with change in body image.

DOCUMENTATION

- Words patient uses to describe self, prostheses, adaptive equipment, and limitations
- Body parts that patient focuses on or ignores
- Patient's statements about appearance, ability, and age
- Interventions directed toward improving patient's body image
- Observations related to change in structure or function of body part
- Observed responses of patient to change in body part, such as touching or not touching
- Health education or counseling provided to help patient cope with altered body image
- Patient's response to nursing interventions
- Evaluations for expected outcomes

REFERENCES

Duchesne, A.-P., Lalande, D., Émond, C., Lalande, G., Dion, J., Bégin, C., & McDuff, P. (2017). Body dissatisfaction and psychological distress in adolescents: Is self-esteem a mediator? *Journal of Health Psychology, 22*(12), 1563–1569.

Lewer, M., Bauer, A., Hartmann, A. S., & Vocks, S. (2017). Different facets of body image disturbance in binge eating disorder: A review. *Nutrients, 9*(12), 1–24.

Moffitt, R. L., Neumann, D. L., & Williamson, S. P. (2018). Comparing the efficacy of a brief self-esteem and self-compassion intervention for state body dissatisfaction and self-improvement motivation. *Body Image, 27*, 67–76.

Morris, L. L., Lupei, M., & Afifi, M. S. (2017). Body image perception after tracheostomy. *ORL—Head and Neck Nursing, 35*(4), 13–18.

Impaired Bowel Continence

DEFINITION

Inability to hold stool, to sense the presence of stool in the rectum, to relax and store stool when having a bowel movement is not convenient

RELATED FACTORS (R/T)

- Avoidance of nonhygienic toilet use
- Constipation

- Dependency for toileting
- Diarrhea
- Difficulty finding the bathroom
- Difficulty obtaining timely assistance to bathroom
- Embarrassment regarding toilet use in social situations
- Environmental constraints that interfere with continence
- Generalized decline in muscle tone
- Impaired physical mobility
- Impaired postural balance
- Inadequate dietary habits
- Inadequate motivation to maintain continence
- Incomplete emptying of bowel
- Laxative misuse
- Stressors

ASSOCIATED CONDITIONS

- Anal trauma
- Congenital abnormalities of the digestive system
- Diabetes mellitus
- Neurocognitive disorders
- Neurological diseases
- Physical inactivity
- Prostatic diseases
- Rectum trauma
- Spinal cord injuries
- Stroke

ASSESSMENT

- Age and developmental stage
- History of neurologic or psychiatric disorder
- Activity status, including type of exercise, frequency, and duration
- Fluid and electrolyte status, including intake and output, skin turgor, urine specific gravity, and mucous membranes
- Gastrointestinal status, including usual bowel elimination habits, change in bowel habits, stool characteristics (color, amount, size, and consistency), pain or discomfort, inspection of abdomen, auscultation of bowel sounds, palpation for masses and tenderness, percussion for tympany and dullness, and laxative and enema use
- Characteristics of incontinence, including frequency, time of day, before or after meals, relationship to activity, and behavior pattern (restlessness)
- Neurologic status, including orientation, level of consciousness, memory, and cognitive ability

DEFINING CHARACTERISTICS

- Abdominal discomfort
- Bowel urgency
- Fecal staining
- Impaired ability to expel formed stool despite recognition of rectal fullness
- Inability to delay defecation
- Inability to hold flatus
- Inability to reach toilet in time

- Inattentive to urge to defecate
- Silent leakage of stool during activities

EXPECTED OUTCOMES

- Patient will establish and maintain a regular pattern of bowel care.
- Patient will not experience bowel incontinent episodes.
- Patient will state understanding of bowel care routine.
- Patient or caregiver will demonstrate skill in carrying out bowel care routine with help from nurse.
- Patient or caregiver will demonstrate increasing skill in performing bowel care routine independently.

Suggested NOC Outcomes

Bowel Continence; Bowel Elimination; Cognition; Self-Care: Toileting; Tissue Integrity: Skin & Mucous Membranes

INTERVENTIONS AND RATIONALES

PCC
- Establish a regular pattern for bowel care; for example, after breakfast every other day, place patient on commode chair and allow patient to remain upright for 30 minutes for maximum response; then clean anal area. *Following a routine encourages regular physiologic function.*
- Monitor and record incontinent episodes; keep baseline record for 3 to 7 days *to track effectiveness of toileting routine.*
- Discuss bowel care routine with family or caregiver *to foster compliance.*

EBP
- Demonstrate bowel care routine to family or caregiver *to reduce anxiety from lack of knowledge or involvement in care.*
- Arrange for return demonstration of bowel care routine *to help establish therapeutic relationship with patient and family or caregiver.*
- Establish a date when family or caregiver will carry out bowel care routine with supportive assistance; *this will ensure that patient receives dependable care.*

EBP
- Instruct family or caregiver on need to regulate foods and fluids that cause diarrhea or constipation *to encourage helpful nutritional habits.*

PCC
- Maintain diet log *to identify irritating foods* and then eliminate them from patient's diet.

S
- Clean and dry perianal area after each incontinent episode *to prevent infection and promote comfort.*

PCC
- Maintain patient's dignity by using protective padding under clothing, by removing patient from group activity after incontinent episode, and by cleaning and returning patient to group without undue attention. *These measures prevent odor, skin breakdown, and embarrassment and promote patient's positive self-image.*

Suggested NIC Interventions

Bowel Incontinence Care; Bowel Management; Perineal Care; Skin Surveillance

EVALUATIONS FOR EXPECTED OUTCOMES

- Patient establishes and maintains regular pattern of bowel care.
- Patient states understanding of bowel care routine.

▓ Patient or caregiver demonstrates competence in performing bowel care routine with assistance from nurse.
▓ Patient or caregiver carries out bowel routine independently.
▓ Patient's skin remains clean, dry, and intact.
▓ Patient's episodes of incontinence decrease by 50%.
▓ Patient expresses positive self-image.

DOCUMENTATION

▓ Bowel care routine and administration of suppositories and enemas
▓ Description of incontinent episodes, including known precipitating factors, time of day, and other relevant details
▓ Patient's and caregivers' skills in bowel care
▓ Patient's level of awareness, response to incontinent episodes, and acceptance of bowel care routine
▓ Family's or caregiver's response to incontinence and to establishment and implementation of a bowel care routine
▓ Observation of effects of bowel care routine, episodes of incontinence, stool characteristics, and condition of skin
▓ Family's or caregiver's skill in carrying out bowel care routine and modifying diet
▓ Evaluations for expected outcomes

REFERENCES

Gu, P., Kuenzig, M. E., Kaplan, G. G., Pimentel, M., & Rezaie, A. (2018). Fecal incontinence in inflammatory bowel disease: A systematic review and meta-analysis. *Inflammatory Bowel Diseases, 24*(6), 1280–1290. doi:10.1093/ibd/izx109
Kelly, A. M. (2019). What can community nurses do for older adults who experience faecal incontinence? *British Journal of Community Nursing, 24*(1), 28–31. doi:10.12968/bjcn.2019.24.1.28
Keogh, A., & Burke, M. (2017). Faecal incontinence, anxiety and depression in inflammatory bowel disease. *Gastrointestinal Nursing, 15*(4), 18–27. doi:10.12968/gasn.2017.15.4.18
Nazarko, L. (2019). Faecal incontinence: Investigation and treatment. *Practice Nursing, 30*(2), 69–74. doi:10.12968/pnur.2019.30.2.69

Insufficient Breast Milk Production

DEFINITION

Inadequate supply of maternal breast milk to support nutritional state of an infant or child

RELATED FACTORS (R/T)

▓ Ineffective latching on to breast
▓ Ineffective sucking reflex
▓ Insufficient opportunity for suckling at the breast
▓ Insufficient suckling time at breast
▓ Maternal alcohol consumption
▓ Maternal insufficient fluid volume
▓ Maternal malnutrition
▓ Maternal smoking
▓ Maternal treatment regimen
▓ Rejection of breast

ASSOCIATED CONDITIONS

▥ Pregnancy

ASSESSMENT

▥ Maternal status, including age and maturity, parity, level of prenatal breastfeeding preparation, past breastfeeding experience, previous postpartum history, physical condition (actual or perceived inadequate milk supply and comfort level), and psychosocial factors (apprehension level, body image, stress from family and career, sociocultural views of breastfeeding, and emotional support from significant others)
▥ Neonatal status, including satisfaction and contentment, growth rate, age–weight relationship, urine output, quantity and characteristics of stools, and ability to latch on to breasts

DEFINING CHARACTERISTICS

▥ Absence of milk production with nipple stimulation
▥ Breast milk expressed is less than prescribed volume for infant
▥ Delay in milk production
▥ Infant constipation
▥ Infant frequently crying
▥ Infant frequently seeks to suckle at breast
▥ Infant refuses to suckle at breast
▥ Infant voids small amounts of concentrated urine
▥ Infant weight gain <500 g in a month
▥ Prolonged breastfeeding time
▥ Unsustained suckling at the breast

EXPECTED OUTCOMES

▥ Mother will produce sufficient milk to satisfy the growth needs of the neonate.
▥ Mother will *perceive* that she is producing sufficient milk for her baby.
▥ Mother and baby will achieve successful and sustained breastfeeding sessions.
▥ Mother will be free of emotions related to low self-esteem, poor body image, and guilt.

Suggested NOC Outcomes

Knowledge: Infant Care; Newborn Adaptation; Breastfeeding Establishment: Infant; Breast-feeding Establishment: Maternal; Nutritional Status: Nutrition Intake; Parent-Infant Attachment; Self-Esteem

INTERVENTIONS AND RATIONALES

EBP ▥ Position the mother/baby properly for baby to latch on to nipple and suckle. *The couplet may need direction in assuming the best position of comfort for suckling.*
PCC ▥ Assess to see if the neonate is able to latch properly to the nipple to suckle. *Ensuring the baby has latched to the nipple instead of the areola aids in milk expression.*
▥ Evaluate whether there is adequate milk removal from each breast at each session. *Milk production is stimulated and increases by suckling and milk removal.*
▥ Do a physical examination of the breast every shift; check nipples for inversion and for pore openings, *as anatomic conditions will limit the ability of the milk to flow to the newborn.*

S ▪ Examine the breasts for engorgement, inflammation, infection, or pain. *These conditions cause discomfort and limit the tolerance of the mother to breastfeed; the mother must remain healthy to continue breastfeeding; inflammation and infection need to be treated.*

S ▪ Assess exhaustion level and the rest and sleep patterns of mother. *Exhaustion and inability to rejuvenate depress milk production.*

S ▪ Assess the neonate's mouth to determine normal anatomy of tongue and palate; assess the neonate's mouth for *Candida* infection. *Anatomic imperfections and thrush infection affect the neonate's ability to suckle.*

S ▪ Assess the neonate's nose for patency to allow for breathing during suckling. *Neonates are nose breathers and must have patent nares in order to suckle.*

S ▪ Monitor the neonate's weight gain daily. *Sufficient nutrition from breast milk will allow weight gain.* Weigh the neonate before and after breastfeeding session. *When used, this can provide an indicator that the breast milk is sufficient.*

S ▪ Monitor the neonate's diaper for urine output (number per day, concentration of urine). *Urine output amount and color are indicators of hydration.* Check fluid–electrolyte status of neonate (urine characteristics and amount; stool output). *These measures guide the health care provider in determining the hydration status of the neonate.*

S ▪ Monitor the neonate for clinical presence of jaundice. *Breastfed neonates have lower rates of jaundice; if jaundice develops, it may be an indicator of insufficient milk intake.*

▪ Provide adequate nourishment and fluid intake to the mother (>150 mL/kg/day). *This is the minimum amount of fluid intake to sustain the mother and provide extra fluid for milk production.*

PCC ▪ Provide quiet uninterrupted time for breastfeeding. *Distractions and interruptions interfere with milk production, milk ejection, and the neonate's focus on suckling.*

PCC ▪ Encourage the mother to talk about emotions, including frustration and disappointment. *Allowing others to help the mother through emotional barriers may assist in creating peaceful emotions that aid in milk production and milk letdown.* Listen carefully to the mother's concerns for clues to emotions and coping with disappointment and guilt; these are early signs of depression and stress. *Early intervention allows emotional healing and allows the mother to focus on the neonate and breastfeeding.*

PCC ▪ Provide rest and sleep intervals for the mother. *Rest and sleep rejuvenate the mother and promote milk production.*

EBP ▪ Reduce nipple pain; ensure proper position as the neonate latches on to the nipple; check for *Candida* infection, and apply prescribed medication and nipple ointment; air-dry nipples. *Identifying and treating common conditions in the mother who is breastfeeding are important to sustain breastfeeding.*

EBP ▪ Instruct the mother about:

   ▪ Milk production may take a week before a sufficient amount is produced. *Understanding expectations improves confidence and reduces anxiety.*

   ▪ Suckle the neonate at least eight times a day to stimulate milk production; the goal is eight to 12 times daily. *Understanding expectations improves confidence and reduces anxiety.*

   ▪ Express milk or pump breasts regularly if the neonate is unable to suckle. *The breasts must be stimulated frequently to stimulate milk production.*

   ▪ Provide the mother and family unit nutritional instructions for best foods and fluids for intake to support breast milk production. *Adequate and proper nutrition will aid the mother in recovery from labor and delivery and provide important nutrients to the neonate.*

   ▪ Teach the mother techniques to keep the neonate awake during the feeding sessions. *The neonate often needs stimulation to remain awake at the breast to suckle sufficient milk.*

S ▣ *Check with health care provider about substances and medications that can suppress milk production (i.e., caffeine, tobacco, nicotine, pseudoephedrine, diuretics, contraception pills). To improve and sustain milk production, avoidance of substances that depress or limit milk production is important.*

T&C ▣ Use a multidisciplinary team approach to support the mother for breast milk production—registered nurse, lactation specialist, certified nurse midwife, pediatrician, registered dietitian, social worker. *A team approach brings expertise to address the needs of the mother and promotes health and well-being for the family unit.*

Suggested NIC Interventions

Breastfeeding Assistance; Active Listening; Newborn Care; Parent Education: Infant; Teaching: Infant Nutrition; Lactation Counseling; Sleep Enhancement

EVALUATIONS FOR EXPECTED OUTCOMES

▣ Mother's production of breast milk becomes sufficient.
▣ Neonate experiences no loss of weight, jaundice, or dehydration.
▣ Mother expresses satisfaction with breastfeeding.
▣ Parents report improved ability to cope with stress of caring for infant.
▣ Mother–infant experience success in breastfeeding.

DOCUMENTATION

▣ Assessment of factors that may enhance or retard breastfeeding
▣ Mother's expressions of satisfaction or problems with breastfeeding
▣ Nursing interventions and mother–infant's response to them
▣ Evaluations for expected outcomes

REFERENCES

de Almeida Carreiro, J., Amorim Francisco, A., Freitas de Vilhena Abrão, A. C., Oliveira Marcacine, K., de Sá Vieira Abuchaim, E., & Pereira Coca, K. (2018). Breastfeeding difficulties: Analysis of a service specialized in breastfeeding. *Acta Paulista de Enfermagem, 31*(4), 430–438.
Gianni, M. L., Bezze, E. N., Sannino, P., Baro, M., Roggero, P., Muscolo, S., ... Mosca, F. (2018). Maternal views on facilitators of and barriers to breastfeeding preterm infants. *BMC Pediatrics, 18*(1), 283. doi:10.1186/s12887-018-1260-2
Nona, S., & Srijana, K. (2018). Perceptions and practices regarding breastfeeding among postnatal mothers. *International Journal of Nursing Education, 10*(4), 128–133.
Shukri, N. H. M., Wells, J., Mukhtar, F., Lee, M. H. S., & Fewtrell, M. (2017). Study protocol: An investigation of mother-infant signalling during breastfeeding using a randomised trial to test the effectiveness of breastfeeding relaxation therapy on maternal psychological state, breast milk production and infant behaviour and growth. *International Breastfeeding Journal, 12*, 33.

Ineffective Breastfeeding

DEFINITION

Difficulty feeding milk from the breasts, which may compromise nutritional status of the infant/child

RELATED FACTORS (R/T)

▣ Delayed stage II lactogenesis
▣ Inadequate milk supply

- Insufficient family support
- Insufficient opportunity for suckling at the breast
- Insufficient parental knowledge regarding breastfeeding techniques
- Insufficient parental knowledge regarding importance of breastfeeding
- Interrupted breastfeeding
- Maternal ambivalence
- Maternal anxiety
- Maternal breast anomaly
- Maternal fatigue
- Maternal obesity
- Maternal pain
- Pacifier use
- Poor infant sucking reflex
- Supplemental feedings with artificial nipple

ASSOCIATED CONDITIONS

- Oropharyngeal defect

ASSESSMENT

- Maternal status, including age and maturity, relationships with significant others, previous bonding history, parity, level of prenatal breastfeeding preparation, knowledge or previous breastfeeding experience, physical condition (actual or perceived inadequate milk supply, nipple shape, and comfort level), and psychosocial factors (apprehension level, body image and perceptions, stress from family and career, sociocultural views of breastfeeding, and emotional support from significant others)
- Neonatal status, including satisfaction and contentment, growth rate, and age–weight relationship

DEFINING CHARACTERISTICS

- Inadequate infant stooling
- Infant arching at breast
- Infant crying at the breast
- Infant crying within the first hour after breastfeeding
- Infant fussing within 1 hour of breastfeeding
- Infant inability to latch on to maternal breast correctly
- Infant resisting latching on to breast
- Infant unresponsive to other comfort measures
- Insufficient emptying of each breast per feeding
- Insufficient infant weight gain
- Insufficient signs of oxytocin release
- Perceived inadequate milk supply
- Sore nipples persisting beyond first week
- Sustained infant weight loss
- Unsustained suckling at the breast

EXPECTED OUTCOMES

- Mother will express physical and psychological comfort with breastfeeding techniques and practice.
- Mother will show decreased anxiety and apprehension.

- Neonate will feed successfully on both breasts and appear satisfied for at least 2 hours after feeding.
- Neonate will grow and thrive.
- Mother will state at least one resource for breastfeeding support.

Suggested NOC Outcomes

> *Breastfeeding Establishment: Infant; Breastfeeding Establishment: Maternal; Breastfeeding Maintenance; Fluid Balance; Hydration; Knowledge: Breastfeeding*

INTERVENTIONS AND RATIONALES

EBP ▪ Educate the mother in breast care and breastfeeding techniques. *This reduces anxiety and enhances proper nutrition of the neonate.*

PCC ▪ Be available, yet discreet, during breastfeeding. *Assessment of the mother's technique can reveal problem areas.* Encourage the mother to ask questions *to increase understanding and reduce anxiety.*

EBP ▪ Teach techniques for encouraging the letdown reflex, including:
  - warm shower
  - breast massage
  - physically caring for the neonate
  - holding the neonate close to the breasts

  These measures reduce anxiety and promote the letdown reflex.

PCC ▪ Provide the mother and infant with a quiet, private, comfortable environment with decreased external stressors *to promote successful breastfeeding.*

PCC ▪ Encourage the expression of fears and anxieties between the mother and significant other *to reduce anxiety and increase the mother's sense of control.*

EBP ▪ Offer information about the importance of adequate nutrition and fluid intake while breastfeeding *in order to meet the infant's demand for breast milk.*

T&C ▪ Offer written information, a reading list, or information about breastfeeding support groups *to help meet the mother's emotional and learning needs.*

Suggested NIC Interventions

> *Breastfeeding Assistance; Emotional Support; Lactation Counseling; Nutrition Management; Parent Education: Infant; Support Group*

EVALUATIONS FOR EXPECTED OUTCOMES

- Mother expresses physical and psychological comfort with breastfeeding techniques and practice.
- Mother displays decreased anxiety and apprehension.
- Neonate feeds successfully on both breasts and appears satisfied for at least 2 hours after feeding.
- Neonate grows and thrives.
- Mother states at least one available resource for breastfeeding support.

DOCUMENTATION

- Mother's expressions of comfort with breastfeeding ability
- Observations of bonding and breastfeeding process

- Teaching and instructions given
- Referrals to support groups
- Neonate growth and weight
- Evaluations for expected outcomes

REFERENCES

Bentley, J. P., Nassar, N., Porter, M., Vroome, M., Yip, E., & Ampt, A. J. (2017). Formula supplementation in hospital and subsequent feeding at discharge among women who intended to exclusively breastfeed: An administrative data retrospective cohort study. *Birth: Issues in Perinatal Care, 44*(4), 352–362.

Gustafsson, I., Nyström, M., & Palmér, L. (2017). Midwives' lived experience of caring for new mothers with initial breastfeeding difficulties: A phenomenological study. *Sexual & Reproductive HealthCare, 12*, 9–15.

Sansone-Southwood, A. (2018). When the breast says no the missing link: A case study. *Journal of Prenatal and Perinatal Psychology and Health, 32*(4), 318–338.

Sipsma, H. L., Ruiz, E., Jones, K., Magriples, U., & Kershaw, T. (2018). Effect of breastfeeding on postpartum depressive symptoms among adolescent and young adult mothers. *Journal of Maternal-Fetal & Neonatal Medicine, 31*(11), 1442–1447.

Interrupted Breastfeeding

DEFINITION

Break in the continuity of feeding milk from the breasts, which may compromise breastfeeding success and/or nutritional status of the infant/child

RELATED FACTORS (R/T)

- Maternal employment
- Maternal–infant separation
- Need to abruptly wean infant

ASSOCIATED CONDITIONS

- Contraindications to breastfeeding
- Infant illness
- Maternal illness

ASSESSMENT

- Maternal status, including age and maturity, employment hours, relationship with significant other, parity, level of prenatal breastfeeding knowledge or experience, and physical condition (comfort level, nipple shape, presence of infection, and use of medication)
- Neonatal status, including age–weight relationship, growth rate, neurologic status, respiratory status, suck reflex, and factors that interfere with proper sucking (such as cleft lip or palate)

DEFINING CHARACTERISTICS

- Nonexclusive breastfeeding

EXPECTED OUTCOMES

* Mother will express her understanding of factors that necessitate interruption in breastfeeding.
* Mother will express comfort with her decision about whether to resume breastfeeding.
* Mother will express and store breast milk appropriately.
* Mother will resume breastfeeding when interfering factors cease.
* Mother will have adequate milk supply when breastfeeding resumes.
* Mother will obtain relief from discomfort associated with engorgement.
* Infant's nutritional needs will be met.

Suggested NOC Outcomes

Breastfeeding Maintenance; Knowledge: Breastfeeding; Motivation; Parent–Infant Attachment; Parenting Performance; Role Performance

INTERVENTIONS AND RATIONALES

PCC * Assess the mother's understanding of reasons for interrupting breastfeeding *to evaluate the need for additional instruction.*

PCC * Reassure the mother that the neonate's nutritional needs will be met through other methods *to allay her anxiety.*

* Assess the mother's desire to resume breastfeeding *to help plan interventions.*

EBP * Provide appropriate educational materials, including audiovisual aids and written materials. *Audiovisual aids demonstrate proper expressing and storing techniques; written material allows the mother to review information at her own pace.*

EBP * Instruct the mother in techniques for expressing and storing breast milk *to ensure adequate milk supply.*

S * Recommend the use of a breast pump according to the following guidelines *to provide maximum stimulation and prolactin production*:
    * Initiate pumping 24 to 48 hours after delivery.
    * Pump a minimum of five times a day.
    * Pump a minimum of 100 minutes/day.
    * Pump long enough to soften the breasts each time, regardless of duration.

S * Encourage the mother to save her breast milk in a sterile container and store it in the refrigerator or freezer for future feedings. *Preserving breast milk ensures that the neonate receives maternal antibodies and helps encourage maternal involvement in neonatal care.*

EBP * If the mother must pump for a prolonged period, encourage her to use a piston-style electric pump. *Using an electric pump rather than a hand pump produces milk with a higher fat content.*

EBP * If the mother intends to resume breastfeeding, instruct her in ways to relieve breast engorgement *to prevent discomfort that may keep the neonate from sucking effectively.*

EBP * If appropriate, instruct the mother in the use of devices such as a nipple shield, *which is designed to alter flat or inverted nipples, a condition that may interfere with successful breastfeeding.*

PCC * Review the mother's daily routine *to advise her on how to incorporate breastfeeding into her schedule.*

T&C * Provide the mother with information about breastfeeding support groups. *A support group can help the mother obtain needed emotional support and continue learning.*

▦ If the mother doesn't intend to resume breastfeeding, advise her to wear a supportive bra, apply ice, and take a mild analgesic, such as acetaminophen, *to alleviate discomfort associated with engorgement.*

Suggested NIC Interventions

Attachment Promotion; Bottle-Feeding; Emotional Support; Lactation Counseling; Parent Education: Infant; Teaching: Individual

EVALUATIONS FOR EXPECTED OUTCOMES

▦ Mother describes factors that necessitate interruption in breastfeeding.
▦ Mother expresses comfort with her decision about whether to resume breastfeeding.
▦ Mother demonstrates proper milk expression and storage techniques.
▦ Mother resumes breastfeeding when interrupting factors are eliminated.
▦ Mother has adequate milk supply when breastfeeding resumes.
▦ Mother obtains relief from discomfort associated with engorgement.
▦ Infant's nutritional needs are met, as evidenced by appropriate weight gain (e.g., 1 oz [28.3 g]/day for first 6 months of life).

DOCUMENTATION

▦ Factors that necessitated interruption in breastfeeding (reassessed periodically to determine status)
▦ Mother's expression of feelings about the need to interrupt breastfeeding
▦ Mother's decision whether to continue breastfeeding when possible
▦ Mother's efforts to ensure adequate milk supply
▦ Mother's responses to nursing interventions
▦ Neonate's growth, weight, and output
▦ Referrals to support groups
▦ Evaluations for expected outcomes

REFERENCES

Clark, A., Baker, S. S., McGirr, K., & Harris, M. (2018). Breastfeeding peer support program increases breastfeeding duration rates among middle- to high-income women. *Breastfeeding Medicine, 13*(2), 112–115.
Simon, J. A., Carabetta, M., Rieth, E. F., & Barnett, K. M. (2018). Perioperative care of the breastfeeding patient. *AORN Journal, 107*(4), 465–474.
Wood, N. K., & Woods, N. F. (2018). Outcome measures in interventions that enhance breastfeeding initiation, duration, and exclusivity: A systematic review. *MCN: The American Journal of Maternal Child Nursing, 43*(6), 341–347.
Zilanawala, A. (2017). Maternal nonstandard work schedules and breastfeeding behaviors. *Maternal & Child Health Journal, 21*(6), 1308–1317.

Readiness for Enhanced Breastfeeding

DEFINITION

A pattern of feeding milk from the breasts to an infant or child, which may be strengthened

- Maternal status, including age and maturity, parity, level of prenatal breastfeeding preparation, past breastfeeding experience, previous postpartum history, physical condition (actual or perceived inadequate milk supply and comfort level), and psychosocial factors (apprehension level, body image, stress from family and career, sociocultural views of breastfeeding, and emotional support from significant others)
- Neonatal status, including satisfaction and contentment, growth rate, age–weight relationship, urine output, quantity and characteristics of stools, and ability to latch on to breasts

DEFINING CHARACTERISTICS

- Mother expresses desire to enhance ability to exclusively breastfeed
- Mother expresses desire to enhance ability to provide breast milk for child's nutritional needs

EXPECTED OUTCOMES

- Mother will breastfeed neonate successfully and will experience satisfaction with breast-feeding process.
- Neonate will feed successfully on both breasts and appear satisfied.
- Neonate will grow and develop in pace with accepted standards.
- Mother will continue breastfeeding neonate after early postpartum period.

Suggested NOC Outcomes

> Breastfeeding Establishment: Infant; Breastfeeding Establishment: Maternal; Breastfeeding Maintenance; Breastfeeding Weaning; Hydration; Knowledge: Breastfeeding

INTERVENTIONS AND RATIONALES

- **PCC** Assess the mother's knowledge and experience of breastfeeding *to focus teaching on specific learning needs*.
- **EBP** Educate the mother and selected support person about breastfeeding techniques:
  - Clean hands and breasts before nursing.
  - Position the neonate for feeding (the neonate should be able to grasp most of the areola).
  - Change positions to decrease nipple tenderness and use both breasts at each feeding.
  - Remove the neonate from the breast by breaking suction; avoid setting time limits in the early stage.

  Greater understanding of techniques improves chances for success.

- **EBP** Teach the mother how to use warm showers and compresses, relaxation and guided imagery, infant suckling, holding the infant close to breasts, and listening to the infant cry *to stimulate letdown*.
- **EBP** Educate the mother about nutritional needs. She requires a well-balanced diet plus an additional 500 calories and two extra glasses of fluid each day *to maintain an adequate milk supply*. She should limit caffeine and avoid foods that make her uncomfortable.
- **EBP** Teach the mother what to expect from a breastfeeding neonate *to prepare the mother for care of the neonate at home*. The neonate should pass one to six stools and wet six to eight diapers per day. Stools should be soft to liquid and nonodorous. The neonate

should feed every 2 to 3 hours or as needed and appear content and satisfied after feeding. Explain that the neonate also requires nonnutritive sucking.

PCC   ▦   Assist the mother and family in planning for home care. The mother needs to rest when the neonate sleeps, practice self-care, learn techniques for expressing and storing breast milk, and recognize signs of engorgement and infection. Family members should understand the importance of helping and supporting the mother in her desire to breastfeed. *A mother who stops breastfeeding after she returns home and resumes work often does so because of fatigue.*

PCC   ▦   Provide quiet environment and privacy *to enhance development of breastfeeding skills.*

PCC   ▦   Encourage mother to express concerns about breastfeeding *to reduce anxiety.*

T&C   ▦   Offer mother information about breastfeeding support groups *to help meet emotional and learning needs.*

Suggested NIC Interventions

Breastfeeding Assistance; Family Support; Lactation Counseling; Nutrition Management; Parent Education: Infant

EVALUATIONS FOR EXPECTED OUTCOMES

▦   Mother breastfeeds neonate successfully and expresses satisfaction with breastfeeding.

▦   Neonate feeds on both breasts and appears satisfied.

▦   Neonate's weight and length remain consistent and within 10th and 19th percentiles, respectively, on pediatric growth grid.

▦   Mother continues to breastfeed infant after discharge from hospital.

DOCUMENTATION

▦   Mother's expressions about breastfeeding experience

▦   Observations of breastfeeding techniques and mother–infant interaction during breastfeeding

▦   Teaching and instructions given

▦   Neonate's growth and weight

▦   Referral to support groups

▦   Mother's plans for breastfeeding after discharge

▦   Evaluations for expected outcomes

REFERENCES

Al Namir, H. M. A., Brady, A.-M., & Gallagher, L. (2017). Fathers and breastfeeding: Attitudes, involvement and support. *British Journal of Midwifery, 25*(7), 426–440.

Bridges, N., Howell, G., & Schmied, V. (2018). Breastfeeding peer support on social networking sites. *Breastfeeding Review, 26*(2), 17–27.

Cohen, B., & Ayyad, B. (2018). Development of a breastfeeding basics class for women to increase breastfeeding support on the postpartum unit. *Journal of Obstetric, Gynecologic & Neonatal Nursing, 47*, S10–S11.

Johnson, A. M., Kirk, R., Jordan Rooks, A., & Muzik, M. (2017). Enhancing breastfeeding through healthcare support: Results from a focus group study of African American mothers. *MIDIRS Midwifery Digest, 27*(2), 232–233.

Ineffective Breathing Pattern

DEFINITION

Inspiration and/or expiration that does not provide adequate ventilation

RELATED FACTORS (R/T)

- Anxiety
- Body position that inhibits lung expansion
- Fatigue
- Increased physical exertion
- Obesity
- Pain

ASSOCIATED CONDITIONS

- Bony deformity
- Chest wall deformity
- Chronic obstructive pulmonary disease
- Critical illness
- Heart diseases
- Hyperventilation syndrome
- Hypoventilation syndrome
- Increased airway resistance
- Increased serum hydrogen concentration
- Musculoskeletal impairment
- Neurological immaturity
- Neurological impairment
- Neuromuscular diseases
- Reduced pulmonary complacency
- Sleep-apnea syndromes
- Spinal cord injuries

ASSESSMENT

- Age
- Weight
- History of respiratory disorder
- Respiratory status, including rate and depth of respiration, symmetry of chest expansion, use of accessory muscles, presence of cough, anterior–posterior chest diameter, palpation for fremitus, percussion of lung fields, auscultation of breath sounds, and pulmonary function studies
- Cardiovascular status, including heart rate and rhythm, blood pressure, and skin color, temperature, and turgor
- Neurologic and mental status, including level of consciousness and emotional level
- Preexisting conditions
- Knowledge, including current understanding of physical condition and physical, mental, and emotional readiness to learn

DEFINING CHARACTERISTICS

- Abdominal paradoxical respiratory pattern
- Altered chest excursion
- Altered tidal volume
- Bradypnea
- Cyanosis
- Decreased expiratory pressure
- Decreased inspiratory pressure
- Decreased minute ventilation
- Decreased vital capacity
- Hypercapnia
- Hyperventilation
- Hypoventilation
- Hypoxemia
- Hypoxia
- Increased anterior-posterior chest diameter
- Nasal flaring
- Orthopnea
- Prolonged expiration phase
- Pursed-lip breathing
- Subcostal retraction
- Tachypnea
- Uses accessory muscles to breathe
- Uses three-point position

EXPECTED OUTCOMES

- Patient's respiratory rate will stay within 5 breaths/minute of baseline.
- Patient respiratory rate will be within normal limits.
- Arterial blood gas (ABG) levels will return to baseline.
- Patient will demonstrate adequate breathing pattern with easy, unlabored respirations.
- Patient will report feeling comfortable when breathing.
- Patient will report feeling rested each day.
- Patient will demonstrate diaphragmatic pursed-lip breathing.
- Patient will achieve maximum lung expansion with adequate ventilation.
- Patient will demonstrate skill in conserving energy while carrying out activities of daily living (ADLs).

Suggested NOC Outcomes

Mechanical Ventilation Response: Adult; Respiratory Status: Airway Patency; Respiratory Status: Gas Exchange; Respiratory Status: Ventilation; Vital Signs

INTERVENTIONS AND RATIONALES

- **S** Assess and record respiratory rate and depth at least every 4 hours *to detect early signs of respiratory compromise.*
- **S** Auscultate breath sounds at least every 4 hours *to detect decreased or adventitious breath sounds*; report changes.

S ▪ Monitor ABG values and pulse oximetry readings *to evaluate oxygenation and respiratory status.*

S ▪ Observe for signs of respiratory distress (nasal flaring, tachypnea, retractions, grunting, and use of accessory muscles for breathing).

EBP ▪ Assist patient into a comfortable position, for example, by supporting the upper extremities with pillows, providing an overbed table with a pillow to lean on, and elevating head of bed. *These measures promote comfort, chest expansion, and ventilation of basilar lung fields.*

EBP ▪ Perform chest physiotherapy *to aid mobilization and secretion removal* if ordered. Percussion, vibration, and postural drainage enhance airway clearance and respiratory effort.

PCC ▪ Provide rest periods between breathing enhancement measures *to avoid fatigue.*

PCC ▪ Help patient with ADLs as needed *to conserve energy and avoid overexertion and fatigue.*

S ▪ Administer oxygen as ordered. *Supplemental oxygen helps reduce hypoxemia and relieve respiratory distress.*

S ▪ Suction airway as needed. *Retained secretions alter the ventilatory response, thus reducing oxygen, leading to hypoxemia.*

PCC ▪ Schedule necessary activities to provide periods of rest. *This prevents fatigue and reduces oxygen demands.*

EBP ▪ Teach patient about:
  ▪ pursed-lip breathing
  ▪ abdominal breathing
  ▪ performing relaxation techniques
  ▪ taking prescribed medications (ensuring accuracy of dose and frequency and monitoring adverse effects)
  ▪ scheduling activities to avoid fatigue and provide for rest periods
  ▪ smoking cessation. *These measures allow patient to participate in maintaining health status and improve ventilation.*

T&C ▪ Refer patient for evaluation of exercise potential and development of individualized exercise program. *Exercise promotes conditioning of respiratory muscles and patient's sense of well-being.*

Suggested NIC Interventions

Acid–Base Monitoring; Airway Management; Airway Suctioning; Anxiety Reduction; Exercise Promotion; Oxygen Therapy; Progressive Muscle Relaxation; Respiratory Monitoring; Ventilation Assistance

EVALUATIONS FOR EXPECTED OUTCOMES

▪ Patient's respiratory rate remains within established limits.
▪ Patient's ABG levels return to and remain within established limits.
▪ Patient indicates, either verbally or through behavior, feeling comfortable when breathing.
▪ Patient reports feeling rested each day.
▪ Patient performs diaphragmatic pursed-lip breathing.
▪ Patient demonstrates maximum lung expansion with adequate ventilation.
▪ When patient carries out ADLs, breathing pattern remains normal.

DOCUMENTATION

▪ Patient's expressions of comfort in breathing, emotional state, understanding of medical diagnosis, and readiness to learn

- Physical findings from pulmonary assessment
- Interventions carried out and patient's responses to them
- Evaluations for expected outcomes

REFERENCES

Aboussouan, L. S., & Mireles-Cabodevila, E. (2017). Sleep-disordered breathing in neuromuscular disease: Diagnostic and therapeutic challenges. *Chest, 152*(4), 880–892.

Maines, E., Baggio, L., Gugelmo, G., Morandi, G., & Bordugo, A. (2017). Newborn with rhizomelia and difficulty breathing. *Skeletal Radiology, 46*(2), 231.

Rai, S., & Ionescu, A. A. (2017). A 44-year-old, Caucasian, male nonsmoker with worsening difficulty in breathing and decreased exercise tolerance. *Breathe, 13*(2), 117–122.

Ratnovsky, A., Gino, O., & Naftali, S. (2017). The impact of breathing pattern and rate on inspiratory muscles activity. *Technology & Health Care, 25*(5), 823–830.

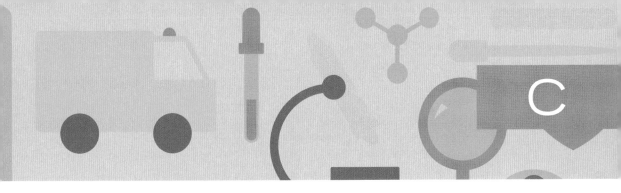

Decreased Cardiac Output

DEFINITION

Inadequate blood pumped by the heart to meet the metabolic demands of the body

RELATED FACTORS

To be developed

ASSESSMENT

- History of cardiac disorder
- Mental status, including orientation, level of consciousness (LOC), sudden mental deterioration accompanied by confusion, agitation, and restlessness
- Cardiovascular status, including history of valvular disorder, capillary heart disease, or myopathy; skin color, temperature, turgor, and capillary refill time; jugular vein distention; hepatojugular reflux; heart rate and rhythm; heart sounds; blood pressure; peripheral pulses; electrocardiogram (ECG); exercise ECG; echocardiogram; and phonocardiogram
- Respiratory status, including respiratory rate and depth, breath sounds, chest x-ray, and arterial blood gas values
- Renal status, including weight, intake and output, and urine specific gravity

ASSOCIATED CONDITIONS

- Altered afterload
- Altered contractility
- Alteration in heart rate
- Alteration in heart rhythm
- Altered preload
- Altered stroke volume

DEFINING CHARACTERISTICS

Altered Heart Rate/Rhythm

- Bradycardia
- Electrocardiogram (ECG) change
- Heart palpitations
- Tachycardia

Altered Preload

- Decreased central venous pressure (CVP)
- Decrease in pulmonary artery wedge pressure (PAWP)

- Edema
- Fatigue
- Heart murmur
- Increase in central venous pressure (CVP)
- Increase in pulmonary artery wedge pressure (PAWP)
- Jugular vein distention
- Weight gain

Altered Afterload

- Abnormal skin color
- Alteration in blood pressure
- Clammy skin
- Decrease in peripheral pulses
- Decrease in pulmonary vascular resistance (PVR)
- Decrease in systemic vascular resistance (SVR)
- Dyspnea
- Increase in pulmonary vascular resistance (PVR)
- Increase in systemic vascular resistance (SVR)
- Oliguria
- Prolonged capillary refill

Altered Contractility

- Adventitious breath sounds
- Coughing
- Decreased cardiac index
- Decrease in ejection fraction
- Decrease in left ventricular stroke work index (LVSMI)
- Decrease in stroke volume index (SVI)
- Orthopnea
- Paroxysmal nocturnal dyspnea
- Presence of S_3 heart sound
- Presence of S_4 heart sound

Behavioral/Emotional

- Anxiety
- Restlessness

EXPECTED OUTCOMES

- Patient will maintain adequate cardiac output.
- Patient's heart rate will be within normal parameters for patient.
- Patient's blood pressure will be within normal parameters for patient.
- Patient will not exhibit arrhythmias.
- Patient's skin will remain warm and dry.
- Patient will not exhibit pedal edema.
- Patient will perform activities within limits of prescribed heart rate with no dyspnea, dizziness, or chest pain.
- Patient will maintain respiratory rate and rhythm within established parameters.
- Patient will perform stress-reduction techniques every 4 hours while awake.

- Patient will verbalize understanding of reportable signs and symptoms.
- Patient will understand diet, medication regimen, and prescribed activity level.

Suggested NOC Outcomes

Cardiac Pump Effectiveness; Circulation Status; Tissue Perfusion: Abdominal Organs; Tissue Perfusion: Peripheral; Fluid Overload Severity; Vital Signs

INTERVENTIONS AND RATIONALES

- **S** Monitor at least every 4 hours and report immediately any irregularities in heart rate, rhythm, and blood pressure. *May indicate impending cardiac failure or other complications.*
- **S** Monitor at least every 4 hours for dyspnea, fatigue, or jugular distention. *May indicate cardiac complications.*
- **S** Monitor and record LOC at least every 4 hours or more often if necessary *to detect hypoxia possibly resulting from decreased cardiac output.*
- Auscultate for heart and breath sounds at least every 4 hours. Report abnormal sounds as soon as they develop. *Extra heart sounds may indicate early cardiac decompensation; adventitious breath sounds may indicate pulmonary congestion and diminished cardiac output.*
- **S** Monitor for dyspnea or shortness of breath every 2 to 4 hours and report changes from baseline. *Patients with silent or painless myocardial infarction may develop dyspnea related to left-sided heart failure.*
- **PCC** Instruct patient to report chest pain right away *because it may signal myocardial hypoxia or injury.*
- Monitor mental status every 2 to 4 hours and report deviations from baseline. *Dizziness, confusion, light-headedness, and restlessness may indicate decreased cerebral blood flow cause by slow carotid sinus reflex.*
- Measure and record intake and output accurately. *Decreased urine output without lowered fluid intake might indicate decreased renal perfusion, possibly from decreased cardiac output.*
- **S** Promptly treat life-threatening arrhythmias as ordered *to avoid crisis.*
- **EBP** Weigh patient daily before breakfast *to detect fluid retention.*
- Inspect for pedal or sacral edema to *detect venous stasis and reduced cardiac output.*
- **EBP** Provide skin care every 4 hours *to enhance skin perfusion and venous flow.*
- **EBP** Gradually increase patient's activities within limits of prescribed heart rate *to allow heart to adjust to increased oxygen demand.* Monitor pulse rate before and after activity *to compare rates and gauge tolerance.*
- **PCC** Plan patient's activities *to avoid fatigue and increased myocardial workload.*
- Administer medication as ordered and observe for adverse reactions. *Especially in older patients, decreased renal and liver function may lead to rapid development of toxicity.*
- Maintain dietary restrictions, as ordered, *to reduce risk of cardiac disease.*
- **EBP** Teach patient stress-reduction techniques *to reduce patient's anxiety and provide a sense of control.*
- **PCC** Explain all procedures and tests to *enhance understanding and reduce anxiety.*
- **PCC** Teach patient and family about reportable symptoms of possible cardiac problems:
  - Dizziness
  - Indigestion
  - Nausea

- Retrosternal pain
- Shortness of breath
- Unusual fatigue and weakness
  Knowing the symptoms of decreased cardiac functioning gives patient a sense of greater control over the situation and encourages compliance with the treatment plan.

EBP
- Instruct patient not to strain during bowel movements, *which may cause stimulation of the vagus nerve, resulting in bradycardia and decreased cardiac output.*

PCC
- Teach patient and family about prescribed diet, medications (name, dosage, frequency, and therapeutic and adverse effects), prescribed activity level, simple methods for lifting and bending, and stress-reduction techniques. *These measures involve patient and family in care.*

PCC
- Reduce stressful elements, such as excessive noise or light in the patient's environment, *to decrease anxiety and restlessness, which may lead to arrhythmias.*
- Administer oxygen, as prescribed, *to increase supply to myocardium.*

Suggested NIC Interventions

Cardiac Precautions; Circulatory Precautions; Fluid Management; Hemodynamic Regulation; Vital Signs Monitoring

EVALUATIONS FOR EXPECTED OUTCOMES

- Patient's pulse rate is within set limits.
- Patient's blood pressure is within set limits.
- Patient doesn't exhibit arrhythmias during monitoring or physical examination.
- Patient's skin is warm and dry to touch.
- Inspection and palpation don't reveal pedal edema.
- Patient carries out activities of daily living (ADLs) without heart rate exceeding or dropping below set limits.
- Patient doesn't indicate, either verbally or through behavior, chest pain, dyspnea, fatigue, or other forms of discomfort after activity.
- Patient performs stress-reduction techniques every 4 hours.
- Patient describes signs and symptoms of decreased cardiac output, such as dizziness, syncope, clammy skin, fatigue, and dyspnea.
- Patient understands importance of following prescribed diet, taking medications as ordered, and maintaining activity level.

DOCUMENTATION

- Patient's symptoms
- Patient's needs and perception of problem
- Observations of physical findings
- Patient's response to activity
- Teaching provided to patient and family members
- Interventions to control or monitor symptoms and patient response
- Development of skills related to diet, medication, activity, and stress management
- Evaluations for expected outcomes

REFERENCES

Abolahrari-Shirazi, S., Kojuri, J., Bagheri, Z., & Rojhani-Shirazi, Z. (2018). Efficacy of combined endurance-resistance training versus endurance training in patients with heart failure after percutaneous coronary intervention: A randomized controlled trial. *Journal of Research in Medical Sciences, 23*, 12.

Albert, N. M., & Kozinn, M. J. (2018). In-hospital initiation of guideline-directed heart failure pharmacotherapy to improve long-term patient adherence and outcomes. *Critical Care Nurse, 38*(5), 16–24.

Jayasena, R., Ding, H., Dowling, A., Shridhar, G. K., Richardson, D., Maiorana, A., & Edwards, I. (2017). Chronic heart failure care model for home monitoring of patients. *International Journal of Integrated Care, 17*(3), 251–252.

Roy, B., Woo, M. A., Wang, D. J. J., Fonarow, G. C., Harper, R. M., & Kumar, R. (2017). Reduced regional cerebral blood flow in patients with heart failure. *European Journal of Heart Failure, 19*(10), 1294–1302.

Risk for Decreased Cardiac Output

DEFINITION

Susceptible to inadequate blood pumped by the heart to meet metabolic demands of the body, which may compromise health

RISK FACTORS

To be developed

ASSESSMENT

- History of cardiac disorder
- Mental status, including orientation and level of consciousness (LOC)
- Cardiovascular status, including history of arrhythmias and syncope, valvular disorder, capillary heart disease, or myopathy; skin color, temperature, turgor, and capillary refill time; serum digoxin levels; jugular vein distention; hepatojugular reflux; heart rate and rhythm; heart sounds; blood pressure; peripheral pulses; electrocardiogram (ECG); exercise ECG; echocardiogram; and phonocardiogram
- Respiratory status, including respiratory rate and depth, breath sounds, chest x-ray, and arterial blood gas values
- Renal status, including weight, intake and output, urine specific gravity, and serum electrolytes

EXPECTED OUTCOMES

- Patient's pulse will be within normal limits.
- Patient's blood pressure will be within normal limits.
- Patient will not exhibit arrhythmias.
- Patient's skin will remain warm and dry.
- Patient will not exhibit pedal edema.
- Patient will show no signs of dizziness or syncope.
- Patient will experience few or no dyspneic episodes.
- Patient will not experience chest pain.
- Patient will express sense of physical comfort after activity.
- Patient will maintain adequate cardiac output.
- Patient will perform stress-reduction techniques.
- Patient will verbalize understanding of reportable signs and symptoms.
- Patient will verbalize understanding of diet, medication, and activity level on cardiac health.

Suggested NOC Outcomes

Cardiac Pump Effectiveness; Circulation Status; Tissue Perfusion: Peripheral; Vital Signs

S ▪ Monitor and record LOC, heart rate and rhythm, and blood pressure and report any abnormal results. *Changes from normal limits may indicate decreased cardiac output.*

S ▪ Monitor patient for dyspnea, fatigue, crackles in lungs, jugular venous distention, or chest pain. *Any or all of these may indicate impending cardiac failure or other complications. Report them immediately.*

▪ Auscultate for heart and breath sounds. Report abnormal sounds as soon as they develop. *Extra heart sounds may indicate early cardiac decompensation; adventitious breath sounds may indicate pulmonary congestion and diminished cardiac output.*

▪ Measure and record intake and output accurately. *Decreased urine output without lowered fluid intake might indicate decreased renal perfusion, possibly from decreased cardiac output.*

S ▪ Promptly treat life-threatening arrhythmias, as ordered, *to avoid crisis.*

EBP ▪ Weigh patient daily before breakfast *to detect fluid retention.*

▪ Inspect for pedal or sacral edema to *detect venous stasis and reduced cardiac output.*

EBP ▪ Provide skin care as needed *to enhance skin perfusion and venous flow.*

▪ Maintain dietary restrictions, as ordered, *to reduce risk of cardiac disease.*

S ▪ Report complaints of dizziness or syncope promptly; *these may indicate cerebral hypoxia resulting from a cardiac rhythm disturbance.*

PCC ▪ Tell patient to report chest pain right away *because it may signal myocardial hypoxia or injury.*

PCC ▪ Teach patient stress-reduction techniques *to reduce patient's anxiety and provide a sense of control.*

PCC ▪ Explain all procedures and tests to *enhance understanding and reduce anxiety.*

PCC ▪ Teach patient and family about chest pain and other reportable symptoms, prescribed diet, medications (name, dosage, frequency, and therapeutic and adverse effects), prescribed activity level, simple methods for lifting and bending, and stress-reduction techniques. *These measures involve patient and family in care.*

▪ Administer oxygen, as prescribed, *to increase supply to myocardium.*

Suggested NIC Interventions

Cardiac Precautions; Circulatory Precautions; Fluid Management; Homodynamic Regulation; Vital Signs Monitoring

▪ Patient's pulse rate remains within set limits.

▪ Patient's blood pressure remains within set limits.

▪ Patient's cardiac output remains adequate.

▪ Patient doesn't exhibit arrhythmias during monitoring or physical examination.

▪ Patient's skin remains warm and dry to touch.

▪ Patient experiences fewer dyspneic episodes.

▪ Patient doesn't experience dizziness or syncope.

▪ Patient doesn't experience chest pain.

▪ Patient will not exhibit pedal edema.

▪ Patient doesn't indicate, either verbally or through behavior, chest pain, dyspnea, fatigue, or other forms of discomfort after activity.

▪ Patient performs stress-reduction techniques as needed.

▪ Patient describes signs and symptoms of decreased cardiac output, such as dizziness, syncope, clammy skin, fatigue, and dyspnea.

▪ Patient understands importance of diet, medications, and activity on cardiac health.

DOCUMENTATION

- Patient's needs and perception of problem
- Observations of physical findings
- Patient's response to activity
- Development of skills related to diet, medication, activity, and stress management
- Incidents of chest pain, including location, character, duration, and treatment
- Interventions to control or monitor symptoms and patient's response
- Patient teaching
- Evaluations for expected outcomes

REFERENCES

Bosch, L., Carluccio, E., Coiro, S., Gong, L., Sim, D., Yeo, D., … Ambrosio, G. (2017). Risk stratification of Asian patients with heart failure and reduced ejection fraction: The effectiveness of the Echo Heart Failure Score. *European Journal of Heart Failure, 19*(12), 1732–1735.

Demissei, B. G., Cotter, G., Prescott, M. F., Felker, G. M., Filippatos, G., Greenberg, B. H., … Voors, A. A. (2017). A multimarker multi-time point-based risk stratification strategy in acute heart failure: Results from the RELAX-AHF trial. *European Journal of Heart Failure, 19*(8), 1001–1010.

Eriksson, B., Wändell, P., Dahlström, U., Näsman, P., Lund, L. H., & Edner, M. (2018). Comorbidities, risk factors and outcome in patients with heart failure and an ejection fraction of more than or equal to 40% in primary care- and hospital care-based outpatient clinics. *Scandinavian Journal of Primary Health Care, 36*(2), 207–215.

Papadaki, A., Martínez-González, M. Á., Alonso-Gómez, A., Rekondo, J., Salas-Salvadó, J., Corella, D., … Arós, F. (2017). Mediterranean diet and risk of heart failure: Results from the PREDIMED randomized controlled trial. *European Journal of Heart Failure, 19*(9), 1179–1185.

Risk for Impaired Cardiovascular Function

DEFINITION

Susceptible to disturbance in substance transport, body homeostasis, tissue metabolic residue removal, and organ function, which may compromise health

RISK FACTORS

- Anxiety
- Average daily physical activity less than recommended for age and gender
- Body mass index above normal range for age and gender
- Excessive accumulation of fat for age and gender
- Excessive alcohol intake
- Excessive stress
- Inadequate dietary habits
- Inadequate knowledge of modifiable factors
- Inattentive to secondhand smoke
- Ineffective blood glucose level management
- Ineffective blood pressure management
- Ineffective lipid balance management
- Smoking
- Substance misuse

ASSOCIATED CONDITIONS

- Depression
- Diabetes mellitus

- Dyslipidemia
- Hypertension
- Insulin resistance
- Pharmaceutical preparations

ASSESSMENT

- Height, weight, gender, and age
- Mental status, anxiety level, and patient perceived stress level
- Cardiovascular status, including history of valvular disorder, capillary heart disease, or myopathy; skin color, temperature, turgor, and capillary refill time; jugular vein distention; hepatojugular reflux; heart rate and rhythm; heart sounds; blood pressure; peripheral pulses; electrocardiogram (ECG); exercise ECG; echocardiogram; and phonocardiogram
- History of cardiac disorders including arrhythmias
- Respiratory status, including respiratory rate and depth, and breath sounds
- Laboratory values for blood glucose and lipid levels
- Diet and dietary habits
- Exercise habits
- Knowledge of modifiable factors for health and wellness
- History of smoking and smoking status
- History of substance misuse

EXPECTED OUTCOMES

- Patient's blood pressure will be within normal limits.
- Patient's blood glucose will be within normal limits.
- Patient will not exhibit arrhythmias.
- Patient will perform stress-reduction techniques.
- Patient will verbalize modifiable factors for health and wellness.
- Patient will verbalize understanding of reportable signs and symptoms.
- Patient will verbalize understanding of diet, medication, and activity level for cardiac health.

Suggested NOC Outcomes

Cardiac Pump Effectiveness; Circulation Status; Tissue Perfusion: Abdominal Organs; Tissue Perfusion: Peripheral; Fluid Overload Severity; Vital Signs

INTERVENTIONS AND RATIONALES

- **S** ▪ Monitor and record LOC, heart rate and rhythm, and blood pressure, and report any abnormal results. *Changes from normal limits may indicate impaired cardiovascular function.*
- **S** ▪ Auscultate for heart and breath sounds. Report abnormal sounds as soon as they develop. *Extra heart sounds may indicate early cardiac decompensation; adventitious breath sounds may indicate pulmonary congestion and diminished cardiac output.*
- **PCC** ▪ Measure and record intake and output accurately. *Decreased urine output without lowered fluid intake might indicate decreased renal perfusion, possibly from decreased cardiac output.*
- **S** ▪ Promptly treat life-threatening arrhythmias, as ordered, *to avoid crisis.*
- **EBP** ▪ Weigh patient daily before breakfast *to detect fluid retention.*

- Inspect for pedal or sacral edema to *detect venous stasis and reduced cardiac output.*
- **EBP** ▪ Provide range of motion as needed *to enhance peripheral perfusion and venous flow.*
- Maintain dietary restrictions, as ordered, *to reduce risk of cardiac disease.*
- **S** ▪ Report complaints of dizziness or syncope promptly; *these may indicate cerebral hypoxia resulting from a cardiac rhythm disturbance.*
- **PCC** ▪ Tell patient to report chest pain right away *because it may signal myocardial hypoxia or injury.*
- **PCC** ▪ Teach patient stress-reduction techniques *to reduce patient's anxiety and provide a sense of control.*
- **PCC** ▪ Teach patient and family about chest pain and other reportable symptoms, prescribed diet, medications (name, dosage, frequency, and therapeutic and adverse effects), prescribed activity level, simple methods for lifting and bending, and stress-reduction techniques. *These measures involve patient and family in care.*

Suggested NIC Interventions

Cardiac Precautions; Circulatory Precautions; Fluid Management; Hemodynamic Regulation; Vital Signs Monitoring

EVALUATIONS FOR EXPECTED OUTCOMES

- Patient's blood pressure remains within normal limits.
- Patient's blood glucose remains within normal limits.
- Patient does not experience arrhythmias.
- Patient participates in stress-reduction techniques.
- Patient seeks out information regarding modifiable factors for health and wellness.
- Patient seeks out information regarding reportable signs and symptoms.
- Patient seeks out information regarding diet, medication, and activity level for cardiac health.

DOCUMENTATION

- Patient's needs and perception of risk
- Observations of physical findings
- Patient's response to activity
- Development of skills related to diet, medication, activity, and stress management
- Interventions to control or monitor symptoms and patient's response
- Patient teaching
- Evaluations for expected outcomes

REFERENCES

Erman, H., Boyuk, B., Cetin, S. I., Sevinc, S., Bulut, U., & Mavis, O. (2021). Beta cell function as an assessment tool for cardiovascular risk in patients with metabolic syndrome. *Journal of Surgery & Medicine (JOSAM)*, 5(10), 1002–1006.

Gigante, A., Proietti, M., Petrillo, E., Mannucci, P. M., Nobili, A., & Muscaritoli, M. (2021). Renal function, cardiovascular diseases, appropriateness of drug prescription and outcomes in hospitalized older patients. *Drugs & Aging*, 38(12), 1097–1105.

Sobhani, S. R., Mortazavi, M., Kazemifar, M., & Azadbakht, L. (2021). The association between fast-food consumption with cardiovascular diseases risk factors and kidney function in patients with diabetic nephropathy. *Journal of Cardiovascular & Thoracic Research*, 13(3), 241–249.

Xue, L., Yuan, X., Zhang, S., & Zhao, X. (2021). Investigating the effects of Dapagliflozin on cardiac function, inflammatory response, and cardiovascular outcome in patients with STEMI complicated with T2DM after PCI. *Evidence-Based Complementary & Alternative Medicine (ECAM)*, 1–6.

Ineffective Childbearing Process

DEFINITION

Inability to prepare for and/or maintain a healthy pregnancy, childbirth process and care of the newborn for ensuring well-being

RELATED FACTORS (R/T)

- Domestic violence
- Inadequate maternal nutrition
- Inconsistent prenatal health visits
- Insufficient cognitive readiness for parenting
- Insufficient knowledge of childbearing process
- Insufficient parental role model
- Insufficient prenatal care
- Insufficient support system
- Low maternal confidence
- Maternal powerlessness
- Maternal psychological distress
- Substance misuse
- Unrealistic birth plan
- Unsafe environment

ASSESSMENT

- Age of patient and partner
- Availability of family members or friends to help
- Planned or unplanned pregnancy
- Family status, including number and ages of other children, usual patterns of interaction among family members, family members' assumed or expected roles, communication patterns, support systems, financial resources, past responses to change, spiritual resources, and living conditions
- Perceived impact of pregnancy on the family unit
- Psychosocial status, including developmental stage, previous experience with childbearing, expectations of the birth process, interest in learning, and current level of knowledge about pregnancy, birth, and recovery
- Ability to learn, including cognitive domain, intellectual and conceptual skills, and attention span
- Support systems, including presence of support person and support person's interest in helping patient and ability to participate in doing so

DEFINING CHARACTERISTICS

During Pregnancy

- Inadequate prenatal care
- Inadequate prenatal lifestyle
- Inadequate preparation of newborn care items
- Inadequate preparation of the home environment
- Ineffective management of unpleasant symptoms in pregnancy
- Insufficient access of support system
- Insufficient respect for unborn baby
- Unrealistic birth plan

During Labor and Delivery

- Decrease in proactivity during labor and delivery
- Inadequate lifestyle for stage of labor
- Inappropriate response to onset of labor
- Insufficient access of support system
- Insufficient attachment behavior

After Birth

- Inadequate baby care techniques
- Inadequate postpartum lifestyle
- Inappropriate baby feeding techniques
- Inappropriate breast care
- Insufficient access of support system
- Insufficient attachment behavior
- Unsafe environment for an infant

EXPECTED OUTCOMES

- Mother will demonstrate a willingness to improve her lifestyle and adhere to medical recommendations for optimal prenatal health.
- Mother will seek and convey confidence in knowledge about pregnancy, the labor and delivery process, and newborn care.
- Mother will cooperate and follow the care directives of the health care team during labor and delivery and the postpartum period.
- Mother will demonstrate coping and emotional strength to adapt to emergent situations during the prenatal, intrapartum, postpartum, and newborn care periods.
- Mother will exhibit maternal interest, attachment, and bonding with the newborn.
- Mother will perform skills for self-care and newborn care, including breastfeeding skills.
- Mother will seek to meet positive self-care needs and to meet the newborn's physical, social, nutritional, and safety needs.

Suggested NOC Outcomes

Fetal Status: Antepartum; Fetal Status: Intrapartum; Newborn Adaptation; Breastfeeding Establishment: Infant; Breastfeeding Establishment: Maternal; Parent-Infant Attachment; Role Performance; Prenatal Health Behavior; Knowledge: Breastfeeding; Knowledge: Infant Care; Knowledge: Labor and Delivery; Maternal Status: Antepartum; Maternal Status: Intrapartum; Maternal Status: Postpartum

INTERVENTIONS AND RATIONALES

- Assess baseline knowledge of prenatal self-care, labor and delivery process, and newborn care *to identify and resolve knowledge deficits.*
- Assess physical and psychological states of the mother during pregnancy *in order to treat medical conditions and develop a patient-centered plan to address needs and deficits.*
- Monitor physiologic vital signs and parameters at each phase of childbearing, *as these aid the clinicians in determining courses of action in response to evolving pathophysiological needs.*

PCC ▪ Monitor the emotional baseline of the mother/family unit *to identify strengths needed to cope with unknown, rapidly changing conditions.*

PCC ▪ Anticipate needs and provide for opportunities for the mother to reach out for assistance and knowledge for her self-care and expectations of labor and delivery and newborn care. *The mother's engagement in the processes demonstrates interest and initiates autonomy.*

PCC ▪ Teach the mother self-care for common prenatal discomforts *to promote patient comfort and autonomy.*

PCC ▪ Teach the mother about the pregnancy and the labor and delivery process. *Understanding expectations improves confidence, reduces anxiety, and aids in creating a trusting relationship.*

PCC ▪ Demonstrate comfort techniques that aid in labor management and delivery. *As the individual is free from discomfort, she can be more accepting of instruction and assist in the labor–delivery processes.*

PCC ▪ Include the mother in planning for changes in the treatment plan during labor and delivery to *indicate respect and reduce anxiety and fear of the unknown.*

EBP ▪ Provide accurate information to the mother/family unit during crisis/emergent situations. *This aids in anxiety reduction, trust establishment, and the family unit's ability to cooperate with the treatment team for the safety of mother and fetus/newborn.*

PCC ▪ Demonstrate techniques that match the mother's abilities to care for the newborn while the newborn is undergoing therapeutic care. *Demonstrate respect and individualization of the plan of care for the mother to meet the physical and emotional needs of the newborn.*

PCC ▪ Provide supportive environment during prenatal, intrapartum, and postpartum periods; *when the mother feels comfortable and cared for, she can focus on self-care, healing, and care of newborn undergoing intensive care management.*

PCC ▪ Provide bonding time between the newborn and mother/family unit; skin-to-skin cuddling; and encourage breastfeeding at delivery *to enhance critical bond development between mother/family unit and newborn.*

PCC ▪ Support the mother/family unit in the recovery and healing process for the mother and the neonate following unplanned, emergent stressful events. *Allowing the mother/family unit to verbalize and explore feelings and emotions aids in the integration process of healing.*

T&C ▪ Arrange for transportation to provider for clinic visit. *Nonadherence to prenatal and postpartum visits may be related to transportation issues.*

EBP ▪ Provide antenatal and postnatal classes on self-care and care of the newborn by a certified childbirth educator. *Advanced knowledge of the childbearing process promotes empowerment and positive maternal outcomes.*

T&C ▪ Coordinate multidisciplinary team—registered nurse, nurse midwife, physician, lactation consultant, registered dietitian, and social worker. *These professionals assess and uniquely meet the needs of the mother and newborn when there are events that interfere with the childbearing process.*

PCC ▪ Assist the family unit to develop the support system/network if management of medical and neonatal conditions warrants extended hospitalization. *Anticipatory guidance in seeking resources and assistance will aid the family to cope and provide autonomy in supporting the family as it supports its members in the hospital.*

Suggested NIC Interventions

Role Enhancement; Parent Education: Infant; Teaching: Infant Safety; Birthing; Infant Care; Family Involvement Promotion; Coping Enhancement

- Mother expresses knowledge of prenatal, labor and delivery, and postnatal processes.
- Mother incorporates suggestions provided.
- Mother/infant bond is established.
- Parents express increased confidence in their ability to perform appropriate feeding techniques.
- Mother demonstrates correct breastfeeding techniques.
- Mother provides adequate care for self and newborn.
- Mother and infant's needs are met.

- Results of assessment
- Instructions given to mother
- Neonate's daily weight
- Parents' knowledge of feeding techniques, involvement with caregiving, and bonding with neonate
- Parents' and neonate's responses to nursing interventions
- Evaluations for expected outcomes

REFERENCES

Chasse, J. D. (2016). Prenatal depression risk reduction & education program. *Journal of Prenatal and Perinatal Psychology and Health, 30*(4), 279–296.
Gedaly, L. R., & Leerkes, E. M. (2016). The role of sociodemographic risk and maternal behavior in the prediction of infant attachment disorganization. *Attachment & Human Development, 18*(6), 554–569.
Gonthier, C., Estellat, C., Deneux-Tharaux, C., Blondel, B., Alfaiate, T., Schmitz, T., ... Azria, E. (2017). Association between maternal social deprivation and prenatal care utilization: The PreCARE cohort study. *BMC Pregnancy and Childbirth, 17*, 126.
Pezaro, S., Pearce, G., & Bailey, E. (2018). Childbearing women's experiences of midwives' workplace distress: Patient and public involvement. *British Journal of Midwifery, 26*(10), 659–669.

Readiness for Enhanced Childbearing Process

A pattern of preparing for and maintaining a healthy pregnancy, childbirth process, and care of the newborn for ensuring well-being, which can be strengthened

- Patient's understanding of health problem and treatment plan
- Patient's health status, support systems, expressed concerns regarding childbirth process

During Pregnancy

- Expresses desire to enhance knowledge of childbearing process
- Expresses desire to enhance management of unpleasant pregnancy symptoms
- Expresses desire to enhance prenatal lifestyle
- Expresses desire to enhance preparation for newborn

During Labor and Delivery

- Expresses desire to enhance lifestyle appropriate for stage of labor
- Expresses desire to enhance proactivity during labor and delivery

After Birth

- Expresses desire to enhance attachment behavior
- Expresses desire to enhance baby care techniques
- Expresses desire to enhance baby feeding techniques
- Expresses desire to enhance breast care
- Expresses desire to enhance environmental safety for the baby
- Expresses desire to enhance postpartum lifestyle
- Expresses desire to enhance use of support system

EXPECTED OUTCOMES

- Patient/childbearing family will demonstrate willingness to maintain/modify lifestyle for optimal prenatal health.
- Patient will convey confidence and knowledge of pregnancy, the labor and delivery process, and newborn care.
- Patient will express appropriate self-control and readily cooperate with recommendations of the health care team during labor and delivery.
- After delivery, parent–newborn attachment will be evident.
- Newborn's physical, social, and nutritional needs will be met.

Suggested NOC Outcomes

Prenatal Health Behavior; Knowledge: Pregnancy; Knowledge: Labor & Delivery; Knowledge: Newborn Care; Parent–Infant Attachment

INTERVENTIONS AND RATIONALES

PCC ▪ Assess baseline knowledge of prenatal self-care, labor and delivery process, and newborn care *to identify and resolve knowledge deficits.*

EBP ▪ Provide written literature on prenatal wellness, labor and delivery expectations, and newborn care. *Providing written materials allows adequate time to synthesize and understand new information.*

PCC ▪ Teach self-care for common prenatal discomforts *to promote patient autonomy.*

PCC ▪ Teach the childbearing family labor and delivery process, and newborn care. *Understanding expectations improves confidence and reduces anxiety.*

PCC ▪ Assist the childbearing family with development of a birth plan. *This allows the childbearing family to participate in managing the birth experience and promotes communication with the health care team.*

PCC ▪ Encourage and support the childbearing family throughout the course of the pregnancy *to improve self-confidence and promote compliance with health recommendations.*

T&C ▪ Refer to certified childbirth educator for classes on prenatal care, labor and delivery (to include cesarean birth), breastfeeding, and newborn care. *Advanced knowledge of the childbearing process promotes empowerment and positive maternal outcomes.*

Suggested NIC Interventions

Anticipatory Guidance; Prenatal Care; Childbirth Preparation; Emotional Support; Parent Education: Infant

EVALUATIONS FOR EXPECTED OUTCOMES

- Childbearing family shows willingness to maintain/modify lifestyle for optimal prenatal health.
- Patient conveys confidence related to the labor and delivery process and newborn care.
- Patient accepts recommendations of the health care team during labor and delivery.
- Newborn's physical, social, and nutritional needs are met.

DOCUMENTATION

- Patient and family statement of lifestyle changes if needed
- Patient's understanding of the labor and delivery process
- Referrals to certified childbirth educator
- Evaluations for expected outcomes

REFERENCES

Haapio, S., Kaunonen, M., Arffman, M., & Åstedt, K. P. (2017). Effects of extended childbirth education by midwives on the childbirth fear of first-time mothers: An RCT. *Scandinavian Journal of Caring Sciences, 31*(2), 293–301.

McCants, B. M., & Greiner, J. R. (2016). Prebirth education and childbirth decision making. *International Journal of Childbirth Education, 31*(1), 24–27.

Meeks, R. C. (2016). Expectation setting during the prenatal period: A key to satisfaction. *International Journal of Childbirth Education, 31*(4), 33–36.

Waller-Wise, R. (2018). Adolescents breastfeeding. *International Journal of Childbirth Education, 33*(1), 44–46.

Risk for Ineffective Childbearing Process

DEFINITION

Susceptible to an inability to prepare for and/or maintain a healthy pregnancy, childbirth process, and care of the newborn for ensuring well-being

RISK FACTORS

- Domestic violence
- Inadequate maternal nutrition
- Inconsistent prenatal health visits
- Insufficient cognitive readiness for parenting
- Insufficient knowledge of childbearing process
- Insufficient parental role model
- Insufficient prenatal care
- Insufficient support system
- Low maternal confidence
- Maternal powerlessness
- Maternal psychological distress
- Substance abuse

- Unrealistic birth plan
- Unwanted pregnancy

ASSESSMENT

- Age of patient and partner
- Planned or unplanned pregnancy
- Family status, including number and ages of other children, usual patterns of interaction among family members, family members' assumed or expected roles, communication patterns, support systems, financial resources, past responses to change, spiritual resources, and living conditions
- Perceived impact of pregnancy on the family unit
- Psychosocial status, including developmental stage, previous experience with childbearing, expectations of the birth process, interest in learning, and current level of knowledge about pregnancy, birth, and recovery
- Ability to learn, including cognitive domain, intellectual and conceptual skills, and attention span
- Support systems, including presence of support person and support person's interest in helping patient and ability to participate in doing so

EXPECTED OUTCOMES

- Patient demonstrates a willingness to improve her lifestyle for optimal prenatal health.
- Patient seeks and conveys confidence in knowledge about pregnancy, the labor and delivery process, and newborn care.
- Patient cooperates and follows the care directives of the health care team during labor and delivery and the postpartum period.
- Patient exhibits maternal interest, attachment, and bonding with the newborn
- Patient performs skills for self-care and newborn care.
- Patient seeks to meet positive self-care needs and to meet the newborn's physical, social, nutritional, and safety needs.

Suggested NOC Outcomes

Fetal Status: Antepartum; Fetal Status: Intrapartum; Newborn Adaptation; Breastfeeding Establishment: Infant; Breastfeeding Establishment: Maternal; Parent-Infant Attachment; Role Performance; Prenatal Health Behavior; Knowledge: Breastfeeding; Knowledge: Infant Care; Knowledge: Labor and Delivery; Maternal Status: Antepartum; Maternal Status: Intrapartum; Maternal Status: Postpartum

INTERVENTIONS AND RATIONALES

- **PCC** Assess baseline knowledge of prenatal self-care, labor and delivery process, and newborn care *to identify and resolve knowledge deficits.*
- **S** Assess physical and psychological states of the mother during pregnancy *in order to treat medical conditions and develop plan to address deficits.*
- **PCC** Analyze cultural beliefs contributing to mother's behavior *since understanding by the health care team can aid in determining a plan of approach and treatment that is patient centered.*
- **PCC** Convey a nonjudgmental attitude *to allow a trusting relationship to develop.*

PCC ▦ Anticipate needs and provide for opportunities for the mother to reach out for assistance and knowledge for her self-care and expectations of labor and delivery and newborn care. *Mother's engagement in the processes demonstrates interest and initiates autonomy.*

EBP ▦ Monitor intrapartum parameters according to accepted standard of practice *to maintain physiologic needs and respond to evolving pathophysiologic needs.*

S ▦ Implement treatment plan prenatally or intrapartum to alleviate medical conditions *to enhance the physiologic condition of the mother.*

PCC ▦ Teach the mother self-care for common prenatal discomforts *to promote patient autonomy.*

PCC ▦ Teach the mother about the pregnancy and the labor and delivery process. *Understanding expectations improves confidence, reduces anxiety, and aids in creating a trusting relationship.*

PCC ▦ Demonstrate comfort techniques that aid in labor management and delivery. *As the individual is free from discomfort, she can be more accepting of instruction and assist in the labor–delivery processes.*

PCC ▦ Include the mother in planning for changes in treatment plan during labor and delivery *to indicate respect and reduce anxiety and fear of the unknown.*

PCC ▦ Demonstrate techniques that match the mother's abilities to care for the newborn. *Demonstrate respect and individualization of the plan of care for the mother.*

PCC ▦ Provide supportive environment during prenatal, intrapartum, and postpartum periods. *When the mother feels comfortable and cared for, she can focus on self-care and care of newborn.*

PCC ▦ Provide bonding time between newborn and mother; skin-to-skin cuddling; and encourage breastfeeding at delivery. *These and other actions enhance critical bond development between mother and newborn.*

EBP ▦ Provide antenatal and postnatal classes on self-care and care of the newborn by a certified childbirth educator. *Advanced knowledge of the childbearing process promotes empowerment and positive maternal outcomes.*

T&C ▦ Coordinate multidisciplinary team—registered nurse, nurse midwife, physician, lactation consultant, registered dietitian, and social worker. *These professionals assess and uniquely meet the needs of the mother and newborn.*

Suggested NIC Interventions

Role Enhancement; Parent Education: Infant; Teaching: Infant Safety; Birthing; Infant Care; Family Involvement Promotion; Coping Enhancement

EVALUATIONS FOR EXPECTED OUTCOMES

▦ Mother expresses knowledge of prenatal, labor and delivery, and postnatal processes.
▦ Mother incorporates suggestions provided.
▦ Mother–infant bond is established.
▦ Parents express increased confidence in their ability to perform appropriate feeding techniques.
▦ Mother demonstrates correct breastfeeding techniques.
▦ Mother provides adequate care for self and newborn.
▦ Mother and infant's needs are met.

DOCUMENTATION

▦ Results of assessment
▦ Instructions given to mother

- Neonate's daily weight
- Parents' knowledge of feeding techniques, involvement with caregiving, and bonding with neonate
- Parents' and neonate's responses to nursing interventions
- Evaluations for expected outcomes

REFERENCES

Alipour, Z., Kheirabadi, G. R., Kazemi, A., & Fooladi, M. (2018). The most important risk factors affecting mental health during pregnancy: A systematic review. *Eastern Mediterranean Health Journal, 24*(6), 549–559.

Charles, J. M., Rycroft-Malone, J., Aslam, R., Hendry, M., Pasterfield, D., & Whitaker, R. (2016). Reducing repeat pregnancies in adolescence: Applying realist principles as part of a mixed-methods systematic review to explore what works, for whom, how and under what circumstances. *BMC Pregnancy & Childbirth, 16*, 1–10.

Khajehei, M., & Finch, L. (2016). The role of residential early parenting services in increasing parenting confidence in mothers with a history of infertility. *International Journal of Fertility & Sterility, 10*(2), 175–183.

Liu, W., Mumford, E., & Petras, H. (2016). Maternal alcohol consumption during the perinatal and early parenting period: A longitudinal analysis. *Maternal and Child Health Journal, 20*(2), 376–385.

Impaired Comfort

DEFINITION

Perceived lack of ease, relief, and transcendence in physical, psychospiritual, environmental, cultural, and/or social dimensions

RELATED FACTORS (R/T)

- Insufficient environmental control
- Insufficient privacy
- Insufficient resources
- Insufficient situational control
- Noxious environmental stimuli

ASSOCIATED CONDITIONS

- Illness-related symptoms
- Treatment regimen

ASSESSMENT

- Patient's understanding of health problem and treatment plan
- Coping mechanisms, problem-solving ability, decision-making competencies
- Quality of relationships, support systems
- Changes in sleep patterns, appetite, and activity level

DEFINING CHARACTERISTICS

- Alteration in sleep pattern
- Anxiety
- Crying
- Discontent with situation
- Distressing symptoms
- Fear

- Feeling cold
- Feeling of discomfort
- Feeling of hunger
- Feeling warm
- Inability to relax
- Irritability
- Itching
- Moaning
- Restlessness
- Sighing
- Uneasy in situation

EXPECTED OUTCOMES

- Patient's heart rate, rhythm, and respiration rate will remain within expected range during rest and activity.
- Patient will maintain muscle mass and strength.
- Patient will report pain using pain scale.
- Patient will report periods of restful sleep.

Suggested NOC Outcomes

Comfort Status; Coping; Knowledge: Health Promotion; Pain Control

INTERVENTIONS AND RATIONALES

- **S** Monitor pain level using a scale of 1 to 10. Assess vital signs during times of discomfort, including blood pressure, heart rate and rhythm, and respirations.
- Assess sleeping patterns in response to discomfort.
- **PCC** Provide a quiet and relaxing atmosphere. Encourage active exercise *to increase a feeling of well-being.*
- **PCC** Provide pain medications as ordered.
- **PCC** Teach relaxation exercises and techniques *to promote reduced pain levels, sleep, and reduce anxiety.*
- **PCC** Include patient in plan of action *to promote self-care.*
- **PCC** Teach medication administration and schedule *to facilitate pain relief.*
- **PCC** Teach massage therapy to caregiver *to promote comfort.*
- **T&C** Refer to pain management clinic if pain cannot be controlled through relaxation and exercise.
- **T&C** Refer to physical therapist *to accommodate patient's level of activity.* Refer to massage therapist *to promote relaxation.*

Suggested NIC Interventions

Active Listening; Aroma Therapy; Calming Technique; Coping Enhancement

EVALUATIONS FOR EXPECTED OUTCOMES

- Patient's vital signs remained within expected range for rest and activity.
- Patient maintained muscle mass and strength.
- Patient used pain scale when reporting episodes of pain.
- Patient reported periods of restful sleep.

- Patient record of vital signs
- Patient reports of pain on a scale of 1 to 10
- Patient reports of restful sleep
- Evaluations for expected outcomes

REFERENCES

Cayley, W. E., Jr. (2018). Four evidence-based communication strategies to enhance patient care. *Family Practice Management, 25*(5), 13–17.

Dreher, B. S. (2017). All the comforts of home: Transformation to a comfort environment in critical care. *Critical Care Nurse, 37*(1), 78–80.

Parks, M. D., Morris, D. L., Kolcaba, K., & McDonald, P. E. (2017). An evaluation of patient comfort during acute psychiatric hospitalization. *Perspectives in Psychiatric Care, 53*(1), 29–37.

Shu Hua, N. G. (2017). Application of Kolcaba's comfort theory to the management of a patient with hepatocellular carcinoma. *Singapore Nursing Journal, 44*(1), 16–23.

Readiness for Enhanced Comfort

A pattern of ease, relief, and transcendence in physical, psychospiritual, environmental, and/or social dimensions, which can be strengthened

- Patient's perception of current state of comfort
- Patient's responsibility for actions taken to maintain a state of comfort
- Support systems, including family members, friends, and clergy
- Attitude of contentment
- Reliance on health care system to resolve complaints

- Expresses desire to enhance comfort
- Expresses desire to enhance feeling of contentment
- Expresses desire to enhance relaxation
- Expresses desire to enhance resolution of complaints

- Patient will express positive perception of nursing assistance to perform activities that promote comfort.
- Patient will experience physical and psychological ease.
- Patient will develop plans to optimize level of comfort.
- Patient will report an increase in relaxation.

Suggested NOC Outcomes

Client Satisfaction; Comfort Level; Comfortable Death; Hope; Personal Autonomy; Personal Well-Being; Quality of Life

`PCC` ▪ Assess the patient's satisfaction with the amount of assistance the nurse is currently offering *to determine whether the patient perceives self as performing own physical, psychosocial, and spiritual activities at a level that's comfortable for the patient.*

`PCC` ▪ Assist the patient in developing plan for increasing comfort *to maximize the patient's level of contentment and rest.*

`QI` `PCC` ▪ Implement a program to promote resolution of complaints *to prevent or alleviate the patient's stress or discomfort.*

`T&C` ▪ Involve staff, family, and community in promoting the patient's comfort *to include all resources that can contribute to the patient's comfort and well-being.*

`PCC` ▪ Teach the patient methods of deep breathing, meditation, and guided imagery *in order to reduce anxiety and promote enhanced comfort.*

▪ Provide pharmacologic relief when ordered to relieve symptoms related to discomfort. *Making the patient comfortable helps the patient cooperate in a more positive way with treatment.*

Suggested NOC Outcomes

Coping Enhancement; Emotional Support; Environmental Management: Comfort; Touch

▪ Patient expresses positive perception of nursing assistance with activities that promote comfort.

▪ Patient reports feelings of encouragement, acceptance, and reassurance during times of stress.

▪ Patient develops plan to adapt to perceived stressors, changes, and interferences with a state of comfort.

▪ Patient expresses an increase in relaxation and level of comfort.

▪ Patient's perception of level of comfort
▪ Patient's plan for increasing comfort
▪ Community resources that exist to increase patient comfort
▪ Future plans to address comfort and contentment
▪ Evaluations for expected outcomes

REFERENCES

Chou, L., Ranger, T. A., Peiris, W., Cicuttini, F. M., Urquhart, D. M., Briggs, A. M., & Wluka, A. E. (2018). Patients' perceived needs for allied health, and complementary and alternative medicines for low back pain: A systematic scoping review. *Health Expectations, 21*(5), 824–847.

Nuraini, T., Gayatri, D., & Rachmawati, I. N. (2017). Comfort assessment of cancer patient in palliative care: A nursing perspective. *International Journal of Caring Sciences, 10*(1), 209–215.

Serrano, B., Baños, R. M., & Botella, C. (2016). Virtual reality and stimulation of touch and smell for inducing relaxation: A randomized controlled trial. *Computers in Human Behavior, 55*, 1–8. doi:10.1016/j.chb.2015.08.007

Readiness for Enhanced Communication

DEFINITION

A pattern of exchanging information and ideas with others, which can be strengthened

ASSESSMENT

- Gender and age as variables in communication patterns
- Developmental history of communication patterns and practices
- Effect of stress on communication
- Family history of communication patterns
- Cultural and religious communication patterns
- Knowledge of difference between passive, aggressive, and assertive patterns of communication

DEFINING CHARACTERISTICS

Expresses desire to enhance communication

EXPECTED OUTCOMES

- Patient will express message clearly as evidenced by feedback that receiver understood the message.
- Patient will express an increased sense of confidence in communicating thoughts and feelings to nurse, family, health care teams, and any kind of reference groups in which an individual participates (e.g., friends, school groups, community groups, faith groups) throughout the life span and the continuum of care.
- Patient will report enhanced ability to respond assertively to individuals who relate with passive or aggressive communication styles.
- Patient will report feelings of confidence in social encounters because of enhanced communication skills.
- Patient will gain practice in applying enhanced communication techniques with individuals, family, and groups.
- Patient communication will be enhanced by nonverbal means, such as use of electronic mail and internet connections, pictures, and drawings.
- Patient will use enhanced communication skills to negotiate and advocate for self with health care providers and in conflict situations.

Suggested NOC Outcomes

Communication: Expressive; Communication: Receptive; Health-Seeking Behaviors

INTERVENTIONS AND RATIONALES

- Establish a clear purpose for interaction. *This provides the patient with goals and a time frame for interaction.*
- PCC • Provide environment that diminishes physical space between nurse and patient to eliminate barriers to communications such as noise and lack of privacy. *Reducing barriers to communication nonverbally communicates to patient that the nurse wants to be involved with patient.*

PCC ◼ Use verbal and nonverbal communication patterns that integrate warmth, genuineness, empathy, and respect to facilitate patient empowerment and relationship building. *Therapeutic nurse–patient relationship building increases patient's feeling of security. The nurse modeling caring behaviors encourages patient to incorporate the same attitudes.*

PCC ◼ Provide support through active listening, appropriate periods of silence, reflection of feelings, and paraphrasing and summarizing comments. *Active listening techniques encourage increased patient participation in communication.*

EBP ◼ Incorporate questions that are open-ended and start with such words as "what," "how," and "could," rather than "why." *Open-ended, nonthreatening questioning encourages patient to discuss issues of concern and improve communication skills.*

◼ Refrain from interrupting, changing subject, revealing too much personal information about self, or responding too quickly to questions during interactions. *Skillful role modeling of positive communication skills keeps focus on patient.*

EBP ◼ Encourage patient verbally and nonverbally to explore strategies to enhance self-advocacy communication skills with health care providers. *Self-advocacy communication skills can guide patient toward autonomy, confidence, and independence.*

◼ Avoid critical, overprotective, or overcontrolling communication patterns when working with patient. *Positive communication patterns reflect respect and facilitate development of patient trust and relationship building.*

EBP ◼ Include role-playing as a teaching strategy to model methods of enhanced verbal and nonverbal communication skills. *Role-playing of verbal and nonverbal communication methods in a nonthreatening, safe environment can enhance communication skills.*

◼ Explore and discuss thoughts and feelings regarding any overuse of negative cognitions and expressions on the part of the patient by suggesting strategies such as rubber band on wrist to snap every time negative expressions start. *Exploration and discussion of negative cognitions may provide an opportunity to explore alternative ways of dealing with negative thoughts and feelings.*

EBP ◼ Teach theory of assertive behavior, and role-play assertive communication approaches. *Assertiveness training can decrease passive or aggressive communication patterns.*

PCC ◼ Listen for themes presented during nurse–patient interactions *because themes can provide areas of focus for patient discussions with caregiver.*

◼ Schedule frequent treatment team meetings regarding communication skill development with patient. *Team meetings with patient can ensure continuity of care and the development of communication patterns, facilitating patient's coping with health and illness.*

PCC ◼ Communicate a plan to patient regarding mutual decision-making (partnering) toward goals and direction of future encounters *to reinforce patient's role within the relationship.*

◼ Consider factors such as age, gender, culture, religion, and spirituality in communicating with patient *to facilitate the provision of holistic and individual care.*

◼ Communicate use of positive self-talk to patient *to enhance confidence in communication.*

Suggested NIC Interventions

Active Listening; Animal-Assisted Therapy; Anticipatory Guidance; Art Therapy; Assertiveness Training; Behavioral Modification: Social Skills; Complex Relationship Building; Music Therapy; Socialization Enhancement

EVALUATIONS FOR EXPECTED OUTCOMES

◼ Patient expresses message clearly as evidenced by feedback that receiver understood the message.

◼ Patient expresses satisfaction with feedback received from caregivers and others.

- Patient reports that nurse and other health care team members provide an increased sense of security through verbal and nonverbal communication.
- Patient reports less anxiety and guilt and more control in providing assertive responses when relating to individuals with passive or aggressive communication styles.
- Patient expresses belief that nurse uses interactions that convey respect, warmth, empathy, and genuineness that can result in enhanced communication skill building.
- Patient discloses feelings of confidence and increased life quality related to enhanced communication skills with family, groups, health care team, and confrontational persons.
- Patient describes enhanced ability to advocate for self in coping with chronic and acute illness.
- Patient reports successful negotiations within health care milieu.

DOCUMENTATION

- Efforts made by nurse to provide didactic information on communication theory and to role model enhanced communication skills, such as assertiveness training
- Patient's response to didactic discussions and strategies, such as role-playing and interactive videos
- Nursing interventions regarding coaching and supporting patient progress toward enhanced communication patterns
- Patient's expressed thoughts and feelings about personal progress toward enhanced communication responses
- Revisions to treatment plan
- Evaluations for expected outcomes

REFERENCES

Baddley, D. (2018). Enhancing effective communication among non-verbal patients. *Pediatric Nursing, 44*(3), 144–146.

Brouwers, M., Rasenberg, E., Weel, C., Laan, R., & Weel, B. E. (2017). Assessing patient-centred communication in teaching: A systematic review of instruments. *Medical Education, 51*(11), 1103–1117.

Liermann, K., & Norton, C. (2016). Enhancing family communication: Examining the impact of a therapeutic wilderness program for struggling teens and parents. *Contemporary Family Therapy: An International Journal, 38*(1), 14–22. doi:10.1007/s10591-015-9371-5

Prouty, A., Fischer, J., Purdom, A., Cobos, E., & Helmeke, K. (2016). Spiritual coping: A gateway to enhancing family communication during cancer treatment. *Journal of Religion and Health, 55*(1), 269–287.

Acute Confusion

DEFINITION

Reversible disturbances of consciousness, attention, cognition, and perception that develop over a short period of time, and which last less than 3 months

RELATED FACTORS (R/T)

- Alteration in sleep–wake cycle
- Dehydration
- Impaired mobility
- Inappropriate use of restraints
- Malnutrition
- Pain
- Sensory deprivation
- Substance misuse
- Urinary retention

ASSOCIATED CONDITIONS

- Alteration in cognitive functioning
- Delirium
- Dementia
- Impaired metabolic functioning
- Infect
- Pharmaceutical agent

ASSESSMENT

- Age, gender, level of education, occupation, and recent immigration status
- Health history, including use of medications, recent surgery, allergies, history of alcoholism, drug abuse, and depression
- Neurologic status, including level of consciousness (LOC); orientation; thought and speech; mood; affect; memory; visual and spatial ability; judgment and insight; psychomotor activity; perceptions; delusions, illusions, and hallucinations; pain level; recent behavioral changes; and history of transient ischemic attacks, head injury, early dementia, AIDS, or schizophrenia
- Cardiovascular status, including vital signs, skin color, auscultation of carotid artery and heart sounds, and history of coronary artery disease or hypertension
- Respiratory status, including rate, depth, and pattern of respirations; auscultation for breath sounds; smoking history; shortness of breath; and history of chronic obstructive pulmonary disease, cancer, or tuberculosis
- Sensory status, including results of vision and hearing examination, use of corrective lenses or hearing aid, and history of eye or ear disorders
- Nutritional status, including typical daily food intake and weight loss
- Sleep status, including recent change in sleep pattern or environment (recent hospitalization)

DEFINING CHARACTERISTICS

- Agitation
- Alteration in cognitive functioning
- Alteration in LOC
- Alteration in psychomotor functioning
- Hallucinations
- Inability to initiate goal-directed behavior
- Inability to initiate purposeful behavior
- Insufficient follow-through with goal-directed behavior
- Insufficient follow-through with purposeful behavior
- Misperception
- Restlessness

EXPECTED OUTCOMES

- Patient will experience no injury.
- Patient's neurologic status will remain stable.
- Family members will report an improved ability to cope with the patient's confused state.
- Patient will start to participate in activities of daily living (ADLs).
- Patient will report feeling increasingly calm.
- Patient and family members will state the causes of acute confusion.
- Patient and family members will express an understanding of the importance of informing other health care providers about episodes of acute confusion.

Suggested NOC Outcomes

Anxiety Level; Cognition; Cognitive Orientation; Distorted Thought Self-Control; Information Processing; Neurologic Status: Consciousness; Safe Home Environment; Sleep

INTERVENTIONS AND RATIONALES

- Assess patient's LOC and changes in behavior *to provide baseline for comparison with ongoing assessment findings.*
- **S** Have a staff member stay at patient's bedside, if necessary, *to protect patient from harm as long as patient is confused.*
- **PCC** Enlist the aid of family member *to help calm patient.*
- **PCC** Limit noise and environmental stimulation *to prevent patient from becoming more confused. Environmental stimulation tends to exacerbate confused states.*
- **S** Monitor neurologic status on a regular basis *to detect any improvement or decline in patient's neurologic function.*
- **S** Use appropriate safety measures *to protect patient from injury.* Avoid physical restraints *to prevent agitating patient.*
- **PCC** Address patient by name and tell your name *to foster patient's awareness of self and environment.*
- Give patient short, simple explanations each time you perform a procedure or task *to decrease confusion.*
- **PCC** Schedule nursing care to provide quiet times for patient *to help avoid sensory overload.*
- Mention time, place, and date frequently throughout day. Have a clock and a calendar where patient can easily see them. Refer to these aids frequently when orienting patient *to foster awareness of self and environment.*
- **EBP** Keep patient's possessions in the same place as much as possible. *A consistent, stable environment reduces confusion and frustration and aids completion of ADLs.*
- **PCC** Ask family members to bring labeled family photos and other favorite articles *to create a more secure environment for patient.*
- Plan patient's routine and be as consistent as possible in following it. *A consistent routine aids task completion and reduces confusion.*
- Speak slowly, clearly, and allow patient ample time to respond *to reduce frustration and promote task completion.*
- **PCC** Encourage patient to perform ADLs, dividing tasks into small, critical units. Be patient and specific in providing instructions. Allow time for patient to perform each task. *These measures enhance self-esteem as well as help prevent complications related to inactivity.*
- **PCC** Encourage family members to share stories and discuss familiar people and events with patient. *Sharing stories and familiar subjects promotes a sense of continuity, aids memory, and creates a sense of security and comfort.* Note that even if patient's short-term memory is impaired, remote memory still may be intact.
- **PCC** Support family members' attempts to interact with patient *to provide positive reinforcement.*
- **PCC** Allow time before and after visits for family members to express feelings. *Listening to family members in an open and nonjudgmental manner helps them cope with patient's illness. Listening to their opinions may also help you assess and monitor patient's condition.*
- **PCC** Reassure patient and family that confusion will be temporary *to help relieve their anxiety.* Always include patient in discussions.
- **T&C** Confer with physician about diagnostic test results, patient's progress in behavior, and patient's LOC. *A collaborative approach to treatment helps ensure high-quality care and continuity of care.*

▣ Discuss episodes of acute confusion with patient and family members *to make sure they understand the cause of confusion.*

EBP ▣ Review supportive measures family members can take at home if patient begins to exhibit signs of confusion. Tell them to give patient short explanations of activities; repeat time, place, and date frequently; speak slowly and clearly and allow patient time to respond; and provide patient with a consistent routine. *Teaching empowers patient and family members to take greater responsibility for their health care needs.*

▣ Stress to patient and family that, in the future, they should inform health care providers about episodes of acute confusion *to help ensure continuity of care.*

Suggested NIC Interventions

Behavior Management: Overactivity/Inattention; Cognitive Stimulation; Delirium Management; Fall Prevention; Hallucination Management; Medication Management; Reality Orientation; Sleep Enhancement

EVALUATIONS FOR EXPECTED OUTCOMES

▣ Patient doesn't experience injury during episodes of acute confusion.
▣ Patient exhibits a mental status within his or her normal range.
▣ Family members report an increased ability to cope with patient's confused state.
▣ Patient performs ADLs to the extent possible.
▣ Patient reports feelings of increased calm.
▣ Patient and family members express an understanding of the causes of acute confusion.
▣ Patient and family members express an understanding of the importance of telling all health care providers about episodes of acute confusion.

DOCUMENTATION

▣ Description of episodes of acute confusion
▣ Factors that precipitate and ameliorate periods of acute confusion
▣ Teaching sessions and referrals
▣ Evaluations for expected outcomes

REFERENCES

Cahill, A., Pearcy, C., Agrawal, V., Sladek, P., & Truitt, M. S. (2017). Delirium in the ICU: What about the floor? *Journal of Trauma Nursing, 24*(4), 242–244.

Phelps, A., Kingston, B., Wharton, R. M., & Pendlebury, S. T. (2017). Routine screening in the general hospital: What happens after discharge to those identified as at risk of dementia? *Clinical Medicine, 17*(5), 395–400.

Thompson, C., Brienza, V. J. M., Sandre, A., Caine, S., Borgundvaag, B., & McLeod, S. (2018). Risk factors associated with acute in-hospital delirium for patients diagnosed with a hip fracture in the emergency department. *Canadian Journal of Emergency Medicine, 80*(6), 911–919.

Risk for Acute Confusion

DEFINITION

Susceptible to reversible disturbances of consciousness, attention, cognition, and perception that develop over a short period of time, which may compromise health

- Alteration in sleep–wake cycle
- Dehydration
- Impaired mobility
- Inappropriate use of restraints
- Malnutrition
- Pain
- Sensory deprivation
- Substance abuse
- Urinary retention

ASSOCIATED CONDITIONS

- Alteration in cognitive functioning
- Delirium
- Dementia
- Impaired metabolic functioning
- Infection
- Pharmaceutical agent

ASSESSMENT

- Age, gender, level of education, occupation, and recent immigration status
- Health history, including use of medications, especially with known cognitive and psychotropic adverse effects; recent surgery; allergies; and history of alcoholism, drug abuse, and depression
- Neurologic status, including level of consciousness (LOC), orientation, thought and speech, mood, affect, memory, visual and spatial ability, judgment and insight, psychomotor activity, and perceptions; delusions, illusions, and hallucinations; pain level; recent behavioral changes; electrolyte imbalances; and history of transient ischemic attacks, head injury, early dementia, AIDS, or schizophrenia
- Cardiovascular status, including vital signs, skin color, auscultation of carotid artery and heart sounds, and history of coronary artery disease or hypertension
- Respiratory status, including rate, depth, and pattern of respirations; auscultation for breath sounds; smoking history; shortness of breath; and history of chronic obstructive pulmonary disease, cancer, or tuberculosis
- Sensory status, including results of vision and hearing examination, use of corrective lenses or hearing aid, and history of eye or ear disorders
- Nutritional status, including typical daily food intake and weight loss
- Sleep status, including recent change in sleep pattern or environment (recent hospitalization)
- Elimination status, including history of urinary tract infection (UTI) and patterns of elimination

EXPECTED OUTCOMES

- Patient's neurologic status will remain stable.
- Patient will obtain adequate amounts of sleep.
- Patient will maintain optimal hydration and nutrition.
- Patient will participate in activities of daily living (ADLs).
- Patient will report feeling increasingly calm.
- Patient and family will state the causes of acute confusion.
- Patient and family will express an understanding of the importance of informing other health care providers about episodes of acute confusion.

Suggested NOC Outcomes

Cognitive Orientation; Distorted Thought Self-Control; Information Processing; Memory; Neurological Status; Personal Safety Behavior; Sleep

INTERVENTION AND RATIONALES

S ▦ Assess patient's LOC and changes in behavior *to provide baseline for comparison with ongoing assessment findings.*

S ▦ Have a staff member stay at patient's bedside, if necessary, *to protect patient from harm.*

S ▦ Enlist the aid of family member *to help calm patient.*

PCC ▦ Limit noise and environmental stimulation *to prevent patient from becoming more confused.*

S ▦ Monitor neurologic status on a regular basis *to detect improvement or decline in patient's neurologic function.*

S ▦ Use appropriate safety measures *to protect patient from injury.* Avoid physical restraints *to prevent agitating patient.*

PCC ▦ Address patient by name and mention your name *to foster patient's awareness of self and environment.*

EBP ▦ Give patient short, simple explanations each time you perform a procedure or task *to decrease confusion.*

▦ Establish or maintain elimination pattern *to assist in maintaining elimination, orientation, and patient safety.*

PCC ▦ Schedule nursing care to provide quiet times for patient *to help avoid sensory overload.*

▦ Mention time, place, and date frequently throughout day. Have a large clock and a calendar where patient can easily see them. Refer to those aids when orienting patient *to foster awareness of self and environment.*

EBP ▦ Keep patient's possessions in the same place as much as possible. *A consistent, stable environment reduces confusion and frustration and aids completion of ADLs.*

PCC ▦ Ask family to bring labeled family photos and other favorite articles *to create a more secure environment for patient.*

▦ Plan patient's routine, and be as consistent as possible in following it. *A consistent routine aids task completion and reduces confusion.*

PCC ▦ Speak slowly and clearly, and allow patient ample time to respond *to reduce sense of frustration and promote task completion.*

▦ Encourage patient to perform ADLs, dividing tasks into small, critical units. Be patient and specific in providing instructions. Allow time for patient to perform each task. *These measures enhance self-esteem as well as help prevent complications related to inactivity.*

PCC ▦ Encourage family to share stories and discuss familiar people and events with patient. *Sharing stories and familiar subjects promotes a sense of continuity, aids memory, and creates a sense of security and comfort.* Note that even if patient's short-term memory is impaired, remote memory still may be intact.

T&C ▦ Confer with physician about diagnostic test results, patient's progress in behavior, and patient's LOC. *A collaborative approach to treatment helps ensure high-quality care and continuity of care.*

▦ Discuss episodes of acute confusion with patient and family members *to make sure they understand the cause of confusion.*

EBP ▦ Review supportive measures family can take at home if patient begins to exhibit signs of confusion. Tell them to give patient short explanations of activities; repeat time, place, and date frequently; speak slowly and clearly and allow patient ample time to respond;

and provide patient with a consistent routine. *Teaching empowers patient and family to take greater responsibility for their health care needs.*

▨ Stress to patient and family that, in the future, they should inform health care providers about episodes of acute confusion *to help ensure continuity of care.*

Suggested NIC Interventions

Behavior Management: Overactivity/Inattention; Cognitive Stimulation; Delirium Management; Hallucination Management; Reality Orientation; Sleep Enhancement

EVALUATIONS FOR EXPECTED OUTCOMES

▨ Patient exhibits a mental status within his or her normal range.
▨ Patient performs ADLs to the extent possible.
▨ Patient reports feelings of increased calm.
▨ Patient and family members express an understanding of the causes of acute confusion.
▨ Patient and family members express an understanding of the importance of telling all health care providers about episodes of acute confusion.

DOCUMENTATION

▨ Description of episodes of acute confusion
▨ Factors that precipitate and ameliorate periods of acute confusion
▨ Teaching sessions and referrals
▨ Evaluations for expected outcomes

REFERENCES

Balková, M., & Tomagová, M. (2018). Use of measurement tools for screening of postoperative delirium in nursing practice. *Central European Journal of Nursing and Midwifery, 9*(3), 897–904.

DiLibero, J. (2018). Improving the accuracy of delirium assessments in neuroscience patients: Scaling a quality improvement program to improve nurses' skill, compliance, and accuracy in the use of the confusion assessment method in the intensive care unit tool. *Dimensions of Critical Care Nursing, 37*(1), 26–34.

Khan, B. A., Perkins, A. J., Campbell, N. L., Gao, S., Khan, S. H., Wang, S., … Kesler, K. (2018). Preventing postoperative delirium after major noncardiac thoracic surgery—A randomized clinical trial. *Journal of the American Geriatrics Society, 66*(12), 2289–2297.

Kivipelto, M., Mangialasche, F., & Ngandu, T. (2018). Lifestyle interventions to prevent cognitive impairment, dementia and Alzheimer disease. *Nature Reviews Neurology, 14*(11), 653–666.

Chronic Confusion

DEFINITION

Irreversible, progressive, insidious disturbances of consciousness, attention, cognition, and perception, which last more than 3 months

RELATED FACTORS (R/T)

▨ Chronic sorrow
▨ Sedentary lifestyle
▨ Substance misuse

- Central nervous system diseases
- Human immunodeficiency virus infections
- Mental disorders
- Neurocognitive disorders
- Stroke

- Age and gender
- Neurologic status, including level of consciousness (LOC), orientation, thought and speech, mood, affect, memory, visual and spatial ability, judgment and insight, psychomotor activity, and perceptions; recent behavior changes; lethargy, restlessness, short- or long-term memory loss, and sleep disturbance; and history of multiple infarctions, transient ischemic attacks, Parkinson's disease, cerebral infarctions, seizures, and alcohol or drug abuse
- Self-care status, including ability to perform instrumental or routine activities of daily living (ADLs)
- Family status, including marital status, economic status, living arrangements, presence of caregiver and relationship to patient, and caregiver's perception of patient's abilities

- Altered personality
- Difficulty retrieving information when speaking
- Difficulty with decision-making
- Impaired executive functioning skills
- Impaired psychosocial functioning
- Inability to perform at least one daily activity
- Incoherent speech
- Long-term memory loss
- Marked change in behavior
- Short-term memory loss

- Patient will exhibit no signs of depression.
- Patient will function at maximal cognitive level.
- Patient will participate in selected activities to fullest extent possible.
- Patient will remain free from harm.

Suggested NOC Outcomes

Client Satisfaction: Safety; Cognition; Cognitive Orientation; Concentration; Decision-Making; Distorted Thought Self-Control; Identity; Information Processing; Memory

- Assess patient's cognitive abilities and changes in behavior *to provide baseline data for comparison with ongoing assessment findings.*
- **PCC** ▪ Encourage family members to watch you perform mental status assessments *to give them a more accurate view of patient's abilities.*

S ▪ Evaluate patient's ability in regard to self-care as well as to function alone and drive a car. *Safety is a primary concern.*

▪ Assess patient for depression *to determine need for treatment.*

▪ Weigh patient, document your findings, and include instructions for regular weighing as part of care plan *to monitor patient's nutritional status.*

PCC ▪ Ask family members about their ability to provide care for patient *to assess their need for assistance.* Project an attentive, nonjudgmental attitude when listening to them *to help ensure that you receive accurate information.*

EBP ▪ Take steps to provide a stable physical environment and consistent daily routine for patient. *Stability and consistency enhance functioning.*

EBP ▪ Teach family members or caregiver strategies to help patient cope:
  ▪ Place an identification bracelet on patient *to promote safety.*
  ▪ Touch patient *to convey acceptance.*
  ▪ Avoid unfamiliar situations when possible *to help ensure a consistent environment.*
  ▪ Provide structured rest periods *to prevent fatigue and reduce stress.*
  ▪ Avoid asking questions patient can't answer—for example, questions that test the patient's orientation to time, place, person, or situation—*to avoid causing frustration.*
  ▪ Provide finger foods if patient won't sit and eat *to ensure adequate nutrition.*
  ▪ Select activities based on patient's interests and abilities, and praise patient for participating in activities *to enhance the sense of self-worth.*
  ▪ Use television and radio carefully *to avoid sensory overload, which may exacerbate confusion.*
  ▪ Limit choices patient has to make *to provide structure and avoid confusion.*
  ▪ Label familiar photos with names of individuals pictured *to provide a sense of security.*
  ▪ Use symbols, rather than written signs, to identify patient's room, bathroom, and other facilities *to help patient identify surroundings.*
  ▪ Place patient's name in large block letters on clothing and other belongings *to help patient recognize personal belongings and prevent them from becoming lost.*

S ▪ If possible, make a home visit *to assess safety of patient's living environment.*

T&C ▪ Assist family members in contacting appropriate community services. If necessary, act as an advocate for patient within health care system *to help secure services needed for ongoing care.*

T&C ▪ Provide family members with information concerning long-term health care facilities. If necessary, assist family members in moving patient to a nursing home or other long-term care setting. *A patient with chronic confusion may require ongoing skilled nursing care.*

PCC ▪ If patient is to be moved to a long-term care facility, explain the reason for the decision in as simple and gentle terms as possible *to facilitate comprehension.* Allow patient to express feelings regarding the move *to facilitate grieving over loss of independence.* Provide psychological support to patient and family members *to alleviate stress they may experience during relocation.*

T&C ▪ Communicate all aspects of the discharge plan to staff members at patient's new residence, including measures to ensure a stable environment and consistent routine; need to monitor patient's ongoing ability to perform ADLs; measures to ensure adequate nutrition; and interventions to provide emotional support to patient and family members. *Documenting a discharge plan and communicating it to caregivers helps ensure continuity of care. Interventions should ensure patient's dignity and rights.*

Suggested NIC Interventions

Anxiety Reduction; Area Restriction; Calming Technique; Cognitive Stimulation; Dementia Management; Emotional Support; Energy Management; Family Involvement Promotion; Medication Management; Reality Orientation; Sleep Enhancement

EVALUATIONS FOR EXPECTED OUTCOMES

- Patient experiences no injury because of chronic confusion.
- Patient exhibits no sign of depression.
- Patient eats enough to maintain weight.
- Family members discuss openly their ability to provide for the patient.
- Patient functions to maximum ability in a stable and structured environment.
- Family members describe strategies to help patient cope with chronic confusion.
- Patient participates in appropriate activities.
- Family maintains a safe environment in the home.
- Patient and family members receive adequate information regarding long-term care options to help them make informed decisions regarding patient's future.

DOCUMENTATION

- Assessment of patient's cognitive abilities, behavior, and self-care status
- Changes in patient's mental status as they occur
- Assistance given to family to help them cope with patient's confusion
- Any plans made to move patient to long-term care facility
- Teaching sessions and referrals
- Evaluations for expected outcomes

REFERENCES

Fredriksen-Goldsen, K. I., Jen, S., Bryan, A. E. B., & Goldsen, J. (2018). Cognitive impairment, Alzheimer's disease, and other dementias in the lives of lesbian, gay, bisexual and transgender (LGBT) older adults and their caregivers: Needs and competencies. *Journal of Applied Gerontology, 37*(5), 545–569.

Meléndez, J. C., Satorres, E., Redondo, R., Escudero, J., & Pitarque, A. (2018). Wellbeing, resilience, and coping: Are there differences between healthy older adults, adults with mild cognitive impairment, and adults with Alzheimer-type dementia? *Archives of Gerontology & Geriatrics, 77*, 38–43.

Stites, S. D., Harkins, K., Rubright, J. D., & Karlawish, J. (2018). Relationships between cognitive complaints and quality of life in older adults with mild cognitive impairment, mild Alzheimer Disease dementia, and normal cognition. *Alzheimer Disease & Associated Disorders, 32*(4), 276–283.

Constipation

DEFINITION

Infrequent or difficult evacuation of feces

RELATED FACTORS (R/T)

- Altered regular routine
- Average daily physical activity is less than recommended for age and gender
- Cognitive dysfunction
- Communication barriers
- Habitually suppresses urge to defecate
- Impaired physical mobility
- Impaired postural balance
- Inadequate knowledge of modifiable factors
- Inadequate toileting habits
- Insufficient fiber intake
- Insufficient fluid intake
- Insufficient privacy
- Stressors
- Substance misuse

- Blockage in the colon
- Blockage in the rectum
- Depression
- Developmental disabilities
- Digestive system diseases
- Endocrine system diseases
- Heart diseases
- Mental disorders
- Muscular diseases
- Nervous system diseases
- Neurocognitive disorders
- Pelvic floor disorders
- Pharmaceutical preparations
- Radiotherapy
- Urogynecological disorders

ASSESSMENT

- History of bowel disorder or surgery
- Gastrointestinal (GI) status, including nausea and vomiting, usual bowel elimination habits, change in bowel elimination habits, laxative use, stool characteristics (color, amount, size, and consistency), pain, inspection of abdomen, auscultation of bowel sounds, palpation for masses and tenderness, and percussion for tympany and dullness
- Oral status, including inspection of oral cavity (gums, tongue, and dentition), pain or discomfort, and salivation
- Activity status, including type, duration, and frequency of exercise; lifestyle; and access to toilet facilities during work and leisure
- Nutritional status, including appetite, dietary intake, amount and type of dietary fiber, fluid intake, food likes and dislikes, meal pattern, access to food supply and storage facilities, access to shopping and transportation, and financial resources available for food
- Fluid status, including fluid intake, urine output, urine specific gravity, and skin turgor
- Knowledge, including ability and motivation to change current patterns and understanding of relationship between intake, bulk, and constipation
- Drug history, including use of constipating agents (such as aluminum-based antacids, anticholinergics, antidepressants, iron supplements, laxatives, and opioids) and history of laxative abuse
- History of ingesting nonfood items (in psychiatric patients)

DEFINING CHARACTERISTICS

- Evidence of symptoms in standardized diagnostic criteria
- Hard stools
- Lumpy stools
- Need for manual maneuvers to facilitate defecation
- Passing fewer than three stools a week
- Sensation of anorectal obstruction

- Sensation of incomplete evacuation
- Straining with defecation

- Patient will participate in the development of bowel program.
- Patient will report urge to defecate, as appropriate.
- Patient will report easy and complete evacuation of stools.
- Patient's elimination pattern will return to a normal pattern for the patient.
- Patient will experience bowel movement every ____ day(s).
- Patient will consume high-fiber or high-bulk diet, unless contraindicated.
- Patient will maintain oral fluid intake of 2,500 mL daily, unless contraindicated.
- Patient will state understanding of relationship of dietary intake and bulk to constipation.
- Patient will list foods needed to prevent recurrence of problem, such as fruit, fruit juices, whole grain bread, and cereals.

Suggested NOC Outcomes

Bowel Elimination; Comfort Level; Hydration; Nutritional Status: Food & Fluid Intake; Symptom Control

- Monitor and record frequency and characteristics of stools. *Careful monitoring forms the basis of an effective treatment plan.*
- Monitor and record patient's fluid intake and output accurately. *Inadequate fluid intake contributes to dry, hard feces. Monitoring fluid balance ensures adequate fluid intake and promotes elimination.*
- **EBP** Unless contraindicated, encourage fluid intake of 2,500 mL daily *to ensure adequate fluid intake.*
- **PCC** Provide privacy for elimination *to promote physiologic functioning.*
- **PCC** Include patient in planning and implementing an individualized bowel regimen *to establish a regular elimination schedule.*
- Walk patient to toilet facilities or place patient on bedpan or commode at specific times daily, as close as possible to usual evacuation time (if known), *to aid adaptation to routine physiologic function.*
- **EBP** Emphasize to patient the importance of responding to the urge to defecate. Be alert for any mental status changes that may impair patient's ability to recognize or attend to the need to defecate or to report the need to caregiver. A timely response to the urge to defecate is necessary to maintain normal physiologic functioning and to avoid pressure and discomfort in the lower GI tract.
- Plan and implement an exercise routine, such as walking, leg raising, abdominal muscle strengthening, and Kegel exercises. Exercise promotes the abdominal and pelvic muscle tone necessary for normal elimination.
- **EBP** Encourage the intake of high-fiber foods. Many older patients have reduced intestinal muscle tone and decreased strength in abdominal muscles, resulting in slower peristalsis, dry feces, and decreased ability to exert pressure for evacuation. High-fiber foods supply bulk for normal elimination and improve intestinal muscle tone.

- Administer laxative or enema, as ordered, *to promote elimination of solids and gases from GI tract.* Monitor effectiveness.
EBP - Teach patient to gently massage along the transverse and descending colon *to stimulate bowel's spastic reflex and aid stool's passage.*
T&C - Consult with dietitian about increasing fiber and bulk in diet to maximum prescribed by physician. *This will improve intestinal muscle tone and promote comfortable elimination.*
EBP - Instruct patient and family in the relationship of diet, exercise, and fluid intake to constipation. Develop plan and provide for mild exercise periods. *These measures promote muscle tone and circulation and discourage deviation from prescribed diet.*

Suggested NIC Interventions

Bowel Management; Constipation/Impaction Management; Exercise Promotion; Fluid Management; Nutrition Management

EVALUATIONS FOR EXPECTED OUTCOMES

- Patient resumes regular bowel elimination schedule.
- Patient participates in planning and implementing bowel program.
- Patient reports urge to defecate, as appropriate.
- Patient reports easy and complete evacuation of stools.
- Patient achieves routine bowel function without excessive use of laxatives, enemas, straining, or discomfort.
- Patient consumes fruit, bran, and other high-fiber foods, unless contraindicated.
- Patient drinks 2,500 mL of fluid daily, unless contraindicated.
- Patient expresses understanding of the effects of diet and fluid intake on constipation.
- Patient names foods that will help prevent recurrence of constipation.
- Patient makes adaptations to lifestyle to ensure maintenance of bowel function.

DOCUMENTATION

- Patient's bowel movements and stool characteristics
- Patient's expressions of concern about constipation, dietary changes, laxative use, and bowel pattern
- Observations of food and fluid intake
- Patient's expression of understanding of relationship between constipation and dietary intake of fluid and bulk
- Patient's response to nursing interventions
- Evaluations for expected outcomes

REFERENCES

Bardsley, A. (2017). Assessment and treatment options for patients with constipation. *British Journal of Nursing, 26*(6), 312–318.
Barrie, M. (2017). Treatment interventions for bowel dysfunction: Constipation. *Journal of Community Nursing, 31*(5), 52–57.
Martin-Marcotte, N. (2018). Functional constipation in children: Which treatment is effective and safe? An evidence-based case report. *Journal of Clinical Chiropractic Pediatrics, 17*(3), 1485–1489.
Martinez de Andino, N. (2018). Current treatment paradigm and landscape for the management of chronic idiopathic constipation in adults: Focus on plecanatide. *Journal of the American Association of Nurse Practitioners, 30*(7), 412–420.

Risk for Constipation

DEFINITION

Susceptible to infrequent or difficult evacuation of feces, which may compromise health

RISK FACTORS

- Altered regular routine
- Average daily physical activity is less than recommended for age and gender
- Cognitive dysfunction
- Communication barriers
- Habitually suppresses urge to defecate
- Impaired physical mobility
- Impaired postural balance
- Inadequate knowledge of modifiable factors
- Inadequate toileting habits
- Insufficient fiber intake
- Insufficient fluid intake
- Insufficient privacy
- Stressors
- Substance misuse

ASSOCIATED CONDITIONS

- Blockage in the colon
- Blockage in the rectum
- Depression
- Developmental disabilities
- Digestive system diseases
- Endocrine system diseases
- Heart diseases
- Mental disorders
- Muscular diseases
- Nervous system diseases
- Neurocognitive disorders
- Pelvic floor disorders
- Pharmaceutical preparations
- Radiotherapy
- Urogynecological disorders

ASSESSMENT

- Age and gender
- Vital signs
- Health history, including bowel disorder or surgery, diabetic gastroparesis, immobility or inactivity, chronic debilitating disease, and episodes characterized by inability to swallow food and fluids
- Gastrointestinal (GI) status, including nausea and vomiting, usual bowel habits, change in bowel habits, laxative use, stool characteristics (color, amount, size, and consistency), pain, inspection of abdomen, auscultation of bowel sounds, palpation for masses and tenderness, and percussion for tympany and dullness

■ Nutritional status, including dietary intake, appetite, current weight, and changes from normal diet
■ Fluid status, including intake and output and skin turgor
■ Musculoskeletal status, including functional mobility, joint mobility, paralysis, paresis, and activity and exercise status
■ Psychosocial status, including understanding of risk of constipation; motivation to change health habits; and understanding of relationship between intake, bulk, activity and mobility, and constipation

EXPECTED OUTCOMES

■ Patient will experience no constipation.
■ Patient will maintain bowel movement every _____ day(s).
■ Patient will consume a high-fiber or high-bulk diet, unless contraindicated.
■ Patient will maintain fluid intake of _____ mL daily (specify).
■ Patient will express understanding of the relationship between constipation and dietary intake, bulk, and activity.
■ Patient will express understanding of preventive measures, such as eating fruit and whole grain breads and cereals and engaging in mild activity, if appropriate.

Suggested NOC Outcomes

Bowel Elimination; Self-Care: Toileting

INTERVENTIONS AND RATIONALES

■ Assess bowel sounds and check patient for abdominal distention. Monitor and record frequency and characteristics of stools *to develop an effective treatment plan for preventing constipation and fecal impaction.*
■ Record intake and output accurately *to ensure accurate fluid replacement therapy.*
EBP ■ Encourage fluid intake of 2.5 L daily, unless contraindicated, *to promote fluid replacement therapy and hydration.*
PCC ■ Initiate bowel program. Place patient on a bedpan or commode at specific times daily, as close to usual evacuation time (if known) as possible, *to aid adaptation to routine physiologic function.*
■ Administer a laxative, an enema, or suppositories, as prescribed, *to promote elimination of solids and gases from GI tract.* Monitor effectiveness.
EBP ■ Teach patient to gently massage along the transverse and descending colon *to stimulate the bowel's spastic reflex and aid in stool passage.*
T&C ■ Consult with a dietitian about how to increase fiber and bulk in patient's diet to the maximum amount prescribed by the physician *to improve intestinal muscle tone and promote comfortable elimination.*
EBP ■ Instruct patient, family member, or caregiver in the relationship between diet, activity and exercise, and fluid intake and constipation *to discourage departure from prescribed diet and assist in promoting elimination.*
■ Include a program of mild exercise in your care plan *to promote muscle tone and circulation.*
PCC ■ Review care plan with patient, family member, or caregiver, emphasizing the relationship between the risk factors for constipation and preventive measures *to foster understanding.*

Suggested NIC Interventions

Anxiety Reduction; Bowel Management; Constipation/Impaction Management; Exercise Promotion; Fluid Management; Fluid Monitoring; Nutrition Management

EVALUATIONS FOR EXPECTED OUTCOMES

■ Patient doesn't experience constipation.
■ Patient has bowel movement every _____ day(s).
■ Patient consumes a high-fiber or high-bulk diet, unless contraindicated.
■ Patient maintains fluid intake of _____ mL daily (specify).
■ Patient expresses understanding of the relationship between constipation and dietary intake, bulk, and activity.
■ Patient expresses understanding of preventive measures, such as eating fruit and whole grain breads and cereals and engaging in mild activity, if appropriate.

DOCUMENTATION

■ Patient's, family members', or caregivers' statements regarding risk of constipation
■ Presence of risk factors for constipation
■ Observations of food and fluid intake, urine output, and stool characteristics
■ Instructions regarding preventive care
■ Patient's, family members', or caregivers' statements indicating understanding of instructions
■ Patient's response to preventive interventions
■ Implementation, alteration, or continuation of bowel program
■ Patient's, family members', or caregivers' demonstrated ability to implement preventive measures
■ Evaluations for expected outcomes

REFERENCES

Ferrara, L. R., & Saccomano, S. J. (2017). Constipation in children: Diagnosis, treatment, and prevention. *Nurse Practitioner, 42*(7), 30–34.
Osuafor, C. N., Enduluri, S. L., Travers, F., Bennett, A. M., Deveney, E., Ali, S., ... Fan, C. W. (2018). Preventing and managing constipation in older inpatients. *International Journal of Health Care Quality Assurance, 31*(5), 415–419.
Trads, M., Deutch, S. R., & Pedersen, P. U. (2018). Supporting patients in reducing postoperative constipation: Fundamental nursing care—A quasi-experimental study. *Scandinavian Journal of Caring Sciences, 32*(2), 824–832.

Chronic Functional Constipation

DEFINITION

Infrequent or difficult evacuation of feces, which has been present for at least three of the prior 12 months

RELATED FACTORS (R/T)

■ Decrease in food intake
■ Dehydration
■ Depression
■ Diet disproportionally high in fat
■ Diet disproportionally high in protein

- Frail elderly syndrome
- Habitually suppresses urge to defecate
- Impaired mobility
- Insufficient dietary intake
- Insufficient fluid intake
- Insufficient knowledge of modifiable factors
- Low caloric intake
- Low-fiber diet
- Sedentary lifestyle

ASSOCIATED CONDITIONS

- Amyloidosis
- Anal fissure
- Anal stricture
- Autonomic neuropathy
- Cerebral vascular accident
- Chronic intestinal pseudo-obstruction
- Chronic renal insufficiency
- Colorectal cancer
- Dementia
- Dermatomyositis
- Diabetes mellitus
- Extra-intestinal mass
- Hemorrhoids
- Hirschsprung's disease
- Hypothyroidism
- Inflammatory bowel disease
- Ischemic stenosis
- Multiple sclerosis
- Myotonic dystrophy
- Panhypopituitarism
- Paraplegia
- Parkinson's disease
- Pelvic floor dysfunction
- Perineal damage
- Pharmaceutical agent
- Polypharmacy
- Porphyria
- Postinflammatory stenosis
- Pregnancy
- Proctitis
- Scleroderma
- Slow colon transit time
- Spinal cord injury
- Surgical stenosis

ASSESSMENT

- Health history, including history of bowel disorder or surgery and age of onset of symptoms
- Gastrointestinal status, including nausea and vomiting, usual bowel elimination habits, changes in bowel elimination habits, laxative use, stool characteristics (color, amount, size and consistency), duration of symptoms, and pain

- Abdominal assessment, including inspection of abdomen, auscultation of bowel sounds, percussion for tympany or dullness, and palpation for tenderness or masses
- Results of diagnostic test such as x-ray, anorectal manometry, colonic manometry, barium enema, and sigmoidoscopy
- Nutritional status, including dietary intake, fiber intake, and appetite, current weight, and change from normal weight
- Fluid and electrolyte status, including intake and output, skin turgor, urine specific gravity, and serum electrolytes
- Detailed medication history
- Activity status

DEFINING CHARACTERISTICS

ADULT: Presence of ≥2 of the following symptoms of Rome III classification system:
- Lumpy or hard stools in ≥25% defecations
- Straining during ≥25% of defecations
- Sensation of incomplete evacuation for ≥25% of defecations
- Sensation of anorectal obstruction/blockage for ≥25% of defecations
- Manual maneuvers to facilitate ≥25% of defecations (digital manipulation, pelvic floor support)
- ≤3 evacuations/week

CHILD > 4 years: Presence of ≥2 criteria on Rome III Pediatric classification system for ≥2 months:
- ≤2 defecations per week
- ≥1 episode of fecal incontinence per week
- Stool retentive posturing
- Painful or hard bowel movements
- Presence of large fecal mass in the rectum
- Large diameter stools that may obstruct the toilet

CHILD ≤4 years: Presence of ≥2 criteria on Rome III Pediatric classification system for ≥1 month:
- ≤2 defecations per week
- ≥1 episode of fecal incontinence per week
- Stool retentive posturing
- Painful or hard bowel movements
- Presence of large fecal mass in the rectum
- Large diameter stools that may obstruct the toilet

  General
- Distended abdomen
- Fecal impaction
- Leakage of stool with digital stimulation
- Pain with defecation
- Palpable abdominal mass
- Positive fecal occult blood test
- Prolonged straining
- Type 1 or 2 on Bristol Stool Chart

EXPECTED OUTCOMES

- Patient will maintain a normal bowel pattern.
- Patient will maintain fluid balance.
- Patient will display normal bowel sounds.
- Patient will express adequate pain relief.

- Patient or caregiver will identify measures to maintain normal bowel pattern.
- Patient or caregiver will demonstrate willingness to adhere to treatment measures.

Suggested NIC Interventions

Adherence Behavior; Bowel Elimination; Comfort Level; Health Beliefs; Hydration; Knowledge: Health Behavior; Nutritional Status: Food & Fluid Intake; Symptom Control

INTERVENTIONS AND RATIONALES

- Monitor and record frequency and characteristics of stool *to determine extent of the problem.*
- **PCC** Instruct the patient or parents if child is too young to keep a daily bowel diary *to gather more reliable information about the child's bowel habits since memory recall can be inaccurate.*
- **EBP** Assure patient is getting the recommended amounts of fiber in diet *as fiber intake below normal limits has been associated with functional constipation.*
- Keep an accurate intake and output record *to evaluate fluid intake status.*
- **EBP** Assure patient is receiving recommended daily fluid intake as per age and weight. *Adequate hydration aids in normal bowel elimination pattern.*
- **EBP** Encourage daily physical activity *to strengthen muscles and promote circulation.*
- Instruct parents of children to begin a toilet training system. This involves sitting on the toilet for 5 minutes after each meal to actively try to defecate. *This takes advantage of the gastrocolic reflex that increases colonic peristalsis, facilitating defecation.*
- **PCC** Teach patient to locate public restrooms and to wear easily removable clothing on outings *to promote normal bowel functioning.*
- **EBP** A footstool may be necessary for patients whose feet do not touch the floor to facilitate a relaxed posture during defecation. *This ensures child has the best posture to aid in defecation.*
- **EBP** Educate patient and caregivers about any prescribed pharmacologic treatments. *It is important for the parents to understand how and when to administer the prescribed medications and any side effects to watch for.*

Suggested NOC Outcomes

Bowel Management; Bowel Training; Constipation/Impaction Management; Counseling; Exercise Promotion; Fluid Management; Health Education; Nutrition Management

EVALUATIONS FOR EXPECTED OUTCOMES

- Patient exhibits a normal bowel pattern.
- Patient drinks adequate amount of fluids.
- Patient displays normal bowel sounds.
- Patient states pain relief measures are adequate.
- Patient or caregiver identifies measures to maintain normal bowel pattern.
- Patient or caregiver states willingness to adhere to treatment measures.

DOCUMENTATION

- Physical assessment findings of the abdomen, including bowel sounds and inspection, palpation, and percussion findings

* Fluid balance status, including intake and output, skin turgor, specific gravity, and mucous membranes
* Frequency and characteristics of stool
* Patient participation in care
* Evaluation for expected outcomes

REFERENCES

Currò, D., Ianiro, G., Pecere, S., Bibbò, S., & Cammarota, G. (2017). Probiotics, fibre and herbal medicinal products for functional and inflammatory bowel disorders. *British Journal of Pharmacology, 174*(11), 1426–1449.

Martin-Marcotte, N. (2018). Functional constipation in children: Which treatment is effective and safe? An evidence-based case report. *Journal of Clinical Chiropractic Pediatrics, 17*(3), 1485–1489.

Martínez-Ochoa, M. J., González-Iglesias, J., Ricard, F., Oliva-Pascual-Vaca, Á., Fernández-Domínguez, J. C., & Morales-Asencio, J. M. (2018). Effectiveness of an osteopathic abdominal manual intervention in pain thresholds, lumbopelvic mobility, and posture in women with chronic functional constipation. *Journal of Alternative and Complementary Medicine, 24*(8), 816–824.

Shen, Q., Zhu, H., Jiang, G., & Liu, X. (2018). Nurse-led self-management educational intervention improves symptoms of patients with functional constipation. *Western Journal of Nursing Research, 40*(6), 874–888.

Risk for Chronic Functional Constipation

DEFINITION

Susceptible to infrequent or difficult evacuation of feces, which has been present nearly three of the prior 12 months, which may compromise health

RISK FACTORS

* Decrease in food intake
* Dehydration
* Depression
* Diet disproportionally high in fat
* Diet disproportionally high in protein
* Frail elderly syndrome
* Habitually suppresses urge to defecate
* Impaired mobility
* Insufficient dietary intake
* Insufficient fluid intake
* Insufficient knowledge of modifiable factors
* Low caloric intake
* Low-fiber diet
* Sedentary lifestyle

ASSOCIATED CONDITIONS

* Amyloidosis
* Anal fissure
* Anal stricture
* Autonomic neuropathy
* Cerebral vascular accident

- Chronic intestinal pseudo-obstruction
- Chronic renal insufficiency
- Colorectal cancer
- Dementia
- Dermatomyositis
- Diabetes mellitus
- Extra-intestinal mass
- Hemorrhoids
- Hirschsprung's disease
- Hypercalcemia
- Hypothyroidism
- Inflammatory bowel disease
- Ischemic stenosis
- Multiple sclerosis
- Myotonic dystrophy
- Panhypopituitarism
- Paraplegia
- Parkinson's disease
- Pelvic floor dysfunction
- Perineal damage
- Pharmaceutical agent
- Polypharmacy
- Porphyria
- Postinflammatory stenosis
- Pregnancy
- Proctitis
- Scleroderma
- Slow colon transit time
- Spinal cord injury
- Surgical stenosis

ASSESSMENT

- Health history, including history of bowel disorder or surgery and age of onset of symptoms
- Gastrointestinal status, including nausea and vomiting, usual bowel elimination habits, changes in bowel elimination habits, laxative use, stool characteristics (color, amount, size, and consistency), duration of symptoms, and pain
- Abdominal assessment, including inspection of abdomen, auscultation of bowel sounds, percussion for tympany or dullness, and palpation for tenderness or masses
- Results of diagnostic test such as x-ray, anorectal manometry, colonic manometry, barium enema, and sigmoidoscopy
- Nutritional status, including dietary intake, fiber intake, and appetite, current weight, and change from normal weight
- Fluid and electrolyte status, including intake and output, skin turgor, urine specific gravity, and serum electrolytes
- Detailed medication history
- Activity status

- Patient will maintain a normal bowel pattern.
- Patient will maintain fluid balance.
- Patient will display normal bowel sounds.
- Patient will express adequate pain relief.
- Patient or caregiver will identify measures to maintain normal bowel pattern.
- Patient or caregiver will demonstrate willingness to adhere to treatment measures.

Suggested NIC Interventions

Adherence Behavior; Bowel Elimination; Comfort Level; Health Beliefs; Hydration; Knowledge: Health Behavior; Nutritional Status: Food & Fluid Intake; Symptom Control

- Assess and monitor frequency and characteristics of stool *to determine if there is a potential problem.*
- **PCC** Instruct patient or parents if child is too young to keep a daily bowel diary *to gather more reliable information about child's bowel habits since memory recall can be inaccurate.*
- **EBP** Assure patient is getting the recommended amounts of fiber in diet *as fiber intake below normal limits has been associated with functional constipation.*
- Keep an accurate intake and output record *to evaluate fluid intake status.*
- **EBP** Assure patient is receiving recommended daily fluid intake as per age and weight. *Adequate hydration aids in normal bowel elimination pattern.*
- **EBP** Encourage daily physical activity *to strengthen muscles and promote circulation.*
- **EBP** A footstool may be necessary for patients whose feet do not touch the floor to facilitate a relaxed posture during defecation. *This ensures the child has the best posture to aid in defecation.*
- **EBP** Educate patient and caregivers about any prescribed pharmacologic treatments. *It is important for the parents to understand how and when to administer the prescribed medications and any side effects to watch for.*

Suggested NOC Outcomes

Bowel Management; Bowel Training; Constipation/Impaction Management; Counseling; Exercise Promotion; Fluid Management; Health Education; Nutrition Management

- Patient exhibits a normal bowel pattern.
- Patient drinks adequate amount of fluids.
- Patient displays normal bowel sounds.
- Patient states pain relief measures are adequate.
- Patient or caregiver identifies measures to maintain normal bowel pattern.
- Patient or caregiver states willingness to adhere to treatment measures.

- Physical assessment findings of the abdomen, including bowel sounds and inspection, palpation, and percussion findings
- Fluid balance status, including intake and output, skin turgor, specific gravity, and mucous membranes
- Frequency and characteristics of stool
- Patient participation in care
- Evaluation for expected outcomes

REFERENCES

Barnes, J., Coleman, B., Hwang, S., Stolic, A., Bousvaros, A., Nurko, S., & Salinas, G. D. (2018). Educational needs in the diagnosis and management of pediatric functional constipation: A US survey of specialist and primary care clinicians. *Postgraduate Medicine, 130*(4), 428–435.

Fujitani, A., Sogo, T., Inui, A., & Kawakubo, K. (2018). Prevalence of functional constipation and relationship with dietary habits in 3- to 8-year-old children in Japan. *Gastroenterology Research and Practice, 2018*, 1–8.

George, S. E., & Borello-France, D. F. (2017). Perspective on physical therapist management of functional constipation. *Physical Therapy, 97*(4), 478–493.

Perceived Constipation

DEFINITION

Self-diagnosis of infrequent or difficult evacuation of feces combined with abuse of methods to ensure a daily bowel movement

RELATED FACTORS (R/T)

- Cultural health beliefs
- Deficient knowledge about normal evacuation patterns
- Disturbed thought processes
- Family health beliefs

ASSESSMENT

- Age and gender
- Family history of constipation
- History of psychiatric disorders
- Fluid and electrolyte status, including intake and output, skin turgor, urine specific gravity, and mucous membranes
- Gastrointestinal status, including bowel elimination habits, change in bowel elimination habits, stool characteristics (color, amount, size, and consistency), pain, auscultation of bowel sounds, laxative or enema use (time and duration), family habits concerning bowel movements, and rectal examination
- Nutritional status, including dietary intake and appetite
- Activity status
- Psychosocial status, including personality, stressors (finances, job, marital discord, and coping mechanisms), support systems (family and others), lifestyle, and knowledge level

DEFINING CHARACTERISTICS

- Enema misuse
- Expects bowel movement at same time daily

- Laxative misuse
- Suppository misuse

EXPECTED OUTCOMES

- Patient will decrease use of laxatives, enemas, or suppositories.
- Patient will state understanding of normal bowel function.
- Patient will discuss feelings about elimination pattern.
- Patient's elimination pattern will return to normal.
- Patient will experience bowel movement every _____ day(s) without laxatives, enemas, or suppositories.
- Patient will state understanding of factors causing constipation.
- Patient will get regular exercise.
- Patient will describe changes in personal habits to maintain normal elimination pattern.
- Patient will state intent to use appropriate resources to help resolve emotional or psychological problems.

Suggested NOC Outcomes

Adherence Behavior; Bowel Elimination; Health Beliefs; Health Beliefs: Perceived Threat; Knowledge: Health Behavior

INTERVENTIONS AND RATIONALES

- **EBP** Modify patient's dietary habits to include adequate fluids, fresh fruits and vegetables, and whole grain cereals and breads, *which supply necessary bulk for normal elimination.*
- **PCC** Encourage patient to engage in daily exercise, such as brisk walking, *to strengthen muscle tone and stimulate circulation.*
- **PCC** Encourage patient to evacuate at regular times *to aid adaptation and routine physiologic function.*
- Urge patient to avoid taking laxatives, if possible, or to gradually decrease their use *to avoid further trauma to intestinal mucosa.*
- Inform patient not to expect a bowel movement every day or even every other day *to avoid use of poor health practices to stimulate elimination.*
- **EBP** If not contraindicated, increase patient's fluid intake to about 3 L daily *to increase functional capacity of bowel elimination.*
- **PCC** Explain normal bowel elimination habits so patient *can better understand normal and abnormal body functions.*
- Reassure patient that normal bowel function is possible without laxatives, enemas, or suppositories *to give patient the necessary confidence for compliance.*
- **T&C** Give information about self-help groups, as appropriate, *to provide additional resources for patient and family.*
- Establish and implement an individualized bowel elimination regimen based on patient's needs. *Knowledge of normal body functions will improve patient's understanding of problem.*
- Instruct patient to avoid straining during elimination *to avoid tissue damage, bleeding, and pain.*
- **EBP** Instruct patient that abdominal massage may help relieve discomfort and promote defecation *because it triggers bowel's spastic reflex.*

Suggested NIC Interventions

Anxiety Reduction; Bowel Management; Counseling; Health Education; Nutrition Management; Teaching: Individual

- Patient decreases use of laxatives, enemas, or suppositories.
- Patient describes normal bowel function and how fluid consumption, high-fiber diet, and exercise affect function.
- Patient expresses feelings about changes in elimination pattern.
- Patient's elimination pattern returns to normal.
- Without using laxatives, enemas, or suppositories, patient has bowel movement every ____ day(s).
- Patient lists factors that may cause constipation.
- Patient engages in regular exercise.
- Patient states plans to make changes in personal habits to prevent constipation.
- Patient makes contact with appropriate resources to help resolve psychological conflicts.

DOCUMENTATION

- Patient's expressions of concern about change in diet, activity level, laxative and enema use, and bowel pattern
- Observations of diet, stool characteristics, and activity tolerance
- Patient teaching about diet, exercise, and constipation management
- Evaluations for expected outcomes

REFERENCES

Barrie, M. (2017). Treatment interventions for bowel dysfunction: Constipation. *Journal of Community Nursing, 31*(5), 52–57.

Clark, K., Lam, L. T., Talley, N. J., Phillips, J. L., & Currow, D. C. (2017). Identifying factors that predict worse constipation symptoms in palliative care patients: A secondary analysis. *Journal of Palliative Medicine, 20*(5), 528–532.

Robertson, J., Baines, S., Emerson, E., & Hatton, C. (2018). Constipation management in people with intellectual disability: A systematic review. *Journal of Applied Research in Intellectual Disabilities, 31*(5), 709–724.

Werth, B. L., Williams, K. A., & Pont, L. G. (2017). Laxative use and self-reported constipation in a community-dwelling elderly population. *Gastroenterology Nursing, 40*(2), 134–141.

Contamination

DEFINITION

Exposure to environmental contaminants in doses sufficient to cause adverse health effects

RELATED FACTORS (R/T)

External

- Carpeted flooring
- Chemical contamination of food
- Chemical contamination of water
- Flaking, peeling surface in the presence of young children
- Inadequate breakdown of contaminant
- Inadequate household hygiene practices
- Inadequate municipal services
- Inadequate personal hygiene practices
- Inadequate protective clothing

- Ingestion of contaminated material
- Playing where environmental contaminants are used
- Unprotected exposure to chemical
- Unprotected exposure to heavy metal
- Unprotected exposure to radioactive material
- Use of environmental contaminant in the home
- Use of noxious material in insufficiently ventilated area
- Use of noxious material without effective protection

Internal

- Concomitant exposure
- Inadequate nutrition
- Smoking

ASSOCIATED CONDITIONS

- Preexisting disease
- Pregnancy

ASSESSMENT

- Community demographics, including age and sex distribution, education and income levels, and ethnic, racial, and religious groups
- Community health status, including prevalence of health problems in community, environmental pollutants, pesticide usage, biologic or radiation hazards, availability of health care services, community members' use of health care services, and beliefs, values, and attitudes about health and illness
- Living conditions, including number of occupants, sanitation, and ventilation
- Occupation and work history

DEFINING CHARACTERISTICS

Pesticides

- Dermatologic effects of pesticide exposure
- Gastrointestinal effects of pesticide exposure
- Neurologic effects of pesticide exposure
- Pulmonary effects of pesticide exposure
- Renal effects of pesticide exposure

Chemicals

- Dermatologic effects of chemical exposure
- Gastrointestinal effects of chemical exposure
- Immunologic effects of chemical exposure
- Neurologic effects of chemical exposure
- Pulmonary effects of chemical exposure
- Renal effects of chemical exposure

Biological

- Dermatologic effects of biologic exposure
- Gastrointestinal effects of biologic exposure

- Neurologic effects of biologic exposure
- Pulmonary effects of biologic exposure
- Renal effects of biologic exposure

Pollution

- Neurologic effects of pollution exposure
- Pulmonary effects of pollution exposure

Waste

- Dermatologic effects of waste exposure
- Gastrointestinal effects of waste exposure
- Hepatic effects of waste exposure
- Pulmonary effects of waste exposure

Radiation

- Genetic effects of radiation exposure
- Immunological effects of radiation exposure
- Neurological effects of radiation exposure
- Oncological effects of radiation exposure

Suggested NOC Outcomes

Anxiety Level; Community Health Status; Fear Level; Community Disaster Readiness

EXPECTED OUTCOMES

- Community members will have minimized health effects associated with contamination.
- Community members will utilize health surveillance data system to monitor for contamination incidents.
- Community members will utilize disaster plan to evacuate and triage affected members.
- Community members will minimize exposure to contaminants.

INTERVENTIONS AND RATIONALES

S ▪ Triage, stabilize, transport, and treat affected community members. *Accurate triage and early treatment provide the best chance of survival to affected persons.*

S ▪ Monitor individuals for therapeutic effects, side effects, and compliance with post-exposure drug therapy. *Drug therapy may extend over a long period of time and will require monitoring for compliance as well as therapeutic and side effects.*

PCC ▪ Help individuals cope with contamination incident; use groups that have survived terrorist attacks as useful resource for victims *to aid in support; those with experience can share reactions and useful coping mechanisms.*

PCC ▪ Help individuals deal with feelings of fear, vulnerability, and grief *to minimize risk of traumatic stress.*

S ▪ Decontaminate persons, clothing, and equipment using approved procedure. Victims may first require decontamination before entering health facility *to receive care in order to prevent the spread of contamination.*

EBP ▦ Use appropriate isolation precautions, including universal, airborne, droplet, and contact isolation. *Proper use of isolation precautions prevents cross-contamination.*

EBP ▦ Provide accurate information on risks involved, preventive measures, and use of antibiotics and vaccines *to enhance the use of protective measures.*

PCC ▦ Encourage individuals to talk to others about their fears. *Interventions aimed at supporting an individual's coping can help the person deal with feelings of fear, helplessness, and loss of control that are normal reactions in a crisis situation.*

T&C **I** ▦ Collaborate with other agencies (local health department, emergency medical services, state and federal agencies). *Communication and collaboration among agencies increase ability to handle crises efficiently and correctly.*

Suggested NIC Interventions

Anxiety Reduction; Crisis Intervention; Environmental Management; Infection Control; Health Education; Triage

EVALUATIONS FOR EXPECTED OUTCOMES

▦ There is no evidence of contamination.
▦ Health surveillance data are negative for contamination.
▦ Community participates in disaster planning efforts.
▦ Community's exposure to contaminants is minimized.

DOCUMENTATION

▦ Results of health surveillance data
▦ Evaluation of simulated disaster plans
▦ Evaluations for expected outcomes

REFERENCES

Fung, F., Wang, H., & Menon, S. (2018). Food safety in the 21st century. *Biomedical Journal, 41*(2), 88–95.

Knox, J., Sullivan, S. B., Urena, J., Miller, M., Vavagiakis, P., Shi, Q., ... Lowy, F. D. (2016). Association of environmental contamination in the home with the risk for recurrent community-associated, methicillin-resistant *Staphylococcus aureus* infection. *JAMA Internal Medicine, 176*(6), 807.

Marino, F., & Nunziata, L. (2018). Long-term consequences of the Chernobyl radioactive fallout: An exploration of the aggregate data. *The Milbank Quarterly, 96*(4), 814–857.

Zahra, N., Kalim, I., Mahmood, M., & Naeem, N. (2017). Perilous effects of heavy metals contamination on human health. *Pakistan Journal of Analytical & Environmental Chemistry, 18*(1), 1–17.

Risk for Contamination

DEFINITION

Susceptible to exposure to environmental contaminants, which may compromise health

RISK FACTORS

External

▦ Carpeted flooring
▦ Chemical contamination of food

- Chemical contamination of water
- Flaking, peeling surface in the presence of young children
- Inadequate breakdown of contaminant
- Inadequate household hygiene practices
- Inadequate municipal services
- Inadequate personal hygiene practices
- Inadequate protective clothing
- Inappropriate use of protective clothing
- Ingestion of contaminated material
- Playing where environmental contaminants are used
- Unprotected exposure to chemical
- Unprotected exposure to radioactive material
- Use of environmental contaminant in the home
- Use of noxious material in insufficiently ventilated area
- Use of noxious material without effective protection

Internal

- Concomitant exposure
- Inadequate nutrition
- Smoking

ASSOCIATED CONDITIONS

- Preexisting disease
- Pregnancy

ASSESSMENT

- Community demographics, including age and sex distribution, education and income levels, and ethnic, racial, and religious groups
- Community health status, including prevalence of health problems in community, environmental pollutants, pesticide usage, biologic or radiation hazards, availability of health care services, community members' use of health care services, and beliefs, values, and attitudes about health and illness
- Living conditions, including number of occupants, sanitation, and ventilation
- Occupation and work history

EXPECTED OUTCOMES

- Community will remain free from adverse effects of contamination.
- Community will utilize health surveillance data system to monitor for contamination incidents.
- Community will participate in mass casualty and disaster readiness drills.
- Community will remain free from contamination-related health effects.
- Community will have minimal exposure to contaminants.

Suggested NOC Outcomes

Community Disaster Readiness; Community Health Status; Health Beliefs: Perceived Threat; Knowledge: Health Behavior; Knowledge: Health Resources; Risk Control

S ▪ Monitor individuals for therapeutic effects, side effects, and compliance with post-exposure drug therapy. *Drug therapy may extend over a long period of time and will require monitoring for compliance as well as therapeutic and side effects.*

S **I** ▪ Conduct surveillance for environmental contamination; notify agencies authorized to protect the environment of contaminants in the area. *Early surveillance and detection are critical components of preparation.*

S ▪ Assist individuals in relocating to safer environment *to decrease their risk of contamination.*

S ▪ Modify environment to minimize risk. *Modification of the environment will decrease the risk of actual contamination.*

S ▪ Implement decontamination of persons, clothing, and equipment by using approved procedure. Victims may first require decontamination before entering health facility *to receive care in order to prevent the spread of contamination.*

EBP ▪ Use appropriate isolation precautions: universal, airborne, droplet, and contact isolation. *Proper use of isolation precautions prevents cross-contamination by contaminating agent.*

EBP ▪ Provide accurate information on risks involved, preventive measures, use of antibiotics and *vaccines to reduce anxiety and increase compliance.*

PCC ▪ Assist community members with feelings of fear and vulnerability. *Interventions aimed at supporting an individual's coping help the person deal with feelings of fear, helplessness, and loss of control that are normal reactions in a crisis situation.*

T&C **I** ▪ In conjunction with other health care providers, schedule mass casualty and disaster readiness drills. *Practice in handling contamination occurrences will decrease the risk of exposure during actual contamination events.*

Suggested NIC Interventions

Bioterrorism Preparedness; Communicable Disease Management; Community; Community Disaster Preparedness; Environmental Management: Safety; Environmental Risk Protection; Health Education; Health Policy Monitoring; Health Screening; Immunization/Vaccination Management; Risk Identification; Surveillance: Safety

▪ No evidence of contamination.
▪ Health surveillance data are negative for contamination.
▪ Community participates in disaster planning efforts.
▪ Community exposure to contaminants is minimized.

▪ Results of health surveillance data
▪ Evaluation of simulated disaster plans
▪ Evaluations for expected outcomes

REFERENCES

McCann, R. S., van den Berg, H., Takken, W., Chetwynd, A. G., Giorgi, E., Terlouw, D. J., & Diggle, P. J. (2018). Reducing contamination risk in cluster-randomized infectious disease-intervention trials. *International Journal of Epidemiology, 47*(6), 2015–2024.

Ng, W., Faheem, A., McGeer, A., Simor, A. E., Gelosia, A., Willey, B. M., … Katz, K. (2017). Community- and healthcare-associated methicillin-resistant *Staphylococcus aureus* strains: An investigation into household transmission, risk factors, and environmental contamination. *Infection Control & Hospital Epidemiology, 38*(1), 61–67.

Seo, S., Wan, Y. L., Dal, N. L., Kim, J. U., Cha, E. S., Ye, J. B., ... Young, W. J. (2018). Assessing the health effects associated with occupational radiation exposure in Korean radiation workers: Protocol for a prospective cohort study. *BMJ Open, 8*(3), e017359.

Sinclair, R., Russell, C., Kray, G., & Vesper, S. (2018). Asthma risk associated with indoor mold contamination in Hispanic communities in Eastern Coachella Valley, California. *Journal of Environmental & Public Health, 2018*, 1–7.

Defensive Coping

DEFINITION

Repeated projection of falsely positive self-evaluation based on a self-protective pattern that defends against underlying perceived threats to positive self-regard

RELATED FACTORS (R/T)

- Conflict between self-perception and value system
- Fear of failure
- Fear of humiliation
- Fear of repercussions
- Insufficient confidence in others
- Insufficient resilience
- Insufficient self-confidence
- Insufficient support system
- Uncertainty
- Unrealistic self-expectations

ASSESSMENT

- Age and gender
- Family system, including marital status and sibling position
- Reason for hospitalization
- Past experience with illness
- Patient's perception of health problem
- Patient's perception of self, including self-worth, body image, problem-solving ability, and coping mechanisms
- Mental status, including general appearance, affect, mood, cognitive and perceptual functioning, and behavior
- Social interaction pattern
- Support systems, such as family and friends

DEFINING CHARACTERISTICS

- Alteration in reality testing
- Denial of problems
- Denial of weaknesses
- Difficulty establishing relationships
- Difficulty maintaining relationships
- Grandiosity
- Hostile laughter
- Hypersensitivity to a discourtesy

- Hypersensitivity to criticism
- Insufficient follow-through with treatment
- Insufficient participation in treatment
- Projection of blame
- Projection of responsibility
- Rationalization of failures
- Reality distortion
- Ridicule of others
- Superior attitude toward others

EXPECTED OUTCOMES

- Patient will recognize need for coping strategies.
- Patient will verbally describe self, including concept, body image, successes, and positive aspects to live events.
- Patient will participate in self-care.
- Patient will engage in decision-making about treatment.
- Patient will accept responsibility for own behavior.
- Patient will establish realistic goals for coping.
- Patient will demonstrate follow-through in decisions related to health care.
- Patient will interact with others in a socially acceptable manner.

Suggested NOC Outcomes

Acceptance: Health Status; Coping; Self-Esteem; Social Interaction Skills

INTERVENTIONS AND RATIONALES

PCC — Encourage patient to evaluate self, possibly by making a written list of positive and negative traits. Encourage patient to use "I" when referring to these traits. *This helps patient identify aspects of self and relate changes to specific variables.*

PCC — Have patient perform self-care to the extent possible *to promote independence and provide a sense of control.*

EBP — Provide a structured daily routine *to provide patient with alternatives to self-absorption.*

PCC — Help patient make treatment-related decisions and encourage follow-through. *Ability to make decisions is the principal component of autonomy.*

- Provide an opportunity for patient to meet with someone who's successfully coping with a similar problem. *This may encourage patient to work toward a positive outcome.*

- Arrange for interaction between patient and others, and observe interaction pattern. *Studying patient's verbal and nonverbal interactions with others gives clues to patient's ability to communicate effectively.*

PCC — Assist patient in identifying successes *to emphasize patient's ability to problem-solve and achieve goals.*

PCC — Assist patient in identifying individuals who are supportive. *Support from others fosters self-confidence.*

- Provide positive feedback when patient assumes responsibility for own behavior *to reinforce effective coping behaviors.*

T&C — Refer patient to a mental health specialist or social worker for follow-up treatment after hospitalization. *Continuing therapy is usually necessary to assist patient to cope with health care status.*

Suggested NIC Interventions

Coping Enhancement; Counseling; Emotional Support; Patient Contracting; Self-Awareness Enhancement; Self-Responsibility Facilitation

EVALUATIONS FOR EXPECTED OUTCOMES

- Patient develops appropriate coping strategies.
- Patient uses at least two positive terms to describe self.
- Patient initiates and completes at least two self-care activities daily.
- Each day, patient makes at least one decision related to activities of daily living, self-care, or treatment.
- Patient establishes realistic long-term and short-term goals.
- Patient expresses responsible attitude toward own behavior.
- Patient reports specific instances of following through on health care decisions.
- Each day, patient socializes with others in an acceptable manner.

DOCUMENTATION

- Patient's perception of self
- Behavioral responses
- Social interaction patterns
- Patient's use of defense mechanisms
- Interventions used to facilitate effective coping
- Patient's responses to nursing interventions
- Evaluations for expected outcomes

REFERENCES

Obrębska, M., & Zinczuk-Zielazna, J. (2017). Explainers as an indicator of defensive attitude to experienced anxiety in young women differing in their styles of coping with threatening stimuli. *Psychology of Language and Communication, 21*(1), 34–50.

Sege, C. T., Bradley, M. M., & Lang, P. J. (2018). Avoidance and escape: Defensive reactivity and trait anxiety. *Behaviour Research and Therapy, 104,* 62.

Simi, Z., Makhlough, M., Jamali, S. K., & Ghasemi, N. (2018). The correlation between attachment styles and defense mechanisms with mental health in diabetic patients. *Qom University of Medical Sciences Journal, 11*(12), 43–51.

Ineffective Coping

DEFINITION

A pattern of invalid appraisal of stressors, with cognitive and/or behavioral efforts, that fails to manage demands related to well-being

RELATED FACTORS (R/T)

- High degree of threat
- Inability to conserve adaptive energies
- Inaccurate threat appraisal
- Inadequate confidence in ability to deal with a situation
- Inadequate opportunity to prepare for stressor

- Inadequate resources
- Ineffective tension release strategies
- Insufficient sense of control
- Insufficient social support

ASSESSMENT

- Psychosocial status, including age, developmental stage, health beliefs, and attitudes
- Current health status
- Diversional activities
- Motivation to learn and obstacles to learning
- Financial resources
- Occupation
- Patient's perception of present health problem or crisis
- Coping techniques that have worked for the patient in the past
- Usual problem-solving techniques/behaviors used to cope with life problems
- Physical or emotional impairment
- Family members' understanding of the client's health status
- Problem-solving techniques usually employed by the family to cope with life problems
- Support systems, including family, companion, friends, and clergy

DEFINING CHARACTERISTICS

- Alteration in concentration
- Alteration in sleep pattern
- Change in communication pattern
- Destructive behavior toward others
- Destructive behavior toward self
- Difficulty organizing information
- Fatigue
- Frequent illness
- Inability to ask for help
- Inability to attend to information
- Inability to deal with a situation
- Inability to meet basic needs
- Inability to meet role expectation
- Ineffective coping strategies
- Insufficient access to social support
- Insufficient goal-directed behavior
- Insufficient problem resolution
- Insufficient problem-solving skills
- Risk-taking behavior
- Substance abuse

EXPECTED OUTCOMES

- Patient will express need to develop better coping behaviors.
- Patient will express understanding of the relationship between emotional state and behavior.
- Patient will communicate feelings about the present situation.
- Patient will be actively involved in planning own care.

- Patient will demonstrate ability to use newly learned coping skills.
- Patient will express feeling of having greater control over present situation.
- Patient will use available support systems, such as family and friends, to aid in coping.
- Patient will reduce use of manipulative behavior to gratify needs.
- Patient will accept responsibility for behavior.
- Patient will demonstrate ability to cope with unexpected changes.
- Patient will identify effective and ineffective coping techniques.
- Patient will identify and demonstrate ability to use at least two healthy coping behaviors.

Suggested NOC Outcomes

Aggression Self-Control; Acceptance of Health Status; Adaptation to Physical Disability; Coping; Decision-Making; Impulse Self-Control; Information Processing; Knowledge: Health Resources; Role Performance; Social Interaction Skills; Social Support

INTERVENTIONS AND RATIONALES

EBP ■ If possible, assign a consistent care provider to patient *to provide continuity of care and promote development of therapeutic relationship.*

PCC ■ Arrange to spend uninterrupted periods of time with patient. Encourage open expression of feelings. Try to identify factors that cause or exacerbate patient's inability to cope, such as fear of loss of health or job. *Devoting time to listening helps patient express emotions, grasp situation, and cope effectively.*

PCC ■ Identify and reduce unnecessary stimuli in environment to *avoid subjecting patient to sensory or perceptual overload.*

PCC ■ Explain all treatments and procedures, and answer patient's questions *to allay fear and allow patient to regain sense of control.*

PCC ■ Have patient increase self-care performance levels gradually *to allow self-paced progress.*

■ Praise patient for making decisions and performing activities *to reinforce coping behaviors.*

■ Establish an environment of mutual trust and respect *to enhance the patient's learning.*

■ Negotiate with patient to develop learning goals *to promote cooperation and foster a sense of control.*

PCC ■ As patient becomes able to express feelings more openly, discuss the relationship between feelings and behavior. *To change, patient must understand this relationship.*

PCC ■ Discourage dependent behavior by assisting patient only when necessary. Provide positive reinforcement for independent behavior *to enhance self-esteem, encourage repetition of desired behavior, and promote effective coping.*

PCC ■ Encourage the patient to make decisions about care *to reduce feelings of helplessness and enhance the patient's sense of mastery over the current situation.*

■ Set limits on manipulative behavior. Provide patient with clear expectations for behavior and describe the consequences if limits are violated. *If patient can't curb inappropriate behavior, consistent limit-setting imposes external controls.*

PCC ■ Help patient recognize and accept responsibility for own actions. Discourage patient from unfairly placing blame on others. *Developing a sense of responsibility is necessary before change can occur.*

PCC ■ Help patient recognize and feel good about positive personal qualities and accomplishments. Provide rewards to reinforce acceptable coping behaviors. *As self-esteem increases, patient will feel less need to manipulate others.*

PCC ■ Praise patient for identifying and using effective coping techniques *to reinforce appropriate behavior.*

- Suggest alternatives to ineffective behaviors identified by patient. Encourage patient to determine what new behaviors can be effectively incorporated into the lifestyle. *Fostering patient participation in care promotes feelings of independence.*

PCC - Select teaching strategies (discussion, demonstration, role-playing, and visual materials) appropriate for patient's learning style *to encourage compliance.*

EBP - Teach strategies that patient can use to develop coping skills. *Knowing different strategies gives patient options in stressful situations.*

EBP - Teach patient relaxation techniques of deep breathing and guided imagery. *Relaxation can assist to reduce anxiety and feelings of anger.*

PCC - Encourage patient to use support systems to assist with coping, *thereby helping restore psychological equilibrium and prevent crisis.*

- Help patient look at current situation and evaluate various coping behaviors *to encourage a realistic view of crisis.*

- Encourage patient to try coping behaviors. *A patient in crisis tends to accept interventions and develops new coping behaviors more easily than at other times.*

PCC - Request feedback from patient about behaviors that seem to work *to encourage patient to evaluate effect of these behaviors.*

T&C - Refer patient for professional psychological counseling. *If patient's maladaptive behavior has high crisis potential, formal counseling helps ease nurse's frustration, increases objectivity, and fosters collaborative approach to patient's care.*

Suggested NIC Interventions

Anger Control Assistance; Anxiety Reduction; Coping Enhancement; Counseling; Decision-Making Support; Environmental Management: Violence Prevention; Impulse Control Training; Learning Facilitation; Role Enhancement; Support System Enhancement

EVALUATIONS FOR EXPECTED OUTCOMES

- Patient states need for better coping behaviors.
- Patient discusses recent stressful event and describes related emotions.
- Patient describes emotions triggered by illness or personal crisis and usual coping behaviors.
- Patient cooperates with nurse to plan care.
- Patient describes one difficult interpersonal situation that was solved by identifying the problem, choosing alternative ways to communicate, and taking action.
- Patient identifies problems, makes plans, and takes action.
- Patient requests assistance from family and friends.
- Patient demonstrates ability to cope with unexpected change.
- Patient identifies and uses at least two healthy coping behaviors such as relaxation techniques.

DOCUMENTATION

- Patient's perception of present situation and what it means
- Patient's verbal expression of feelings indicating comfort or discomfort
- Patient's expressions indicating his or her motivation to learn
- Patient's learning objectives
- Methods used to teach patient
- Information taught and skills demonstrated to patient

- Observations of patient's behaviors
- Interventions to help patient cope
- Patient's responses to interventions
- Evaluations for expected outcomes

REFERENCES

Evans, C., Cotter, K., & Smokowski, P. (2017). Giving victims of bullying a voice: A qualitative study of post bullying reactions and coping strategies. *Child & Adolescent Social Work Journal, 34*(6), 543–555.
Ito, M., & Matsushima, E. (2017). Presentation of coping strategies associated with physical and mental health during health check-ups. *Community Mental Health Journal, 53*(3), 297–305.
Lim, R. H., & Sharmeen, T. (2018). Medicines management issues in dementia and coping strategies used by people living with dementia and family carers: A systematic review. *International Journal of Geriatric Psychiatry, 33*(12), 1562–1581.
Suzuki, M., Furihata, R., Konno, C., Kaneita, Y., Ohida, T., & Uchiyama, M. (2018). Stressful events and coping strategies associated with symptoms of depression: A Japanese general population survey. *Journal of Affective Disorders, 238*, 482–488.

Readiness for Enhanced Coping

DEFINITION

A pattern of valid appraisal of stressors with cognitive and/or behavioral efforts to manage demands related to well-being, which can be strengthened

ASSESSMENT

- Age
- Usual coping mechanisms
- Perceived coping ability
- Role responsibilities
- Social support
- Spiritual resources

DEFINING CHARACTERISTICS

- Awareness of possible environmental change
- Expresses desire to enhance knowledge of stress management strategies
- Expresses desire to enhance management of stressors
- Expresses desire to enhance social support
- Expresses desire to enhance use of emotion-oriented strategies
- Expresses desire to enhance use of problem-oriented strategies
- Expresses desire to enhance use of spiritual resource

EXPECTED OUTCOMES

- Patient will identify major issues that require ongoing enhancement of coping strategies.
- Patient will express feelings associated with present coping strategies.
- Patient will demonstrate readiness to develop enhanced strategies.
- Patient will identify support persons and activities that will assist in goal attainment.

Suggested NOC Outcomes

Coping; Quality of Life

INTERVENTIONS AND RATIONALES

PCC   ▪ Establish a trusting relationship with patient. *Building trust will allow patient to be more open.*

▪ Begin discussions at patient's level of comfort. *If patient wants to discuss feelings, it won't benefit patient or nurse to begin presenting strategies that require logical reasoning.*

PCC   ▪ Determine from listening to patient options that might be attractive to patient in reaching new goals for coping; for example, support group, spiritual direction, and journaling. *Patient will strive to enhance coping skills using those opportunities to which patient feels best suited.*

PCC   ▪ Arrange to meet with patient regularly to assist in helping patient focus on goals and evaluate progress. *Recognizing even small attempts at successful coping encourages patient to increase own efforts.*

Suggested NIC Interventions

Active Listening; Coping Enhancement

EVALUATIONS FOR EXPECTED OUTCOMES

▪ Patient has successfully articulated major areas where enhanced coping strategies are needed.

▪ Patient expresses feelings associated with current coping strategies.

▪ Patient demonstrates readiness to develop enhanced strategies.

▪ Patient identifies the person(s) perceived as being able to support therapeutically in the patient's efforts.

▪ Patient identifies with group support or attends class or session to learn more about coping.

DOCUMENTATION

▪ Patient's assessment of coping skills

▪ Patient's goals for enhanced coping

▪ Actions taken by patient to cope from situation to situation

▪ Patient's response to nursing interventions

▪ Evaluations for expected outcomes

REFERENCES

Bettis, A. H., Coiro, M. J., England, J., Murphy, L. K., Zelkowitz, R. L., Dejardins, L., ... Compas, B. E. (2017). Comparison of two approaches to prevention of mental health problems in college students: Enhancing coping and executive function skills. *Journal of American College Health*, 65(5), 313–322.

Innes, S. I. (2017). The relationship between levels of resilience and coping styles in chiropractic students and perceived levels of stress and well-being. *Journal of Chiropractic Education*, 31(1), 1–7.

Rodkjaer, L. O., Laursen, T., Seeberg, K., Drouin, M., Johansen, H., Dyrehave, C., ... Ostergaard, L. (2017). The effect of a mind-body intervention on mental health and coping self-efficacy in HIV-infected individuals: A feasibility study. *Journal of Alternative and Complementary Medicine*, 23(5), 326–330.

Satorres, E., Viguer, P., Fortuna, F. B., & Meléndez, J. C. (2018). Effectiveness of instrumental reminiscence intervention on improving coping in healthy older adults. *Stress & Health: Journal of the International Society for the Investigation of Stress*, 34(2), 227–234.

Ineffective Community Coping

DEFINITION

A pattern of community activities for adaptation and problem solving that is unsatisfactory for meeting the demands or needs of the community

RELATED FACTORS (R/T)

- Inadequate resources for problem-solving
- Insufficient community resources
- Nonexistent community systems

ASSESSMENT

- Community demographics, including age and sex distribution, education and income levels, and ethnic, racial, and religious groups
- Family status, including family composition (percentage of single-parent families in community), responsibilities assumed by teenagers in caring for siblings, and ability of families to meet their physical, social, emotional, and economic needs
- Community health status, including prevalence of health problems in community, attitudes toward sex and sexuality, availability of health care services, community members' use of health care services, and beliefs, values, and attitudes about health and illness
- Education system, including availability of sex education in schools, availability of programs to help pregnant teens complete their education, and willingness of parents to allow children to participate
- Political system, including government officials' support for or opposition to sex education
- Attitude of religious groups toward sex and sexuality and religious groups' influence on educators
- Transportation availability to clinics and other social services and recreation opportunities for adolescents
- Welfare and health care system and reliance of teen mothers on welfare for support

DEFINING CHARACTERISTICS

- Community does not meet expectation of its members
- Deficient community participation
- Elevated community illness rate
- Excessive community conflict
- Excessive stress
- High incidence of community problems
- Perceived community powerlessness
- Perceived community vulnerability

EXPECTED OUTCOMES

- Community members will express desire to develop improved communication among community members.
- Community members will express need for plan to improve community functioning.
- Community members express desire to develop and implement plans to strengthen community resources.

- Community members will express willingness to participate in problem-solving strategies.
- Community members will evaluate success of plan in meeting goals and objectives and will continue to revise it, as necessary.

Suggested NOC Outcomes

Community Competence; Community Health Status; Risk Control

INTERVENTIONS AND RATIONALES

PCC Work with the community to assess and develop needed programs *to provide community members with information about risks, problems, and complications of community needs.*

PCC Work closely with community to assess strengths and weaknesses of community functioning *to assess their needs and provide care.*

EBP Implement an outreach and health promotion program *to raise community members' awareness of community problems.* Consider these steps:
  - Work with teachers, school psychologists, counselors, school nurses, students, and the parent–teacher association *to determine the needs among the child and adolescent population.*
  - Encourage local youth groups, religious organizations, and social service organizations to feature guest speakers on community issues at their meetings. *Speakers with expertise in the area of community dynamics are able to provide information that helps community members build stronger resources.*
  - Contact representatives of local corporations *to ask for funding for educational programs.*
  - Help community members establish work groups for organization and collaboration. *Organizing community teams will foster problem-solving.*
  - Provide education on community issues and problems. *Access to information allows for greater problem-solving.*

PCC Encourage community members to establish work groups or a task force *to develop and implement needed programs within the community.*

PCC Work with community members to evaluate the effectiveness of the programs and assist with modifying programs, as needed, *to ensure the program's effectiveness and promote use of the program as a model for preventive health.*

I **QI** Collect statistical data as needed *to help evaluate the effectiveness of programs.*

Suggested NIC Interventions

Community Health Development; Health Education; Health Screening; Program Development; Consultation; Family Planning: Contraception; Referral

EVALUATIONS FOR EXPECTED OUTCOMES

- Community members have improved communication among community members.
- Community members develop plan to improve community functioning.
- Community members develop and implement plan to strengthen community resources.
- Community members participate in problem-solving strategies.
- Community members evaluate success of plan and revise it, as needed.

- Community perception of problem
- Statistics that support existence of problem
- Community resources that already exist to alleviate problem
- Future plans to deal with problem
- Evaluations for expected outcomes

REFERENCES

Agarwal, G., Angeles, R., Pirrie, M., McLeod, B., Marzanek, F., Parascandalo, J., & Thabane, L. (2018). Evaluation of a community paramedicine health promotion and lifestyle risk assessment program for older adults who live in social housing: A cluster randomized trial. *CMAJ, 190*(21), E638–E647.

Berenguera, A., Pons, V. M., Moreno, P. P., March, S., Ripoll, J., Rubio, V. M., ... Pujol, R. E. (2017). Beyond the consultation room: Proposals to approach health promotion in primary care according to health-care users, key community informants and primary care centre workers. *Health Expectations, 20*(5), 896–910.

Hammerback, K., Hannon, P. A., Parrish, A. T., Allen, C., Kohn, M. J., & Harris, J. R. (2018). Comparing strategies for recruiting small, low-wage worksites for community-based health promotion research. *Health Education and Behavior, 45*(5), 690–696.

Nickel, S., Süß, W., Lorentz, C., & Trojan, A. (2018). Long-term evaluation of community health promotion: Using capacity building as an intermediate outcome measure. *Public Health, 162*, 9–15.

Readiness for Enhanced Community Coping

DEFINITION

A pattern of community activities for adaptation and problem solving for meeting the demands or needs of the community, which can be strengthened

ASSESSMENT

- Community demographics, including age and gender distribution, ethnic groups, racial groups, religious groups, and education and income levels
- Community health status, including availability of health care services, use of health care services, prevalence of childhood illnesses in the community, epidemiologic statistics, and beliefs, values, and attitudes about health and illness
- Education system, including educational level of adult population and state law or school system's requirements for immunization before school attendance
- Religious institutions and their support for, or objections to, immunization
- Social services, including availability of clinics and other social services, access to health care, welfare system, and parents' dependence on welfare for support

DEFINING CHARACTERISTICS

- Expresses desire to enhance availability of community recreation programs
- Expresses desire to enhance availability of community relaxation programs
- Expresses desire to enhance communication among community members
- Expresses desire to enhance communication between aggregates and larger community
- Expresses desire to enhance community planning for predictable stressors
- Expresses desire to enhance community resources for managing stressors
- Expresses desire to enhance community responsibility for stress management
- Expresses desire to enhance problem-solving for identified issue

■ Community members will express understanding of problems associated with failure to immunize population and will recognize need for plan to reduce number of children and adults who aren't immunized.

■ Community members will establish plan to increase rate of immunization and ensure adequate protection from communicable diseases.

■ Community members will work to reduce spread of communicable diseases and increase rate of immunization within community.

■ Community members will evaluate established plans for ensuring that all children become immunized and will make changes to plans as needed.

Suggested NOC Outcomes

Community Competence; Community Health Status; Community Health Status: Immunity; Community Risk Control: Communicable Disease

PCC ■ Work with community members to pinpoint potential problems associated with inadequate immunization of the population *to ensure adequate protection against communicable diseases*. Consider taking these steps:

 ■ Identify new members of the community, such as immigrants and refugees, *to help reach parents who need information about immunization.*

 ■ Identify parents who don't follow-through with the required series of immunizations *to protect children from incomplete immunization.*

I **QI** ■ Encourage community members to implement a program to disseminate information about problems associated with inadequate immunization *to educate residents and promote the community's established immunization program.*

EBP ■ Provide extensive education about communicable diseases and the importance of immunizations *to empower community residents and help decrease the risk of communicable diseases.*

T&C **I** **QI** ■ Encourage health departments, clinics, and practitioners' offices to provide information on the recommended childhood immunization schedule to the public *to foster education about immunization.*

PCC ■ Contact parents of children who aren't immunized in person or by handwritten note. Make it clear that your purpose in promoting immunization is to protect child from illness *to build parents' trust in immunization programs.*

EBP ■ Provide immunization information in the parents' first language *to overcome a lack of understanding caused by language barriers.*

I **QI** ■ Develop a list of referrals for the parents of children who aren't immunized. Include information on low-cost health insurance, city health centers, and well-baby clinics *to encourage compliance.*

T&C ■ Coordinate with local nursing schools, health department nurses, and other interested nursing groups to provide the necessary number of professionals to deliver adequate immunizations *to reduce the risk of communicable disease.*

EBP ■ Conduct a follow-up survey on immunization rates *to measure the effectiveness of educational efforts.*

I **QI** ■ Collect statistical data from community sources, such as health department and schools, *to continue to identify children who haven't been immunized.*

Suggested NIC Interventions

Communicable Disease Management; Community Health Development; Health Education; Health Policy Monitoring; Immunization/Vaccination Management

EVALUATIONS FOR EXPECTED OUTCOMES

- Community members understand risks of failing to immunize population and recognize need for plan.
- Community members put forth plan to meet community's immunization needs, which contains definite actions yet allows for modifications.
- Community members implement plan to reduce spread of communicable diseases and increase rate of immunization.
- Community members evaluate plan and make changes, as needed, to help solve problems and further the goal of meeting community's immunization needs.

DOCUMENTATION

- Evidence of need for immunization program
- Statistical data documenting problem
- Written plan to resolve problem
- Efforts made to disseminate written information to community
- Evaluations for expected outcomes

REFERENCES

Cole, E. (2018). A grassroots approach to health promotion. *Nursing Standard, 33*(7), 22–25.
Garry, B., & Boran, S. (2017). Promotion of oral health by community nurses. *British Journal of Community Nursing, 22*(10), 496–502.
Kimhi, S. (2016). Levels of resilience: Associations among individual, community, and national resilience. *Journal of Health Psychology, 21*(2), 164–170. doi:10.1177/1359105314524009
Marcellus, L., & Shahram, S. Z. (2017). Starting at the beginning: The role of public health nursing in promoting infant and early childhood mental health. *Nursing Leadership, 30*(3), 43–53.
Roll, A. E., & Bowers, B. J. (2017). Promoting healthy aging of individuals with developmental disabilities. *Western Journal of Nursing Research, 39*(2), 234–251.

Compromised Family Coping

DEFINITION

An usually supportive primary person (family member, significant other, or close friend) provides insufficient, ineffective, or compromised support, comfort, assistance, or encouragement that may be needed by the client to manage or master adaptive tasks related to his or her health challenge

RELATED FACTORS (R/T)

- Coexisting situations affecting the support person
- Exhaustion of support person's capacity
- Family disorganization
- Insufficient information available to support person
- Insufficient reciprocal support
- Insufficient support given by client to support person

- Insufficient understanding of information by support person
- Misinformation obtained by support person
- Misunderstanding of information by support person
- Preoccupation by support person with concern outside of family

ASSESSMENT

- Family's perception of situation
- Family status, including normal pattern of interaction among family members, family's understanding and knowledge of patient's present condition, support systems available (financial, social, and spiritual), family's response to past crises, including coping behaviors and problem-solving techniques; recreational activities; and communication patterns used to express anger, affection, and confrontation
- Patient's health care resources, including hospital, community resources, health care providers such as therapists, and case manager (outpatient)
- Patient's illness, including its progression and severity, patient's perception of health problem, and problem-solving techniques used by patient to cope with life problems
- Possible impact of patient's health status on family's future structure and lifestyle
- Degree of difficulty imposed by care of patient

DEFINING CHARACTERISTICS

- Assistive behaviors by support person produce unsatisfactory results
- Client complaint about support person's response to health problem
- Client concern about support person's response to health problem
- Limitation in communication between support person and client
- Protective behavior by support person incongruent with client's abilities
- Protective behavior by support person incongruent with client's need for autonomy
- Support person reports inadequate understanding that interferes with effective behaviors
- Support person reports insufficient knowledge that interferes with effective behaviors
- Support person reports preoccupation with own reaction to client's need
- Support person withdraws from client

EXPECTED OUTCOMES

- Family will discuss patient's illness and its impact on family functioning.
- Family will designate a spokesperson to receive information regarding the patient's illness.
- Family will establish a visiting routine beneficial to patient and family.
- Family members will engage in healthy coping behaviors.
- Family will state understanding of patient's health status.
- Family members will become involved in planning for and providing patient's care.
- Family members will identify and use available support systems.
- Family members will set realistic goals for patient.
- Family members will express feeling of having greater control over their situation.
- Family will identify and use available support systems.

Suggested NOC Outcomes

Caregiver Emotional Health; Caregiver–Patient Relationship; Caregiver Stressors; Caregiving Endurance Potential; Family Coping; Family Normalization

- Assess effects of patient's disease on family functioning *to plan interventions that enhance long-term well-being of family and patient.*
- Identify the spokesperson for the family *to avoid creating communication conflicts within family.*
- **PCC** Encourage family members to identify strengths and weaknesses in the family system. Help them explore values, beliefs, perceived changes, and actual role changes related to older patient's altered physical or emotional condition *to enhance insight.*
- **PCC** Assist patient and family members in developing short-term and long-term goals and contingency plans *to increase a sense of control and direction for the future.*
- **EBP** Evaluate and rectify any knowledge deficit that family members have about patient's disease and treatment. Experience doesn't guarantee correct knowledge. *Lack of knowledge can exacerbate frustration and tension within the family.*
- **PCC** Provide an outlet for family members to express their frustrations about their present caregiving responsibilities. *Being able to talk about what they are presently experiencing will allow the opportunity to stand back and see what is happening in their relationship with patient.*
- **EBP** Help family members explore coping strategies used effectively during past crises and discuss how to apply these strategies to the present situation *to make family members aware of their demonstrated ability to adapt to change.*
- **PCC** Maintain a nonjudgmental attitude while working with family members. Some families may hesitate to accept outside help. Other families may be unwilling to make even small sacrifices to care for an older relative. Remember that if family members haven't been supportive or close to the patient before, you're unlikely to change their attitudes. *A nonjudgmental outlook benefits the patient and family members. Learning to accept your limitations will help you avoid burnout.*
- **PCC** Facilitate family conferences; help family members identify key issues and select support services, if needed. *Involving patient and family in care planning promotes open communication throughout illness.*
- **T&C** Suggest using a care manager to help with the ongoing coordination of patient's needs. Help family identify a care manager they can relate to. *A care manager may help simplify decision-making and limit family conflict.*
- Help patient and family establish a visiting routine that won't tax their resources. Each family member may be responsible for a day or period of time, if desired. Use patient's daily routine to aid in planning; for example, no visiting during treatments or periods of uninterrupted sleep. *This enhances family's sense of contributing to patient's overall care.*
- Provide family with clear, concise information about patient's condition. Be aware of what family has been told, and help them interpret information. *This ensures clear, uncluttered communication between patient, family, and caregivers.*
- **PCC** Ensure privacy during patient and family visits. *This demonstrates respect and fosters open communication between family members.*
- **T&C** Help family support patient's independence. Encourage attendance at therapy sessions, and allow patient to demonstrate new skills and abilities *to help family members learn how they can help promote patient's independence and self-care.*
- **PCC** Provide emotional support to family by being available to answer questions. *This demonstrates your willingness to help family seek health-related information.*
- **T&C** Help patient and family members identify appropriate community services, such as adult day care, respite care, and geriatric outreach services, *to provide access to additional sources of support.*

T&C ▦ Coordinate referrals to other health care professionals, such as a social worker or physical therapist, *to ensure clear communication among health care providers, which enables the patient to receive appropriate comprehensive care.*

T&C ▦ Encourage family members to participate in appropriate support groups *to help them obtain social support and information and to provide an opportunity to express feelings.*

T&C ▦ Encourage family members to contact and use appropriate community agencies *to help prevent burnout among family members after patient leaves the hospital.* Families may need encouragement to use support and respite care services if past efforts to use such services proved unsuccessful.

▦ Remain supportive and understanding if patient or family members are reluctant to use needed community resources, such as adult day care, respite care, and home health care services. *An older patient may feel that using outside resources means sacrificing independence; family members may feel that asking for help indicates lack of caring.*

Suggested NIC Interventions

Caregiver Support; Coping Enhancement; Conflict Mediation; Decision-Making Support; Emotional Support; Family Involvement Promotion; Family Mobilization; Family Support; Learning Facilitation; Respite Care; Spiritual Support; Support Group

EVALUATIONS FOR EXPECTED OUTCOMES

▦ Family members discuss feelings about patient's illness and its impact on family functioning.
▦ Family members designate spokesperson to receive and communicate information regarding the patient's illness.
▦ Family members accurately describe patient's health status.
▦ Family members voice their feelings about patient's condition.
▦ Family members identify and use at least two healthy coping behaviors.
▦ Family members demonstrate ability to plan for and provide patient's care.
▦ Family members identify and use available support systems.
▦ Family members set realistic goals for patient.
▦ Family members demonstrate improved capacity for short-term and long-term planning.
▦ Family members express feeling of increased control over their situation.

DOCUMENTATION

▦ Family's response to patient's illness
▦ Family's current understanding of patient's illness
▦ Family members' perceptions of patient's health and long-term implications
▦ Family members' statements indicating their feelings toward patient
▦ Observations about family's interaction with patient and acceptance of current situation
▦ Assessment of family functioning (including family's level of insight into their behavior)
▦ Content of family conferences
▦ Teaching and referrals given to family members
▦ Family members' abilities to meet patient's physical and emotional needs
▦ Consultations with other health care team members
▦ Interventions to help family members cope
▦ Family members' responses to nursing interventions
▦ Referrals to community agencies
▦ Community resources used, their effectiveness, and recommendations for future use (indicate family's level of acceptance of nurse's recommendations)
▦ Evaluations for expected outcomes

REFERENCES

Kleinrock, M. (2018). The importance of clinical and economic support systems for caregivers. *American Health & Drug Benefits, 11*(8), 402–403.

Machado, B. M., Ferreira Dahdah, D., & Martins Kebbe, L. (2018). Caregivers of family members with chronic diseases: Coping strategies used in everyday life. *Brazilian Journal of Occupational Therapy, 26*(2), 219–313.

McCann, T. V., & Lubman, D. I. (2018). Adaptive coping strategies of affected family members of a relative with substance misuse: A qualitative study. *Journal of Advanced Nursing, 74*(1), 100–109.

Nabors, L., Cunningham, J. F., Lang, M., Wood, K., Southwick, S., & Stough, C. O. (2018). Family coping during hospitalization of children with chronic illnesses. *Journal of Child and Family Studies, 27*(5), 1482–1491.

Disabled Family Coping

DEFINITION

Behavior of primary person (family member, significant other, or close friend) that disables his or her capacities and the client's capacities to effectively address tasks essential to either person's adaptation to the health challenge

RELATED FACTORS (R/T)

- Ambivalent family relationship
- Chronically unexpressed feelings to support person
- Differing coping styles between support person and client
- Differing coping styles between support persons
- Inconsistent management of family's resistance to treatment

ASSESSMENT

- Patient's illness, including its course, severity, and effect on family members
- Patient's health care resources, including hospital, community resources, and health care providers, such as therapists and case managers
- Family resources (financial, social, and spiritual)
- Demands on family imposed by patient's condition
- Family process, including number of members, usual patterns of interaction, roles of each family member, communication patterns, relationship changes (such as separation, divorce, or remarriage), and past response to crisis
- Family status, including involvement with patient, quality of relationships, communication patterns, coping strategies, family's understanding of patient's illness, family's feelings about patient's illness, willingness of family members to commit time to patient care, and family's ability to provide care
- Transportation limitations, including geographic distances to health resources

DEFINING CHARACTERISTICS

- Abandonment
- Adopts illness symptoms of client
- Aggression
- Agitation
- Client dependence
- Depression
- Desertion
- Disregard for client's needs
- Distortion of reality about client's health problem

- Family behaviors detrimental to well-being
- Hostility
- Impaired ability to structure a meaningful life
- Impaired individualism
- Intolerance
- Neglect of basic needs of client
- Neglect of relationship with family member
- Neglect of treatment regimen
- Performing routines without regard for client's needs
- Prolonged hyperfocus on client
- Psychosomatic symptoms
- Rejection

EXPECTED OUTCOMES

- To the extent possible, family members will participate in aspects of patient's care without evidence of increased conflict.
- Family members will express feelings and individual needs.
- Patient will express confidence in being able to make decisions, despite pressure from family members.
- Patient will contact appropriate sources of support outside the family.
- Patient will take steps to ensure that care needs are met despite family's shortcomings.
- Patient will express greater understanding of emotional limitations of family members.
- Family members will identify factors that trigger stress and inappropriate behavior.
- Family members will make use of appropriate sources of support.
- Family members will interact appropriately with staff members and each other.

Suggested NOC Outcomes

Caregiver Emotional Health; Caregiver–Patient Relationship; Caregiving Endurance Potential; Family Coping; Family Health Status; Family Social Climate; Family Support During Treatment

INTERVENTIONS AND RATIONALES

- Assess effects of patient's disease on family functioning. *A thorough assessment of the family's coping behaviors is necessary to developing a therapeutic action plan.*
- Assess family history *to identify family's strengths and limitations.*
- **PCC** Determine if family members are prepared to accept help. *Changes in behavior won't take place until family members are ready.*
- Encourage family members to participate in patient care as much as possible. *Family members should have an opportunity to overcome dysfunctional behavior.*
- **PCC** Help family identify which tasks to tackle now and which to put off until the stress level decreases. *Performing easy, familiar activities decreases discomfort during times of stress.*
- **PCC** Identify instances of successful communication among family members *to single out and encourage positive behavior.*
- Assist family members to identify situations that trigger inappropriate behavior. *Family members must learn to recognize their tolerance threshold to react appropriately.*
- **PCC** Assist family members to identify coping mechanisms used successfully in the *past to enable them to develop appropriate responses without learning new behaviors.*
- **PCC** Assist family members to identify options when confronted with difficult decisions. *Members of dysfunctional families commonly believe they lack choices.*

◾ Maintain objectivity when dealing with family conflicts. Don't become embroiled in the dynamics of a dysfunctional family in order *to maintain your ability to intervene objectively and effectively.*

PCC ◾ If patient and family members appear incapable of taking steps to heal their relationships, focus on being a patient advocate. Reaffirm patient's right to make own decisions without interference from family members. Provide necessary information to patient to facilitate decision-making. *Dysfunctional family coping patterns evolve over many years and are unlikely to change just because patient has a serious illness. Accepting your limitations when working with family members will help you to avoid burnout and better meet patient's needs.*

T&C ◾ Encourage patient to seek emotional support that the family can't provide by participating in a support group. Help patient select support group that best meets the patient's personal needs and outlook. Consider recommending Codependents Anonymous, a group for individuals who have difficulty maintaining healthy relationships as a result of being raised in a dysfunctional family. *Participation in a support group may improve patient's ability to cope as well as provide an opportunity to form meaningful relationships.*

T&C ◾ Refer patient to a home health care agency, homemaker service, Meals on Wheels, or other appropriate outside agencies for assistance and follow-up. *Use of various community services may help to make up for shortcomings in family's ability to provide care.*

PCC ◾ Listen openly to patient's expressions of pain over unresolved conflicts with family members. Patient may have to grieve over a future with no "ideal" family, capable of fully meeting the patient's emotional needs. *Therapeutic listening helps patient to understand self and family better and to understand how past conflicts affect present behavior.*

Suggested NIC Interventions

Anger Control Assistance; Caregiver Support; Family Involvement Promotion; Family Mobilization; Family Support; Family Therapy; Mutual Goal Setting; Normalization Promotion; Support Group

EVALUATIONS FOR EXPECTED OUTCOMES

◾ Family members demonstrate improved willingness to cooperate in patient's care.
◾ Family members state specific factors that lead to inappropriate behavior.
◾ Family members express feelings and try to meet each other's emotional needs.
◾ Patient expresses increased confidence in being able to make decisions.
◾ Patient contacts at least one support group in an effort to form meaningful relationships outside family.
◾ Family members state their plans for contacting sources of support.
◾ Patient takes steps to meet personal care needs.
◾ Patient indicates, either verbally or through behavior, a better understanding of family members and an increased ability to accept their emotional limitations.

DOCUMENTATION

◾ Family's response to patient's illness
◾ Observation of family members' interactions with each other and with outsiders
◾ Observations of family members' reactions to stress
◾ Examples of communication between family members
◾ Interventions performed to help improve family members' coping skills
◾ Referrals made to support groups and community services

▪ Patient's expressions of grief, anger, and disappointment over unresolved conflicts with family members
▪ Evaluations for expected outcomes

REFERENCES

Gibbs, T. A. (2018). 42.4 Interventions to engage and support the family system. *Journal of the American Academy of Child & Adolescent Psychiatry, 57*, S61.
Salehi-Tali, S., Ahmadi, F., Zarea, K., & Fereidooni, M. M. (2018). Commitment to care: The most important coping strategies among family caregivers of patients undergoing haemodialysis. *Scandinavian Journal of Caring Sciences, 32*(1), 82–91.
Thomas, C., Turner, M., Payne, S., Milligan, C., Brearley, S., Seamark, D., ... Blake, S. (2018). Family carers' experiences of coping with the deaths of adults in home settings: A narrative analysis of carers' relevant background worries. *Palliative Medicine, 32*(5), 950–959.
Xu, Y., Lin, X., Chen, S., Liu, Y., & Liu, H. (2018). Ageism, resilience, coping, family support, and quality of life among older people living with HIV/AIDS in Nanning, China. *Global Public Health, 13*(5), 612–625.

Readiness for Enhanced Family Coping

DEFINITION

A pattern of management of adaptive tasks by primary person (family member, significant other, or close friend) involved with the client's health challenge, which can be strengthened

ASSESSMENT

▪ Family process, including normal pattern of interaction among family members, family's understanding and knowledge of patient's present condition, support systems available (financial, social, and spiritual), family's past response to crises (coping patterns), and communication patterns used to express anger, affection, and confrontation
▪ Patient's illness, including progression and severity of illness, patient's perception of health problem, and problem-solving techniques used by patient to cope with life problems

DEFINING CHARACTERISTICS

▪ Expresses desire to acknowledge growth impact of crisis
▪ Expresses desire to choose experiences that optimize wellness
▪ Expresses desire to enhance connection with others who have experienced a similar situation
▪ Expresses desire to enhance enrichment of lifestyle
▪ Expresses desire to enhance health promotion

EXPECTED OUTCOMES

▪ Family members will discuss impact of patient's illness and feelings about it.
▪ Family members will participate in treatment plan.
▪ Family members will establish a visiting routine beneficial to patient and themselves.
▪ Family members will demonstrate care needed to maintain patient's health status.
▪ Family members will identify and use available support systems.

Suggested NOC Outcomes

Family Coping; Family Normalization; Family Participation in Professional Care

INTERVENTIONS AND RATIONALES

PCC   ▨ Allow time for family members to discuss impact of patient's illness and their feelings. Encourage expression of feelings *to allow family members to realistically adjust to the patient's problems.*

PCC   ▨ Encourage family conferences; help family members identify key issues and select support services, if needed, *to develop sense of shared responsibility and feelings of safety, adequacy, and comfort.*

▨ Help patient and family establish a visiting routine that won't tax patient's or family's resources. Use patient's daily routine to aid in planning—for example, no visiting during treatments or during periods of uninterrupted sleep. *Involving family members reassures patient of their care and reduces family's fear and anxiety.*

▨ Reinforce family members' efforts to care for the patient *to let them know they're doing their best and to ease adaptation and grieving process.*

PCC   ▨ Demonstrate care procedures and encourage participation in treatment and planning decisions (such as selecting times for pulmonary toilet for the patient with cystic fibrosis). *Meeting others' needs promotes self-esteem.*

EBP   ▨ Provide family members with clear, concise information about patient's condition. Be aware of what they have been told, and help them interpret information. *This information will help alleviate their concerns.*

PCC   ▨ Ensure privacy for patient and family during visits *to foster open communication.*

▨ Help family support the patient's independence. Encourage attendance at therapy sessions and allow the patient to demonstrate new skills and abilities. *Independence helps patient reach maximum functional level.*

PCC   ▨ Provide emotional support to family by being available to answer questions. *Attentive listening conveys empathy, recognition, and respect for a person.*

PCC   ▨ Inform family of community resources and support groups available to assist in managing the patient's illness and providing emotional or financial support to caretakers, such as Easterseals Association, Visiting Nurse Association, and Meals on Wheels. *Community resources may help the patient develop potential, independence, and self-reliance.*

Suggested NIC Interventions

Caregiver Support; Family Involvement Promotion; Health Education; Self-Modification Assistance

EVALUATIONS FOR EXPECTED OUTCOMES

▨ Family members acknowledge their feelings about patient's illness.
▨ Family members spend adequate time with patient and seek to participate in care.
▨ Family members establish a visiting routine beneficial to patient and themselves.
▨ Family members display competence in caring for patient through return demonstration and provide adequate level of care to maintain patient's health.
▨ Family members make contact with support resources available in their community.

DOCUMENTATION

▨ Family's response to patient's illness
▨ Family's current understanding of patient's illness
▨ Observations about family's interaction with patient and acceptance of current situation
▨ Evaluations for expected outcomes

REFERENCES

Ahmad, S., Ishtiaq, S. M., & Mustafa, M. (2017). The role of socio-economic status in adoption of coping strategies among adolescents against domestic violence. *Journal of Interpersonal Violence, 32*(18), 2862–2881.

Azman, A., Jamir Singh, P. S., & Sulaiman, J. (2017). Caregiver coping with the mentally ill: A qualitative study. *Journal of Mental Health, 26*(2), 98–103.

Machado, B. M., Ferreira Dahdah, D., & Martins Kebbe, L. (2018). Caregivers of family members with chronic diseases: Coping strategies used in everyday life. *Brazilian Journal of Occupational Therapy, 26*(2), 219–313.

McCann, T. V., & Lubman, D. I. (2018). Adaptive coping strategies of affected family members of a relative with substance misuse: A qualitative study. *Journal of Advanced Nursing, 74*(1), 100–109.

D

Death Anxiety

Emotional distress and insecurity, generated by anticipation of death and the process of dying of oneself or significant others, which negatively affects one's quality of life

RELATED FACTORS (R/T)

- Anticipation of adverse consequences of anesthesia
- Anticipation of impact of death on others
- Anticipation of pain
- Anticipation of suffering
- Awareness of imminent death
- Depressive symptoms
- Discussions on the topic of death
- Impaired religiosity
- Loneliness
- Low self-esteem
- Nonacceptance of own mortality
- Spiritual distress
- Uncertainty about encountering a higher power
- Uncertainty about life after death
- Uncertainty about the existence of a higher power
- Uncertainty of prognosis
- Unpleasant physical symptoms

ASSOCIATED CONDITIONS

- Depression
- Stigmatized illnesses with high fear of death
- Terminal illness

ASSESSMENT

- Age
- History of present illness
- Mental status, including level of consciousness, orientation, cognition, memory, and insight
- Self-care status, including ability to carry out activities of daily living
- Sleep pattern
- Pain assessment, including location, quality, intensity on a scale of 1 to 10, temporal factors, sources of provocation, and relief

- Psychological status, including reaction to illness and dying, and expressions of fear, anger, hope, and anxiety
- Spiritual status, including that which gives purpose or meaning in life, religious affiliation, current perception of faith, religious practices, changes in religious beliefs or practices brought on by illness, and evidence of unmet spiritual needs (meaning and purpose, love and relatedness, forgiveness)
- Cultural norms associated with illness and death
- Family status, including marital status, family roles, family communications, family's ability to meet patient's physical and emotional needs, extent to which religion defines family's value system, and changes patient's illness and impending death will make in family functioning

DEFINING CHARACTERISTICS

- Dysphoria
- Expresses concern about caregiver strain
- Expresses concern about the impact of one's death on significant other
- Expresses deep sadness
- Expresses fear of developing terminal illness
- Expresses fear of loneliness
- Expresses fear of loss of mental abilities when dying
- Expresses fear of pain related to dying
- Expresses fear of premature death
- Expresses fear of prolonged dying process
- Expresses fear of separation from loved ones
- Expresses fear of suffering related to dying
- Expresses fear of the dying process
- Expresses fear of the unknown
- Expresses powerlessness
- Reports negative thoughts related to death and dying

EXPECTED OUTCOMES

- Patient will identify need for time with others and need for time alone.
- Patient will identify comfort measures that enhance feelings of well-being.
- Patient will communicate important thoughts and feelings to family members.
- Patient will obtain the requested level of spiritual support.
- Patient will use available support systems to cope with dying.
- Patient will express feelings of comfort and peacefulness.
- Patient will experience dying with dignity, sensitivity, and love.

Suggested NOC Outcomes

Acceptance: Health Status; Anxiety Level; Depression Level; Dignified Life Closure; Fear Self-Control; Hope; Spiritual Well-Being

INTERVENTIONS AND RATIONALES

- **PCC** Assess how much help patient wants. *Patient may need a higher degree of independence than caregiver wants to allow.*
- **PCC** Offer to spend time either reading to patient or just sitting there quietly. *Typically, patient approaching death desires the presence of another but isn't interested in conversing.*

`PCC` ▨ If patient is confused, provide reassurance by telling patient who's in the room. *This information may help to reduce anxiety.*

`PCC` ▨ Provide comfort measures—bathing, massage, regulation of environmental temperature, mouth care, administration of ice chips or wet washcloth—according to patient's preferences. *Some patients may prefer not to be bothered unless they specifically request comfort measures.*

`PCC` ▨ Help family members identify, discuss, and resolve issues related to patient's dying. *Patient needs the support of family members. Family members may need help removing emotional blocks that prevent them from providing full support to patient.*

`PCC` ▨ Demonstrate to patient your willingness to discuss spiritual aspects of death and dying *to foster open discussion.* Keep conversation focused on patient's spiritual values and the role they play in coping with dying *to ensure that your interaction with patient remains therapeutic.*

`T&C` ▨ Refer patient to a priest, minister, rabbi, or spiritual counselor according to patient's preference *to show respect for patient's beliefs and provide expert spiritual care.*

`PCC` ▨ Ask if there's a prayer or words of spiritual comfort that are especially meaningful to patient, and recite this special prayer together if patient seems comfortable with your request. *Doing so will demonstrate support for patient's spiritual needs and convey caring and acceptance.*

`PCC` ▨ Help patient cope by listening actively and communicating acceptance of patient's thoughts and feelings. *Dying patients need the opportunity to express their feelings.*

`PCC` ▨ Provide simple physical gestures of support such as holding hands with patient. Encourage family members to do the same. Verify with patient that your actions aren't intrusive. *As patients begin to let go, they sometimes want to experience less touching.*

`PCC` ▨ Reassure patient that he or she won't be left alone; however, respect patient's requests to be alone. *For some patients, asking to be alone is part of the process of letting go.*

Suggested NIC Interventions

Active Listening; Anticipatory Guidance; Family Involvement Promotion; Pain Management; Spiritual Support; Touch

EVALUATIONS FOR EXPECTED OUTCOMES

▨ Patient expresses satisfaction with private time and time spent with others.
▨ Patient uses those comfort measures that enhance individual well-being and reduce physical symptoms associated with anxiety.
▨ Patient engages in conversation and activities with family, caregivers, and other support people.
▨ Patient expresses satisfaction with spiritual support that is offered.
▨ Patient makes appropriate use of available support systems to cope with the dying process.
▨ Patient exhibits sense of comfort and overall peace.
▨ Patient dies in a dignified manner in an environment of sensitivity and love.

DOCUMENTATION

▨ Behavioral manifestations of anxiety
▨ Patient's expressions of feelings related to death and dying
▨ Patient's requests for visitors or expression of desire for solitude
▨ Conferences with family members

- Patient's requests for comfort measures and their effectiveness
- Referrals to clergy, spiritual advisors, or others
- Patient's response to nursing interventions
- Evaluations for expected outcomes

REFERENCES

Aan de Stegge, B. M., Tak, L. M., Rosmalen, J. G. M., & Oude Voshaar, R. C. (2018). Death anxiety and its association with hypochondriasis and medically unexplained symptoms: A systematic review. *Journal of Psychosomatic Research, 115*, 58–65.

Jo, K.-H., & An, G.-J. (2018). Effects of a group reminiscence program on self-forgiveness, life satisfaction, and death anxiety among institutionalized older adults. *Korean Journal of Adult Nursing, 30*(5), 546–554.

Lau, B. H., Wong, D. F. K., Fung, Y. L., Zhou, J., Chan, C. L. W., Chow, A. Y. M., & Lau, B. H.-P. (2018). Facing death alone or together? Investigating the interdependence of death anxiety, dysfunctional attitudes, and quality of life in patient-caregiver dyads confronting lung cancer. *Psycho-Oncology, 27*(8), 2045–2051.

Sharpe, L., Curran, L., Butow, P., & Thewes, B. (2018). Fear of cancer recurrence and death anxiety. *Psycho-Oncology, 27*(11), 2559–2565.

Readiness for Enhanced Decision-Making

DEFINITION

A pattern of choosing a course of action for meeting short- and long-term health-related goals, which can be strengthened

ASSESSMENT

- Patient's perception of own ability to make decisions
- Patient's expression of desire to align decisions with personal values and goals
- Patient's expression of desire to improve congruence between decisions and sociocultural values and goals
- Patient's desire to evaluate the efficacy of own decisions
- Patient's need for reliable information on which to base own decisions

DEFINING CHARACTERISTICS

- Expresses desire to enhance congruency of decisions with sociocultural goals
- Expresses desire to enhance congruency of decisions with sociocultural values
- Expresses desire to enhance congruency of decisions with goals
- Expresses desire to enhance congruency of decisions with values
- Expresses desire to enhance decision-making
- Expresses desire to enhance risk–benefit analysis of decisions
- Expresses desire to enhance understanding of choices for decision-making
- Expresses desire to enhance understanding of the meaning of choices
- Expresses desire to enhance use of reliable evidence for decisions

EXPECTED OUTCOMES

- Patient will express desire to make effective decisions to meet short- and long-term goals.
- Patient will share decision-making goals and concerns.
- Patient will discuss measures used to evaluate quality of decisions made.

- Patient will make decisions that promote maximal physical, mental, social, and psychological well-being.
- Patient will involve family, community, friends, and clergy in health care decisions.

Suggested NOC Outcomes

Decision-Making; Participation in Health Care Decisions; Self-Care: Instrumental Activities of Daily Living (IADLs)

INTERVENTIONS AND RATIONALES

PCC - Assess patient's ability to make decisions that affect patient's well-being *to determine patient's level of ability to participate in health care decisions.*
PCC - Work with patient to enhance patient's decision-making capabilities *to promote personal actions of a competent individual to exercise governance in life decisions.*
PCC - Provide patient with decision-making support *to enhance self-care and well-being of the patient and family.*
PCC - Assist patient with decisions that involve family, community, friends, and clergy *to provide opportunities for shared decision-making and enhanced support for the patient.*

Suggested NOC Outcomes

Decision-Making Support; Health System Guidance; Self-Responsibility Facilitation

EVALUATIONS FOR EXPECTED OUTCOMES

- Patient expresses desire to make effective decisions to meet short- and long-term goals.
- Patient shares decision-making goals and concerns.
- Patient discusses measures used to evaluate the quality of decisions made.
- Patient makes decisions that promote maximal physical, mental, social, and psychological well-being.
- Patient involves family, community, friends, and clergy in health care decisions.

DOCUMENTATION

- Patient's perception of decision-making abilities
- Patient's involvement of family, community, friends, and clergy in decision-making
- Future plans to make decisions that improve physical, mental, social, and psychological well-being
- Evaluations for expected outcomes

REFERENCES

Cadet, M. J. (2018). An overview of prostate cancer screening recommendations and shared decision-making process model to guide nursing practice. *MEDSURG Nursing, 27*(5), 301–304.

Jay, A., Thomas, H., & Brooks, F. (2018). Induction of labour: How do women get information and make decisions? Findings of a qualitative study. *British Journal of Midwifery, 26*(1), 22–29.

Johnson, R. A., Huntley, A., Hughes, R. A., Cramer, H., Turner, K. M., Perkins, B., & Feder, G. (2018). Interventions to support shared decision making for hypertension: A systematic review of controlled studies. *Health Expectations, 21*(6), 1191–1207.

Rhynas, S. J., Garrido, A. G., Logan, G., MacArthur, J., & Burton, J. K. (2018). New care home admission following hospitalisation: How do older people, families and professionals make decisions about discharge destination? A case study narrative analysis. *International Journal of Older People Nursing, 13*(3), 1.

Decisional Conflict

DEFINITION

Uncertainty about course of action to be taken when choice among competing actions involves risk, loss, or challenge to values and beliefs

RELATED FACTORS (R/T)

- Conflict with moral obligation
- Conflicting information sources
- Inexperience with decision-making
- Insufficient information
- Insufficient support system
- Interference in decision-making
- Moral principle supports mutually inconsistent actions
- Moral rule supports mutually inconsistent actions
- Moral value supports mutually inconsistent actions
- Perceived threat to value system
- Unclear personal beliefs
- Unclear personal values

ASSESSMENT

- Age and gender
- Sexual orientation
- Perception of health care options
- Developmental stage, including physical maturity, cognition, beliefs, values, and ethics
- Marital status
- Family system (nuclear, extended role, and sibling position)
- Sociocultural factors, including educational level, occupation, socioeconomic status, ethnic group, sexual preference, and religious beliefs
- Psychological status, including level of function, coping mechanisms, support systems, self-image, self-esteem, and attitude toward physical appearance
- History of sexual experiences, including experimentation, trauma, and other experiences
- Level of functioning (cognitive, emotional, and behavioral)
- Coping mechanisms
- Past experience with decision-making
- Available support system

DEFINING CHARACTERISTICS

- Delay in decision-making
- Distress while attempting a decision
- Physical sign of distress
- Physical sign of tension
- Questioning of moral principle while attempting a decision
- Questioning of moral rule while attempting a decision
- Questioning of moral values while attempting a decision
- Questioning of personal beliefs while attempting a decision
- Questioning of personal values while attempting a decision
- Recognizes undesired consequences of actions being considered
- Self-focused

- Uncertainty about choices
- Vacillating among choices

EXPECTED OUTCOMES

- Patient will describe feelings about current situation.
- Patient will discuss benefits and drawbacks of treatment options.
- Patient will make decisions related to daily activities.
- Patient will express feelings about morals and decision-making.
- Patient will discuss conflicts between personal values and social pressures.
- Patient will identify desirable and undesirable consequences of undesired activity.
- Patient will accept assistance from family, friends, clergy, and other people.
- Patient will practice progressive muscle relaxation to decrease tension created by decisional conflict.
- Patient will report feeling comfortable about ability to make an appropriate, rational choice.

Suggested NOC Outcomes

Coping; Decision-Making; Family Functioning; Information Processing; Participation in Health Care Decisions; Personal Autonomy

INTERVENTIONS AND RATIONALES

PCC ▪ Encourage expressions of feelings about social patterns and society norms *to improve recognition of feelings and foster open discussion.*

▪ Assure patient that you're willing to discuss all topics. Assure patient that all information will be kept confidential *to encourage honest discussion of concerns.*

PCC ▪ Encourage the patient to explore feelings related to vital topics *to promote trust and provide time when the patient can discuss feelings confidentially.*

PCC ▪ Listen to patient's concerns about difficulties in making a decision. Use a nonjudgmental approach and encourage expression of feelings *to demonstrate acceptance of patient and respect for the patient's culture, beliefs, and value system.*

PCC ▪ Assist patient with the process of decision-making in relation to daily activities. *Learning the process will provide the patient with a framework for decision-making and enhance patient's feelings of self-confidence when making more difficult health care decisions.*

PCC ▪ Help patient make decisions about daily activities *to enhance feelings of autonomy.*

PCC ▪ Encourage visits with family, friends, and clergy; provide privacy during visits *to foster emotional support.*

EBP ▪ Teach progressive muscle relaxation techniques *to decrease physical and psychological signs of tension.*

T&C ▪ Help patient identify decision-making areas that require assistance from others and provide appropriate referrals. *Providing referrals will ensure ongoing support. Putting patient in touch with appropriate community resources will help promote feeling that others are genuinely interested in patient's well-being.*

T&C ▪ Refer patient for long-term counseling if necessary. *Long-standing emotional conflicts may require in-depth intervention.*

Suggested NIC Interventions

Active Listening; Assertiveness Training; Counseling; Decision-Making Support; Learning Facilitation; Mutual Goal Setting; Patient Contracting; Self-Responsibility Facilitation; Support System Enhancement

- Patient expresses anxiety, tension, and other feelings related to difficult medical treatment decisions.
- Patient discusses peer pressure, family conflict, or other factors that may be influencing undesirable behaviors.
- Patient describes benefits and drawbacks of treatment options.
- Patient makes minor decisions related to daily activities.
- Patient identifies available sources of emotional support and requests help, if needed.
- Patient accepts assistance from family, friends, clergy, and other people.
- Patient practices progressive muscle relaxation to decrease tension created by decisional conflict.
- Patient reports feeling at ease with ability to choose treatment option that's appropriate for him or her.

- Patient's statements that provide insight into conflict regarding treatment options
- Cognitive, emotional, and behavioral functioning
- Interventions to assist patient with resolving decisional conflict
- Patient's response to nursing interventions
- Evaluations for expected outcomes

REFERENCES

Boland, L., Kryworuchko, J., Saarimaki, A., & Lawson, M. L. (2017). Parental decision making involvement and decisional conflict: A descriptive study. *BMC Pediatrics, 17*, 146.

Chen, N., Lin, Y., Liang, S., Tung, H., Tsay, S., & Wang, T. (2018). Conflict when making decisions about dialysis modality. *Journal of Clinical Nursing, 27*(1/2), e138–e146.

Lamahewa, K., Mathew, R., Iliffe, S., Wilcock, J., Manthorpe, J., Sampson, E. L., & Davies, N. (2018). A qualitative study exploring the difficulties influencing decision making at the end of life for people with dementia. *Health Expectations, 21*(1), 118–127.

Vella, L., Ring, H. A., Aitken, M. R. F., Watson, P. C., Presland, A., & Clare, I. C. H. (2018). Understanding self-reported difficulties in decision-making by people with autism spectrum disorders. *Autism: The International Journal of Research & Practice, 22*(5), 549–559.

Ineffective Denial

Conscious or unconscious attempt to disavow the knowledge or meaning of an event to reduce anxiety and/or fear, leading to the detriment of health

- Anxiety
- Excessive stress
- Fear of death
- Fear of losing autonomy
- Fear of separation
- Ineffective coping strategies
- Insufficient emotional support
- Insufficient sense of control
- Perceived inadequacy in dealing with strong emotions
- Threat of unpleasant reality

- Age
- Activity patterns, including sudden interest or participation in activities that may be dangerous
- Perception of present health state, including awareness of diagnosis, perception of personal relevance or impact on life pattern, and description of symptoms
- Mental status, including general appearance, affect, mood, memory, orientation, communication, thinking process, perception, abstract thinking, judgment, and insight
- Coping behaviors
- Problem-solving strategies
- Support systems, including family, friends, clergy, and financial resources
- Belief system, including values, norms, and religion
- Self-concept, including self-esteem and body image

DEFINING CHARACTERISTICS

- Delay in seeking health care
- Denies fear of death
- Denies fear of invalidism
- Displaces fear of impact of the condition
- Displaces source of symptoms
- Does not admit impact of disease on life
- Does not perceive relevance of danger
- Does not perceive relevance of symptoms
- Inappropriate affect
- Minimizes symptoms
- Refusal of health care
- Use of dismissive comments when speaking of distressing event
- Use of dismissive gestures when speaking of distressing event
- Use of treatment not advised by health care professional

EXPECTED OUTCOMES

- Patient will describe knowledge and perception of present health problem or event.
- Patient will describe life pattern and report any recent changes.
- Patient will express knowledge and perception of present health on ability to participate in hobbies and other activities.
- Patient will participate in the planned health care regimen.
- Patient will demonstrate behaviors associated with grief process.
- Patient will discuss present health problem with physician, nurses, and family members.
- Patient will express a more positive view of the aging process.
- Patient will express a more positive view of the distressing event.
- Patient will indicate, either verbally or through behavior, an increased awareness of reality.

Suggested NOC Outcomes

Acceptance: Health Status; Anxiety Level; Coping; Fear Self-Control; Health Beliefs; Health Beliefs: Perceived Threat; Symptom Control

INTERVENTIONS AND RATIONALES

PCC ■ Provide for a specific amount of uninterrupted, non–care-related time with patient each day. *This allows patient to discuss knowledge, feelings, and concerns.*

PCC ▪ Encourage patient to express feelings related to present problem, its severity, and its potential impact on life pattern. *This helps patient express doubts and resolve concerns.*

T&C ▪ Maintain frequent communication with physician to assess what patient has been told about illness. *This fosters consistent, collaborative approach to patient's care.*

PCC ▪ Listen to patient with nonjudgmental acceptance *to demonstrate positive regard for patient as a person worthy of respect.*

EBP ▪ Help patient learn the stages of anticipatory grieving *to increase understanding and ability to cope.*

▪ As patient is ready and receptive, teach patient about health problem and treatment regimen. Reinforce learning as patient becomes receptive. *While in a state of denial, patients are often either unwilling or unable to assimilate factual information about health issues.*

PCC ▪ Encourage patient to communicate with others, asking questions and clarifying concerns based on readiness. *Patient fixated in denial may isolate and withdraw from others.*

PCC ▪ Visit more frequently as patient begins to accept reality; alleviate fears when necessary. *This helps reduce patient's fear of being alone and fosters accurate reality testing.*

Suggested NIC Interventions

Anxiety Reduction; Behavior Modification; Calming Technique; Coping Enhancement; Counseling; Decision-Making Support; Health Education; Mutual Goal Setting; Reality Orientation; Truth Telling

EVALUATIONS FOR EXPECTED OUTCOMES

▪ Patient describes present health problem or event.
▪ Patient describes life pattern and reports recent changes.
▪ Patient expresses positive and negative feelings about illness or event.
▪ Patient communicates understanding of stages of grieving.
▪ Patient demonstrates behavior appropriate to present phase of grieving process.
▪ When ready, patient discusses health problem with physician, nurses, and family members.
▪ Patient displays increasing awareness of reality, either verbally or through behavior.

DOCUMENTATION

▪ Patient's perception of health problem or event
▪ Mental status (baseline and ongoing)
▪ Evidence of patient adjusting to the event
▪ Patient's knowledge of illness or event
▪ Patient's behavioral responses
▪ Interventions implemented to assist patient
▪ Patient's response to nursing interventions
▪ Evaluations for expected outcomes
▪ Referrals provided

REFERENCES

Blumenthal-Barby, J. S., & Ubel, P. A. (2018). In defense of "denial": Difficulty knowing when beliefs are unrealistic and whether unrealistic beliefs are bad. *American Journal of Bioethics, 18*(9), 4–15.

Martin-Joy, J. S., Malone, J. C., Cui, X.-J., Johansen, P.-Ø., Hill, K. P., Rahman, M. O., ... Vaillant, G. E. (2017). Development of adaptive coping from mid to late life: A 70-year longitudinal study of defense maturity and its psychosocial correlates. *Journal of Nervous & Mental Disease, 205*(9), 685–691.

Renz, M., Reichmuth, O., Bueche, D., Traichel, B., Mao, M. S., Cerny, T., & Strasser, F. (2018). Fear, pain, denial, and spiritual experiences in dying processes. *American Journal of Hospice & Palliative Medicine, 35*(3), 478–491.

Talepasand, S., & Mahfar, F. (2018). Relationship between defense mechanisms and the quality of life in women with breast cancer. *International Journal of Cancer Management, 11*(1), e11116.

Impaired Dentition

DEFINITION

Disruption in tooth development/eruption patterns or structural integrity of individual teeth

RELATED FACTORS (R/T)

- Barrier to self-care
- Difficulty accessing dental care
- Excessive intake of fluoride
- Excessive use of abrasive oral cleaning agents
- Habitual use of staining substances
- Inadequate dietary habits
- Inadequate oral hygiene
- Insufficient knowledge of dental health
- Malnutrition

ASSOCIATED CONDITIONS

- Bruxism
- Chronic vomiting
- Oral temperature sensitivity
- Pharmaceutical agent

ASSESSMENT

- Age and gender
- Dental health history, including primary and secondary tooth development; frequency of visits to the dentist; frequency of brushing; condition of teeth (such as presence of caries, extractions, plaque, malocclusion, and evulsion), gums, lips, tongue, and mucous membranes; and signs of salivary dysfunction (such as fissuring at corners of mouth, sore mucous membranes, dryness and cracking of lips, crusting of tongue and palate, and paresthesia of tongue or mucous membrane)
- Health history, including medication history, x-ray treatments, infection, allergies, trauma, lead poisoning, rubella, nephrotic illness, and malnutrition
- Use of abrasive oral cleaning agents on the teeth or gums
- Nutritional status, including amount of sugar in diet
- Socioeconomic conditions, including access to dental health care
- Environmental conditions, including lack of fluoride in drinking water
- Willingness and ability to perform dental health measures and to attend dental appointments

- Abraded teeth
- Absence of teeth
- Dental caries
- Enamel discoloration
- Erosion of enamel
- Excessive oral calculus
- Excessive oral plaque
- Facial asymmetry
- Halitosis
- Incomplete tooth eruption for age
- Loose tooth
- Malocclusion
- Premature loss of primary teeth
- Root caries
- Tooth fracture
- Tooth misalignment
- Toothache

- Patient will brush teeth at least once per day.
- Patient will demonstrate good brushing technique.
- Patient won't show evidence of dental caries, periodontal disease, or malocclusion.
- Patient will reduce quantity of cariogenic food in diet.
- Patient's teeth will show evidence of good daily oral hygiene.

Suggested NOC Outcomes

Oral Hygiene; Self-Care: Oral Hygiene

EBP ■ Teach patient principles of good dental hygiene using teaching methods appropriate to age group *to foster compliance.*

EBP ■ Demonstrate good brushing technique. Stress the importance of having teeth feel clean rather than the need to follow a specific procedure. Help patient establish a schedule for brushing. If necessary, provide direct assistance as well as demonstrations *to reinforce good dental hygiene habits.*

EBP ■ Teach patient about the relationship between diet and dental health. Identify examples of foods that promote good dental health (such as milk) and foods that promote tooth decay (such as those containing refined sugar, honey, or molasses). Teach patient to identify and avoid products with excessive sucrose *to increase the awareness of cariogenic foods and encourage better eating habits and more frequent brushing.*

PCC ■ Alert patient if assessment reveals evidence of dental caries, periodontal disease, malocclusion, or other conditions requiring dental care *to ensure awareness of impaired dentition and the need for follow-up care.* Provide a referral to a dentist *to ensure professional care.*

PCC ■ Assess whether patient is able and willing to meet needs regarding dental health. Provide referrals to community resources that may help patient obtain dental care. *The high cost of dental care may cause some families to neglect dental care needs.*

EBP ■ If patient is prone to dental problems, emphasize the need for more meticulous home dental care *to avoid further deterioration of patient's teeth and gums.*

PCC ■ Schedule an appointment to determine whether patient has followed up on the referral to a dentist *to ensure continuity of care.*

Suggested NOC Outcomes

Oral Health Maintenance; Oral Health Promotion; Teaching: Individual

EVALUATIONS FOR EXPECTED OUTCOMES

- Patient assumes responsibility for brushing teeth.
- Patient demonstrates good brushing technique.
- Patient shows no evidence of dental caries, periodontal disease, or malocclusion.
- Patient reduces quantity of cariogenic foods in diet.
- Patient's teeth show evidence of good daily oral hygiene.

DOCUMENTATION

- Dental health history
- Evidence of dental problems
- Teaching sessions with patient
- Evidence of improvement in patient's dental hygiene
- Patient's response to nursing interventions
- Evaluations for expected outcomes

REFERENCES

Barker, T. S., Smith, C. A., Waguespack, G. M., Mercante, D. E., & Gunaldo, T. P. (2018). Collaborative skill building in dentistry and dental hygiene through intraprofessional education: Application of a quality improvement model. *Journal of Dental Hygiene, 92*(5), 14–21.

Elani, H. W., Simon, L., Ticku, S., Bain, P. A., Barrow, J., & Riedy, C. A. (2018). Systematic review: Does providing dental services reduce overall health care costs? A systematic review of the literature. *Journal of the American Dental Association, 149*(8), 696–703.

Stein, C., Santos, N. M. L., Hilgert, J. B., & Hugo, F. N. (2018). Effectiveness of oral health education on oral hygiene and dental caries in schoolchildren: Systematic review and meta-analysis. *Community Dentistry & Oral Epidemiology, 46*(1), 30–37.

Weintraub, J. A., Zimmerman, S., Ward, K., Wretman, C. J., Sloane, P. D., Stearns, S. C., ... Preisser, J. S. (2018). Improving nursing home residents' oral hygiene: Results of a cluster randomized intervention trial. *Journal of the American Medical Directors Association, 19*(12), 1086–1091.

Delayed Child Development

DEFINITION

Child who continually fails to achieve developmental milestones within the expected time frame

Infant or Child Factors

- Inadequate access to health care provider
- Inadequate attachment behavior
- Inadequate stimulation
- Unaddressed abuse
- Unaddressed psychological neglect

Caregiver Factors

- Anxiety
- Decreased emotional support availability
- Depressive symptoms
- Excessive stress
- Unaddressed domestic violence

- Family process, including number and ages of children, usual patterns of interaction, roles of parents and children, communication patterns, relationship changes (such as separation, divorce, or remarriage), and past response to crisis
- Parental status, including perception of child's behavior, past responses to stress, child care provisions, history of inappropriate parenting, and history of destructive behavior or substance abuse
- Alteration in child's growth and development resulting from illness or dysfunctional parenting
- Developmental level (physical, cognitive, psychosocial, and linguistic) and learning needs
- Growth history, including changes in child's size and form, current height and weight, percentile on pediatric growth grid, body proportions, bone development (determined through X-ray examination), tooth development, organ systems development, neuroendocrine function (growth hormone, thyroid hormone, and androgen levels), genetic abnormalities that may affect growth, prenatal influences (fetal exposure to alcohol or illicit drugs, maternal smoking, or malnutrition), birth trauma (possible oxygen deprivation or nerve injuries), and breast-feeding or bottle-feeding
- Cultural information, including nationality, ethnicity, religious affiliation, and beliefs and practices regarding health and child rearing
- Psychosocial status, including family's resources, health beliefs and attitudes, interest in learning, knowledge and skill regarding current health problem, obstacles to learning, support systems (willingness and ability of others to help the child), and usual coping pattern

- Consistent difficulty performing cognitive skills typical of age group
- Consistent difficulty performing language skills typical of age group
- Consistent difficulty performing motor skills typical of age group
- Consistent difficulty performing psychosocial skills typical of age group

- Child will demonstrate cognitive skills typical of age group.
- Child will demonstrate language skills typical of age group.

- Child will demonstrate motor skills typical of age group.
- Child will demonstrate psychosocial skills typical of age group.
- Child will participate in activities and be provided with a supervised, unconfined environment that includes age-appropriate toys and fosters interaction with child's development.
- Parents will express understanding of measures to reduce child's risk for delayed development.
- Parents will identify risk factors that may interfere with child's development.

Suggested NOC Outcomes

Family Functioning; Growth; Parenting Performance; Personal Health Status; Risk Control

INTERVENTIONS AND RATIONALES

PCC ■ Assess family's developmental stage; family roles; family rules; socioeconomic status; family health history; history of substance abuse; history of sexual abuse of spouse or children; problem-solving and decision-making skills; religious affiliation; ethnicity. *Assessment information will aid in developing a workable plan of care.*

EBP ■ Educate parents about child's need for quality interaction with family members and others.

EBP ■ Inform parents about age-appropriate activities and toys as well as potential playmates for a child of specific age. Emphasize importance of providing an unconfined, supervised environment in which the child can *play to encourage play that encourages the child to move freely.*

EBP ■ Educate parents about risk factors that may lead to delayed development, such as lack of supportive interactions or age-appropriate activities. *The ability to recognize risk factors will promote getting help for the parents and child sooner.*

EBP ■ Teach coping skills to parents *to enable them to deal effectively with the child's needs.*

PCC ■ Encourage parents to listen to the child and communicate in a loving, supportive way *in order to allow the child to maintain a positive attitude.*

PCC ■ Encourage parents to identify preventive measures they may initiate at home to ensure continuity of care. *Consistency in providing care will help the child understand that the plan carries over to all aspects of child's life.*

PCC ■ Provide parents with a copy of child's teaching plan. *This helps to reinforce what the child is learning.*

T&C ■ Refer to case manager/social worker *to ensure that a home assessment is done.*

Suggested NIC Interventions

Nutrition Management; Family Process Maintenance; Coping Enhancement; Family Integrity Promotion; Maintenance; Normalization Promotion; Substance Use Prevention; Substance Use Treatment; Risk Identification

EVALUATIONS FOR EXPECTED OUTCOMES

- Child participates in activities that stimulate cognitive skills typical of age group.
- Child participates in activities that stimulate language skills typical of age group.
- Child participates in activities that stimulate motor skills typical of age group.
- Child participates in activities that stimulate psychosocial skills typical of age group.
- Child meets developmental milestones.

- Child participates in activities appropriate for age and developmental stage.
- Parents' expression of normal developmental stages and measures to reduce developmental delays.

DOCUMENTATION

- Observations of developmental assessments—cognitive skills, language skills, motor skills, and psychosocial skills
- Interventions to provide supportive care and child's response
- Instructions given on developmental stages and measures to reduce developmental delay

REFERENCES

Gmmash, A. S., Effgen, S. K., Skubik-Peplaski, C., & Lane, J. D. (2021). Parental adherence to home activities in early intervention for young children with delayed motor development. *Physical Therapy*, *101*(4), 1–11.

Prado, E. L., Maleta, K., Caswell, B. L., George, M., Oakes, L. M., DeBolt, M. C., Bragg, M. G., Arnold, C. D., Iannotti, L. L., Lutter, C. K., & Stewart, C. P. (2020). Early child development outcomes of a randomized trial providing 1 egg per day to children age 6 to 15 months in Malawi. *Journal of Nutrition*, *150*(7), 1933–1942.

Tan, S., Mangunatmadja, I., & Wiguna, T. (2019). Risk factors for delayed speech in children aged 1–2 years. *Paediatrica Indonesiana*, *59*(2), 55–62.

Witt, S., Weitkämper, A., Neumann, H., Lücke, T., & Zmyj, N. (2018). Delayed theory of mind development in children born preterm: A longitudinal study. *Early Human Development*, *127*, 85–89.

Risk for Delayed Child Development

DEFINITION

Child who is susceptible to failure to achieve developmental milestones within the expected time frame

RISK FACTORS

Infant or Child Factors

- Inadequate access to health care provider
- Inadequate attachment behavior
- Inadequate stimulation
- Unaddressed psychological neglect

Caregiver Factors

- Anxiety
- Decreased emotional support availability
- Depressive symptoms
- Excessive stress
- Unaddressed domestic violence

ASSOCIATED CONDITIONS

- Antenatal pharmaceutical preparations
- Congenital disorders
- Depression

- Inborn genetic diseases
- Maternal mental disorders
- Maternal physical illnesses
- Prenatal substance misuse
- Sensation disorders

ASSESSMENT

- Family process, including number and ages of children, usual patterns of interaction, roles of parents and children, communication patterns, relationship changes (such as separation, divorce, or remarriage), and past response to crisis
- Parental status, including perception of child's behavior, past responses to stress, child care provisions, history of inappropriate parenting, and history of destructive behavior or substance abuse
- Alteration in child's growth and development resulting from illness or dysfunctional parenting
- Developmental level (physical, cognitive, psychosocial, and linguistic) and learning needs
- Growth history, including changes in child's size and form, current height and weight, percentile on pediatric growth grid, body proportions, bone development (determined through x-ray examination), tooth development, organ systems development, neuroendocrine function (growth hormone, thyroid hormone, and androgen levels), genetic abnormalities that may affect growth, prenatal influences (fetal exposure to alcohol or illicit drugs, maternal smoking, or malnutrition), birth trauma (possible oxygen deprivation or nerve injuries), and breastfeeding or bottle-feeding
- Cultural information, including nationality, ethnicity, religious affiliation, and beliefs and practices regarding health and child rearing
- Psychosocial status, including family's resources, health beliefs and attitudes, interest in learning, knowledge and skill regarding current health problem, obstacles to learning, support systems (willingness and ability of others to help the child), and usual coping pattern

EXPECTED OUTCOMES

- Child will continue to grow and gain weight in accordance with growth chart of age and sex.
- Child will consume _____ calories and _____ mL of fluids representing _____ servings (specify for each food group).
- Child will participate in activities and be provided with a supervised, unconfined environment that includes age-appropriate toys and fosters interaction with child's development.
- Parents will express understanding of measures to reduce child's risk for delayed development.
- Parents will identify risk factors that may interfere with child's development.

Suggested NOC Outcomes

Family Functioning; Growth; Parenting Performance; Personal Health Status; Risk Control

INTERVENTIONS AND RATIONALES

- Assess family's developmental stage; family roles; family rules; socioeconomic status; family health history; history of substance abuse; history of sexual abuse of spouse or children; problem-solving and decision-making skills; religious affiliation; ethnicity. *Assessment information will aid in developing a workable plan of care.*

- Weigh and measure child. Review growth chart *to establish current height and weight values.* Establish a meal program *to meet child's nutritional needs.*

PCC - Create an environment in which family members can express themselves openly and honestly. Establish rules for communication during meetings with family. *Having rules allows everyone to participate and keep the discussion on the designated topic.*

EBP - Teach parents about nutritional requirements needed for child of specific weight and age. Discuss various meal choices available to child. *Providing instruction in writing simplifies parents' role in selecting healthy foods.*

EBP - Educate parents about child's need for quality interaction with family members and others.

EBP - Inform parents about age-appropriate activities and toys as well as potential playmates for a child of specific age. Emphasize importance of providing an unconfined, supervised environment in which child can *play to encourage play that encourages child to move freely.*

EBP - Educate parents about risk factors that may lead to delayed development, such as lack of supportive interactions or age-appropriate activities. *The ability to recognize risk factors will promote getting help for parents and child sooner.*

EBP - Teach coping skills to parents *to enable them to deal effectively with child's needs.*

- Encourage parents to listen to child and communicate in a loving, supportive way *in order to allow child to maintain a positive attitude.*

- Encourage parents to identify preventive measures they may initiate at home to ensure continuity of care. *Consistency in providing care will help child understand that the plan carries over to all aspects of child's life.*

PCC - Provide parents with a copy of child's teaching plan. *This helps to reinforce what child is learning.*

T&C - Refer to case manager/social worker *to ensure that a home assessment is done.*

T&C - Refer to nutritionist *for follow-up with food issues.*

Suggested NIC Interventions

Nutrition Management; Family Process Maintenance; Coping Enhancement; Family Integrity Promotion; Maintenance; Normalization Promotion; Substance Use Prevention; Substance Use Treatment; Risk Identification

EVALUATIONS FOR EXPECTED OUTCOMES

- Child meets developmental milestones.
- Child consumes adequate food and fluid to maintain normal weight.
- Child participates in activities appropriate for age and developmental stage.
- Parents' expression of normal developmental stages and measures to reduce developmental delays.

DOCUMENTATION

- Observations of developmental assessments
- Interventions to provide supportive care and patient's response
- Instructions given to patient and family members on developmental stages and measures to reduce developmental delay
- Child's weight
- Evaluations for expected outcomes

REFERENCES

Dees, W. L., Hiney, J. K., & Srivastava, V. K. (2017). Alcohol and puberty: Mechanisms of delayed development. *Alcohol Research: Current Reviews, 38*(2), e1–e6.

Reeves, L., Hartshorne, M., Black, R., Atkinson, J., Baxter, A., & Pring, T. (2018). Early talk boost: A targeted intervention for three year old children with delayed language development. *Child Language Teaching and Therapy, 34*(1), 53–62.

Witt, S., Weitkämper, A., Neumann, H., Lücke, T., & Zmyj, N. (2018). Delayed theory of mind development in children born preterm: A longitudinal study. *Early Human Development, 127*, 85–89.

Zeng, N., Ayyub, M., Sun, H., Wen, X., Xiang, P., & Gao, Z. (2017). Effects of physical activity on motor skills and cognitive development in early childhood: A systematic review. *BioMed Research International, 2017*, 1–13.

Delayed Infant Motor Development

DEFINITION

Individual who consistently fails to achieve developmental milestones related to the normal strengthening of bones and muscles and ability to move and touch one's surroundings

RELATED FACTORS (R/T)

Infant Factors

- Difficulty with sensory processing
- Insufficient curiosity
- Insufficient initiative
- Insufficient persistence

Caregiver Factors

- Anxiety about infant care
- Carries infant in arms for excessive time
- Does not allow infant to choose physical activities
- Does not allow infant to choose toys
- Does not encourage infant to grasp
- Does not encourage infant to reach
- Does not encourage sufficient infant play with other children
- Does not engage infant in games about body parts
- Does not teach movement words
- Insufficient fine motor toys for infant
- Insufficient gross motor toys for infant
- Insufficient time between periods of infant stimulation
- Limits infant experiences in the prone position
- Maternal postpartum depressive symptoms
- Negative perception of infant temperament
- Overstimulation of infant
- Perceived infant care incompetence

ASSOCIATED CONDITIONS

- 5-minute Appearance, Pulse, Grimace, Activity, & Respiration (APGAR) score <7
- Antenatal pharmaceutical preparations
- Complex medical conditions
- Failure to thrive

- Maternal anemia in late pregnancy
- Maternal mental health disorders in early pregnancy
- Maternal prepregnancy obesity
- Neonatal abstinence syndrome
- Neurodevelopmental disorders
- Postnatal infection of preterm infant
- Sensation disorders

ASSESSMENT

- Infant's development milestones; smiling, crying, babbling, response to affection, reaching, holding head up, bringing hand up to mouth, pushing up to elbows when lying on stomach
- Developmental level (physical, cognitive, psychosocial, and linguistic) and learning needs
- Family process, including number and ages of children, usual patterns of interaction, roles of parents and children, communication patterns, relationship changes (such as separation, divorce, or remarriage), and past response to crisis
- Parental status, including perception of child's behavior, past responses to stress, child care provisions, history of inappropriate parenting, and history of destructive behavior or substance abuse
- Alteration in infant's growth and development resulting from illness or dysfunctional parenting
- Growth history, including changes in infant's size and form, current height and weight, percentile on pediatric growth grid, body proportions, bone development (determined through X-ray examination), tooth development, organ systems development, neuroendocrine function (growth hormone, thyroid hormone, and androgen levels), genetic abnormalities that may affect growth, prenatal influences (fetal exposure to alcohol or illicit drugs, maternal smoking, or malnutrition), birth trauma (possible oxygen deprivation or nerve injuries), and breast-feeding or bottle-feeding
- Cultural information, including nationality, ethnicity, religious affiliation, and beliefs and practices regarding health and child rearing
- Psychosocial status, including family's resources, health beliefs and attitudes, interest in learning, knowledge and skill regarding current health problem, obstacles to learning, support systems (willingness and ability of others to help the child), and usual coping pattern

DEFINING CHARACTERISTICS

- Difficulty lifting head
- Difficulty maintaining head position
- Difficulty picking up blocks
- Difficulty pulling self to stand
- Difficulty rolling over
- Difficulty sitting with support
- Difficulty sitting without support
- Difficulty standing with assistance
- Difficulty transferring objects
- Difficulty with hand-and-knee crawling
- Does not engage in activities
- Does not initiate activities

- Infant will demonstrate expected developmental milestone; lifting head, maintaining head position, picking up blocks, pulling self to stand, rolling over, sitting with support, sitting without support, standing with assistance, transferring objects, hand-and-knee crawl, engage in activities, initiate activities.
- Infant will participate in activities and be provided with a supervised, unconfined environment that includes age-appropriate toys and fosters interaction with infant's development.
- Parents will express understanding of measures to reduce infant's risk for delayed development.
- Parents will identify risk factors that may interfere with infant's development.

Suggested NOC Outcomes

Child Development: 1 Month; Child Development: 2 Months; Child Development: 4 Months; Child Development: 6 Months; Newborn Adaptation; Parent–Infant Attachment; Parenting Performance

- **PCC** Assess family's developmental stage; family roles; family rules; socioeconomic status; family health history; history of substance abuse; history of sexual abuse of spouse or children; problem-solving and decision-making skills; religious affiliation; ethnicity. *Assessment information will aid in developing a workable plan of care.*
- **PCC** Create an environment in which family members can express themselves openly and honestly. Establish rules for communication during meetings with the family. *Having rules allows everyone to participate and keep the discussion on the designated topic.*
- **EBP** Educate parents about infant's need for quality interaction with family members and others.
- **EBP** Inform parents about age-appropriate activities and toys as well as potential playmates for an infant of specific age. Emphasize importance of providing an unconfined, supervised environment in which the infant can *play to encourage play that encourages the infant to move freely.*
- **EBP** Educate parents about risk factors that may lead to delayed development, such as lack of supportive interactions or age-appropriate activities. *The ability to recognize risk factors will promote getting help for the parents and infant sooner.*
- **EBP** Teach coping skills to parents *to enable them to deal effectively with the infant's needs.*
- **PCC** Encourage parents to interact with the infant and communicate in a loving, supportive way *nurturing environment encourages infant development.*
- **T&C** Refer to case manager/social worker *to ensure that a home assessment is done.*

Suggested NIC Interventions

Developmental Enhancement: Infant; Infant Care; Infant Care: Newborn; Teaching: Infant Stimulation 0–4 Months; Teaching: Infant Stimulation 5–8 Months; Teaching: Infant Stimulation 9–12 Months

- Infant meets developmental milestones.
- Infant participates in activities appropriate for age and developmental stage.
- Parents' expression of normal developmental stages and measures to reduce developmental delays.

DOCUMENTATION

- Observations of developmental assessments
- Interventions to provide supportive care and infant's response
- Instructions given to patient and family members on developmental stages and measures to reduce developmental delay
- Evaluations for expected outcomes

REFERENCES

Baptista, J., Belsky, J., Marques, S., Silva, J. R., Martins, C., & Soares, I. (2019). Early family adversity, stability and consistency of institutional care and infant cognitive, language and motor development across the first six months of institutionalization. *Infant Behavior & Development*, 57, N.PAG.

Valla, L., Slinning, K., Kalleson, R., Wentzel, L. T., & Riiser, K. (2020). Motor skills and later communication development in early childhood: Results from a population-based study. *Child: Care, Health & Development*, 46(4), 407–413.

Viana Cardoso, K. V., Marques de Carvalho, C., Marques de Carvalho Letícia Helene Mendes Ferreira, C., Mendes Ferreira, L. H., & de Castro Ferracioli Gama, M. (2021). Infants motor development in parental intervention during childcare: Case series. *Fisioterapia e Pesquisa*, 28(2), 172–178.

Zhang, H., Tian, Y., Zhang, S., Wang, S., Yao, D., Shao, S., Li, J., Li, S., Li, H., & Zhu, Z. (2020). Homocysteine-mediated gender-dependent effects of prenatal maternal depression on motor development in newborn infants. *Journal of Affective Disorders*, 263, 667–675.

Risk for Delayed Infant Motor Development

DEFINITION

Individual susceptible to failure to achieve developmental milestones related to the normal strengthening of bones, muscles and ability to move and touch one's surroundings

RISK FACTORS

Infant Factors

- Difficulty with sensory processing
- Insufficient curiosity
- Insufficient initiative
- Insufficient persistence

Caregiver Factors

- Anxiety about infant care
- Carries infant in arms for excessive time
- Does not allow infant to choose toys
- Does not encourage infant to grasp
- Does not encourage infant to reach
- Does not encourage sufficient infant play with other children
- Does not engage infant in games about body parts
- Does not teach movement words
- Insufficient fine motor toys for infant
- Insufficient gross motor toys for infant
- Insufficient time between periods of infant stimulation
- Limits infant experiences in the prone position

- Maternal postpartum depressive symptoms
- Negative perception of infant temperament
- Overstimulation of infant
- Perceived infant care incompetence

ASSOCIATED CONDITIONS

- 5-minute Appearance, Pulse, Grimace, Activity, & Respiration (APGAR) score <7
- Antenatal pharmaceutical preparations
- Complex medical conditions
- Failure to thrive
- Maternal anemia in late pregnancy
- Maternal mental health disorders in early pregnancy
- Maternal prepregnancy obesity
- Neonatal abstinence syndrome
- Neurodevelopmental disorders
- Postnatal infection of preterm infant
- Sensation disorders

ASSESSMENT

- Infant's development milestones; smiling, crying, babbling, response to affection, reaching, holding head up, bringing hand up to mouth, pushing up to elbows when lying on stomach
- Developmental level (physical, cognitive, psychosocial, and linguistic) and learning needs
- Family process, including number and ages of children, usual patterns of interaction, roles of parents and children, communication patterns, relationship changes (such as separation, divorce, or remarriage), and past response to crisis
- Parental status, including perception of child's behavior, past responses to stress, child care provisions, history of inappropriate parenting, and history of destructive behavior or substance abuse
- Alteration in infant's growth and development resulting from illness or dysfunctional parenting
- Growth history, including changes in infant's size and form, current height and weight, percentile on pediatric growth grid, body proportions, bone development (determined through X-ray examination), tooth development, organ systems development, neuroendocrine function (growth hormone, thyroid hormone, and androgen levels), genetic abnormalities that may affect growth, prenatal influences (fetal exposure to alcohol or illicit drugs, maternal smoking, or malnutrition), birth trauma (possible oxygen deprivation or nerve injuries), and breast-feeding or bottle-feeding
- Cultural information, including nationality, ethnicity, religious affiliation, and beliefs and practices regarding health and child rearing
- Psychosocial status, including family's resources, health beliefs and attitudes, interest in learning, knowledge and skill regarding current health problem, obstacles to learning, support systems (willingness and ability of others to help the child), and usual coping pattern

EXPECTED OUTCOMES

- Infant will demonstrate expected developmental milestone; lifting head, maintaining head position, picking up blocks, pulling self to stand, rolling over, sitting with support, sitting without support, standing with assistance, transferring objects, hand-and-knee crawl, engage in activities, initiate activities.

- Infant will participate in activities and be provided with a supervised, unconfined environment that includes age-appropriate toys and fosters interaction with infant's development.
- Parents will express understanding of measures to reduce infant's risk for delayed development.
- Parents will identify risk factors that may interfere with infant's development.

Suggested NOC Outcomes

Child Development: 1 Month; Child Development: 2 Months; Child Development: 4 Months; Child Development: 6 Months; Newborn Adaptation; Parent–Infant Attachment; Parenting Performance

INTERVENTIONS AND RATIONALES

PCC ▪ Assess family's developmental stage; family roles; family rules; socioeconomic status; family health history; history of substance abuse; history of sexual abuse of spouse or children; problem-solving and decision-making skills; religious affiliation; ethnicity. *Assessment information will aid in developing a workable plan of care.*

PCC ▪ Create an environment in which family members can express themselves openly and honestly. Establish rules for communication during meetings with the family. *Having rules allows everyone to participate and keep the discussion on the designated topic.*

EBP ▪ Educate parents about infant's need for quality interaction with family members and others.

EBP ▪ Inform parents about age-appropriate activities and toys as well as potential playmates for an infant of specific age. Emphasize importance of providing an unconfined, supervised environment in which the infant can *play to encourage play that encourages the infant to move freely.*

EBP ▪ Educate parents about risk factors that may lead to delayed development, such as lack of supportive interactions or age-appropriate activities. *The ability to recognize risk factors will promote getting help for the parents and infant sooner.*

EBP ▪ Teach coping skills to parents *to enable them to deal effectively with the infant's needs.*

PCC ▪ Encourage parents to interact with the infant and communicate in a loving, supportive way *nurturing environment encourages infant development.*

T&C ▪ Refer to case manager/social worker *to ensure that a home assessment is done.*

Suggested NIC Interventions

Developmental Enhancement: Infant; Infant Care; Infant Care: Newborn; Teaching: Infant Stimulation 0–4 Months; Teaching: Infant Stimulation 5–8 Months; Teaching: Infant Stimulation 9–12 Months

EVALUATIONS FOR EXPECTED OUTCOMES

- Infant meets developmental milestones.
- Infant participates in activities appropriate for age and developmental stage.
- Parents' expression of normal developmental stages and measures to reduce developmental delays.

DOCUMENTATION

▦ Observations of developmental assessments
▦ Risk factors associated with developmental assessments
▦ Interventions to provide supportive care and infant's response
▦ Instructions given to patient and family members on developmental stages and measures to reduce developmental delay
▦ Evaluations for expected outcomes

REFERENCES

Baptista, J., Belsky, J., Marques, S., Silva, J. R., Martins, C., & Soares, I. (2019). Early family adversity, stability and consistency of institutional care and infant cognitive, language and motor development across the first six months of institutionalization. *Infant Behavior & Development*, 57, N.PAG.

Valla, L., Slinning, K., Kalleson, R., Wentzel, L. T., & Riiser, K. (2020). Motor skills and later communication development in early childhood: Results from a population-based study. *Child: Care, Health & Development*, 46(4), 407–413.

Viana Cardoso, K. V., Marques de Carvalho, C., Marques de Carvalho Letícia Helene Mendes Ferreira, C., Mendes Ferreira, L. H., & de Castro Ferracioli Gama, M. (2021). Infants motor development in parental intervention during childcare: Case series. *Fisioterapia e Pesquisa*, 28(2), 172–178.

Zhang, H., Tian, Y., Zhang, S., Wang, S., Yao, D., Shao, S., Li, J., Li, S., Li, H., & Zhu, Z. (2020). Homocysteine-mediated gender-dependent effects of prenatal maternal depression on motor development in newborn infants. *Journal of Affective Disorders*, 263, 667–675.

Diarrhea

DEFINITION

Passage of three or more loose or liquid stools per day

RELATED FACTORS (R/T)

▦ Anxiety
▦ Early formula feeding
▦ Inadequate access to safe drinking water
▦ Inadequate access to safe food
▦ Inadequate knowledge about rotavirus vaccine
▦ Inadequate knowledge about sanitary food preparation
▦ Inadequate knowledge about sanitary food storage
▦ Inadequate personal hygiene practices
▦ Increased stress level
▦ Laxative misuse
▦ Malnutrition
▦ Substance misuse

ASSOCIATED CONDITIONS

▦ Critical illness
▦ Endocrine system diseases
▦ Enteral nutrition
▦ Gastrointestinal diseases
▦ Immunosuppression
▦ Infections

- Pharmaceutical preparations
- Treatment regimen

- History of bowel disorder or surgery
- Gastrointestinal (GI) status, including nausea and vomiting, usual bowel elimination habits, change in bowel elimination habits, stool characteristics (color, amount, size, and consistency), pain, inspection of abdomen, auscultation of bowel sounds, palpation for masses and tenderness, percussion for tympany and dullness, laxative and enema use, medications (especially antibiotics), and results of stool culture, upper GI series, and barium enema
- Nutritional status, including dietary intake, change from normal diet, appetite, current weight, change from normal weight, food irritants and contaminants, and serum albumin levels
- Fluid and electrolyte status, including intake and output, urine specific gravity, skin turgor, mucous membranes, serum potassium and sodium levels, and blood urea nitrogen
- Psychosocial status, including personality, stressors (such as finances, job, marital discord, and disease process), coping mechanisms, support systems, lifestyle, and recent travel

- Abdominal cramping
- Abdominal pain
- Bowel urgency
- Dehydration
- Hyperactive bowel sounds

- Patient's diarrheal episodes will decline or disappear.
- Patient will control diarrhea with medication.
- Patient will resume usual bowel pattern.
- Patient will maintain fluid and electrolyte balance.
- Patient will maintain weight.
- Patient's skin will remain intact.
- Patient will identify causative factors, preventive measures, and changed body image.
- Patient will acknowledge relationship of stress and anxiety to episodes of diarrhea.
- Patient will state plans to use stress-reduction techniques (specify).
- Patient will seek out persons with similar conditions or join a support group.

Suggested NOC Outcomes

Bowel Continence; Bowel Elimination; Electrolyte & Acid–Base balance; Fluid Balance; Hydration; Symptom Control; Symptom Severity

- **S** Assess and monitor frequency and characteristics of stools, auscultate bowel sounds, and record results at least every shift *to monitor treatment effectiveness.*
- **S** Tell patient to notify staff of each episode of diarrhea *to promote comfort and maintain communication.*

- Administer antidiarrheal medications, as ordered, *to improve body function, promote comfort, and balance body fluids, salts, and acid–base levels.* Monitor and report medications' effectiveness.
- **S** Monitor and record patient's intake and output, including number of stools. Report imbalances. *Monitoring ensures correct fluid replacement therapy.*
- **S** Provide replacement fluids and electrolytes as prescribed. Maintain accurate records *to ensure balanced fluid intake and output.*
- **T&C** Request dietary consult and if ordered, offer the patient the BRAT (banana, rice, apple, and toast) diet *to help meet nutritional needs without exacerbating diarrhea.*
- **S** Check skin daily *to detect and prevent breakdown.* Report decreased skin turgor or excoriation of perianal area.
- Weigh patient daily until diarrhea is controlled *to detect fluid loss or retention.*
- **EBP** Teach patient about:
  - causative and preventive factors *to promote understanding of problem.*
  - cleaning of perianal area, including use of powders and lotions, *to promote comfort and skin integrity.*
  - dietary restrictions *to control diarrhea, such as a lactose-free diet, which reduces residual waste and decreases intestinal irritation and spasms.*
  - use relaxation techniques *to reduce muscle tension and nervousness.*
  - recognize and reduce intake of diarrhea-producing foods or substances (such as dairy products and fruit) *to reduce residual waste matter and decrease intestinal irritation.*
- **PCC** Identify stressors and help patient solve problems *to provide more realistic approach to care.*
- **EBP** Teach stress-reduction techniques and help patient perform them daily by providing time, privacy, and needed equipment. *This temporarily relieves emotional distress.*
- **PCC** Encourage and assist patient to practice relaxation techniques *to reduce tension and promote self-knowledge and growth.*

Suggested NIC Interventions

Anxiety Reduction; Bowel Management; Coping Enhancement; Diarrhea Management; Electrolyte Management; Emotional Support; Energy Management; Fluid Management; Medication Management; Nutrition Management; Skin Care: Topical Treatments; Weight Management

EVALUATIONS FOR EXPECTED OUTCOMES

- Patient doesn't experience diarrhea.
- Patient's diarrheal episodes decline by at least 50%.
- Patient resumes usual bowel elimination pattern.
- Patient maintains fluid and electrolyte balance.
- Patient maintains weight.
- Patient's skin remains intact.
- Patient explains cause of diarrhea and steps to prevent recurrence.
- Patient demonstrates successful use of stress-reduction techniques.
- Patient attends a support group for individuals with a similar condition.
- Patient explains how stress may contribute to diarrhea.
- Patient explains plan to use stress-reduction techniques.
- Patient describes and demonstrates at least one stress-reduction technique.

DOCUMENTATION

- Frequency and characteristics of stool
- Patient's expressions of concern about diarrhea, causative factors, surgery, and adaptation to changes in body image
- Observations of effects of medications, intake and output, weight, stool characteristics, and skin condition
- Observations of effects of relaxation and stress-reduction techniques and dietary management on diarrhea
- Evaluations for expected outcomes

REFERENCES

Chandra, K. A., & Wanda, D. (2017). Traditional method of initial diarrhea treatment in children. *Comprehensive Child & Adolescent Nursing, 40,* 128–136.

Jafarnejad, S., Shab-Bidar, S., Speakman, J. R., Parastui, K., Daneshi-Maskooni, M., & Djafarian, K. (2016). Probiotics reduce the risk of antibiotic-associated diarrhea in adults (18–64 years) but not the elderly (>65 years). *Nutrition in Clinical Practice, 31*(4), 502–513.

Lacy, B. E. (2018). Practical evaluation and management of irritable bowel syndrome with diarrhea: A case study approach. *Journal of Family Practice, 67,* S31–S36.

Risk for Disuse Syndrome

DEFINITION

Susceptible to deterioration of body systems as the result of prescribed or unavoidable musculoskeletal inactivity, which may compromise health

RISK FACTORS

- Pain

ASSOCIATED CONDITIONS

- Alteration in level of consciousness
- Mechanical immobility
- Paralysis
- Prescribed immobility

ASSESSMENT

- Condition leading to prolonged inactivity or immobility
- Age
- Neurologic status, including mental status, level of consciousness (LOC), and sensory and motor ability
- Cardiovascular status, including blood pressure, heart rate, temperature, peripheral pulses, capillary refill, clotting profile, skin temperature and color, presence of edema, and chest pain or discomfort
- Respiratory status, including rate and rhythm, depth of inspiration, chest symmetry, use of accessory muscles, cough and sputum, percussion of lung fields, auscultation of breath sounds, chest pain or discomfort, and arterial blood gas (ABG) levels
- Gastrointestinal (GI) status, including inspection of abdomen, auscultation of bowel sounds, palpation for tenderness and masses, percussion for areas of dullness, usual

bowel habits, change in bowel habits, laxative use, pain or discomfort, and characteristics of stools (color, size, amount, and consistency)

▦ Nutritional status, including dietary intake, appetite, current weight, and change from normal weight

▦ Fluid status, including intake and output, urine specific gravity, mucous membranes, serum electrolyte levels, blood urea nitrogen (BUN), and creatinine level

▦ Genitourinary status, including voiding pattern, characteristics of urine (color, odor, sediment, and amount), history of urinary problems or infections, palpation of bladder, pain or discomfort, use of urinary assistive device, urinalysis, and urine cultures

▦ Musculoskeletal status, including range of motion (ROM); muscle size, strength, and tone; coordination; and functional mobility scale:
0 = completely independent
1 = requires use of equipment or device
2 = requires help, supervision, or teaching from another person
3 = requires help from another person and equipment or device
4 = dependent; doesn't participate in activity

▦ Integumentary status, including skin color, texture, turgor, temperature, elasticity, sensation, moisture, hygiene, and lesions

▦ Psychosocial factors, including family support, coping style, current understanding of prescribed inactivity, willingness to cooperate with treatment, mood, behavior, motivation, and stressors (such as inactivity, finances, job, and marital discord)

EXPECTED OUTCOMES

▦ Patient won't display evidence of altered mental, sensory, or motor ability.

▦ Patient won't have evidence of thrombus formation, venous stasis, or altered cardiovascular function.

▦ Patient won't show evidence of decreased chest movement, cough stimulus, or depth of ventilation.

▦ Patient won't show pooling of secretions or signs of infection.

▦ Patient won't have evidence of constipation and will maintain normal bowel elimination patterns.

▦ Patient will maintain adequate dietary intake, hydration, and weight.

▦ Patient won't show evidence of urine retention, infection, or renal calculi.

▦ Patient will maintain muscle strength and tone and joint ROM.

▦ Patient won't show evidence of contractures or subluxations.

▦ Patient won't show evidence of skin breakdown.

▦ Patient will maintain normal neurologic, cardiovascular, respiratory, GI, nutritional, genitourinary, musculoskeletal, and integumentary functioning during period of inactivity.

▦ Patient will express feelings about prolonged inactivity.

Suggested NOC Outcomes

Comfort Level; Coordinated Movement; Endurance; Immobility Consequences: Physiologic; Immobility Consequences: Psycho-Cognitive; Mobility; Pain Level; Risk Control

INTERVENTIONS AND RATIONALES

T&C ▦ Provide frequent contact with staff, diversionary materials (magazines, radio, and television), and orienting mechanisms (clock and calendar). *Reality orientation fosters patient awareness of environment.*

EBP ▪ Avoid positions that put prolonged pressure on body parts and compress blood vessels. Patient should change positions at least every 2 hours within prescribed limits. *These measures enhance circulation and help prevent tissue or skin breakdown.*

S ▪ Inspect skin every shift and protect areas subject to irritation. Follow facility policy for prevention of pressure ulcers *to prevent or mitigate skin breakdown.*

EBP ▪ Use pressure-reducing or pressure-equalizing equipment, as indicated or ordered (flotation pad, air pressure mattress, sheepskin pads, or special bed). *This helps prevent skin breakdown by relieving pressure.*

S ▪ Apply antiembolism stockings; remove for 1 hour every 8 hours. *Stockings promote venous return to heart, prevent venous stasis, and decrease or prevent swelling of lower extremities.*

S ▪ Monitor clotting profile. Administer and monitor anticoagulant therapy, if ordered, and monitor for signs and symptoms of bleeding *because anticoagulant therapy may cause hemorrhage.*

S ▪ Monitor temperature, blood pressure, pulse, and respirations at least every 4 hours *to assess for indications of infection or other complications.*

S ▪ Teach and monitor deep breathing, coughing, and use of incentive spirometer. Maintain regimen every 2 hours. *These measures help clear airways, expand lungs, and prevent respiratory complications.*

▪ Encourage fluid intake of 2.5 to 3.5 L daily, unless contraindicated, *to maintain urine output and aid bowel elimination.* Weigh daily and monitor hydration status (serum electrolyte, BUN, creatinine levels, and intake and output).

S ▪ Monitor breath sounds and respiratory rate, rhythm, and depth at least every 4 hours *to rule out respiratory complications.* Monitor ABG levels or pulse oximetry, if indicated, *to assess oxygenation, ventilation, and metabolic status.*

S ▪ Suction airway, as needed and ordered, *to clear airway and stimulate cough reflex*; note secretion characteristics.

S ▪ Establish baseline *to compare elimination patterns and habits.* Elevate head of bed and provide privacy to allow comfortable elimination.

EBP ▪ Instruct patient to avoid straining during bowel movements; administer stool softeners, suppositories, or laxatives, as ordered, and monitor effectiveness. *Straining during bowel movements may be hazardous to patients with cardiovascular disorders and increased intracranial pressure.*

▪ Provide small, frequent meals of favorite foods to increase dietary intake. Increase fiber content to enhance bowel elimination. Increase protein and vitamin C *to promote wound healing. Limit calcium to reduce risk of renal and bladder calculi.*

S ▪ Monitor urine characteristics and patient's subjective complaints typical of urinary tract infection (UTI), such as burning, frequency, and urgency. Obtain urine cultures, as ordered. *These measures aid early detection of UTI.*

PCC ▪ Identify level of functioning to provide baseline for future assessment and encourage appropriate participation in care *to prevent complications of immobility and increase patient's feelings of self-esteem.*

EBP ▪ Perform active or passive ROM exercises at least once per shift. Teach and monitor appropriate isotonic and isometric exercises. *These measures prevent joint contractures, muscle atrophy, and other complications of prolonged inactivity.*

PCC ▪ Provide or help with daily hygiene; keep skin dry and lubricated *to prevent cracking and possible infection.*

PCC ▪ Encourage patient and family to ventilate frustration. Allow open expression of all feelings associated with prolonged inactivity *to help patient and family cope with treatment.*

Suggested NIC Interventions

Activity Therapy; Body Mechanics Promotion; Cognitive Stimulation; Energy Management; Exercise Promotion; Exercise Therapy: Ambulation; Fluid Management; Nutrition Management

EVALUATIONS FOR EXPECTED OUTCOMES

▪ Patient doesn't exhibit altered LOC, mental status, sensory ability, or motor ability.
▪ Patient doesn't exhibit evidence of thrombus formation, venous stasis, or altered cardiovascular function.
▪ Patient shows no evidence of decreased chest movement, cough stimulus, or depth of ventilation.
▪ Patient maintains clear breath sounds bilaterally and doesn't show evidence of fever, chills, cough, purulent sputum, pooled secretions, or rapid, shallow respirations.
▪ Patient's bowel elimination pattern remains normal.
▪ Patient maintains adequate dietary intake, daily fluid intake, and weight.
▪ Patient doesn't exhibit evidence of distended bladder, fever, chills, frequent burning or painful urination, urgency, hematuria, flank pain, or urine retention.
▪ Patient's muscle strength and tone and joint ROM remain stable.
▪ Patient doesn't exhibit evidence of joint contractures.
▪ Patient doesn't experience skin breakdown.
▪ Patient maintains neurologic, cardiovascular, respiratory, GI, nutritional, genitourinary, musculoskeletal, and integumentary functioning.
▪ Patient openly expresses frustration, anger, despondency, and other feelings associated with prolonged inactivity.

DOCUMENTATION

▪ Patient's concerns or perceptions of circumstances necessitating inactivity; willingness to accept and participate in treatment
▪ Assessment of body systems at risk for deterioration
▪ Interventions to provide preventive or supportive care and prescribed treatment
▪ Treatment given to patient and patient's understanding and demonstrated ability to carry out instructions
▪ Patient's response to nursing interventions
▪ Evaluations for expected outcomes

REFERENCES

Bettis, T., Kim, B.-J., & Hamrick, M. W. (2018). Impact of muscle atrophy on bone metabolism and bone strength: Implications for muscle-bone crosstalk with aging and disuse. *Osteoporosis International, 29*(8), 1713–1720.
Kawahara, K., Suzuki, T., Yasaka, T., Nagata, H., Okamoto, Y., Kita, K., & Morisaki, H. (2017). Evaluation of the site specificity of acute disuse muscle atrophy developed during a relatively short period in critically ill patients according to the activities of daily living level: A prospective observational study. *Australian Critical Care, 30*(1), 29–36.
Lin, W.-C. (2017). A nursing experience of a burn patient at risk for disuse syndrome. *Tzu Chi Nursing Journal, 16*(4), 119–128.
Than, C., Tosovic, D., Seidl, L., & Mark Brown, J. (2016). The effect of exercise hypertrophy and disuse atrophy on muscle contractile properties: A mechanomyographic analysis. *European Journal of Applied Physiology, 116*(11/12), 2155–2165.

Decreased Diversional Activity Engagement

DEFINITION

Reduced stimulation, interest, or participation in recreational or leisure activities

RELATED FACTORS (R/T)

- Current setting does not allow engagement in activity
- Impaired mobility
- Environmental barrier
- Insufficient energy
- Insufficient motivation
- Physical discomfort
- Insufficient diversional activity

ASSOCIATED CONDITIONS

- Prescribed immobility
- Psychological distress
- Therapeutic isolation

ASSESSMENT

- Physical status, including level of comfort, mobility, and activity tolerance
- Cardiovascular status, including heart rate and rhythm, blood pressure sitting and standing, history of murmurs, cardiac disease
- Respiratory status, including respiratory rate and rhythm—resting and with activity, shortness of breath, cyanosis, and wheezing
- Neurologic status, including level of consciousness, orientation, mood, behavior, memory, and coordination
- Psychosocial status, including presence of family and friends, hobbies, and interests; social interaction, cultural and ethnic background; favorite music, television, and reading material; and changes or adaptations needed to carry out activities
- Environment, including isolation and availability of diversional activities
- Developmental level (physical, cognitive, psychosocial, and linguistic) and learning needs

DEFINING CHARACTERISTICS

- Alteration in mood
- Boredom
- Discontent with situation
- Flat affect
- Frequent naps
- Physical deconditioning

EXPECTED OUTCOMES

- Patient will express interest in using leisure time meaningfully.
- Patient will express interest in activities that can be provided.

- Patient will participate in chosen activity.
- Patient will watch selected television program or listen to radio program or selected music daily.
- Patient will report satisfaction with use of leisure time.
- Patient or caregiver will modify environment to provide maximum stimulation, such as by hanging posters or cards and moving bed next to a window.

Suggested NOC Outcomes

Leisure Participation; Motivation; Social Involvement; Personal Well-Being

INTERVENTIONS AND RATIONALES

PCC ▪ Encourage discussion of previously enjoyed hobbies, interests, or skills *to direct planning of new activities.* Suggest performing an activity helpful to others or otherwise productive *to promote self-fulfillment.*

PCC ▪ Obtain radio, CD player, iPod, or television (if desired) and allow patient to select programs. Communicate patient's desires to coworkers. Turn on television set at ____ (time) to ____ (channel). *Use of selective television, radio, and so on can help pass time.*

T&C ▪ Ask volunteers (friends, family, or hospital volunteer) to read newspapers, books, or magazines to patient at specific times. *Personal contact helps alleviate boredom.*

PCC ▪ Work with patient and family to find ways to carry out desired activities. Use imagination and creativity; for example, a former carpenter may adapt to carving small objects rather than building large ones. *Adaptive equipment helps patient pursue previous activities within new limits.*

PCC ▪ Engage patient in conversation while carrying out routine care. Discuss patient's favorite topics as much as possible. *Conversation conveys caring and recognition of patient's worth.*

PCC ▪ Provide various supplies and activities for the patient's use. Make sure items are appropriate to the patient's age, developmental level, and environment. *Ready access to diversional activities entices patient to make use of time alone. Age-appropriate items should be geared to the cognitive, motor, and safety needs.*

PCC ▪ Avoid scheduling procedures during patient's leisure time *to promote quality of life.*

- Provide talking books or CDs if available. *These provide low-effort sources of enjoyment for bedridden patient.*

- Obtain an adapter for television *to provide captions for hearing-impaired patient.*

PCC ▪ Encourage visitors to involve patient in favorite activities through discussion, reading, and attendance at programs, if appropriate, *to reduce boredom.*

PCC ▪ Encourage patient's family or caregiver to bring personal articles (posters, cards, and pictures) to help make environment more stimulating. *Patient may respond better to objects with personal meaning.*

T&C ▪ Make referral to recreational, occupational, or physical therapist for consultation on adaptive equipment to carry out desired activity; arrange for therapy sessions. *Adaptive equipment allows patient to continue enjoying activities or may stimulate interest in new activities.*

- Provide plants for patient to tend to. *Caring for live plants may stimulate interest.*

- Change scenery when possible; for example, take patient outside in wheelchair *to help reduce boredom.*

PCC ▪ Identify type of music patient prefers; seek help from family and hospital resources to provide selected music daily. *Music may relieve boredom and stimulate interest.*

Suggested NIC Interventions

Activity Therapy; Art Therapy; Energy Management; Recreation Therapy; Self-Responsibility Facilitation; Socialization Enhancement; Therapeutic Play; Visitation Facilitation

EVALUATIONS FOR EXPECTED OUTCOMES

- Patient expresses desire to participate in activities during leisure time.
- Patient discusses recent activity with staff members, family, or others.
- Patient engages in activity.
- Patient discusses content of television or radio program.
- Patient reports reduced feelings of boredom.
- Patient (or caregiver) has modified environment, thereby increasing stimulation.

DOCUMENTATION

- Patient's expression of boredom, frustration, and desire to carry out leisure activity
- Patient's interests and ability to carry out activity and necessary modifications required to accomplish activity
- Observations of patient's skill level and extent of participation in activity
- Patient's expression of satisfaction with use of unoccupied time
- Evaluations for expected outcomes

REFERENCES

Andrews, N. E., Strong, J., Meredith, P. J., & Branjerdporn, G. S. (2018). Approach to activity engagement and differences in activity participation in chronic pain: A five-day observational study. *Australian Occupational Therapy Journal, 65*(6), 575–585.

Hess, T. M., Growney, C. M., O'Brien, E. L., Neupert, S. D., & Sherwood, A. (2018). The role of cognitive costs, attitudes about aging, and intrinsic motivation in predicting engagement in everyday activities. *Psychology & Aging, 33*(6), 953–964.

Jones, B. A., Arcelus, J., Bouman, W. P., & Haycraft, E. (2017). Barriers and facilitators of physical activity and sport participation among young transgender adults who are medically transitioning. *International Journal of Transgenderism, 18*(2), 227–238.

Knibbe, T. J., Mcpherson, A. C., Gladstone, B., & Biddiss, E. (2018). "It's all about incentive": Social technology as a potential facilitator for self-determined physical activity participation for young people with physical disabilities. *Developmental Neurorehabilitation, 21*(8), 521–530.

Risk for Dry Eye

DEFINITION

Susceptible to inadequate tear film, which may cause eye discomfort and/or damage ocular surface, which may compromise health

RISK FACTORS

- Air conditioning
- Air pollution
- Caffeine consumption
- Decreased blinking frequency
- Excessive wind

- Inadequate knowledge of modifiable factors
- Inappropriate use of contact lenses
- Inappropriate use of fans
- Inappropriate use of hairdryer
- Inattentive to secondhand smoke
- Insufficient fluid intake
- Low air humidity
- Omega-3 fatty acid deficiency
- Smoking
- Sunlight exposure
- Use of products with benzalkonium chloride preservatives
- Vitamin A deficiency

ASSOCIATED CONDITIONS

- Artificial respiration
- Autoimmune diseases
- Chemotherapy
- Decreased blinking
- Decreased level of consciousness
- Hormonal change
- Incomplete eyelid closure
- Leukocytosis
- Metabolic diseases
- Neurological injury with sensory or motor reflex loss
- Neuromuscular blockade
- Oxygen therapy
- Pharmaceutical preparations
- Proptosis
- Radiotherapy
- Reduced tear volume
- Surgical procedures

ASSESSMENT

- Age
- Gender
- Physical condition of eye and surrounding tissue
- Health history, including accidents, allergies, exposure to pollutants, falls, hyperthermia, hypothermia, poisoning, sensory or perceptual changes (auditory, gustatory, kinesthetic, olfactory, tactile, and visual), and trauma
- Use of glasses or contact lenses
- Complaints and concerns about eyes

EXPECTED OUTCOMES

- Patient will not experience dry eyes.
- Patient will not experience eye irritation.
- Patient will state personal risk factors for dry eye.
- Patient will take steps to minimize risk factors.
- Patient will understand need for collaboration with health care team if signs/symptoms occur/persist.

Suggested NOC Outcomes

Risk Control; Risk Detection; Tissue Integrity: Skin/Mucous Membranes; Knowledge: Health Behavior

INTERVENTIONS AND RATIONALES

- Identify use of systemic medications that may decrease tear production and lifestyle behaviors that may potentiate dry eye conditions. *Assessment data may influence interventions.*
- Assess for history of medical conditions *to determine underlying risks for dry eye syndrome.*
- Modify physical environment to increase humidity, minimize excessive air movement, and control dust, *which can decrease tear production.*
- Administer artificial tears as indicated *to relieve symptoms.*
- **S** Perform protective measures such as preservative-free artificial tears or polyethylene eye cover for critically ill patients *to prevent eye damage due to dry eye syndrome.*
- **EBP** Teach about simple environmental modifications *to reduce evaporation of tears.* Encourage patient to take frequent breaks from visually demanding activities *to help minimize risk factors.* Suggest diet rich in omega-3 fatty acid or dietary supplement. *Diet low in omega-3 fatty acids can increase risk of dry eye syndrome.*
- **S** Instruct patient on the use of sunglasses *to limit exposure to light.*
- Instruct patient to try over-the-counter artificial tears *for temporary relief of dry eye.*
- **EBP** Encourage adherence to lifestyle modifications, *which will improve quality of life and decrease the risk of eye damage.*
- **T&C** Refer to an eye specialist if symptoms persist *for further evaluation and continued care.*
- Collaborate with primary care provider regarding possible changes in medications *that may be contributing to dry eye condition.*
- **T&C** Encourage annual eye examination *to monitor for any changes.*
- Offer written treatment guidelines as needed *to reinforce learning.*

Suggested NIC Interventions

Risk Management; Risk Identification; Behavior Management

EVALUATIONS FOR EXPECTED OUTCOMES

- Patient expresses relief of eye dryness.
- Patient expresses decrease in eye irritation.
- Patient states risk factors for dry eye.
- Patient recognizes possibility of adverse reaction to dry eye.
- Patient collaborates with health care team members.

DOCUMENTATION

- Patient's expressions of concern about adverse reaction and symptoms of previous episodes of dry eye
- Observations of physiological and behavioral manifestations of dry eye
- Interventions performed to allay adverse reaction
- Patient's response to interventions
- Evaluations for expected outcomes

REFERENCES

Bağbaba, A., Şen, B., Delen, D., & Uysal, B. S. (2018). An automated grading and diagnosis system for evaluation of dry eye syndrome. *Journal of Medical Systems, 42*(11), 227.

Clayton, J. A. (2018). Dry eye. *New England Journal of Medicine, 378*(23), 2212–2223.

de Lima Fernandes, A. P. N., de Medeiros Araújo, J. N., Botarelli, F. R., Pitombeira, D. O., Ferreira Júnior, M. A., & Vitor, A. F. (2018). Dry eye syndrome in intensive care units: A concept analysis. *Revista Brasileira de Enfermagem, 71*(3), 1162–1169.

Marshall, L. L., & Roach, J. M. (2016). Treatment of dry eye disease. *Consultant Pharmacist, 31*(2), 96–106.

Ineffective Dry Eye Self-Management

DEFINITION

Unsatisfactory management of symptoms, treatment regimen, physical, psychosocial, and spiritual consequences and lifestyle changes inherent in living with inadequate tear film

RELATED FACTORS (R/T)

- Cognitive dysfunction
- Competing demands
- Competing lifestyle preferences
- Conflict between health behaviors and social norms
- Decreased perceived quality of life
- Difficulty accessing community resources
- Difficulty managing complex treatment regimen
- Difficulty navigating complex health care systems
- Difficulty with decision-making
- Inadequate commitment to a plan of action
- Inadequate health literacy
- Inadequate knowledge of treatment regimen
- Inadequate number of cues to action
- Inadequate role models
- Inadequate social support
- Limited ability to perform aspects of treatment regimen
- Low self-efficacy
- Negative feelings toward treatment regimen
- Nonacceptance of condition
- Perceived barrier to treatment regimen
- Perceived social stigma associated with condition
- Unrealistic perception of seriousness of condition
- Unrealistic perception of susceptibility to sequelae
- Unrealistic perception of treatment benefit

ASSOCIATED CONDITIONS

- Allergies
- Autoimmune diseases
- Chemotherapy

- Developmental disabilities
- Graft versus host disease
- Incomplete eyelid closure
- Leukocytosis
- Metabolic diseases
- Neurological injury with motor reflex loss
- Neurological injury with sensory reflex loss
- Oxygen therapy
- Pharmaceutical preparations
- Proptosis
- Radiotherapy
- Reduced tear volume
- Surgical procedures

ASSESSMENT

- Age
- Gender
- Physical condition of eye and surrounding tissue
- Health history, including accidents, allergies, exposure to pollutants, falls, hyperthermia, hypothermia, poisoning, sensory or perceptual changes (auditory, gustatory, kinesthetic, olfactory, tactile, and visual), and trauma
- Use of glasses or contact lenses
- Complaints and concerns about eyes

DEFINING CHARACTERISTICS

Dry Eye Signs

- Chemosis
- Conjunctival hyperemia
- Epiphora
- Filamentary keratitis
- Keratoconjunctival staining with fluorescein
- Low aqueous tear production according to Schirmer I Test
- Mucous plaques

Dry Eye Symptoms

- Expresses dissatisfaction with quality of life
- Reports blurred vision
- Reports eye fatigue
- Reports feeling of burning eyes
- Reports feeling of ocular dryness
- Reports feeling of ocular foreign body
- Reports feeling of ocular itching
- Reports feeling of sand in eye

Behaviors

- Difficulty performing eyelid care
- Difficulty reducing caffeine consumption

- Inadequate maintenance of air humidity
- Inadequate use of eyelid closure device
- Inadequate use of prescribed medication
- Inappropriate use of contact lenses
- Inappropriate use of fans
- Inappropriate use of hairdryer
- Inappropriate use of moisture chamber goggles
- Inattentive to dry eye signs
- Inattentive to dry eye symptoms
- Inattentive to second hand smoke
- Insufficient dietary intake of omega-3 fatty acids
- Insufficient dietary intake of vitamin A
- Insufficient fluid intake
- Nonadherence to recommended blinking exercises
- Nonadherence to recommended eye breaks
- Use of products with benzalkonium chloride preservatives

EXPECTED OUTCOMES

- Patient will take steps to minimize dry eyes.
- Patient will not experience eye irritation.
- Patient will state personal risk factors for dry eye.
- Patient will collaborate with health care team for signs/symptoms of dry eyes.

Suggested NOC Outcomes

Risk Control; Risk Detection; Tissue Integrity: Skin/Mucous Membranes; Knowledge: Health Behavior

INTERVENTIONS AND RATIONALES

EBP
- Identify use of systemic medications that may decrease tear production and lifestyle behaviors that may potentiate dry eye conditions. *Assessment data may influence interventions.*

PCC
- Assess for history of medical conditions *to determine underlying risks for dry eye syndrome.*

PCC
- Modify physical environment to increase humidity, minimize excessive air movement, and control dust, *which can decrease tear production.*

- Administer artificial tears as indicated *to relieve symptoms.*

S
- Perform protective measures such as preservative-free artificial tears or polyethylene eye cover for critically ill patients *to prevent eye damage due to dry eye syndrome.*

EBP
- Teach about simple environmental modifications *to reduce evaporation of tears.* Encourage patient to take frequent breaks from visually demanding activities *to help minimize risk factors.* Suggest diet rich in omega-3 fatty acid or dietary supplement. *Diet low in omega-3 fatty acids can increase risk of dry eye syndrome.*

S
- Instruct patient on the use of sunglasses *to limit exposure to light.*

- Instruct patient to try over-the-counter artificial tears *for temporary relief of dry eye.*

EBP
- Encourage adherence to lifestyle modifications, *which will improve quality of life and decrease the risk of eye damage.*

T&C ▒ Refer to eye specialist if symptoms persist *for further evaluation and continued care.*
▒ Collaborate with primary care provider regarding possible changes in medications *that may be contributing to dry eye condition.*
T&C ▒ Encourage annual eye exam *to monitor for any changes.*
▒ Offer written treatment guidelines as needed *to reinforce learning.*

Suggested NIC Interventions

Risk Management; Risk Identification; Behavior management

EVALUATIONS FOR EXPECTED OUTCOMES

▒ Patient will take steps to minimize dry eyes.
▒ Patient will not experience eye irritation.
▒ Patient will state personal risk factors for dry eye.
▒ Patient will understand need for collaboration with health care team for signs/symptoms of dry eyes.
▒ Patient expresses confidence ability to perform activities in plan of care.
▒ Patient expresses willingness to participate in plan of care.
▒ Patient expresses relief of eye dryness.
▒ Patient expresses decrease in eye irritation.
▒ Patient states risk factors for dry eye.
▒ Patient recognizes adverse reactions due to eye dryness.
▒ Patient seeks assistance from health care team members as needed.

DOCUMENTATION

▒ Patient's expressions of confidence in self-care for symptoms of dry eye
▒ Patient's expressions of concern about adverse reaction and symptoms of previous episodes of dry eye
▒ Observations of physiologic and behavioral manifestations of dry eye
▒ Interventions performed to allay adverse reaction
▒ Patient's response to interventions
▒ Evaluations for expected outcomes

REFERENCES

de Araujo, D. D., Silva, D. V. A., Rodrigues, C. A. O., Silva, P. O., Macieira, T. G. R., & Chianca, T. C. M. (2019). Effectiveness of nursing interventions to prevent dry eye in critically ill patients. *American Journal of Critical Care, 28*(4), 299–306.

Establishing a Protocol for the Management of Dry Eye Disease. (2021). *Ocular Surgery News,* 3–11.

Ross, E., Furniss, E., Chandramohan, N., & Markoulli, M. (2021). The multi-faceted approach to dry eye disease. *Clinical & Experimental Optometry, 104*(3), 417–420.

Shin, Y. J. (2019). Recent treatment of dry eye. *Journal of the Korean Medical Association/Taehan Uisa Hyophoe Chi, 62*(4), 218–223.

Risk for Dry Mouth

DEFINITION

Susceptible to discomfort or damage to the oral mucosa due to reduced quantity or quality of saliva to moisten the mucosa, which may compromise health

RISK FACTORS

- Dehydration
- Depression
- Excessive stress
- Excitement
- Smoking

ASSESSMENT

- Age
- Gender
- Oral status, including inspection of oral cavity (gums and tongue), pain or discomfort, and salivation
- Health history including current illness and medications
- History of pathologic conditions known to cause dehydration such as diabetes mellitus
- Nutritional status, including current weight, change from normal weight, and dietary pattern
- Psychosocial status, including change in financial status, coping skills, habits (smoking and alcohol intake), patient's perception of health problem, and recent traumatic event
- Oxygen therapy
- Ability to feed self and perform oral hygiene

ASSOCIATED CONDITIONS

- Chemotherapy
- Fluid restriction
- Inability to feed orally
- Oxygen therapy
- Pharmaceutical agent
- Pregnancy
- Radiation therapy to the head and neck
- Systemic diseases

EXPECTED OUTCOMES

- Patient will have intact oral mucosa.
- Patient will have pink, moist oral mucous membranes.
- Patient will have minimal, if any, complications.
- Patient will participate with appropriate oral care.
- Patient will demonstrate oral hygiene practices.

Suggested NOC Outcomes

Hydration; Nutritional Status; Oral Health; Self-Care: Oral Hygiene; Tissue Integrity: Skin & Mucous Membranes

INTERVENTIONS AND RATIONALES

S   Inspect patient's oral cavity every shift. Describe and document condition; report any change in status. *Regular assessments can anticipate or alleviate problems.*

S ▪ Perform the prescribed treatment regimen with artificial saliva product *to improve the condition of patient's mucous membranes*. Monitor progress, reporting favorable and adverse responses to the treatment regimen.

EBP ▪ Provide supportive measures, as indicated:
  ▪ Assist with oral hygiene before and after meals *to promote a feeling of comfort and well-being*.
  ▪ Position patient in High Fowler's (unless contraindicated) to perform oral care *to reduce risk of aspiration*.
  ▪ Use a toothbrush with suction if patient can't spit out water *to minimize risk of aspiration*.
  ▪ Provide mouthwash or gargles, as ordered, *to increase patient comfort and maintain moisture in the mouth*.
  ▪ Lubricate patient's lips frequently with water-based lubricant *to prevent cracked, irritated skin*.

EBP ▪ Instruct patient in oral hygiene practices, if necessary. Have patient return a demonstration of the oral care routine.
  ▪ Use a soft-bristled toothbrush.
  ▪ Brush with a circular motion away from the gums.
  ▪ Include the tongue when brushing.

EBP ▪ Instruct patient to chew gum or suck on sugarless hard candy *to stimulate salivation*.

EBP ▪ Instruct patient to use alcohol-free mouthwash. *Products containing alcohol have a drying effect on the mucous membranes*.

EBP ▪ Discuss precipitating factors, if known, and work to prevent future episodes. For example, encourage patient to stay hydrated and to report effects of medication. *Patient's increased awareness of causative factors will help prevent recurrence*.

PCC ▪ Encourage adherence to other aspects of health care management (controlling diabetes, changing dietary habits, and avoiding alcoholic beverages) *to control or minimize effects on mucous membranes*.

Suggested NIC Interventions

Oral Health Maintenance; Oral Health Promotion; Oral Health Restoration; Self-Care Assistance

EVALUATIONS FOR EXPECTED OUTCOMES

▪ Patient's mucous membranes remain moist, pink, and free from cuts and abrasions.
▪ Patient doesn't develop complications related to extended dehydration of mucous membranes.
▪ Patient discusses possible causes of alteration in oral mucous membranes, such as dehydration and reactions to medication.
▪ Patient discusses and demonstrates preventive measures such as regular oral hygiene.

DOCUMENTATION

▪ Observations of condition, healing, and response to treatment
▪ Interventions to provide supportive care and patient's response to supportive care
▪ Instructions given, patient's understanding of instructions, and patient's demonstrated skill in carrying out prescribed oral care measures
▪ Evaluations for expected outcomes

REFERENCES

Appleby, N. J., Temple-Smith, M. J., Stacey, M. A., Bailey, D. L., Deveny, E. M., & Pirotta, M. (2016). General practitioners' knowledge and management of dry mouth—A qualitative study. *Australian Family Physician, 45*(12), 902–906.

Epstein, J. B., Villines, D. C., Singh, M., & Papas, A. (2017). Management of dry mouth: Assessment of oral symptoms after use of a polysaccharide-based oral rinse. *Oral Surgery, Oral Medicine, Oral Pathology & Oral Radiology, 123*(1), 76–83.

Gadalla, H. (2018). Treating dry mouth: Dry mouth/xerostomia are common conditions that need a multifaceted approach to mitigate symptoms. *Dimensions of Dental Hygiene, 16*(7), 25–30.

Villa, A., Nordio, F., & Gohel, A. (2016). A risk prediction model for xerostomia: A retrospective cohort study. *Gerodontology, 33*(4), 562–568.

Ineffective Adolescent Eating Dynamics

Altered eating attitudes and behaviors resulting in over or under eating patterns that compromise nutritional health

- Altered family dynamics
- Anxiety
- Changes to self-esteem upon entering puberty
- Depression
- Eating disorder
- Eating in isolation
- Excessive family mealtime control
- Excessive stress
- Inadequate choice of food
- Irregular mealtime
- Media influence on eating behaviors of high caloric unhealthy foods
- Media influence on knowledge of high caloric unhealthy foods
- Negative parental influences on eating behaviors
- Psychological abuse
- Psychological neglect
- Stressful mealtimes

- Physical challenge with eating
- Physical challenge with feeding
- Physical issues of parents
- Psychological health issues of parents

- Health history, including previous eating disorders; dieting; physical, emotional, or sexual abuse; and episodes of emesis and self-induced emesis
- History of weight loss or gain of 2 lb/week
- Cardiovascular status, including skin color and temperature, heart rate and rhythm, blood pressure, and complete blood count
- Nutritional status, including daily food intake, food likes and dislikes, meal preparation, and knowledge of dietary requirements; height and weight (and weight fluctuations) over past year; serum albumin, lymphocyte, and electrolyte levels; and signs of malnutrition or dehydration

- Psychological status, including expressions of need for control or perceived loss of self-control, behavioral changes, expressions of helplessness, recent emotional crisis, stress, and body image
- Family status, including role performance, perception of role within family, and attitudes and perceptions related to food, body image, success, and control

DEFINING CHARACTERISTICS

- Avoids participation in regular mealtimes
- Complains of hunger between meals
- Food refusal
- Frequent snacking
- Frequently eating from fast food restaurants
- Frequently eating poor quality food
- Frequently eating processed food
- Over eating
- Poor appetite
- Under eating

EXPECTED OUTCOMES

Adolescent will:
- comply with prescribed treatment.
- express feelings associated with food, exercise, weight loss, and medical condition.
- describe perception of personal daily caloric needs.
- express understanding that current eating and exercise patterns are self-destructive.
- consume appropriate number of calories each day.
- ask for help in controlling destructive behavior.
- participate in decisions about care and participate in support group for people with eating disorders.
- express insight into reasons behind current eating patterns and other self-destructive behaviors.

Suggested NOC Outcomes

Body Image; Child Development: Adolescence; Nutritional Status; Psychosocial Adjustment: Life Change; Self-Esteem; Weight: Body Mass

INTERVENTIONS AND RATIONALES

S ▦ Monitor and record adolescent's vital signs, weight, and electrolyte levels *to detect abnormal values and prevent complications.*

T&C ▦ Obtain a referral for dietary consultation *to identify caloric intake, necessary diet modifications, and goals for weight gain and stabilization.*

PCC ▦ Encourage adolescent to participate in self-care and, as appropriate, to make decisions about therapy *to foster a sense of control and involvement in restoring health.*

EBP ▦ Teach adolescent about nutritional requirements needed for specific weight and age. Discuss various meal choices available. *Providing instruction in writing simplifies adolescent's role in selecting healthy foods.*

PCC ▦ Encourage adolescent to express feelings about self, eating, and exercise *to correct misconceptions, clarify thoughts, and reinforce realistic self-appraisal.*

PCC ■ Reinforce appropriate behaviors *to encourage the adolescent to comply with therapy and to participate in care.*

EBP ■ Use behavior modification strategies consistently *to enable adolescent to predict consequences of behavior.*

■ Avoid using coercive techniques to make adolescent participate in care or adhere to rules. *Use of coercion may encourage adolescent to view manipulative behavior as acceptable.*

S ■ Monitor food consumption and record intake *to ensure that adolescent consumes prescribed calories.*

S ■ Monitor adolescent in the bathroom *to detect episodes of purging.*

PCC ■ Without conveying an attitude of distrust, watch for signs of noncompliance with the medical regimen. Emphasize that prescribed caloric intake is necessary to maintain health. *This promotes early detection of self-destructive behavior and may improve adolescent's sense of control.*

PCC ■ Encourage adolescent's participation in group discussions with peers who also have eating disorders *to foster insight and group support.*

PCC ■ Encourage parents to demonstrate emotional support for adolescent throughout the course of treatment *to strengthen the family support system.*

PCC ■ Encourage parents to participate in a support group with other parents of adolescents with eating disorders *to provide a forum for expressing feelings and obtaining support from individuals who can understand their concerns.*

EBP ■ Teach parents how to detect signs that their child may be relapsing into self-destructive behaviors *to help them identify the need for early assistance and enhance their confidence in their ability to protect their child from harm.*

Suggested NIC Interventions

Active Listening; Body Image Enhancement; Coping Enhancement; Counseling; Developmental Enhancement: Adolescent; Parent Education: Adolescent; Support Group; Therapy Group

EVALUATIONS FOR EXPECTED OUTCOMES

■ Adolescent complies with prescribed treatment regimen.
■ Adolescent expresses feelings associated with food, exercise, weight loss, and medical condition.
■ Adolescent describes perception of personal daily caloric needs.
■ Adolescent expresses understanding that current eating and exercise patterns are self-destructive.
■ Adolescent consumes appropriate number of calories each day.
■ Adolescent asks for help in controlling destructive behavior.
■ Adolescent participates in decisions related to care and treatment.
■ Adolescent participates in support group for people with eating disorders.
■ Adolescent expresses insight into reasons behind eating patterns and other self-destructive behaviors.
■ Adolescent expresses satisfaction with parental involvement in care.

DOCUMENTATION

■ Vital signs
■ Weight (recorded daily or weekly according to facility's protocol)
■ Amount of food consumed at each meal
■ Adolescent's description of self

- Observations of rituals related to food and exercise
- Adolescent's participation in and response to support group
- Observations of self-destructive behaviors, such as forced emesis or use of laxatives or diuretics
- Exercise patterns
- Behavior modification techniques used by caregivers
- Adolescent's response to treatment protocol
- Adolescent's response to nursing interventions
- Evaluations for expected outcomes

REFERENCES

Forrest, L. N., Smith, A. R., & Swanson, S. A. (2017). Characteristics of seeking treatment among U.S. adolescents with eating disorders. *International Journal of Eating Disorders, 50*(7), 826–833.

Hicks White, A. A., Pratt, K. J., & Cottrill, C. (2018). The relationship between trauma and weight status among adolescents in eating disorder treatment. *Appetite, 129,* 62–69.

Richards, I. L., Subar, A., Touyz, S., & Rhodes, P. (2018). Augmentative approaches in family-based treatment for adolescents with restrictive eating disorders: A systematic review. *European Eating Disorders Review, 26*(2), 92–111.

Simic, M., Stewart, C. S., Eisler, I., Baudinet, J., Hunt, K., O'Brien, J., & McDermott, B. (2018). Intensive treatment program (ITP): A case series service evaluation of the effectiveness of day patient treatment for adolescents with a restrictive eating disorder. *International Journal of Eating Disorders, 51*(11), 1261–1269.

Ineffective Child Eating Dynamics

DEFINITION

Altered attitudes, behaviors and influences on child eating patterns resulting in compromised nutritional health

RELATED FACTORS (R/T)

Eating Habit

- Bribing child to eat
- Consumption of large volumes of food in a short period of time
- Disordered eating habits
- Eating in isolation
- Excessive parental control over child's eating experience
- Excessive parental control over family mealtime
- Forcing child to eat
- Inadequate choice of food
- Lack of regular mealtimes
- Limiting child's eating
- Rewarding child to eat
- Stressful mealtimes
- Unpredictable eating patterns
- Unstructured eating or snacks between meals

Family Process

- Abusive relationship
- Anxious parent–child relationship
- Disengaged parenting style

▓ Hostile parent–child relationship
▓ Insecure parent–child relationship
▓ Over-involved parenting style
▓ Tense parent–child relationship
▓ Under-involved parenting style

Parental

▓ Anorexia
▓ Depression
▓ Inability to divide eating responsibility between parent and child
▓ Inability to divide feeding responsibility between parent and child
▓ Inability to support healthy eating patterns
▓ Ineffective coping strategies
▓ Lack of confidence in child to develop healthy eating habits
▓ Lack of confidence in child to grow appropriately
▓ Substance abuse

Environmental

▓ Media influence on eating behaviors of high caloric unhealthy foods
▓ Media influence on knowledge of high caloric unhealthy foods

ASSOCIATED CONDITIONS

▓ Physical challenge with eating
▓ Physical challenge with feeding
▓ Physical issues of parents
▓ Psychological health issues of parents

ASSESSMENT

▓ Eating habits
▓ Nutritional status, including daily food intake, food likes and dislikes, meal preparation, and knowledge of dietary requirements; height and weight (and weight fluctuations) over past year; serum albumin, lymphocyte, and electrolyte levels; and signs of malnutrition or dehydration
▓ Health history, including previous eating disorders; dieting; physical, emotional, or sexual abuse; and episodes of emesis and self-induced emesis
▓ History of weight loss or gain of 2 lb/week
▓ Cardiovascular status, including skin color and temperature, heart rate and rhythm, blood pressure, and complete blood count
▓ Psychological status, including expressions of need for control or perceived loss of self-control, behavioral changes, expressions of helplessness, recent emotional crisis, stress, and body image
▓ Family status, including role performance, perception of role within family, and attitudes and perceptions related to food, body image, success, and control

DEFINING CHARACTERISTICS

▓ Avoids participation in regular mealtimes
▓ Complains of hunger between meals
▓ Food refusal
▓ Frequent snacking
▓ Frequently eating from fast food restaurants

- Frequently eating poor quality food
- Frequently eating processed food
- Over eating
- Poor appetite
- Under eating

EXPECTED OUTCOMES

Child will:
- participate in regular mealtimes.
- only eat when hungry and stop eating when full.
- identify favorite foods and disliked foods.
- consume appropriate number of calories each day.

Parent(s) will:
- identify appropriate nutritious foods.
- limit purchasing fast foods and convenience foods.
- not restrict child's eating.
- not pressure child to eat.
- participate in meal planning.
- participate in support group for people with eating disorders.
- express insight into reasons behind current eating patterns.

Suggested NOC Outcomes

Appetite; Adherence Behavior: Healthy Diet; Compliance Behavior: Prescribed Diet; Knowledge: Eating Disorder Management; Nutritional Status: Nutrient Intake

INTERVENTIONS AND RATIONALES

S • Monitor and record child's vital signs, weight, and electrolyte levels *to detect abnormal values and prevent complications.*

T&C • Obtain a referral for dietary consultation *to identify caloric intake, necessary diet modifications, and goals for weight gain and stabilization.*

PCC • Assess child's food preferences *to identify foods that will stimulate child's appetite.*

PCC • Encourage child to participate in self-care and, as appropriate, to make decisions about therapy *to foster a sense of control and involvement in restoring health.*

EBP • Assist child in recognizing the feeling of hunger, *learning to differentiate hunger from other feelings assists in preventing eating in the absence of hunger.*

EBP • Teach child's parents about nutritional requirements needed for specific weight and age. Discuss various meal choices available. *Providing instruction in writing simplifies the selecting healthy foods.*

S • Monitor food consumption and record intake *to ensure that the child consumes prescribed calories.*

EBP • Encourage parents to limit when and where child eats *helps to foster healthy eating patterns.*

PCC • Encourage parents to explore their beliefs about food and eating *to develop understanding of parental role in feeding and meal planning.*

PCC • Encourage parents to participate in a support group with other parents of children with eating disorders *to provide a forum for expressing feelings and obtaining support from individuals who can understand their concerns.*

Suggested NIC Interventions

Diet Staging; Feeding; Nutrition Therapy; Nutritional Counseling; Nutritional Monitoring; Weight Management

EVALUATIONS FOR EXPECTED OUTCOMES

Child:
- participates in regular mealtimes.
- only eats when hungry and stops eating when full.
- identifies favorite foods and preferences.
- identifies disliked foods.
- consumes appropriate number of calories each day.

Parent(s):
- identify appropriate nutritious foods.
- limit purchasing fast foods or convenience foods to once per week.
- plan meals that meet caloric needs of child.
- eliminate feeding restrictive behaviors.
- eliminate pressuring child to eat.
- eliminate excessive monitoring of child's eating.
- participate in support group for people with eating disorders.
- discuss reasons behind current family eating patterns.

DOCUMENTATION

- Vital signs
- Child's stated appetite
- Weight (recorded daily or weekly according to facility's protocol)
- Amount of food consumed at each meal
- Observations of rituals related to food and exercise
- Number of convenience meals eaten in a week
- Child's response to treatment protocol
- Child's response to nursing interventions
- Parental use of bribes during meals
- Evaluations for expected outcomes

REFERENCES

Decataldo, A., & Fiore, B. (2018). Is eating in the school canteen better to fight overweight? A sociological observational study on nutrition in Italian children. *Children & Youth Services Review, 94*, 246–256.

Gomes, A. I., Barros, L., Pereira, A. I., & Roberto, M. S. (2018). Effectiveness of a parental school-based intervention to improve young children's eating patterns: A pilot study. *Public Health Nutrition, 21*(13), 2485–2496.

Munkholm, A., Bjorner, J. B., Petersen, J., Micali, N., Olsen, E. M., & Skovgaard, A. M. (2017). Validation of the eating pattern inventory for children in a general population sample of 11- to 12-year-old children. *Assessment, 24*(6), 810–819.

Schmidt, R., Vogel, M., Hiemisch, A., Kiess, W., & Hilbert, A. (2018). Pathological and non-pathological variants of restrictive eating behaviors in middle childhood: A latent class analysis. *Appetite, 127*, 257–265.

Risk for Electrolyte Imbalance

DEFINITION

Susceptible to changes in serum electrolyte levels, which may compromise health

RISK FACTORS

- Diarrhea
- Excessive fluid volume
- Insufficient fluid volume
- Insufficient knowledge of modifiable factors
- Vomiting

ASSOCIATED CONDITIONS

- Compromised regulatory mechanism
- Endocrine regulatory dysfunction
- Renal dysfunction
- Treatment regimen

ASSESSMENT

- Fluid and electrolyte status, weight, intake and output, urine specific gravity, skin turgor, mucous membranes
- Results of laboratory tests including serum electrolytes, blood urea nitrogen
- Vital signs including heart rate and rhythm, blood pressure, pulse
- History of renal, cardiac, and gastrointestinal disorders

EXPECTED OUTCOMES

- Patient will maintain electrolyte levels within normal limits.
- Patient will maintain adequate fluid balance consistent with underlying disease restrictions.
- Patient will identify health situations that increase risk for electrolyte imbalance and verbalize interventions to promote balance.
- Patient will verbalize signs and symptoms that require immediate intervention by health care provider.
- Patient will remain safe from injury associated with electrolyte imbalance.

Suggested NOC Outcomes

Electrolyte & Acid–Base Balance; Fluid Balance

INTERVENTIONS AND RATIONALES

- **S** ▪ Assess patient's fluid status. *Patients who demonstrate fluid volume alterations are likely to have electrolyte alterations as well.*
- **S** ▪ Monitor patient for physical signs of electrolyte imbalance. *Many cardiac, neurologic, and musculoskeletal symptoms are indicative of specific electrolyte abnormalities.*
- **S** ▪ Collect and evaluate serum electrolyte results as ordered *to allow for prompt diagnosis and treatment of any abnormalities.*
- **EBP** ▪ Educate patient and family regarding risks for electrolyte disturbances associated with their particular medical condition and possible interventions if symptoms occur. *Early identification and intervention may prevent life-threatening complications of electrolyte imbalance.*

PCC ▪ Provide support and encouragement to patient and family in their efforts to participate in the management of the condition. *Positive feedback will increase self-confidence and feeling of partnership in care.*

T&C ▪ Coordinate care with other members of the health care team to provide safe environment. *Electrolyte imbalances can cause poor coordination, weakness, and altered gait.*

Suggested NIC Interventions

Electrolyte Management; Electrolyte Monitoring; Fluid–Electrolyte Management; Laboratory Data Interpretation

EVALUATIONS FOR EXPECTED OUTCOMES

▪ Patient's electrolyte levels remain within normal limits.
▪ Patient's fluid balance is consistent with restrictions of underlying disease.
▪ Patient identifies health situations that increase the risk for electrolyte imbalance and interventions to promote balance.
▪ Patient verbalizes signs and symptoms that require immediate interventions by a health care provider.
▪ Patient remains safe from injury associated with electrolyte imbalance.

DOCUMENTATION

▪ Record of patient's electrolyte results and interventions
▪ Record of patient's fluid status
▪ Patient's understanding of signs and symptoms that require intervention of a health care provider
▪ Evaluations for expected outcomes

REFERENCES

Ellison, D., & Cisneros Farrar, F. (2018). Kidney influence on fluid and electrolyte balance. *Nursing Clinics of North America, 53*(4), 469–480.
Giordano, M., Ciarambino, T., Castellino, P., Malatino, L., Di Somma, S., Biolo, G., … Adinolfi, L. E. (2016). Diseases associated with electrolyte imbalance in the ED: Age-related differences. *American Journal of Emergency Medicine, 34*(10), 1923–1926.
Kear, T. M. (2017). Fluid and electrolyte management across the age continuum. *Nephrology Nursing Journal, 44*(6), 491–497.
Walker, M. D. (2016). Fluid and electrolyte imbalances: Interpretation and assessment. *Journal of Infusion Nursing, 39*(6), 382–386.

Risk for Elopement Attempt

DEFINITION

Susceptible to leaving a health care facility or a designated area against recommendation or without communicating to health care professionals or caregivers, which may compromise safety and/or health

RISK FACTORS

▪ Anger behaviors
▪ Dissatisfaction with current situation
▪ Exit-seeking behavior

- Frustration about delay in treatment regimen
- Inadequate caregiver vigilance
- Inadequate interest in improving health
- Inadequate social support
- Perceived complexity of treatment regimen
- Perceived excessive family responsibilities
- Perceived excessive responsibilities in interpersonal relations
- Perceived lack of safety in surrounding environment
- Persistent wandering
- Psychomotor agitation
- Self-harm intent
- Substance misuse

ASSOCIATED CONDITIONS

- Autism spectrum disorder
- Developmental disabilities
- Mental disorders

ASSESSMENT

- Age
- Mental status (anxiety, stress, depression, agitation, fear)
- Cognitive status (dementia, developmental disabilities, altered mental status)
- Legal status of patient (court-ordered treatment/voluntary, minor, adult)
- Expressions of frustration or anger
- History of substance misuse
- Support systems in place

EXPECTED OUTCOMES

- Patient will not leave treatment or residence unattended or without permission.
- Patient will not leave secured area.
- Patient will participate in treatment plan.
- Patient will collaborate with health care team.
- Patient will remain in safe environment.

Suggested NOC Outcomes

Elopement Occurrence; Elopement Propensity Risk

INTERVENTIONS AND RATIONALES

- **PCC** Assess patient's mental status and cognitive function *to determine patient's ability to make decisions.*
- **PCC** Assess patient for signs of intended elopement—verbal expression of wanting to leave, packing belongings, loitering near exits, attempting to open doors *behaviors may indicate patient's intent to leave.*
- **S** Maintain a physically secure environment with alarms *to alert staff of patient's attempt to leave.*
- **S** Supervise patient when not in a secure area *decreases patient anxiety.*

PCC ▓ Encourage patient to seek assistance from health care team for feelings of anxiety, fear, etc. *Allows health care team to develop interventions specific to patient's needs.*

EBP ▓ Discuss with patient the consequences for leaving against medical advice *patient may not fully understand the negative effects of leaving before goals are met.*

PCC EBP ▓ Work with patient to develop plan of care that meets patient's needs *autonomy and/or collaboration increases compliance with plan of care.*

Suggested NIC Interventions

Elopement Precautions

EVALUATIONS FOR EXPECTED OUTCOMES

▓ Patient does not leave treatment or residence unattended or without permission.
▓ Patient does not leave secured area unattended.
▓ Patient participates in treatment plan.
▓ Patient collaborates with health care team.
▓ Patient expresses importance of remaining in safe environment.

DOCUMENTATION

▓ Patients current physical description (height, weight, hair color, eye color, any distinguishing characteristics)
▓ Patient's mental status
▓ Patient's cognitive assessment
▓ Risk factors and behaviors of intent to leave facility
▓ Patient's expressions to remain in a safe environment
▓ Teaching and instructions provided to patient and family member or other caregivers
▓ Evaluations for expected outcomes

REFERENCES

Beaulieu, T., Krishnamoorthy, A., Lima, V., Li, T., Wu, A., Montaner, J., Barrios, R., & Ti, L. (2019). Impact of personality disorders on leaving hospital against medical advice among people living with HIV in British Columbia, Canada. *Social Psychiatry & Psychiatric Epidemiology, 54*(9), 1153–1159.

Haines, K., Freeman, J., Vastaas, C., Rust, C., Cox, C., Kasotakis, G., Fuller, M., Krishnamoorthy, V., Siciliano, M., Alger, A., Montgomery, S., & Agarwal, S. (2020). "I'm Leaving": Factors that impact against medical advice disposition post-trauma. *Journal of Emergency Medicine (0736-4679), 58*(4), 691–697.

Mahajan, R. K., Gautam, P. L., Paul, G., & Mahajan, R. (2019). Retrospective evaluation of patients leaving against medical advice in a tertiary care teaching hospital. *Indian Journal of Critical Care Medicine, 23*(3), 139–142.

Misumida, N., Abdel-Latif, A., Smyth, S. S., Messerli, A. W., Ziada, K. M., Ogunbayo, G. O., & Shrout, T. A. (2019). Trends, management patterns, and predictors of leaving against medical advice among patients with documented noncompliance admitted for acute myocardial infarction. *JGIM: Journal of General Internal Medicine, 34*(4), 486–488.

Impaired Emancipated Decision-Making

DEFINITION

A process of choosing a health care decision that does not include personal knowledge and/ or consideration of social norms, or does not occur in a flexible environment, resulting in decisional dissatisfaction

- Decrease in understanding of all available health care options
- Inability to adequately verbalize perceptions about health care options
- Inadequate time to discuss health care options
- Insufficient confidence to openly discuss health care options
- Insufficient information regarding health care options
- Insufficient privacy to openly discuss health care options
- Insufficient self-confidence in decision-making

ASSESSMENT

- Levels of consciousness and orientation
- Age
- Stage of development
- Presence of cognitive impairment
- Level of education
- Language fluency

DEFINING CHARACTERISTICS

- Delay in enacting chosen health care option
- Distress when listening to other's opinion
- Excessive concern about what others think is the best decision
- Excessive fear of what others think about a decision
- Feeling constrained in describing own opinion
- Inability to choose a health care option that best fits current lifestyle
- Inability to describe how option will fit into current lifestyle
- Limited verbalization about health care option in other's presence

EXPECTED OUTCOMES

- The patient will demonstrate consideration of how available health care choices fit with their values, beliefs, preferences, and lifestyle.
- The patient will express consideration of their own values, beliefs, and preferences, independent of those of others in considering the available health care options.
- The patient will verbalize opinion freely.
- The patient will make a health care choice.
- The patient will verbalize satisfaction with health care choice based on the available options.

Suggested NOC Outcomes

Decision-Making; Information Processing; Participation in Health Care Decisions

INTERVENTIONS AND RATIONALES

PCC ▪ Engage patient in the therapeutic relationship. Demonstrate an attitude of respect, patience, and acceptance. *Persons who feel cared for, understood, and respected in health care situations are better motivated to collaboratively participate in their care.*

PCC ■ Continually assess for readiness to make a health care choice *to promote timely decision-making.*

PCC ■ Ensure privacy for one-to-one interaction between patient and nurse. *Patient's status in relationships with family/loved ones may inhibit frank discussion in their presence.*

PCC ■ Ensure that communications and information provided are at a level consistent with patient's cognitive abilities *to ensure understanding.*

PCC ■ Avoid limiting choices based on health care provider preference, values, or beliefs and avoid encouraging one choice over another. *The health care team is accountable to patient to provide appropriate information on all available options and to promote autonomous decision-making.*

PCC ■ Explore with patient the meaning of experience of making a health care decision. Ask what meanings the current health care situation and having to make a health care decision have for the patient. *The health care need and necessity to make a health care decision may represent a crisis for the patient. Understanding patient's experience of this can direct the identification of other necessary assessments and interventions.*

PCC ■ Discuss patient's emotional experience of needing to make a health care choice. *Patient may feel anger, fear, anxiety, pressured, or overwhelmed by the need to choose or the choices offered.*

PCC ■ Validate patient's experience, and ask permission to discuss patient's thoughts and feelings about own choices. Identify any anxiety or fear related to making a decision. *Fear and anxiety can lead to anger, feeling pressured or overwhelmed, procrastination, and/or excessive seeing of reassurance or opinions from others.*

PCC ■ If fear or anxiety is present, validate patient's experience *to promote self-esteem, strengthen the therapeutic relationship, and promote autonomous decision-making.*

EBP ■ Provide clarifying information about choices if needed. *Misinterpretations of information may lead to difficulty making a decision.*

T&C ■ Refer to professional support to address anxious distorted thoughts if needed. *Counseling may be required to assist patient to work through distorted thoughts and determine own best course of action.*

PCC ■ Share with patient observation of distress when hearing other's opinion. Ask patient to share thoughts that are leading to distress. *Sharing thoughts that lead to distress regarding others' opinions may reveal relationship barriers to decision-making. Indecision may arise from dissonance between patient's own values, beliefs, and preferences and those of loved ones or health care providers.* Validate those thoughts. *Validation of patient's distressing thoughts promotes self-esteem, builds the therapeutic relationship, and promotes autonomous decision-making.*

PCC ■ If needed, clarify perceptions of health care team decisional preference. *Patient may feel pressured to make an unwanted choice by a perceived power differential within the therapeutic relationship.*

PCC ■ Engage patient to use a problem-solving framework to identify and to evaluate the possible available choices. Ask patient to list the advantages and drawbacks to each choice, as well as personal values, goals, and preferences related to each choice. Encourage patient to identify personal and social barriers to enacting any of the choices. Then ask patient to rate the suitability of each choice based on appraisal of each one. *Use of a problem-solving framework in consideration of health care choices encourages patient to consider health care options from the context of own experience and to identify own best choices given patient's life situation.*

Suggested NIC Interventions

Active Listening; Assertiveness Training; Decision-Making Support; Learning Facilitation; Mutual Goal Setting

EVALUATIONS FOR EXPECTED OUTCOMES

- The patient states how available health care choices fit with their values, beliefs, preferences, and lifestyle.
- The patient expresses own values, beliefs, and preferences in making the health care decision, comparing and contrasting how they differ from those of loved ones.
- The patient does not perceive pressure to choose or preference of a choice by the health care team.
- The patient freely verbalizes own opinion.
- The patient chooses health care option and expresses satisfaction with own choice based on the options available.

DOCUMENTATION

- Assessment findings
- Health teaching regarding patient's health need and available health care choices
- Patient verbatim statements regarding perceptions of health care situation and available choices
- Patient verbatim statements regarding own emotional experience of making a health care decision, related interventions undertaken, and patient response
- Observations of patient distress when hearing others' opinions, related interventions enacted, and patient response
- Use of problem-solving framework and patient response to same

REFERENCES

Bradley, E., & Green, D. (2018). Involved, inputting or informing: "Shared" decision making in adult mental health care. *Health Expectations, 21*(1), 192–200.
Jordan, A., Wood, F., Edwards, A., Shepherd, V., & Joseph-Williams, N. (2018). What adolescents living with long-term conditions say about being involved in decision-making about their healthcare: A systematic review and narrative synthesis of preferences and experiences. *Patient Education & Counseling, 101*(10), 1725–1735.
Land, V., Parry, R., & Seymour, J. (2017). Communication practices that encourage and constrain shared decision making in health-care encounters: Systematic review of conversation analytic research. *Health Expectations, 20*(6), 1228–1247.
Wigfall, L. T., & Tanner, A. H. (2018). Health literacy and health-care engagement as predictors of shared decision-making among adult information seekers in the USA: A secondary data analysis of the health information national trends survey. *Journal of Cancer Education, 33*(1), 67–73.

Risk for Impaired Emancipated Decision-Making

DEFINITION

Susceptible to a process of choosing a health care decision that does not include personal knowledge and/or consideration of social norms, or does not occur in a flexible environment, resulting in decisional dissatisfaction

RISK FACTORS

- Decrease in understanding of all available health care options
- Inability to adequately verbalize perceptions about health care options
- Inadequate time to discuss health care options
- Insufficient confidence to openly discuss health care options
- Insufficient information regarding health care options
- Insufficient privacy to openly discuss health care options
- Insufficient self-confidence in decision-making

ASSESSMENT

- Levels of consciousness and orientation
- Age
- Stage of development
- Presence of cognitive impairment
- Level of education
- Language fluency

EXPECTED OUTCOMES

- The patient will verbalize own opinion freely.
- The patient will verbalize own values, beliefs, and preferences.
- The patient will identify any disparities between self and others' values, beliefs, and preferences.
- The patient's information needs will be met.
- The patient will make an autonomous health care choice.

Suggested NOC Outcomes

Decision-Making; Information Processing; Participation in Health Care Decisions

INTERVENTIONS AND RATIONALES

PCC ▪ Engage patient in the therapeutic relationship. Demonstrate an attitude of respect, patience, and acceptance. *Persons who feel cared for, understood, and respected in health care situations are better motivated to collaboratively participate in own care.*

PCC ▪ Ensure privacy for one-to-one interaction between patient and nurse. *Patient's status in relationships with family/loved ones may inhibit frank discussion in their presence.* If necessary, move the interaction, modify the environment, or remove others to ensure privacy.

PCC ▪ Avoid limiting choices based on health care provider preference, values, or beliefs and avoid encouraging one choice over another. *The health care team is accountable to the patient to provide appropriate information on all available options and to promote autonomous decision-making.*

PCC ▪ Ensure that communications and information provided are at a level consistent with the patient's cognitive abilities *to ensure understanding.*

PCC ▪ Ask patient about understanding of patient's health care need and the available choices *to identify any misperceptions.*

PCC ▪ Validate patient's understanding *to promote self-esteem, confidence in knowledge, and strengthen the therapeutic relationship.*

PCC ▪ Accept patient's personal knowledge as relevant to the decision-making process. Discourage patient from discounting personal knowledge and deferring to others' knowledge *to promote self-empowerment, confidence, and self-esteem.*

EBP ▪ Provide education as needed in an accepting, nonjudgmental, supportive manner. Avoid taking a stance of correcting patient; rather, build on patient's knowledge and understanding *to build knowledge capacity while preserving self-esteem.*

PCC ▪ Respectfully inquire as to patient's cultural background, including gender roles, generational roles, and social expectations. *Patient is the best source of knowledge of own particular culture.*

PCC ▪ Encourage patient to explore any cultural considerations in health care decision-making and to share what it is like for patient to include those considerations. *Negative or conflicting emotions, or indecision may arise in the patient due to incongruence between patient's cultural values and beliefs and personal values, beliefs, and preferences.*

PCC ▪ Explore with patient the meaning of experiencing making a health care decision. Ask what meaning the current health care situation and having to make a health care decision has for patient. *The health care need and necessity to make a health care decision may represent a crisis for the patient. Understanding patient's experience of this can direct the identification of other necessary assessments and interventions.*

PCC ▪ Ask patient about strategies used in the past to make decisions. Validate patient's past choices in strategies. Reinforce independent strategies *to identify and draw on personal experiences and strengths in decision-making.*

PCC ▪ If past experience in decision-making is limited, engage patient to use a problem-solving framework to identify and to evaluate the possible available choices. Ask patient to list the advantages and drawbacks to each choice, as well as personal values, goals, and preferences related to each choice. Encourage patient to identify personal and social barriers to enacting any of the choices. Then ask patient to rate the suitability of each choice based on appraisal of each one. *Use of a problem-solving framework in consideration of health care choices encourages patient to consider health care options from the context of own experience and to identify own best choices given the patient's life situation.*

Suggested NIC Interventions

Active Listening; Assertiveness Training; Decision-Making Support; Learning Facilitation; Mutual Goal Setting

EVALUATIONS FOR EXPECTED OUTCOMES

▪ The patient freely verbalizes personal opinions about the available health care choices.
▪ The patient verbalizes how health care choices align with personal values, beliefs, and preferences.
▪ The patient identifies conflicts between own choice and others' values, beliefs, and preferences.
▪ The patient verbalizes feeling informed about own choices.
▪ The patient makes an autonomous health care choice.
▪ The patient verbalizes satisfaction with own health care choice given the available options.

DOCUMENTATION

▪ Assessment findings
▪ Interventions taken to ensure privacy, and patient and loved ones response
▪ Patient verbatim statements regarding the patient's understanding and perceptions of own health care choices, own cultural identification and norms, and the meaning the patient makes of own health concern and the need to make a health care decision; related interventions undertaken and patient response
▪ Past decision-making strategies used and utility for application in current situation
▪ Health teaching regarding health care choices, including patient response
▪ Any use of a problem-solving framework and patient response to same
▪ Patient's decision made and verbatim statements regarding the patient's satisfaction with it given the choices available

REFERENCES

Hawley, S. T., & Morris, A. M. (2017). Cultural challenges to engaging patients in shared decision making. *Patient Education & Counseling, 100*(1), 18–24.

Lin, M.-L., & Chen, C.-H. (2017). Difficulties in surgical decision making and associated factors among elective surgical patients in Taiwan. *Journal of Nursing Research, 25*(6), 464–470.

Lühnen, J., Haastert, B., Mühlhauser, I., & Richter, T. (2017). Informed decision-making with and for people with dementia—Efficacy of the PRODECIDE education program for legal representatives: Protocol of a randomized controlled trial (PRODECIDE-RCT). *BMC Geriatrics, 17*, 1–11.

Papastavrou, E., Efstathiou, G., Tsangari, H., Karlou, C., Patiraki, E., Jarosova, D., … Suhonen, R. (2016). Patients' decisional control over care: A cross-national comparison from both the patients' and nurses' points of view. *Scandinavian Journal of Caring Sciences, 30*(1), 26–36.

Readiness for Enhanced Emancipated Decision-Making

DEFINITION

A process of choosing a health care decision that includes personal knowledge and/or consideration of social norms, which can be strengthened

ASSESSMENT

- Levels of consciousness and orientation
- Age
- Stage of development
- Presence of cognitive impairment
- Level of education
- Language fluency

DEFINING CHARACTERISTICS

- Expresses desire to enhance ability to choose health care options that best fit current lifestyle
- Expresses desire to enhance ability to enact chosen health care option
- Expresses desire to enhance ability to understand all available health care options
- Expresses desire to enhance ability to verbalize own opinion with constraint
- Expresses desire to enhance comfort to verbalize health care options in the presence of others
- Expresses desire to enhance confidence in decision-making
- Expresses desire to enhance confidence to discuss health care options openly
- Expresses desire to enhance decision-making
- Expresses desire to enhance privacy to discuss health care options

EXPECTED OUTCOMES

- The patient will engage with the nurse to meet needs for privacy.
- The patient will openly seek information, and verbalize that the patient's information needs are met.
- The patient will assertively communicate own opinions regarding own health care choices.
- The patient will self-select a health care choice that meets the patient's lifestyle needs and reflects the patient's values, beliefs, and preferences.
- The patient will verbalize satisfaction with own health care decision given the available choices.

Suggested NOC Outcomes

Decision-Making; Information Processing; Participation in Health Care Decisions

INTERVENTIONS AND RATIONALES

PCC ▪ Collaborate with patient to determine strategies to meet patient's needs for privacy *to promote self-care, self-esteem, and decision-making.*

PCC ▪ Provide information proactively in anticipation of patient's needs, as well as upon request by patient. Encourage patient to ask questions and provide meaningful answers to them *to promote psychological readiness to make a decision, self-esteem, and confidence in knowledge.*

PCC ▪ Avoid the use of technical terms when at all possible; explain the meaning of technical terms when they must be used in communication with or in the presence of the patient *to prevent a perceived power differential, which can be a barrier to patient understanding and self-esteem and impede the therapeutic relationship.*

PCC ▪ Ensure that communications and information provided are at a level consistent with patient's cognitive abilities *to ensure understanding.*

PCC ▪ Promote self-esteem through active listening, validation of concerns, knowledge and feelings, conveyance of respect for patient's values, beliefs, and preferences *to promote psychological readiness to make a decision and to strengthen the therapeutic relationship.*

PCC ▪ Use active listening to identify and reflect back to patient the opinions of choices available to patient *to promote autonomous consideration of options the patient and confidence in own opinions.*

PCC ▪ Ask patient to verbalize what lifestyle, social, and other factors patient needs to consider in making a decision, and how these would impact or be impacted by the health care choices available to the patient *to promote consideration of the context of patient's decision-making.*

PCC ▪ Ask patient about strategies used in the past to make decisions. Validate patient's past choices in strategies. Engage patient in realistic appraisal of the applicability of past strategies to current situation *to identify and draw on personal experiences and strengths in decision-making.*

EBP ▪ Teach patient about the utility of problem-solving frameworks to assist in decision-making. As desired, ask patient to use a problem-solving framework to identify and to evaluate the possible choices available. Ask patient to list the advantages and drawbacks to each choice, as well as personal values, goals, and preferences related to each choice. Encourage patient to identify personal and social barriers to enacting any of the choices. Then ask patient to rate the suitability of each choice based on patient's appraisal of each one. *Use of a problem-solving framework in consideration of health care choices encourages the patient to consider health care options from the context of own experience and to identify own best choices given the patient's life situation.*

PCC ▪ As needed, assist patient to practice assertive expression of opinions. Encourage the patient to communicate in a way that is authentic, and simultaneously respectful of own feelings, values, beliefs, and wishes, as well as those of others. *Assertive expression of opinions promotes self-esteem within and after interpersonal interactions.*

EBP ▪ Role playing assertive expression of opinions may be helpful to prepare patient to do so in real-life situations. *Role play can be an effective strategy toward the development of skill mastery.*

Suggested NIC Interventions

Active Listening; Assertiveness Training; Decision-Making Support; Learning Facilitation; Mutual Goal Setting

- The patient collaborates on meeting own needs for privacy.
- The patient openly seeks information.
- The patient verbalizes having sufficient information to make own health care decision.
- The patient communicates own opinions regarding health care choices while remaining respectful of those of others.
- The patient self-selects a health care choice that meets the patient's lifestyle needs and reflects the patient's values, beliefs, and preferences.
- The patient verbalizes satisfaction with health care decision given the available choices.

- Assessment findings
- Patient engagement in planning and enacting interventions to ensure privacy; interventions taken to ensure privacy
- Information sought and health teaching provided, including patient response
- Past decision-making strategies used and patient's verbatim perceptions of utility for application in current situation
- Patient's verbatim opinions of the available health care choices
- Patient response to education regarding problem-solving framework and as appropriate, the patient's use of it in the current situation
- Patient-identified factors in making own health care decision
- As applicable, patient engagement in practice of assertive expression of opinions
- Decision made by patient
- Patient verbalizations regarding satisfaction with choices and own decision

REFERENCES

Goering, E. M., & Krause, A. (2017). From sense making to decision making when living with cancer. *Communication & Medicine, 14*(3), 268–273.

King, L., Harrington, A., Linedale, E., & Tanner, E. (2018). A mixed methods thematic review: Health-related decision-making by the older person. *Journal of Clinical Nursing, 27*(7–8), e1327–e1343.

Robbins, D. A., Mattison, J. E., & Dorrance, K. A. (2018). Person-centricity: Promoting self-determination and responsibility in health and health care. *Military Medicine, 183*, 198–203.

Shatkin, J. P. (2016). 5.4 Not invincible: How adolescents make decisions and why they take risks. *Journal of the American Academy of Child & Adolescent Psychiatry, 55*, S93.

Labile Emotional Control

Uncontrollable outbursts of exaggerated and involuntary emotional expression

- Alteration in self-esteem
- Emotional disturbance
- Fatigue
- Insufficient knowledge about symptom control
- Insufficient knowledge of disease
- Insufficient muscle strength
- Social distress

▦ Stressors
▦ Substance misuse

ASSOCIATED CONDITIONS

▦ Brain injury
▦ Functional impairment
▦ Mood disorder
▦ Musculoskeletal impairment
▦ Pharmaceutical agent
▦ Physical disability
▦ Psychiatric disorder

ASSESSMENT

▦ Physiologic status, including patterns of nutrition, pain, elimination, activity, and rest
▦ Developmental delay or disability
▦ History of or current neurologic disease and/or traumatic brain injury
▦ History of or current exposure to trauma involving own or a loved one's death or the threat of death, serious injury, or sexual violence
▦ History of or current mental illness, including ADHD, mood, anxiety, eating, somato-form, autism spectrum, or borderline personality disorders
▦ History of impulse control disorder
▦ Mental status exam, including appearance, affect, mood, sensorium, cognition, motor (i.e., speech, movements, gait), thought process, thought content, perceptual disturbance
▦ Childhood experience of parental responsiveness to emotional and psychological needs
▦ Substance use, including alcohol, street drugs, and prescription medications used differently than as prescribed, and patient's perceived benefits of substance use
▦ Usual pattern of emotional response. For areas of distress intolerance, specific types of stressors, frequency, and maladaptive response(s)
▦ Presence of rumination on stressors, or a typical pattern of rumination on stressors
▦ Patient's perception of health situation
▦ Patient's perception of own exaggerated and involuntary emotional expression

DEFINING CHARACTERISTICS

▦ Absence of eye contact
▦ Crying
▦ Difficulty in use of facial expressions
▦ Embarrassment regarding emotional expression
▦ Excessive crying without feeling sadness
▦ Excessive laughing without feeling happiness
▦ Expression of emotion incongruent with triggering factor
▦ Involuntary crying
▦ Involuntary laughing
▦ Uncontrollable crying
▦ Uncontrollable laughing
▦ Withdrawal from occupational situation
▦ Withdrawal from social situation

- Patient will identify the personal and social impacts of emotional outbursts and own goals for managing/limiting outbursts.
- Patient will discuss bodily, cognitive, and situational experiences correlating with periods of emotional outbursts.
- Patient will practice strategies to promote emotional control.
- Patient will express positive self-esteem.

Suggested NOC Outcomes

Aggression Control; Anxiety Control; Coping; Impulse Control; Self-Esteem; Self-Mutilation Restraint; Social Interaction Skills

PCC — Do not attempt to teach new skills/information while patient is in the midst of an intense emotional outburst *as patient's cognitive capacity may be reduced at this time.*

EBP — Teach new skills when patient is calm. *Emotional outbursts physiologically are time-limited.*

PCC — During the outburst, use a calm tone and communicate in short, direct, specific statements. Expect that patient may need extra time to process information and that instructions may need to be repeated *as diminished cognitive capacity may impact processing of information.*

PCC — When the outburst has ended, ensure that patient's immediate physiologic needs (i.e., rest, nutrition, hydration, elimination) are addressed before engaging in interventions to reduce and prevent future outbursts. *Basic physiologic needs must be met for patient to be able to engage therapeutically.*

EBP — Teach patient about the social impact of patient's emotional outbursts as needed. Ask patient to identify at least one person, besides self, who has been impacted by emotional outbursts. Ask patient to identify at least one way patient has been impacted socially and one way patient has been impacted occupationally (i.e., work, school) by outbursts *to promote insight and stimulate motivation to engage in strategies to limit outbursts.*

PCC — Use nonjudgmental, matter-of-fact language *to promote self-esteem.*

PCC — Engage patient in discussion of how life would be different if patient had better control over emotional outbursts *to foster motivation and engagement in care.*

PCC — Ask patient to decide at least one reason why patient wants to better control emotional expression *to foster motivation and engagement in interventions, and to promote self-efficacy.*

PCC — Teach patient to practice awareness of bodily sensations *to help learn the early signs of emotional arousal.*

EBP — Assist patient to make linkages between bodily sensations and emotional state. Teach strategies to decrease physiologic arousal *to help the patient to limit unwanted emotional outbursts.*

PCC — Assist patient to identify environmental and situational triggers to physiologic arousal, and engage patient to create a plan to limit physiologic arousal *to promote self-efficacy in proactive management of emotional outbursts.*

PCC — Promote self-esteem. Emphasize therapeutic gains made by patient and encourage nonjudgmental, realistic appraisal of therapeutic challenges. *Higher self-esteem promotes cognitive self-regulatory capacity.*

EBP — Assist patient to identify and practice strategies to manage distressing/exciting situations and strong emotions. Use vicarious learning or role play exercises to practice plan of response to limit emotional outbursts. *Practice of strategies in a safe and controlled environment develops skills in strategies and builds confidence to apply strategies in triggering situations.*

PCC ▥ Involve patient in own care. Provide options and solicit feedback on patient's experience of care. *Partnering with patient promotes self-efficacy and self-esteem and strengthens the therapeutic alliance.*

PCC ▥ Solicit patient's thoughts and experience of bodily sensations during care. Reinforce and support use of adaptive coping strategies to limit emotional outbursts *to help patient further develop awareness of signs and triggers and to promote use of strategies to limit/prevent outbursts.*

PCC ▥ Communicate continuous nonjudgmental acceptance of the patient through verbal and meta-communication *to strengthen the therapeutic alliance, promote self-esteem.*

PCC ▥ Provide patient with specific, simple, step-by-step information on what to expect in care *to reduce/prevent emotional arousal, communicate respect, and engage patient in care.*

PCC ▥ Chunk information according to immediate care requirements, and provide updates as each stage of care ensues. *Chunking information decreases cognitive stress and promotes retention.*

T&C ▥ Assist patient with referral to specialized resources in mindfulness, dialectical behavior therapy, and/or cognitive behavioral therapy as indicated in consultation with the interdisciplinary care team. *Mindfulness improves attention and body awareness, and promotes cognitive control and attentional capability in situations of high emotion. Mindfulness, dialectical behavioral therapy, and cognitive behavior therapy each have applications for improving cognitive control and emotional dysregulation.*

Suggested NIC Interventions

Anger Control Assistance; Anxiety Reduction; Cognitive Restructuring; Coping Enhancement; Impulse Control Training; Support Group

EVALUATIONS FOR EXPECTED OUTCOMES

▥ The patient discusses experience of own emotional outbursts and identifies ways they have affected the patient. There is also discussion on ways emotional outbursts have impacted the patient socially, including the effects on other people, relationships, social, and occupational opportunities. The patient identifies reasons to work toward better control of emotional expression.

▥ The patient identifies bodily sensations/changes, thoughts, and situations antecedent to emotional outbursts. The patient notes any trends in antecedents.

▥ The patient practices strategies to notice own physiologic, cognitive and emotional states, and practices strategies to decrease physiologic and emotional arousal.

▥ The patient identifies achievements inherent in decision to engage in interventions to limit emotional outbursts, setting goals, skills learned, skills practiced, and positive gains made in treatment.

DOCUMENTATION

▥ Food and fluid intake, assessment of pain if present, bowel and bladder activity, sleep patterns, activity, and exercise

▥ Relevant medical, developmental, and psychiatric history

▥ History of trauma

- Substance use if applicable, the patient's reasons for using, and relationship of substance use to emotional outbursts
- Patient, family, and nurse's observations of emotional outbursts, antecedents, impacts of and responses to outbursts
- Interventions implemented to limit uncontrolled emotional outbursts, including patient engagement and response
- Evaluations for expected outcomes
- Referrals to other services

REFERENCES

Abasi, I., Dolatshahi, B., Farazmand, S., Pourshahbaz, A., & Tamanaeefar, S. (2018). Emotion regulation in generalized anxiety and social anxiety: Examining the distinct and shared use of emotion regulation strategies. *Iranian Journal of Psychiatry, 13*(3), 161–167.

Brown, K., & Taghehchian, R. (2016). Bottled up: An experiential intervention for emotional suppression. *Journal of Family Psychotherapy, 27*(4), 302–307.

Callear, A., Harvey, S. T., Bimler, D., & Catto, N. (2018). Profiling children's emotion regulation behaviours. *British Journal of Developmental Psychology, 36*(4), 540–556.

Edwards, M. K., Rhodes, R. E., & Loprinzi, P. D. (2017). A randomized control intervention investigating the effects of acute exercise on emotional regulation. *American Journal of Health Behavior, 41*(5), 534–543.

Thurston, H., Bell, J. F., & Induni, M. (2018). Community-level adverse experiences and emotional regulation in children and adolescents. *Journal of Pediatric Nursing, 42*, 25–33.

Imbalanced Energy Field

DEFINITION

A disruption in the vital flow of human energy that is normally a continuous whole and is unique, dynamic, creative, and nonlinear

RELATED FACTORS (R/T)

- Anxiety
- Discomfort
- Excessive stress
- Interventions that disrupt the energetic pattern or flow
- Pain

ASSOCIATED CONDITIONS

- Illness
- Injury

ASSESSMENT

- Psychological status, including anxiety, fatigue, depression, somatic complaints, and recent lifestyle changes (death of loved one, conflict in a relationship, or loss of job)
- Health status, including presence of disorder that's life-threatening or requires surgery
- Sensory status, including pain and disorders that may affect senses
- Spiritual status, including religious beliefs and affiliation; available support systems; and feelings of helplessness, hopelessness, anger, and withdrawal
- Caregiver's readiness to provide therapeutic healing, including education and training in therapeutic touch or similar treatment technique

- Arrhythmic energy field patterns
- Blockage of the energy flow
- Congested energy field patterns
- Congestion of the energy flow
- Dissonant rhythms of the energy field patterns
- Energy deficit of the energy flow
- Expression of the need to regain the experience of the whole
- Hyperactivity of the energy flow
- Irregular energy field patterns
- Magnetic pull to an area of the energy field
- Pulsating to pounding frequency of the energy field patterns
- Pulsations sensed in the energy flow
- Random energy field patterns
- Rapid energy field patterns
- Slow energy field patterns
- Strong energy field patterns
- Temperature differentials of cold in the energy flow
- Temperature differentials of heat in the energy flow
- Tingling sensed in the energy flow
- Tumultuous energy field patterns
- Unsynchronized rhythms sensed in the energy flow
- Weak energy field patterns

- Patient will feel increasingly relaxed as demonstrated by slower and deeper breathing, skin flushing in treated area, audible sighing, or verbal reports of feeling more relaxed.
- Patient will visualize images that relax him or her.
- Patient will report feeling less tension or pain.
- Patient will use self-healing techniques, such as meditation, guided imagery, yoga, and prayer.
- Patient will express increased sense of personal and spiritual well-being.

Suggested NOC Outcomes

Comfort Level; Health Beliefs; Personal Health Status; Personal Well-Being; Spiritual Health

PCC · Implement measures to promote therapeutic healing. Place your hands 4 to 6 inches (10 to 15 cm) above patient's body. Pass your hands over entire skin surface. *This technique helps you become attuned to patient's energy field, which is the flow of energy that surrounds a person's being.* With experience and training in therapeutic touch or similar treatment, you can identify sensory cues to energy field disturbances, such as heat, cold, tingling, and an electric sensation.

PCC · Try to gain patient's cooperation as you perform healing techniques, such as therapeutic touch, *to enhance effectiveness of healing techniques and foster participation in spiritual aspects of care.*

PCC · Continue to treat patient using therapeutic healing techniques. *One treatment rarely restores a full sense of inner well-being.*

PCC ▥ Suggest that patient use self-healing techniques, such as meditation, guided imagery, yoga, and prayer, *to encourage patient to participate in own care.*

PCC ▥ Familiarize family with the benefits of healing or therapeutic touch *in order for them to support its use after patient is discharged home.*

Suggested NIC Interventions

Communication Enhancement; Energy Management; Environmental Management; Pain Management; Spiritual Support; Relaxation Therapy

EVALUATIONS FOR EXPECTED OUTCOMES

▥ Patient shows evidence of relaxation, such as slower and deeper breathing, flushing in treated area, audible sighing, or verbal reports of feeling more relaxed.
▥ Patient reports experiencing relaxing visual images.
▥ Patient reports reduction in tension or pain.
▥ Patient uses self-healing techniques, such as meditation, guided imagery, yoga, and prayer.
▥ Patient reports an increased sense of well-being.

DOCUMENTATION

▥ Summary of patient's psychosocial status
▥ Patient's progress in learning techniques that enhance relaxation
▥ Patient's perceptions of benefits of healing and self-healing techniques
▥ Family members' reaction to the use of therapeutic touch
▥ Evaluations for expected outcomes

REFERENCES

Cheraghi, M. A., Hosseini, A. S. S., Gholami, R., Bagheri, I., Binaee, N., Matourypour, P., & Ranjbaran, M. (2017). Therapeutic touch efficacy: A systematic review. *Medical-Surgical Nursing Journal, 5*(4), 52–59.

Peck, S., Corse, G., & Lu, D.-F. (2017). Case report: Energy field changes approaching and during the death experience. *Integrative Medicine: A Clinician's Journal, 16*(6), 36–42.

Shields, D., Fuller, A., Resnicoff, M., Butcher, H. K., & Frisch, N. (2017). Human energy field: A concept analysis. *Journal of Holistic Nursing, 35*(4), 352–368.

Readiness for Enhanced Exercise Engagement

DEFINITION

A pattern of attention to physical activity characterized by planned, structured, repetitive body movements, which can be strengthened

ASSESSMENT

▥ Patient's age, height, weight
▥ Patient's perception of exercise's role in health and wellness
▥ Patient's physical condition including respiratory status, cardiovascular status, and musculoskeletal status

▦ Perception, knowledge, and readiness to learn about the need to participate in an exercise routine for maintaining health and wellness

DEFINING CHARACTERISTICS

▦ Expresses desire to enhance autonomy for activities of daily living
▦ Expresses desire to enhance competence to interact with physical and social environments
▦ Expresses desire to enhance knowledge about environmental conditions for participation in physical activity
▦ Expresses desire to enhance knowledge about group opportunities for participation in physical activity
▦ Expresses desire to enhance knowledge about physical settings for participation in physical activity
▦ Expresses desire to enhance knowledge about the need for physical activity
▦ Expresses desire to enhance physical abilities
▦ Expresses desire to enhance physical appearance
▦ Expresses desire to enhance physical conditioning
▦ Expresses desire to maintain motivation to participate in a physical activity plan
▦ Expresses desire to maintain physical abilities
▦ Expresses desire to maintain physical well-being through physical activity
▦ Expresses desire to meet others' expectations about physical activity plans

EXPECTED OUTCOMES

▦ Patient will state desire to adhere to an exercise routine.
▦ Patient will state desire to enhance knowledge in an exercise routine.
▦ Patient will state desire to enhance their physical appearance.
▦ Patient will state desire to improve physical strength and endurance.
▦ Patient will state understanding of the need to increase activity level gradually.
▦ Patient will identify controllable factors that cause injury, musculoskeletal strain, and fatigue.
▦ Patient will state a sense of satisfaction with each new level of activity attained.

Suggested NOC Outcomes

Exercise Participation; Knowledge: Energy Conservation; Knowledge: Health Behavior; Weight Maintenance Behavior

INTERVENTIONS AND RATIONALES

PCC ▦ Assess patient's concerns related to exercise planning and execution *to be able to suggest strategies to overcome challenges.*
PCC ▦ Model effective techniques for planning and executing exercise routine. *Patients who are challenged by planning and executing activities often find it helpful to observe practical approaches instead of solely hearing theoretical information.*
EBP ▦ Teach behavior management strategies *to help patient minimize fears of failure.*
PCC ▦ Encourage patient to set realistic goals. *Unrealistic goals can go unmet leading to frustration and discouragement.*

PCC ▓ Praise successes in any steps of planning or executing activities. *Positive reinforcement enhances self-confidence.*

T&C ▓ Refer or collaborate with exercise therapists in managing the patient's activity. *Colleagues in related disciplines bring valuable additional perspectives to complex clinical situations.*

Suggested NIC Interventions

Exercise Promotion; Exercise Promotion: Strength Training; Exercise Promotion: Stretching; Exercise Therapy: Balance; Exercise Therapy: Joint Mobility; Exercise Therapy: Muscle Control

EVALUATIONS FOR EXPECTED OUTCOMES

▓ Patient participates in regular exercise routine schedule.
▓ Patient seeks out information for exercise appropriate for level of ability.
▓ Patient engages in exercise that increases strength, agility, endurance, and balance.
▓ Patient increases activity gradually to decrease risk of injury.
▓ Patient uses community resources for support.
▓ Patient states satisfaction with each new level of activity attained.

DOCUMENTATION

▓ Patient's perception of need for exercise
▓ Patient's priorities in performing selected activities
▓ Patient's description of physical effects of various activities
▓ Observations of physical findings in response to activity
▓ Teaching activities performed with patient
▓ Evaluations for expected outcomes

REFERENCES

Barstow, B., Thirumalai, M., Mehta, T., Padalabalanarayanan, S., Kim, Y., & Motl, R. W. (2020). Developing a decision support system for exercise engagement among individuals with conditions causing mobility impairment: Perspectives of fitness facility fitness exercisers and adapted fitness center trainer. *Technology & Disability, 32*(4), 295–305.

Shu-Chuan, C., Hsiu-Chen, Y., & Yu-Lun, K. (2020). Scale development and model validation for the process of exercise engagement for people with prediabetes. *Journal of Korean Academy of Nursing, 50*(2), 298–312.

Riciputi, S., McDonough, M. H., Snyder, F. J., & McDavid, M. L. (2020). Staff support promotes engagement in a physical activity-based positive youth development program for youth from low-income families. *Sport, Exercise, and Performance Psychology, 9*(1), 45–57. doi:10.1037/spy0000169

Silveira, S. L., Richardson, E. V., & Motl, R. W. (2020). Social cognitive theory as a guide for exercise engagement in persons with multiple sclerosis who use wheelchairs for mobility. *Health Education Research, 35*(4), 270–282.

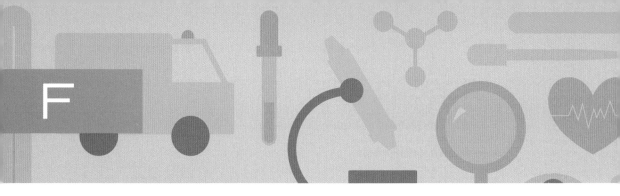

F

Risk for Adult Falls

Adult susceptible to experiencing an event resulting in coming to rest inadvertently on the ground, floor, or other lower level, which may compromise health

RISK FACTORS

Physiologic Factors

- Chronic musculoskeletal pain
- Decreased lower extremity strength
- Dehydration
- Diarrhea
- Faintness when extending neck
- Faintness when turning neck
- Hypoglycemia
- Impaired physical mobility
- Impaired postural balance
- Incontinence
- Obesity
- Sleep disturbances
- Vitamin D deficiency

Psychoneurological Factors

- Agitated confusion
- Anxiety
- Cognitive dysfunction
- Depressive symptoms
- Fear of falling
- Persistent wandering
- Substance misuse

Unmodified Environmental Factors

- Cluttered environment
- Elevated bed surface
- Exposure to unsafe weather-related condition
- Inadequate anti-slip material in bathroom
- Inadequate anti-slip material on floors
- Inadequate lighting

- Inappropriate toilet seat height
- Inattentive to pets
- Lack of safety rails
- Objects out of reach
- Seats without arms
- Seats without backs
- Uneven floor
- Unfamiliar setting
- Use of throw rugs

Other Factors

- Difficulty performing activities of daily living
- Difficulty performing instrumental activities of daily living
- Factors identified by standardized, validated screening tool
- Getting up at night without help
- Inadequate knowledge of modifiable factors
- Inappropriate clothing for walking
- Inappropriate footwear

ASSOCIATED CONDITIONS

- Anemia
- Assistive devices for walking
- Depression
- Endocrine system diseases
- Lower-limb prosthetics
- Major injury
- Mental disorders
- Musculoskeletal diseases
- Neurocognitive disorders
- Orthostatic hypotension
- Pharmaceutical preparations
- Sensation disorders
- Vascular diseases

ASSESSMENT

- Psychosocial status, including age, developmental stage, learning ability, decision-making ability, health beliefs and attitudes, interest in learning, knowledge and skills regarding current health problem, obstacles to learning, financial resources, support systems, and usual coping pattern
- Neurologic status, including level of consciousness, memory, mental status, and orientation
- Physical impairment or limitation, recent joint replacement, other surgery or illness
- Environmental hazards such as throw rugs, carpet edges, stairways, slippery floors, tubs and showers, unsteady handrails

EXPECTED OUTCOMES

- Patient and/or family will identify the factors that increase potential for falls.
- Patient and/or family will assist in identifying and applying safety measures to prevent injury.
- Patient and/or family will make necessary physical changes in the environment to ensure increased safety.

- Patient and/or family will develop strategies to maintain safety.
- Patient will optimize activities of daily living within sensorimotor limitations.

Suggested NOC Outcomes

Fall Prevention Behavior; Falls Occurrence; Mobility; Risk Control; Knowledge: Fall Prevention; Coordinated Movement; Safe Home Environment

INTERVENTIONS AND RATIONALES

S - Identify factors that may cause or contribute to injury from a fall *in order to enhance the patient, family, and caregiver awareness of the risks.*

S - Improve environmental safety factors as needed. *Doing frequent assessments of patient's environment is necessary to make sure new risks have not occurred.*

S - Assess patient's ability to use call bell or other safety emergency system. Remove anything from the environment that will increase the risk of falls; for example, throw rugs, cords, furniture blocking the patient's path to the bathroom. *Patient's immediate environment must be reviewed frequently to prevent unnecessary falls.*

EBP - Teach patient and family about the need for safe illumination. Advise patient to wear sunglasses when outside *to reduce glare.* Suggest the use of contrasting colors in household furnishings *to enable patient to distinguish difference in things when walking and sitting.*

PCC - For patients with hearing loss, encourage the use of a hearing aid *to minimize hearing deficit.*

EBP - Teach patient with unstable gait the proper use of assistive devices. Many patients never learn to use canes, crutches, and so on, properly *to decrease the potential for falling.*

PCC - Review medications with patient and family. Help patient understand which medications put patient at greater risk for falls. Knowing the risk may help patient take more care in moving about. It may also call for reviewing with the primary care physician. *Two or more medications taken by a patient puts the patient at higher risk. Many medications taken by the elderly can cause dizziness, sleepiness, lowered blood pressure, and confusion. Without sufficient instructions, patient may be at a higher risk for falls.*

T&C - Provide additional patient education for household safety. Refer patient to appropriate resources (such as police, fire, home health nurses) for safety education. There is interest in the community for educating the elderly in the area of fall prevention. *Many hospitalizations of elderly people because of trauma are caused by falls.*

Suggested NIC Interventions

Fall Prevention; Environmental Management: Safety; Risk Identification; Medication Management; Exercise Therapy: Balance

EVALUATION FOR EXPECTED OUTCOMES

- Patient and family are able to point out things in the environment that put them at risk.
- Patient and family members assist in making the changes necessary to promote fall prevention.
- Patient demonstrates the ability to move about without falling.
- Patient identifies resources in the community to help the patient with ongoing fall prevention.

DOCUMENTATION

- Statements by the patient and family about potential for injury as a result of sensory or motor deficits

- Interventions to reduce risk of fall by the patient
- Information about sources of risk to the patient
- Patient response to implementation of preventive measures
- Evaluation of expected outcomes

REFERENCES

Choi, Y., Staley, B., Henriksen, C., Xu, D., Lipori, G., Brumback, B., & Winterstein, A. G. (2018). A dynamic risk model for inpatient falls. *American Journal of Health-System Pharmacy, 75*(17), 1293–1303.
Godlock, G., Christiansen, M., & Feider, L. (2016). Implementation of an evidence-based patient safety team to prevent falls in inpatient medical units. *Med Surg Nursing, 25*(1), 17–23.
Leone, R. M., & Adams, R. J. (2016). Safety standards: Implementing fall prevention interventions and sustaining lower fall rates by promoting the culture of safety on an inpatient rehabilitation unit. *Rehabilitation Nursing, 41*(1), 26–32.
Sharif, S. I., Al-Harbi, A. B., Al-Shihabi, A. M., Al-Daour, D. S., & Sharif, R. S. (2018). Falls in the elderly: Assessment of prevalence and risk factors. *Pharmacy Practice (1886–3655), 16*(3), 1–6.

Risk for Child Falls

DEFINITION

Child susceptible to experiencing an event resulting in coming to rest inadvertently on the ground, floor, or other lower level, which may compromise health

RISK FACTORS

Caregiver Factors

- Changes diapers on raised surfaces
- Exhaustion
- Fails to lock wheels of child equipment
- Inadequate knowledge of changes in developmental stages
- Inadequate supervision of child
- Inattentive to environmental safety
- Inattentive to safety devices during sports activities
- Places child in bouncer seat on raised surfaces
- Places child in infant walkers
- Places child in mobile seat on raised surfaces
- Places child in seats without a seat belt
- Places child in shopping cart basket
- Places child on play equipment unsuitable for age group
- Postpartum depressive symptoms
- Sleeps with child in arms without protective measures
- Sleeps with child on lap without protective measures

Physiological Factors

- Cognitive dysfunction
- Decreased lower extremity strength
- Dehydration
- Hypoglycemia
- Hypotension
- Impaired physical mobility

- Impaired postural balance
- Incontinence
- Malnutrition
- Neurobehavioral manifestations
- Obesity
- Sleep disturbances

Unmodified Environmental Factors

- Absence of stairway gate
- Absence of stairway handrail
- Absence of wheel locks on child equipment
- Absence of window guard
- Cluttered environment
- Furniture placement facilitates access to balconies
- Furniture placement facilitates access to windows
- High chairs positioned near tables or counters
- Inadequate antislip material on floors
- Inadequate automobile restraints
- Inadequate lighting
- Inadequate maintenance of play equipment
- Inadequate restraints on elevated surfaces
- Inattentive to pets
- Objects out of reach
- Seats without arms
- Seats without backs
- Uneven floor
- Unfamiliar setting
- Use of furniture without anti-tipping devices
- Use of nonage appropriate furniture
- Use of throw rugs

Other Factors

- Factors identified by standardized, validated screening tool
- Inappropriate clothing for walking
- Inappropriate footwear

ASSOCIATED CONDITIONS

- Assistive devices for walking
- Feeding and eating disorders
- Musculoskeletal diseases
- Neurocognitive disorders
- Pharmaceutical preparations
- Sensation disorders

ASSESSMENT

- Psychosocial status, including age, developmental stage, learning ability, decision-making ability, knowledge about safety, and obstacles to learning
- Neurologic status, including level of consciousness, memory, mental status, and orientation

- Physical impairment or limitation, surgery, or illness
- Environmental hazards such as throw rugs, carpet edges, furniture and furniture placement, lighting, stairways, slippery floors, tubs and showers, window openings, porches, and balconies

EXPECTED OUTCOMES

- Child and/or family will identify the factors that increase potential for falls.
- Child and/or family will assist in identifying and applying safety measures to prevent injury.
- Family will make necessary physical changes in the environment to ensure increased safety.
- Child and/or family will develop strategies to maintain safety.

Suggested NOC Outcomes

Fall Prevention Behavior; Falls Occurrence; Risk Control; Knowledge: Fall Prevention; Safe Home Environment

INTERVENTIONS AND RATIONALES

S ▪ Identify factors that may cause or contribute to injury from a fall *in order to enhance child, family, caregiver awareness of the risks.*

S ▪ Improve environmental safety factors as needed; install window guards, secure furniture to wall, install safety gates at stairways. *Doing frequent assessments of the child's environment is necessary to make sure new risks have not occurred.*

S ▪ Remove objects that provide climbing access to elevated surfaces. *Climbing onto high surfaces increases the risk of falling.*

S ▪ Keep crib siderails in high position when child is unattended *to prevent climbing over or falling over side rails.*

S ▪ Ensure child wears properly fitting shoes *as shoes that are not the appropriate size cause unstable gait.*

EBP ▪ Teach the family about the need for safe illumination. Suggest the use of contrasting colors in household furnishings *to enable the child to distinguish difference in things when walking and sitting.*

PCC ▪ For children with hearing loss, encourage the use of a hearing aid *to minimize hearing deficit.*

EBP ▪ Teach the child the proper use of assistive devices properly, *to decrease the potential for falling.*

PCC ▪ Review medications with the family and provide education about medications that put the child at greater risk for falls. *Many medications taken by children can cause dizziness, sleepiness, and confusion.*

S ▪ Provide education for household safety. Refer family to appropriate resources (such as police, fire, home health nurses) for safety education. *Children may experience trauma requiring emergency services due to falls.*

Suggested NIC Interventions

Fall Prevention; Environmental Management: Safety; Risk Identification; Teaching: Toddler Safety 13 to 18 Months; Teaching: Toddler Safety 19 to 24 Months; Teaching: Toddler Safety 25 to 36 Months

EVALUATIONS FOR EXPECTED OUTCOMES

- Child and/or family review and identify the factors that increase potential for falls.
- Child and/or family participates in identifying and applying safety measures to prevent injury.
- Family makes necessary physical changes in the environment to ensure increased safety.
- Child and/or family develops strategies to maintain safety.

DOCUMENTATION

- Statements by the family about potential for injury
- Interventions to reduce risk of fall by the child
- Information about sources of risk to the child
- Family response to implementation of preventive measures
- Evaluation of expected outcomes

REFERENCES

Flaherty, M. R., Raybould, T., Savarino, J., Yager, P., Mooney, D. P., Farr, B. J., … Cairo, S. (2021). Unintentional window falls in children and adolescents. *Academic Pediatrics*, *1*(3), 497–503.

Gordon, M. D., Walden, M., Braun, C., Hagan, J., & Lovenstein, A. (2021). Parents' perception of fall risk and incidence of falls in the pediatric ambulatory environment. *Journal of Pediatric Nursing*, *61*, 424–432.

Lombard, K. J., Elsbernd, T. A., Bews, K. A., & Klinkner, D. B. (2019). Building a case for pediatric fall prevention. *Journal of Trauma Nursing*, *26*(2), 89–92.

Nguyen, Q.-U. P., Saynina, O., Pirrotta, E. A., Huffman, L. C., & Wang, N. E. (2021). A retrospective observational cohort study: Epidemiology and outcomes of pediatric unintentional falls in US emergency departments. *Injury*, *52*(8), 2244–2250.

Disturbed Family Identity Syndrome

DEFINITION

Inability to maintain an ongoing interactive, communicative process of creating and maintaining a shared collective sense of the meaning of the family

RELATED FACTORS (R/T)

- Ambivalent family relations
- Different coping styles among family members
- Disrupted family rituals
- Disrupted family roles
- Excessive stress
- Inadequate social support
- Inconsistent management of therapeutic regimen among family members
- Ineffective coping strategies
- Ineffective family communication
- Perceived danger to value system
- Perceived social discrimination
- Sexual dysfunction
- Unaddressed domestic violence
- Unrealistic expectations
- Values incongruent with cultural norms

ASSOCIATED CONDITIONS

▒ Infertility treatment regimen

ASSESSMENT

▒ Parental status, including age, marital status, number and ages of dependent children, and knowledge of normal child behavior
▒ Family status, including normal patterns of interaction among family members, family members' and patient's understanding of present situation
▒ Family member's ability to function in family roles, family conflicts, financial status, and rituals during holidays and family celebrations
▒ Coping patterns, including type and number of changes family has recently experienced, usual response to stress, ability to adapt to change, and use of support systems
▒ Family's past response to crises, including coping patterns and communication patterns to express anger, affection, and confrontation
▒ Family health history, including history of mental illness, stress-related illnesses, history of substance abuse, and sexual abuse of spouse or children
▒ Psychological status, including self-image and self-esteem, functional ability, independence level, and problem-solving and decision-making skills
▒ Spiritual status, including affiliation with a religious group and religious practices

DEFINING CHARACTERISTICS

▒ Decisional conflict (00083)
▒ Disabled family coping (00073)
▒ Disturbed personal identity (00121)
▒ Dysfunctional family processes (00063)
▒ Impaired resilience (00210)
▒ Ineffective childbearing process (00221)
▒ Ineffective relationship (00223)
▒ Ineffective sexuality pattern (00065)
▒ Interrupted family processes (00060)

EXPECTED OUTCOMES

▒ Family will establish clearly defined roles, boundaries, and equitable responsibilities for each family member.
▒ Family will exhibit effective decision-making process.
▒ Family will exhibit clear, direct, and honest communication.
▒ Family will identify support systems and participate in assistance from those systems.

Suggested NOC Outcomes

Coping; Decision-Making; Family Coping; Family Environment: Internal; Family Functioning; Family Normalization; Family Resiliency; Family Social Climate; Social Involvement

INTERVENTIONS AND RATIONALES

PCC ▒ Provide education to family members for communication techniques to clearly express their needs. *Open honest communication resolves disputes and set boundaries.*

PCC ▦ Facilitate discussion of ideas and beliefs about family roles and responsibilities *to establish appropriate boundaries and family member roles.*

PCC ▦ Provide an opportunity for family members to discuss conflicts in an open, safe atmosphere *to decrease anxiety and help family members develop confidence in their ability to resolve problems.*

PCC ▦ Assist family members in identifying their strengths and their progress in addressing problems *to build self-esteem.*

PCC ▦ Expedite communication within family to allow members to express their feelings about present situation. *This encourages supportive behavior to meet reciprocal needs in a crisis.*

PCC ▦ Arrange and participate in family conferences, as needed. *Some families may require help to improve interpersonal communication.*

▦ Encourage family members to evaluate communication patterns periodically *to reinforce benefits of effective communication skills.*

PCC ▦ Whenever possible, ensure privacy to family members for their discussions or conferences. *These measures allow you to help family identify and work toward mutual goals and facilitate effective family coping.*

T&C ▦ Encourage family members to seek counseling *to enhance interpersonal skills and strengthen the family unit.*

T&C ▦ Make referrals to social services or community agencies, as appropriate, *to provide family with access to additional coping resources.*

Suggested NIC Interventions

Coping Enhancement; Counseling; Family Mobilization; Family Process Maintenance; Family Support; Family Therapy; Normalization Promotion; Spiritual Support; Support System Enhancement

EVALUATIONS FOR EXPECTED OUTCOMES

▦ Family members discuss problems in an open, safe environment.

▦ Family members acknowledge their strengths and their progress in resolving problems.

▦ Family members state their plans to continue to seek counseling and attend appropriate support group meetings.

▦ Family members verbalize realistic expectations of each member's role.

▦ Family members participate in methods of solving problems and resolving conflicts.

▦ Family members share feelings about issues within the family.

DOCUMENTATION

▦ Family statements of improved self-confidence in task accomplishment

▦ Satisfaction level of family members

▦ Family stated goals for activity planning and execution

▦ Interventions to assist family and family's responses to those interventions

▦ Referrals to outside agencies

▦ Use of support services

▦ Problems and conflicts described by family members

▦ Changes in roles and responsibilities and information about how these changes were negotiated

▦ Evidence of changes in family communication patterns

▦ Evaluations for expected outcomes

REFERENCES

Deal, J. E. (2019). Normativity and desirability in observational assessments of family interaction. *Family Process, 58*(3), 749–760.

Frear, K. A., Paustian-Underdahl, S., Halbesleben, J. R. B., & French, K. A. (2019). Strategies for work–family management at the intersection of career–family centrality and gender. *Archives of Scientific Psychology, 7*(1), 50–59. doi:10.1037/arc0000068

Greenbaum, R. L., Deng, Y., Butts, M. M., Wang, C. S., & Smith, A. N. (2021). Managing my shame: Examining the effects of parental identity threat and emotional stability on work productivity and investment in parenting. *Journal of Applied Psychology.* doi:10.1037/apl0000597

Misra, S., Johnson, K. A., Parnarouskis, L. M., Koenen, K. C., Williams, D. R., Gelaye, B., & Borba, C. P. C. (2020). How early life adversities influence later life family interactions for individuals with Schizophrenia in outpatient treatment: A qualitative analysis. *Community Mental Health Journal, 56*(6), 1188–1200.

Risk for Disturbed Family Identity Syndrome

DEFINITION

Susceptible to an inability to maintain an ongoing interactive, communicative process of creating and maintaining a shared collective sense of the meaning of the family, which may compromise family members' health

RISK FACTORS

- Ambivalent family relations
- Different coping styles among family members
- Disrupted family rituals
- Disrupted family roles
- Excessive stress
- Inadequate social support
- Inconsistent management of therapeutic regimen among family members
- Ineffective coping strategies
- Ineffective family communication
- Perceived danger to value system
- Perceived social discrimination
- Sexual dysfunction
- Unaddressed domestic violence
- Unrealistic expectations
- Values incongruent with cultural norms

ASSOCIATED CONDITIONS

- Infertility treatment regimen

ASSESSMENT

- Parental status, including age, marital status, number and ages of dependent children, and knowledge of normal child behavior
- Family status, including normal patterns of interaction among family members, family members' and patient's understanding of present situation
- Family member's ability to function in family roles, family conflicts, financial status, and rituals during holidays and family celebrations

- Coping patterns, including type and number of changes family has recently experienced, usual response to stress, ability to adapt to change, and use of support systems
- Family's past response to crises, including coping patterns and communication patterns to express anger, affection, and confrontation
- Family health history, including history of mental illness, stress-related illnesses, history of substance abuse, and sexual abuse of spouse or children
- Psychological status, including self-image and self-esteem, functional ability, independence level, and problem-solving and decision-making skills
- Spiritual status, including affiliation with a religious group and religious practices

EXPECTED OUTCOMES

- Family will maintain clearly defined roles, boundaries, and equitable responsibilities for each family member.
- Family will exhibit effective decision-making process.
- Family will exhibit clear, direct, and honest communication.
- Family will identify support systems and participate in assistance from those systems.

Suggested NOC Outcomes

Coping; Decision-Making; Family Coping; Family Environment: Internal; Family Functioning; Family Normalization; Family Resiliency; Family Social Climate; Social Involvement

INTERVENTIONS AND RATIONALES

- **PCC** Provide education to family members for communication techniques to clearly express their needs. *Open honest communication prevents disputes and set boundaries.*
- **PCC** Facilitate discussion of ideas and beliefs about family roles and responsibilities *to establish appropriate boundaries and family member roles.*
- **PCC** Provide an opportunity for family members to discuss conflicts in an open, safe atmosphere *to decrease anxiety and help family members develop confidence in their ability to resolve problems.*
- **PCC** Assist family members in identifying their strengths and their progress in addressing problems *to build self-esteem.*
- **PCC** Expedite communication within family to allow members to express their feelings about present situation. *This encourages supportive behavior to meet reciprocal needs in a crisis.*
- **PCC** Arrange and participate in family conferences, as needed. *Some families may require help to improve interpersonal communication.*
- Encourage family members to evaluate communication patterns periodically *to reinforce benefits of effective communication skills.*
- **PCC** Whenever possible, ensure privacy to family members for their discussions or conferences. *These measures allow you to help family identify and work toward mutual goals and facilitate effective family coping.*
- **T&C** Encourage family members to seek counseling *to enhance interpersonal skills and strengthen the family unit.*
- **T&C** Make referrals to social services or community agencies, as appropriate, *to provide family with access to additional coping resources.*

Suggested NIC Interventions

Coping Enhancement; Counseling; Family Mobilization; Family Process Maintenance; Family Support; Family Therapy; Normalization Promotion; Spiritual Support; Support System Enhancement

EVALUATIONS FOR EXPECTED OUTCOMES

- Family members identify factors associated with current issue.
- Family members discuss problems in an open, safe environment.
- Family members acknowledge their strengths and their progress in resolving problems.
- Family members state their plans to continue to seek counseling and attend appropriate support group meetings.
- Family members verbalize realistic expectations of each member's role.
- Family members participate in methods of solving problems and resolving conflicts.
- Family members share feelings about issues within the family.

DOCUMENTATION

- Family statements of improved self-confidence in task accomplishment
- Satisfaction level of family members
- Family stated goals for activity planning and execution
- Interventions to assist family and family's responses to those interventions
- Referrals to outside agencies
- Use of support services
- Problems and conflicts described by family members
- Changes in roles and responsibilities and information about how these changes were negotiated
- Evidence of changes in family communication patterns
- Evaluations for expected outcomes

REFERENCES

Deal, J. E. (2019). Normativity and desirability in observational assessments of family interaction. *Family Process, 58*(3), 749–760.

Frear, K. A., Paustian-Underdahl, S., Halbesleben, J. R. B., & French, K. A. (2019). Strategies for work–family management at the intersection of career–family centrality and gender. *Archives of Scientific Psychology, 7*(1), 50–59. doi:10.1037/arc0000068

Greenbaum, R. L., Deng, Y., Butts, M. M., Wang, C. S., & Smith, A. N. (2021). Managing my shame: Examining the effects of parental identity threat and emotional stability on work productivity and investment in parenting. *Journal of Applied Psychology.* doi:10.1037/apl0000597

Misra, S., Johnson, K. A., Parnarouskis, L. M., Koenen, K. C., Williams, D. R., Gelaye, B., & Borba, C. P. C. (2020). How early life adversities influence later life family interactions for individuals with Schizophrenia in outpatient treatment: A qualitative analysis. *Community Mental Health Journal, 56*(6), 1188–1200.

Dysfunctional Family Processes

DEFINITION

Family functioning which fails to support the well-being of its members

RELATED FACTORS (R/T)

- Addictive personality
- Ineffective coping strategies
- Insufficient problem-solving skills
- Substance misuse

ASSOCIATED CONDITIONS

- Biological factors
- Intimacy dysfunction
- Surgical procedure

ASSESSMENT

- Family status, including alcoholic family member's ability to function in occupational and family roles, ability of other family members to function in their roles, family conflicts, financial status, and rituals during holidays and family celebrations
- Coping patterns, including type and number of changes family has recently experienced, usual response to stress, ability to adapt to change, and use of support systems
- Family health history, including medication use, mental illness, stress-related illnesses, history of alcohol or drug abuse, and evidence of emotional, physical, or sexual abuse of spouse or children
- Parental status, including age, marital status, number and ages of dependent children, and knowledge of normal child behavior
- Drinking pattern, including continuous or binge drinking, periods of abstinence and relapse, use of other substances, symptoms of withdrawal, and past drinking patterns and treatment
- Psychological status, including self-image and self-esteem, functional ability, independence level, and problem-solving and decision-making skills
- Spiritual status, including affiliation with a religious group and religious practices

DEFINING CHARACTERISTICS

Behavioral

- Agitation
- Alteration in concentration
- Blaming
- Broken promises
- Chaos
- Complicated grieving
- Conflict avoidance
- Contradictory communication pattern
- Controlling communication pattern
- Criticizing
- Decrease in physical contact
- Denial of problems
- Dependency
- Difficulty having fun
- Difficulty with intimate relationship
- Difficulty with life-cycle transition
- Disturbances in academic performance in children
- Enabling substance use pattern
- Escalating conflict
- Failure to accomplish developmental tasks
- Harsh self-judgment
- Immaturity
- Inability to accept a wide range of feelings
- Inability to accept help
- Inability to adapt to change
- Inability to deal constructively with traumatic experiences
- Inability to express a wide range of feelings
- Inability to meet emotional needs of its members
- Inability to meet the security needs of its members

- Inability to meet spiritual needs of its members
- Inability to receive help appropriately
- Inappropriate anger expression
- Ineffective communication skills
- Insufficient knowledge about substance abuse
- Insufficient problem-solving skills
- Lying
- Manipulation
- Nicotine addiction
- Orientation favors tension relief rather than goal attainment
- Paradoxical communication pattern
- Power struggles
- Rationalization
- Refusal to get help
- Seeking of affirmation
- Seeking of approval
- Self-blame
- Social isolation
- Special occasions centered on substance use
- Stress-related physical illnesses
- Substance misuse
- Unreliable behavior
- Verbal abuse of children
- Verbal abuse of parent
- Verbal abuse of partner

Feelings

- Abandonment
- Anger
- Anxiety
- Confuses love and pity
- Confusion
- Depression
- Dissatisfaction
- Distress
- Embarrassment
- Emotional isolation
- Emotionally controlled by others
- Failure
- Fear
- Feeling different from others
- Feeling misunderstood
- Feeling unloved
- Frustration
- Guilt
- Hopelessness
- Hostility
- Hurt
- Insecurity
- Lingering resentment
- Loneliness

- Loss
- Loss of identity
- Low self-esteem
- Mistrust
- Moodiness
- Powerlessness
- Rejection
- Repressed emotions
- Shame
- Taking responsibility for substance misuser's behavior
- Tension
- Unhappiness
- Vulnerability
- Worthlessness

Roles and Relationships

- Change in role function
- Chronic family problems
- Closed communication system
- Conflict between partners
- Deterioration in family relationships
- Diminished ability of family members to relate to each other for mutual growth and maturation
- Disruption in family rituals
- Disruption in family roles
- Disturbance in family dynamics
- Economically disadvantaged
- Family denial
- Inconsistent parenting
- Ineffective communication with partner
- Insufficient cohesiveness
- Insufficient family respect for autonomy of its members
- Insufficient family respect for individuality of its members
- Insufficient relationship skills
- Neglect of obligation to family member
- Pattern of rejection
- Perceived insufficient parental support
- Triangulating family

EXPECTED OUTCOMES

- Family members will acknowledge that there's dysfunction within the family.
- Alcoholic family member will sign a contract stating that the person agrees to abstain from alcohol.
- Family members will sign contracts stating that they won't engage in abusive behavior.
- Family members will communicate their needs using "I" statements.
- Parents will take steps to reassert appropriate boundaries with children and resume parental responsibilities.
- Family members will discuss problems in an open, safe environment.
- Family members will acknowledge their strengths and their progress in resolving problems.

- Number and intensity of family crises will diminish.
- Family members will state their plans to continue to seek counseling and attend appropriate support group meetings.

Suggested NOC Outcomes

Family Coping; Family Functioning; Family Normalization; Role Performance; Substance Addiction Consequences

INTERVENTIONS AND RATIONALES

PCC ▪ Encourage family members to acknowledge that alcoholism is a problem within the family *to break through family denial.* Encourage individual family members to take responsibility for their problems. *Problems can't be addressed until family members take responsibility for them.*

PCC ▪ Inform alcoholic family member that he or she will have to address alcoholism before progress can be made in rebuilding family relations. Tell the person that abstinence with the help of a support group such as Alcoholics Anonymous is the only proven effective treatment for alcoholism *to establish abstinence as the basis for treatment.*

▪ Ask the alcoholic family member to sign a contract stating he or she will abstain from alcohol *to help him or her take responsibility for own behavior.*

S ▪ Help family members evaluate the consequences of abusive and violent behavior. Inform them that any suspected abuse will be reported. Ask family members to sign contracts stating they won't abuse each other *to help ensure the safety of family members.*

PCC ▪ Teach family members to communicate their needs assertively. Encourage family members to use "I" statements to express feelings, for example, "I'm mad because you didn't show up for the school play like you promised," *to help family members get in touch with and talk about their feelings.*

PCC ▪ Discuss with parents their ideas and beliefs regarding parental authority. Ask if they feel they have abdicated authority. Work with parents to develop steps to reassert parental authority *to reestablish appropriate boundaries and relieve children of the need to assume parental roles.*

PCC ▪ Provide an opportunity for family members to discuss conflicts in an open, safe atmosphere *to decrease anxiety and help family members develop confidence in their ability to resolve problems.*

PCC ▪ Assist family members in identifying their strengths and their progress in addressing problems *to build self-esteem.*

T&C ▪ Encourage family members to continue to seek counseling *to enhance interpersonal skills and strengthen the family unit.*

T&C ▪ Encourage family members to participate in Al-Anon or Alateen *to foster recovery.*

Suggested NIC Interventions

Coping Enhancement; Family Process Maintenance; Family Support; Substance Use Prevention; Substance Use Treatment

EVALUATIONS FOR EXPECTED OUTCOMES

- Family members acknowledge that there is dysfunction in the family.
- Alcoholic family member signs a contract stating that the person agrees to abstain from alcohol.

- Family members sign contracts stating that they won't engage in abusive behavior.
- Family members communicate their needs using "I" statements.
- Parents take steps to reassert appropriate boundaries with children and to resume parental responsibilities.
- Family members discuss problems in an open, safe environment.
- Family members acknowledge their strengths and the progress they have made in resolving problems.
- Number and intensity of family crises diminish.
- Family members state their plans to continue to seek counseling and attend appropriate support groups.

DOCUMENTATION

- Family's reactions to and experience with alcoholism
- Interventions to assist family and family's response to them
- Referrals to community agencies
- Evaluations for expected outcomes

REFERENCES

Kivelä, S., Leppäkoski, T., Helminen, M., & Paavilainen, E. (2018). A cross-sectional descriptive study of the family functioning, health and social support of hospital patients with family violence backgrounds. *Scandinavian Journal of Caring Sciences, 32*(3), 1083–1092.

Sleczka, P., Braun, B., Grüne, B., Bühringer, G., & Kraus, L. (2018). Family functioning and gambling problems in young adulthood: The role of the concordance of values. *Addiction Research & Theory, 26*(6), 447–456.

Tramonti, F., Bonfiglio, L., Bongioanni, P., Belviso, C., Fanciullacci, C., Rossi, B., … Carboncini, M. C. (2019). Caregiver burden and family functioning in different neurological diseases. *Psychology, Health & Medicine, 24*(1), 27–34.

Zhang, Y. (2018). Family functioning in the context of an adult family member with illness: A concept analysis. *Journal of Clinical Nursing, 27*(15–16), 3205–3224.

Interrupted Family Processes

DEFINITION

Break in the continuity of family functioning which fails to support the well-being of its members

RELATED FACTORS (R/T)

- Changes in interaction with community
- Power shift among family members
- Shift in family roles

ASSOCIATED CONDITION

- Shift in health status of a family member

ASSESSMENT

- Age of family members
- Family status, including normal patterns of interaction among family members, family members' and patient's understanding of present situation, and support systems available (financial, social, and spiritual)
- Family health history, including history of mental illness, stress-related illnesses, history of substance abuse, and sexual abuse of spouse or children

- Psychological status, including self-image and self-esteem, functional ability, independence level, and problem-solving and decision-making skills
- Family's past response to crises, including coping patterns and communication patterns to express anger, affection, and confrontation

DEFINING CHARACTERISTICS

- Alteration in availability for affective responsiveness
- Alteration in family conflict resolution
- Alteration in family satisfaction
- Alteration in intimacy
- Alteration in participation for problem-solving
- Change in communication pattern
- Change in somatization
- Change in stress-reduction behavior
- Changes in expressions of conflict with community resources
- Changes in expressions of isolation from community resources
- Changes in participation for decision-making
- Changes in available emotional support
- Decrease in mutual support
- Ineffective task completion
- Power alliance change
- Ritual change

EXPECTED OUTCOMES

- Family members will agree on who's the primary decision maker.
- Family members will develop adaptive responses by assuming duties carried out by ill member, for example, meal preparation, transportation, shopping, laundry, cleaning, and providing emotional support to other family members.
- Family members will identify support systems to assist them and will participate in mobilizing those systems.
- Patient and family members will voice realistic expectations of each member's role.
- Family members will express need to assume new or altered roles and adapt to changes within family structure.
- Family members won't experience verbal, physical, emotional, or sexual abuse.
- Family members will communicate clearly, honestly, consistently, and directly.
- Family members will establish clearly defined roles and equitable responsibilities.
- Family members will express understanding of rules and expectations.
- Family members will report that methods of solving problems and resolving conflicts have improved.
- Family members will report a decrease in the number and intensity of family crises.
- Family members will contact a community agency or support group for continued assistance (depending on type, severity, and prognosis of illness), for example, American Cancer Society, American Lung Association, Arthritis Foundation, Hospice, Myasthenia Gravis Foundation, Multiple Sclerosis Society, or National Kidney Foundation.
- Family members will share feelings about issues within the family.

Suggested NOC Outcomes

Coping; Decision-Making; Family Coping; Family Environment: Internal; Family Functioning; Family Normalization; Family Resiliency; Family Social Climate; Social Involvement

`PCC` ▪ Identify individual assuming role as head of family *to establish family hierarchy and functional ability.*

`EBP` ▪ Provide head of family with information necessary for decision-making, such as updated information on patient's condition. *This avoids potential for misinterpretation and places responsibility for communication within family unit.*

`PCC` ▪ Help head of family decide which support systems need to be mobilized and used. *This allows opportunity to evaluate head of family's management ability and family's problem-solving ability.*

`PCC` ▪ Provide emotional support to head of family regarding altered role and additional responsibilities. *This encourages family member to express feelings, ask questions, seek help, and make decisions.*

`PCC` ▪ Expedite communication within family to allow members to express their feelings about present situation. *This encourages supportive behavior to meet reciprocal needs in a crisis.*

`PCC` ▪ Arrange and participate in family conferences as needed. *Some families may require help to improve interpersonal communication.*

`PCC` ▪ Arrange with family to spend as much time as possible with patient to allow them to participate in providing care where it is appropriate. *This accommodation may fulfill both patient's and family's needs for participation.*

▪ Hold adults accountable for their alcohol or substance abuse and have them sign a "Use Contract" *to decrease denial, increase trust, and promote change.*

`S` ▪ Assist family to set limits on abusive behaviors and have them sign "Abuse Contracts" *to foster feelings of safety and trust.*

`PCC` ▪ Teach family to communicate clearly and honestly to increase their ability *to express thoughts and feelings in a positive way.*

▪ Encourage family members to evaluate communication patterns periodically *to reinforce benefits of effective communication skills.*

`PCC` ▪ Whenever possible, ensure privacy to family members for their discussions or conferences. *These measures allow you to help family identify and work toward mutual goals and facilitate effective family coping.*

`T&C` ▪ Make referrals to social services or community agencies, as appropriate, *to provide family with access to additional coping resources.*

▪ Include patient in family conferences and family interaction as often as possible.

Suggested NIC Interventions

Coping Enhancement; Counseling; Family Mobilization; Family Process Maintenance; Family Support; Family Therapy; Normalization Promotion; Spiritual Support; Support System Enhancement

▪ Family members identify family member to be primary decision maker, serving as head of family.

▪ Family members describe clearly defined roles and responsibilities.

▪ Family members demonstrate understanding of roles and responsibilities.

▪ Family members openly share feelings about present situation.

▪ Family members don't experience any type of abuse.

▪ Family members report that family communication is clear, honest, and respectful.

▪ Patient and family members voice realistic expectations about emotional and financial impact on family structure.

▦ Family members identify problems and work together to solve them.
▦ Family members report fewer family crises.
▦ Family members recognize the need for professional assistance.
▦ Family members identify and contact available resources, as needed.
▦ Family members contact community support groups and associations and attend at least two meetings.

DOCUMENTATION

▦ Observations of family's reactions to situation
▦ Interventions to assist family and family's responses to those interventions
▦ Referrals to outside agencies
▦ Patient's and family's responses to nursing interventions
▦ Problems and conflicts described by family members
▦ Behavioral contracts signed by family members
▦ Changes in roles and responsibilities and information about how these changes were negotiated
▦ Evidence of changes in family communication patterns
▦ Evaluations for expected outcomes

REFERENCES

Conway, E. R., Watson, B., Tatangelo, G., McCabe, M., Haapala, I., Biggs, S., & Kurrle, S. (2018). Is it all bleak? A systematic review of factors contributing to relationship change in dementia. *International Psychogeriatrics, 30*(11), 1619–1637.

D'Ippolito, I. M., Aloisi, M., Azicnuda, E., Silvestro, D., Giustini, M., Verni, F., … Bivona, U. (2018). Changes in caregivers lifestyle after severe acquired brain injury: A preliminary investigation. *BioMed Research International, 2018*, 1–14.

Monk, J. K., Oseland, L. M., Nelson Goff, B. S., Ogolsky, B. G., & Summers, K. (2017). Integrative intensive retreats for veteran couples and families: A pilot study assessing change in relationship adjustment, posttraumatic growth, and trauma symptoms. *Journal of Marital & Family Therapy, 43*(3), 448–462.

Taylor, J. O., Hartzler, A. L., Osterhage, K. P., Demiris, G., & Turner, A. M. (2018). Monitoring for change: The role of family and friends in helping older adults manage personal health information. *Journal of the American Medical Informatics Association, 25*(8), 989–999.

Readiness for Enhanced Family Processes

DEFINITION

A pattern of family functioning to support the well-being of family members, which can be strengthened

ASSESSMENT

▦ Family structure, including perception of self and family, family composition, social roles of family members, family developmental stages, socioeconomics, education, occupation, ethnicity, and cultural and religious beliefs
▦ Family health pattern, including perception of health, health management, family developmental tasks, coping mechanisms, health beliefs and values, health status, stressors, and safety
▦ Family function, including family interactions, use of resources, decision-making, growth and development, responses to affection and concerns

DEFINING CHARACTERISTICS

- Expresses desire to enhance balance between autonomy and cohesiveness
- Expresses desire to enhance communication pattern
- Expresses desire to enhance energy level of family to support activities of daily living
- Expresses desire to enhance family adaptation to change
- Expresses desire to enhance family dynamics
- Expresses desire to enhance family resilience
- Expresses desire to enhance growth of family members
- Expresses desire to enhance interdependence with community
- Expresses desire to enhance maintenance of boundaries between family members
- Expresses desire to enhance respect for family members
- Expresses desire to enhance safety of family members

EXPECTED OUTCOMES

- Family members will identify family goals and structured directions.
- Family members will express enjoyment and satisfaction in their roles in the family.
- Family members will regularly participate in traditional family activities.
- Family members will maintain open and positive communications.
- Family members will maintain a safe home environment.
- Family members will contact community resources for help, if needed.
- Family members will seek regular health screenings and immunizations.
- Family members will identify and acknowledge risk factors.
- Family members will make plans for dealing with life changes and unexpected events.
- Family members will maintain healthy lifestyles by exercising regularly, eating a well-balanced diet, avoiding substance abuse, and using proven holistic health strategies.

Suggested NOC Outcomes

Community Competence; Community Health Status; Compliance Behavior; Decision-Making; Family Coping; Family Functioning; Family Health Status; Family Integrity; Family Normalization; Family Participation in Professional Care; Health Beliefs: Perceived Ability to Perform; Health Beliefs: Perceived Control; Health Orientation; Health Promoting Behavior; Hope; Identity; Risk Detection

INTERVENTIONS AND RATIONALES

PCC ■ Encourage family members to identify individual and family goals and structured directions. *Individual and family goals set the boundaries that are respected by family members. Family functioning with structured direction should enhance family members' ability to meet their physical, social, and psychological needs.*

PCC ■ Encourage family members to express enjoyment and satisfaction in their roles in the family *to enhance family dynamics and strengthen family bonds.*

EBP ■ Assist family members in coping with changes related to growth and development. *Each transition stage of growth and development is a stressful life event.*

PCC ■ Explore with family members traditional activities that all family members will enjoy doing together. *Sharing traditional family activities increases loyalty, security, and a sense of belonging for family members.*

- Assess measures taken to maintain open and positive communications. *Healthy communications bridge the gap between members of the family.*
- **PCC** Assist family to clarify family values and beliefs regarding health and health practices by helping family identify their values, restate the values, and identify conflicts between values and action. *Values guide actions and have power to motivate behaviors. Value conflicts could lead to noncompliant health practices and interrupt the well-being of family members.*
- **S** Assess measures taken to maintain safety in the home environment. *Environments that are free from environmental hazards, both chemical and physical, assure a sense of security.*
- **PCC** Assess the stress-coping ability of family members, individually and as a whole, to determine the strength and weakness status of the individual's and family's stress-coping pattern. Help family make realistic plans for dealing with life changes and unexpected events. *Preparation for stress enhances the use of coping mechanisms and minimizes the threat.*
- **T&C** Provide family with information on social support and community resources. *Social support and community resources enhance the family process, reinforce family strength, and assist when families are experiencing stresses.*
- **EBP** Provide family with information on recommended health screenings and immunizations and encourage them to schedule regular checkups according to their growth and developmental stages. *Screening is a valuable tool to enhance preventive interventions.*
- **EBP** Help family develop a genogram to identify genetic risk factors. *Information from a genogram highlights a family's health patterns, provides knowledge leading to early identification of genetically related diseases, and may delay disease onset.*
- **EBP** Educate and encourage family members to exercise regularly, eat a well-balanced diet, avoid substance abuse, and use proven holistic health strategies. *Health promotion behaviors could maintain optimum health.*

Suggested NIC Interventions

Active Listening; Anticipatory Guidance; Attachment Promotion; Behavior Modification: Social Skills; Coping Enhancement; Emotional Support; Environmental Management: Attachment Process; Environmental Management: Comfort; Environmental Management: Safety; Environmental Management: Violence Prevention; Exercise Promotion; Family Involvement Promotion; Family Mobilization; Family Process Maintenance; Family Support; Health Education; Health Screening; Health System Guidance; Hope Instillation; Humor; Meditation Facilitation; Risk Identification; Role Enhancement; Security Enhancement; Self-Esteem Enhancement; Self-Responsibility Facilitation; Socialization Enhancement; Spiritual Support; Support System Enhancement; Truth Telling; Values Clarification

EVALUATIONS FOR EXPECTED OUTCOMES

- Family functions in a structured and goal-oriented direction.
- Family members state enjoyment and satisfaction in their roles in the family.
- Family members regularly participate in traditional family activities.
- Family members maintain open and positive communications.
- Family members maintain a safe home environment.
- Family utilizes various available social support venues as well as community resources to meet the needs of the family and individual family members.

▓ Family members participate in regular health screenings and immunizations.

▓ Family members identify and acknowledge risk factors.

▓ Family members have plans for dealing with life changes and unexpected events.

▓ Family members maintain healthy lifestyle by exercising regularly, eating a well-balanced diet, avoiding substance abuse, and using proven holistic health strategies.

DOCUMENTATION

▓ Identification of goals and activities carried out

▓ Satisfaction level of family members

▓ Use of support services

▓ Health visits, patterns of exercise and diet, use of other health-promoting strategies

▓ Evaluations for expected outcomes

REFERENCES

Choi, Y., Kim, T. Y., Noh, S., Lee, J., & Takeuchi, D. (2018). Culture and family process: Measures of familism for Filipino and Korean American parents. *Family Process, 57*(4), 1029–1048.

Khamis, V. (2017). Psychological distress of parents in conflict areas: The mediating role of war atrocities, normative stressors and family resources. *Journal of Mental Health, 26*(2), 104–110.

Kuo, P. X., Volling, B. L., & Gonzalez, R. (2018). Gender role beliefs, work-family conflict, and father involvement after the birth of a second child. *Psychology of Men & Masculinity, 19*(2), 243–256.

Paskewitz, E. A., & Beck, S. J. (2017). When work and family merge: Understanding intragroup conflict experiences in family farm businesses. *Journal of Family Communication, 17*(4), 386–400.

Fatigue

DEFINITION

An overwhelming sustained sense of exhaustion and decreased capacity for physical and mental work at the usual level

RELATED FACTORS (R/T)

▓ Altered sleep–wake cycle

▓ Anxiety

▓ Depressive symptoms

▓ Environmental constraints

▓ Increased mental exertion

▓ Increased physical exertion

▓ Malnutrition

▓ Nonstimulating lifestyle

▓ Pain

▓ Physical deconditioning

▓ Stressors

ASSOCIATED CONDITIONS

▓ Anemia

▓ Chemotherapy

▓ Chronic disease

▓ Chronic inflammation

▓ Dementia

- Fibromyalgia
- Hypothalamus–pituitary–adrenal axis dysregulation
- Myasthenia gravis
- Neoplasms
- Radiotherapy
- Stroke

ASSESSMENT

- History of underlying disease process
- Respiratory status, including dyspnea on exertion and respiratory rate and depth
- Cardiovascular status, including skin color, temperature, turgor, and blood pressure
- Age
- Sleep pattern, including hours slept at night and amount of time awake before becoming tired
- Nutritional status, including appetite, dietary intake, current weight, and change from normal weight
- Neurologic status, including headaches
- Activity status, including type and duration of exercise, occupation, and use of leisure time
- Psychosocial status, including personality stressors (finances, job, or marital discord), coping mechanisms, support systems (family members and others), and lifestyle
- Menstrual history, including length of menses and amount of menstrual flow

DEFINING CHARACTERISTICS

- Altered attention
- Apathy
- Decreased aerobic capacity
- Decreased gait velocity
- Difficulty maintaining usual physical activity
- Difficulty maintaining usual routines
- Disinterested in surroundings
- Drowsiness
- Expresses altered libido
- Expresses demoralization
- Expresses frustration
- Expresses lack of energy
- Expresses nonrelief through usual energy-recovery strategies
- Expresses tiredness
- Expresses weakness
- Inadequate role performance
- Increased physical symptoms
- Increased rest requirement
- Insufficient physical endurance
- Introspection
- Lethargy
- Tiredness

EXPECTED OUTCOMES

- Patient will identify measures to prevent or modify fatigue.
- Patient will incorporate as part of daily activities those measures necessary to modify fatigue.

- Patient will explain relationship of fatigue to disease process and activity level.
- Patient will verbally express increased energy.
- Patient will articulate plan to resolve fatigue problems.
- Patient will employ measures to prevent and modify fatigue.

Suggested NOC Outcomes

Activity Tolerance; Comfort Level; Endurance; Energy Conservation; Nutritional Status: Energy; Psychomotor Energy; Personal Health Status; Personal Well-Being

INTERVENTIONS AND RATIONALES

PCC ▦ Prevent unnecessary fatigue; for example, avoid scheduling two energy-draining procedures on the same day. *Using energy-conserving techniques avoids overexertion and potential for exhaustion.*

▦ Conserve energy through rest, planning, and setting priorities *to prevent or alleviate fatigue.*

EBP ▦ Alternate activities with periods of rest. Encourage activities that can be completed in short periods or divided into several segments; for example, read one chapter of a book at a time. *Scheduling regular rest periods helps decrease fatigue and increase stamina.*

EBP ▦ Discuss effect of fatigue on daily living and personal goals. Explore with patient relationship between fatigue and disease process *to help increase patient compliance with schedule for activity and rest.*

PCC ▦ Reduce demands placed on patient; for example, ask one family member to call at specified times and relay messages to friends and other family members *to reduce physical and emotional stress.*

PCC ▦ Structure patient's environment; for example, set up daily schedule based on patient's needs and desires. *This encourages compliance with treatment regimen.*

EBP ▦ Encourage patient to eat foods rich in iron and minerals, unless contraindicated. *This helps avoid anemia and demineralization.*

▦ Postpone eating when patient is fatigued *to avoid aggravating condition.*

▦ Provide small, frequent feedings *to conserve patient's energy and encourage increased dietary intake.*

EBP ▦ Establish a regular sleeping pattern. *Getting 8 to 10 hours of sleep nightly helps reduce fatigue.*

▦ Encourage avoidance of highly emotional situations *to minimize their impact on fatigue.*

PCC ▦ Encourage patient to explore feelings and emotions with a supportive counselor, clergy member, or other professional *to help cope with illness.*

Suggested NIC Interventions

Activity Therapy; Coping Enhancement; Energy Management; Exercise Promotion; Nutrition Management; Mood Management; Mutual Goal Setting; Sleep Enhancement

EVALUATIONS FOR EXPECTED OUTCOMES

- Patient describes at least three measures to prevent or modify fatigue.
- Patient incorporates at least three measures to modify fatigue into daily routine.
- Patient discusses relationship of fatigue to disease process and activity level; for example, in heart disease, fatigue is a sign that the heart cannot meet increased oxygen demands.
- Patient reports reduced fatigue level.

- Patient describes plan to resolve fatigue problems, including both physiologic and emotional remedies.
- Patient follows measures to prevent and modify fatigue.

DOCUMENTATION

- Patient's ability to describe fatigue and its relationship to disease process and condition
- Patient's ability to decrease fatigue by using various effective methods
- Patient's level of activity in relation to fatigue
- Patient's dietary intake
- Evaluations for expected outcomes

REFERENCES

Cajanding, R. J. (2017). Causes, assessment and management of fatigue in critically ill patients. *British Journal of Nursing, 26*(21), 1176–1181.

James, L., Samuels, C. H., & Vincent, F. (2018). Evaluating the effectiveness of fatigue management training to improve police sleep health and wellness: A pilot study. *Journal of Occupational & Environmental Medicine, 60*(1), 77–82.

Mattioli, D. (2018). Focusing on the caregiver: Compassion fatigue awareness and understanding. *MEDSURG Nursing, 27*(5), 323–327.

McCormack, R. C., O'Shea, F., Doran, M., & Connolly, D. (2018). Impact of a fatigue management in work programme on meeting work demands of individuals with rheumatic diseases: A pilot study. *Musculoskeletal Care, 16*(3), 398–404.

Fear

DEFINITION

Basic, intense emotional response aroused by the detection of imminent threat, involving an immediate alarm reaction (American Psychological Association)

RELATED FACTORS (R/T)

- Communication barriers
- Learned response to threat
- Response to phobic stimulus
- Unfamiliar situation

ASSOCIATION CONDITIONS

- Sensation disorders

ASSESSMENT

- Age and gender
- History of experience with illness, hospitalization, and surgery
- Changes in behavior, eating or sleeping habits, and ability to concentrate
- Developmental status, including cognitive, psychosexual, and psychosocial stages; cognitive and motor capabilities; and communication and socialization skills
- Availability of support systems, including family members, friends, and clergy
- Financial resources

- History of coping with fear
- Physiologic manifestations of fear, including changes in pulse rate, respiratory rate, blood pressure, skin temperature, and quality and pitch of voice
- Psychological manifestations of fear, including changes in behavior, appetite, and sleep pattern

DEFINING CHARACTERISTICS

Physiological Factors

- Anorexia
- Diaphoresis
- Diarrhea
- Dyspnea
- Increased blood pressure
- Increased heart rate
- Increased respiratory rate
- Increased sweating
- Increased urinary frequency
- Muscle tension
- Nausea
- Pallor
- Pupil dilation
- Vomiting
- Xerostomia

Behavioral/Emotional

- Apprehensiveness
- Concentration on the source of fear
- Decreased self-assurance
- Expresses alarm
- Expresses fear
- Expresses intense dread
- Expresses tension
- Impulsive behaviors
- Increased alertness
- Ineffective impulse control
- Nervousness
- Psychomotor agitation

EXPECTED OUTCOMES

- Patient will identify source of fear.
- Patient will communicate feelings about separation from support systems.
- Patient will communicate feelings of comfort or satisfaction.
- Patient will demonstrate effective use of coping mechanisms.
- Patient will use situational supports to reduce fear.
- Patient will integrate into daily behavior at least one fear-reducing coping mechanism, such as asking questions about treatment progress or making decisions about care.

Suggested NOC Outcomes

Anxiety Control; Comfort Level; Coping; Fear Self-Control

PCC ▪ Encourage patient to identify source of fear; try to assess patient's understanding of situation. *Patient's perceptions may be erroneously based.*

PCC ▪ Explain all treatments and procedures, answering any questions patient might have. Present information at patient's level of understanding or acceptance *to reduce patient's anxiety and enhance cooperation.*

▪ Don't dismiss fear or blithely reassure patient that "everything will be alright." *Refusing to acknowledge fear or giving false reassurance impairs coping.*

PCC ▪ Provide patient with accurate information about patient's condition and scheduled procedures and treatments. *Accurate information dispels misconceptions that can fuel fear.*

S ▪ Orient patient to surroundings. Make any adaptations to compensate for sensory deficits. *This enhances patient's ability to orient to time, place, person, and events.*

▪ Assign same nurse to care for patient whenever possible *to provide consistency of care, enhance trust, and reduce threat commonly associated with multiple caregivers.*

PCC ▪ Spend as much time as possible establishing rapport with patient. Communicate at patient's eye level. Speak in a soft, reassuring voice. *Establishing rapport encourages patient to express feelings and provides comfort.*

▪ If patient has no visitors, spend an extra 15 minutes each shift in casual conversation; encourage other staff members to stop for brief visits *to help patient cope with separation.*

PCC ▪ Remain with patient when experiencing a higher than usual level of fear *to provide a source of support.*

▪ Help patient maintain daily contact with family:
  ▪ Arrange for telephone calls.
  ▪ Help write letters.
  ▪ Promptly convey messages to patient from family and vice versa.
  ▪ Encourage patient to have pictures of loved ones.
  ▪ Provide privacy for visits; take patient to day room or other quiet area. *These measures help patient reestablish and maintain social relationships.*

PCC ▪ Involve patient in planning care and setting goals *to renew confidence and give sense of control in a crisis situation.*

EBP ▪ Instruct patient in relaxation techniques, such as imagery and progressive muscle relaxation, *to reduce symptoms of sympathetic stimulation.*

▪ Administer antianxiety medications, as ordered, and monitor effectiveness. *Drug therapy may be needed to manage high anxiety levels or panic disorders.*

▪ Answer questions and help patient understand care *to reduce anxiety and correct misconceptions.*

▪ When feasible and where policies permit, relax visiting restrictions *to reduce patient's sense of isolation.*

▪ Allow a close family member or friend to participate in care *to provide an additional source of support.*

PCC ▪ Support family and friends in their efforts to understand patient's fear and to respond accordingly *to help them understand that patient's emotions are appropriate in context of situation.*

Suggested NIC Interventions

Active Listening; Anxiety Reduction; Cognitive Restructuring; Counseling; Coping Enhancement; Decision-Making Support; Security Enhancement; Presence; Support Group

▪ Patient states causes of fear.
▪ Patient demonstrates effective use of coping mechanisms.

▦ Patient expresses distress caused by separation from support systems.
▦ Patient reports feeling less fearful.
▦ Patient reaches out to others for support through phone calls, letters, or other means.
▦ Patient exhibits marked decrease in physiologic and behavioral manifestations of fear.
▦ Patient demonstrates use of at least one coping mechanism daily to reduce fear.

DOCUMENTATION

▦ Patient's expressions of concern about illness, hospitalization, and separation from support system and overt expressions of fear
▦ Physical manifestations of fear
▦ Observations of physiologic and behavioral manifestations of patient's fear
▦ Interventions performed to reduce patient's fears and encourage healthy coping mechanisms
▦ Patient's response to interventions
▦ Evaluations for expected outcomes

REFERENCES

Ellis, E. M., Klein, W. M. P., Orehek, E., & Ferrer, R. A. (2018). Effects of emotion on medical decisions involving tradeoffs. *Medical Decision Making, 38*(8), 1027–1039.
Fakari, F. R., Simbar, M., & Naz, M. S. G. (2018). The relationship between fear-avoidance beliefs and pain in pregnant women with pelvic girdle pain: A cross-sectional study. *International Journal of Community Based Nursing & Midwifery, 6*(4), 305–313.
Hall, D. L., Luberto, C. M., Philpotts, L. L., Song, R., Park, E. R., & Yeh, G. Y. (2018). Mind-body interventions for fear of cancer recurrence: A systematic review and meta-analysis. *Psycho-Oncology, 27*(11), 2546–2558.
Hofer, J., Busch, H., Šolcová, I. P., & Tavel, P. (2017). Relationship between subjectively evaluated health and fear of death among elderly in three cultural contexts. *International Journal of Aging & Human Development, 84*(4), 343–365.

Ineffective Infant Feeding Dynamics

DEFINITION

Altered parental feeding behaviors resulting in over or under eating patterns

RELATED FACTORS (R/T)

▦ Abusive relationship
▦ Attachment issues
▦ Disengaged parenting style
▦ Lack of confidence in child to develop healthy eating habits
▦ Lack of confidence in child to grow appropriately
▦ Lack of knowledge of appropriate methods of feeding infant for each stage of development
▦ Lack of knowledge of infant's developmental stages
▦ Lack of knowledge of parent's responsibility in infant feeding
▦ Media influence on feeding infant high caloric, unhealthy foods
▦ Media influence on knowledge of high caloric, unhealthy foods
▦ Multiple caregivers
▦ Over-involved parenting style
▦ Under-involved parenting style

ASSOCIATED CONDITIONS

- Chromosomal disorders
- Cleft lip
- Cleft palate
- Congenital heart disease
- Genetic disorder
- Neural tube defects
- Physical challenge with eating
- Physical health issues of parents
- Prolonged enteral feedings
- Psychological health issues of parents
- Sensory integration problems

ASSESSMENT

- Perinatal history, including gestational age and Apgar score
- Parents' knowledge on the importance and correct infant feeding behaviors
- Suck and swallow reflex, including condition of lip and palate
- Nutritional status, including intake (type, amount, and frequency of feedings), output (frequency, amount, and characteristics of urine), current weight, weight change since birth, skin turgor, and signs of dehydration
- Laboratory studies, including glucose and bilirubin levels
- Parental status, including age, maturity level, and previous experience with infant feeding
- Parental history of substance misuse
- Parental engagement with infant

DEFINING CHARACTERISTICS

- Food refusal
- Inappropriate transition to solid foods
- Overeating
- Poor appetite
- Undereating

EXPECTED OUTCOMES

- Infant will exhibit ability to feed sufficiently and correctly.
- Infant will attain the expected milestones during growth and development.
- Infant will not experience weight loss or excessive weight gain.
- Parent(s) will describe the normal feeding pattern of infants.
- Parent(s) will follow the correct feeding pattern.
- Parent(s) will identify factors that interfere with infant establishing effective feeding pattern.
- Parent(s) will express increased confidence in performing appropriate feeding techniques.

Suggested NOC Outcomes

Bottle Feeding Establishment: Infant; Breastfeeding Establishment: Infant; Infant Nutritional Status

- Assess infant's feeding pattern *to monitor for ineffective patterns.*
- **S** ▪ Weigh infant at the same time each day on the same scale *to detect excessive weight loss early.*
- Assess infant's sucking pattern *to monitor for ineffective patterns.*
- Assess parents' knowledge of feeding techniques *to help identify and clear up misconceptions.*
- **PCC** ▪ Assess parents' level of anxiety about infant's feedings. *Anxiety may interfere with parents' ability to learn new techniques.*
- Remain with parents and infant during the feeding *to identify problem areas and direct interventions.*
- **EBP** ▪ Teach parents to place infant in the upright position during feeding *to prevent aspiration.*
- Provide positive reinforcement for parents' efforts to improve their feeding technique *to decrease anxiety and enhance feelings of success.*
- For bottle-feeding, record the amount ingested at each feeding; for breastfeeding, record the number of minutes infant nurses at each breast and the amount of any supplement ingested *to monitor for inadequate caloric and fluid intake.*
- Monitor infant for poor skin turgor, dry mucous membranes, decreased or concentrated urine, and sunken fontanels and eyeballs *to detect possible dehydration and allow for immediate intervention.*
- Record the number of stools and amount of urine voided each shift. *An altered bowel elimination pattern may indicate decreased food intake; decreased amounts of concentrated urine may indicate dehydration.*
- Assess the need for gavage feeding. *Infant may temporarily require alternative means of obtaining adequate fluids and calories.*
- Alternate oral and gavage feeding *to conserve infant's energy.*
- If infant requires IV nourishment, assess the insertion site, amount infused, and infusion rate every hour *to monitor fluid intake and identify possible complications, such as infiltration and phlebitis.*
- Assess infant for neurologic deficits or other pathophysiologic causes of ineffective sucking *to identify the need for more extensive evaluation.*
- **EBP** ▪ Explain to parent(s) the importance of proper nutrition for infants by following the prescribed feeding pattern. *Increases understanding of nutritional needs of infant and promotes appropriate feeding pattern.*
- **PCC** ▪ Assess the stress-coping ability of parent(s), to determine the strength and weakness status of stress-coping pattern. Help parent(s) make realistic plans for feeding schedule and feeding plan. *Preparation for stress enhances the use of coping mechanisms.*
- **T&C** ▪ Provide parent(s) with information on social support and community resources. *Social support and community resources enhance the parenting process, reinforce parenting strength, and assist when parents are experiencing stresses.*

Suggested NIC Interventions

Attachment Promotion; Breastfeeding Assistance; Environmental Management; Lactation Counseling; Nutrition Management; Nutritional Monitoring; Parent Education: Infant

- Infant exhibits ability to feed sufficiently and correctly.
- Infant attains the expected milestones during growth and development.
- Infant does not experience weight loss or excessive weight gain.

- Parent(s) describes the normal feeding pattern of infants.
- Parent(s) follows the correct feeding pattern.
- Parent(s) identifies factors that interfere with infant establishing effective feeding pattern.
- Parent(s) expresses increased confidence in performing appropriate feeding techniques.

DOCUMENTATION

- Frequency, amount, and type of fluid ingested by infant
- Infant's daily weight
- Parents' knowledge of feeding techniques, involvement with caregiving, and bonding with infant
- Frequency of infant's bowel elimination and urination
- Signs of dehydration
- Nursing interventions
- Use of special feeding techniques and equipment
- Parents' and infant's responses to nursing interventions
- Evaluations for expected outcomes

REFERENCES

Gross, R. S., Mendelsohn, A. L., & Messito, M. J. (2018). Additive effects of household food insecurity during pregnancy and infancy on maternal infant feeding styles and practices. *Appetite, 130*, 20–28

Madlala, S., & Kassier, S. (2018). Antenatal and postpartum depression: Effects on infant and young child health and feeding practices. *South African Journal of Clinical Nutrition, 31*(1), 1–7.

Nelson, J. M., Perrine, C. G., Freedman, D. S., Williams, L., Morrow, B., Smith, R. A., & Dee, D. L. (2018). Infant feeding-related maternity care practices and maternal report of breastfeeding outcomes. *Birth: Issues in Perinatal Care, 45*(4), 424–431.

Rodriguez, J., Affuso, O., Azuero, A., Downs, C. A., Turner-Henson, A., & Rice, M. (2018). Infant feeding practices and weight gain in toddlers born very preterm: A pilot study. *Journal of Pediatric Nursing, 43*, 29–35.

Risk for Female Genital Mutilation

DEFINITION

Susceptible to full or partial ablation of the female external genitalia and other lesions of the genitalia, whether for cultural, religious or any other non therapeutic reasons, which may compromise health

RISK FACTORS

- Lack of family knowledge about impact of practice on physical health
- Lack of family knowledge about impact of practice on reproductive health
- Lack of family knowledge about impact of practice on psychosocial health

ASSESSMENT

- Age
- Beliefs about female sexuality
- Marital status

- Role of family members
- Patient's perception of sexual identity and role
- Patient's perception of significance of sexual relationships
- Family beliefs about female sexuality
- Cultural background and ethnic group
- Social and religious practices relating to sexuality

EXPECTED OUTCOMES

- Patient will remain free of non medical alteration of genitalia.
- Patient will not experience complications associated with non medical alteration of genitalia.
- Patient will not experience sexual dysfunction associated with non medical alteration of genitalia.
- Patient will voice feelings about potential or actual changes in sexual activity.

Suggested NOC Outcomes

Abuse Recovery; Abuse Recovery: Emotional; Abuse Recovery: Physical; Abuse Recovery: Sexual; Knowledge: Sexual Functioning; Physical Maturation: Female; Sexual Functioning; Social Support

INTERVENTIONS AND RATIONALES

PCC ▪ Establish a therapeutic relationship with patient *to provide a safe, comfortable atmosphere for discussing sexual concerns.*

S ▪ Screen for risk factors associated with mutilation practices. *Allows for early intervention.*

S ▪ Monitor for signs and symptoms of physical injury. *Patient may not be comfortable notifying health providers.*

PCC ▪ Allow a specific amount of uninterrupted, non–care-related time *to talk with patient to demonstrate your comfort with sexuality issues and reassure patient that personal concerns are acceptable for discussion.*

PCC ▪ Display an accepting, nonjudgmental manner *to encourage patient to discuss concerns about sexuality. A nonjudgmental approach demonstrates unconditional positive regard for patient.*

PCC ▪ Encourage patient to verbalize fears and to ask questions about sexual functioning. *Establishes a knowledge base from which the patient can make decisions.*

EBP ▪ Discuss the effect of sexual health on health and wellness. *Sexual health is a human need.*

PCC ▪ Determine if patient has a functional spiritual network *to assist with needs of belonging, care, and beliefs.*

PCC ▪ Provide positive affirmation of worth *to build self-esteem and rapport.*

EBP ▪ Provide factual information about sexual myths and misinformation that patient or patient family may verbalize. *Evidence allows patient and patient family to make informed decisions.*

PCC ▪ Build and maintain communication with patient family and/or significant other *to identify patterns of behavior, thinking, feelings in which family members exert power or control over sexuality of patient.*

T&C ■ Offer referral for counseling, such as a mental health professional, if indicated. *Referrals provide opportunities for additional ongoing therapy during hospitalization and after discharge.*

Suggested NIC Interventions

Abuse Protection Support; Active Listening; Conflict Mediation; Teaching: Sexuality; Values Clarification

EVALUATIONS FOR EXPECTED OUTCOMES

■ Patient remains free of non medical alteration of genitalia.
■ Patient does not experience complications associated with non medical alteration of genitalia.
■ Patient does not experience sexual dysfunction associated with non medical alteration of genitalia.
■ Patient verbalizes feelings about potential or actual changes in sexual activity.

DOCUMENTATION

■ Patient's verbal and nonverbal behaviors
■ Patient's perception of female genital mutilation
■ Observations of patient's behavior in response to female genital mutilation
■ Interventions performed to assist patient
■ Specific nursing interventions to reduce emotional and behavioral reactions, such as active listening, limit setting, and counseling referrals
■ Interventions to support and educate patient
■ Response to nursing interventions
■ Evaluations for expected outcomes

REFERENCES

Jiménez-Ruiz, I., Almansa-Martínez, P., & Alcón Belchí, C. (2017). Dismantling the man-made myths upholding female genital mutilation. *Health Care for Women International, 38*(5), 478–491.
Klein, E., Helzner, E., Shayowitz, M., Kohlhoff, S., & Smith-Norowitz, T. A. (2018). Female genital mutilation: Health consequences and complications—A short literature review. *Obstetrics & Gynecology International, 2018,* 1–7.
Pastor-Bravo, M. D. M., Almansa-Martínez, P., & Jiménez-Ruiz, I. (2018). Living with mutilation: A qualitative study on the consequences of female genital mutilation in women's health and the healthcare system in Spain. *Midwifery, 66,* 119–126.
Waigwa, S., Doos, L., Bradbury-Jones, C., & Taylor, J. (2018). Effectiveness of health education as an intervention designed to prevent female genital mutilation/cutting (FGM/C): A systematic review. *Reproductive Health, 15*(1), 62.

Deficient Fluid Volume

DEFINITION

Decreased intravascular, interstitial, and/or intracellular fluid. This refers to dehydration, water loss alone without change in sodium

RELATED FACTORS (R/T)

- Difficulty meeting increased fluid volume requirement
- Inadequate access to fluid
- Inadequate knowledge about fluid needs
- Ineffective medication self-management
- Insufficient fluid intake
- Insufficient muscle mass
- Malnutrition

ASSOCIATED CONDITIONS

- Active fluid volume loss
- Deviations affecting fluid absorption
- Deviations affecting fluid elimination
- Deviations affecting fluid intake
- Excessive fluid loss through normal route
- Fluid loss through abnormal route
- Pharmaceutical preparations
- Treatment regimen

ASSESSMENT

- Age
- Height and weight
- Gastrointestinal (GI) status, including usual bowel patterns, changes in bowel patterns, stool characteristics (color, amount, size, consistency, and frequency), auscultation of bowel sounds, and inspection of abdomen
- History of fluid loss, including vomiting, nasogastric tube drainage, diarrhea, or hemorrhage
- Pulse, blood pressure, respirations, and temperature
- Fluid and electrolyte status, including weight, intake and output, urine specific gravity, skin turgor, and mucous membranes
- Neurologic status, including level of consciousness
- Laboratory studies, including serum electrolyte, blood urea nitrogen, hemoglobin levels, hematocrit (HCT), and stool cultures

DEFINING CHARACTERISTICS

- Altered mental status
- Altered skin turgor
- Decreased blood pressure
- Decreased pulse pressure
- Decreased pulse volume
- Decreased tongue turgor
- Decreased urine output
- Decreased venous filling
- Dry mucous membranes
- Dry skin
- Increased body temperature
- Increased heart rate

- Increased serum hematocrit levels
- Increased urine concentration
- Sudden weight loss
- Sunken eyes
- Thirst
- Weakness

EXPECTED OUTCOMES

- Patient's vital signs will remain stable.
- Patient's intake and output will be balanced and within normal limits for age.
- Patient will produce adequate urine volume.
- Patient will have elastic skin turgor and moist mucous membranes.
- Patient's urine specific gravity will remain between 1.005 and 1.010.
- Patient's fluid and blood volume will return to normal.
- Patient will express understanding of factors that caused fluid volume deficit.

Suggested NOC Outcomes

Electrolyte & Acid–Base Balance; Fluid Balance; Hydration; Urinary Elimination; Kidney Function; Nausea and Vomiting Severity; Thermoregulation; Vital Signs

INTERVENTIONS AND RATIONALES

S ■ Monitor and record vital signs every 2 hours or as often as necessary until stable. Then monitor and record vital signs every 4 hours. *Tachycardia, dyspnea, or hypotension may indicate fluid volume deficit or electrolyte imbalance.*

EBP ■ Cover patient lightly. Avoid overheating *to prevent vasodilation, blood pooling in extremities, and reduced circulating blood volume.*

EBP ■ Measure intake and output every 1 to 4 hours. Record and report significant changes. Include urine, stools, vomitus, wound drainage, nasogastric drainage, chest tube drainage, and any other output. *Low urine output and high specific gravity indicate hypovolemia.*

■ Administer fluids, blood or blood products, or plasma expanders as ordered *to replace fluids and whole blood loss and facilitate fluid movement into intravascular space.* Monitor and record effectiveness and any adverse effects.

■ Weigh patient daily at same time for more accurate and consistent data. *Weight is a good indicator of fluid status.*

■ Assess skin turgor and oral mucous membranes every 8 hours *to check for dehydration.* Give meticulous mouth care every 4 hours *to avoid dehydrating mucous membranes.*

■ Test urine specific gravity every 8 hours. *Elevated specific gravity may indicate dehydration.*

S ■ Don't allow patient to sit or stand up quickly as long as circulation is compromised *to avoid orthostatic hypotension and possible syncope.*

■ Measure abdominal girth every 12 hours *to monitor for ascites and third-space shift.* Report changes.

■ Administer and monitor medications *to prevent further fluid loss.*

EBP ■ Explain reasons for fluid loss and teach patient how to monitor fluid volume, for example, by recording daily weight and measuring intake and output. *This encourages patient involvement in personal care.*

Suggested NIC Interventions

Acid–Base Management; Electrolyte Monitoring; Fluid Management; Hypovolemia Management; Nutrition Management; Swallowing Therapy; Vital Signs Monitoring

EVALUATIONS FOR EXPECTED OUTCOMES

- Patient's pulse rate, blood pressure, respirations, and body temperature remain within set limits.
- Patient's fluid volume remains adequate.
- Patient's urine output remains at volume established for patient.
- Patient's skin turgor is elastic.
- Patient's specific gravity remains between 1.005 and 1.010, unless specified otherwise.
- Patient has no signs of dehydration; mucous membranes remain pink and moist.
- Urine output is at least 30 mL/hour or 100 mL in 4 hours.
- Patient and caregiver demonstrate understanding of factors precipitating fluid volume deficit.

DOCUMENTATION

- Patient's complaints of thirst, weakness, dizziness, and palpitations
- Observations of physical findings
- Intake and output (amount and type)
- Patient's weight and abdominal girth
- Interventions performed to control fluid loss
- Nursing interventions performed to maintain adequate fluid intake
- Patient's response to interventions
- Evaluations for expected outcomes

REFERENCES

Akech, S., Rotich, B., Chepkirui, M., Ayieko, P., Irimu, G., English, M., & Clinical Information Network authors. (2018). The prevalence and management of dehydration amongst neonatal admissions to general paediatric wards in Kenya—A clinical audit. *Journal of Tropical Pediatrics*, 64(6), 516–522.

Balakumar, V., Murugan, R., Sileanu, F. E., Palevsky, P., Clermont, G., & Kellum, J. A. (2017). Both positive and negative fluid balance may be associated with reduced long-term survival in the critically ill. *Critical Care Medicine*, 45(8), e749–e757.

Namasivayam-MacDonald, A. M., Slaughter, S. E., Morrison, J., Steele, C. M., Carrier, N., Lengyel, C., & Keller, H. H. (2018). Inadequate fluid intake in long term care residents: Prevalence and determinants. *Geriatric Nursing*, 39(3), 330–335.

Sakr, Y., Birri, P. N. R., Kotfis, K., Nanchal, R., Shah, B., Kluge, S., ... Rubatto Birri, P. N. (2017). Higher fluid balance increases the risk of death from sepsis: Results from a large international audit. *Critical Care Medicine*, 45(3), 386–394.

Risk for Deficient Fluid Volume

DEFINITION

Susceptible to experiencing decreased intravascular, interstitial, and/or intracellular fluid volumes, which may compromise health

RISK FACTORS

- Difficulty meeting increased fluid volume requirement
- Inadequate access to fluid

- Inadequate knowledge about fluid needs
- Ineffective medication self-management
- Insufficient fluid intake
- Insufficient muscle mass
- Malnutrition

ASSOCIATED CONDITIONS

- Active fluid volume loss
- Deviations affecting fluid absorption
- Deviations affecting fluid elimination
- Deviations affecting fluid intake
- Excessive fluid loss through normal route
- Fluid loss through abnormal route
- Pharmaceutical preparations
- Treatment regimen

ASSESSMENT

- Age
- Vital signs
- Respiratory status, including increased respiratory rate
- Level of consciousness
- History of problems that can cause fluid loss, such as vomiting, diarrhea, indwelling tubes, and hemorrhage
- Pulse, blood pressure, respirations, and temperature
- Fluid and electrolyte status, including weight, intake and output, urine specific gravity, skin turgor, and mucous membranes
- Laboratory studies, including serum electrolyte, blood urea nitrogen, and hemoglobin (Hb) levels and hematocrit (HCT)

EXPECTED OUTCOMES

- Patient's vital signs will remain stable.
- Patient will maintain urine output of at least ____ mL/hour.
- Patient's electrolyte values will remain within normal range.
- Patient will maintain intake at ____ mL/24 hours.
- Patient's intake will equal or exceed output.
- Patient will express understanding of need to maintain adequate fluid intake.
- Patient will demonstrate skill in weighing himself or herself accurately and recording weight.
- Patient will measure and record own intake and output.
- Patient will return to appropriate diet.

Suggested NOC Outcomes

Electrolyte & Acid–Base Balance; Fluid Balance; Hydration; Nausea & Vomiting Severity; Nutritional Status: Food & Fluid Intake; Risk Detection; Self-Care Status; Swallowing Status; Urinary Elimination

INTERVENTIONS AND RATIONALES

S ▪ Monitor and record vital signs every 4 hours. *Fever, tachycardia, dyspnea, or hypotension may indicate hypovolemia.*

▪ Maintain accurate record of intake and output *to aid estimation of patient's fluid balance.*

▪ Measure urine output every hour. Record and report an output of less than ____ mL/ hour. *Decreased urine output may indicate reduced fluid volume.*

▪ Measure and record drainage from all tubes and catheters *to take such losses into account when replacing fluid.*

S ▪ When copious drainage appears on dressings, weigh dressings every 8 hours, and record with other output sources. *Excessive wound drainage causes significant fluid imbalances (1 kg dressing equals about 1 L of fluid).*

▪ Test urine specific gravity each shift. Monitor laboratory values and report abnormal findings to physician. *Increased urine specific gravity may indicate dehydration. Elevated hematocrit and hemoglobin level also indicate dehydration.*

S ▪ Monitor serum electrolyte levels and report abnormalities. *Fluid loss may cause significant electrolyte imbalance.*

▪ Obtain and record patient's weight at the same time every day to help ensure accurate data. *Daily weighing helps estimate body fluid status.*

▪ Monitor skin turgor each shift to check for dehydration; report any decrease in turgor. *Poor skin turgor is a sign of dehydration.*

▪ Examine oral mucous membranes each shift. *Dry mucous membranes are a sign of dehydration.*

▪ Cover wounds *to minimize fluid loss and prevent skin excoriation.*

PCC ▪ Determine patient's fluid preferences *to enhance intake.*

▪ Keep oral fluids at bedside within patient's reach and encourage patient to drink. *This gives patient some control over fluid intake and supplements parenteral fluid intake.*

EBP ▪ Instruct patient in maintaining appropriate fluid intake, including recording daily weight, measuring intake and output, and recognizing signs of dehydration. *This encourages patient and caregiver participation and enhances patient's sense of control.*

▪ Force oral fluids when possible and indicated *to enhance replacement of lost fluids.* (Bowel sounds should be present and patient awake before giving oral fluids.)

▪ Administer parenteral fluids as prescribed *to replace fluid losses.* Maintain parenteral fluids or blood transfusions at prescribed rate *to prevent further fluid loss or overload.*

▪ Progress patient to appropriate diet as prescribed *to help achieve fluid and electrolyte balance.*

Suggested NIC Interventions

Acid–Base Management; Fluid Management; Fluid Monitoring; Hypovolemia Management; Nutrition Management; Intravenous (IV) Therapy; Hypovolemia Monitoring; Surveillance

EVALUATIONS FOR EXPECTED OUTCOMES

▪ Patient's temperature, pulse rate, blood pressure, and respirations are within set limits (specify).

▪ Patient's urine output remains at specified volume.

▪ Patient's electrolyte values remain normal.

- Patient's daily fluid intake remains within established limits (specify).
- Patient's cumulative intake equals or exceeds cumulative output.
- Patient demonstrates understanding of importance of maintaining fluid balance.
- Patient weighs himself or herself with same scale at same time each day and records results.
- Patient maintains weight.
- Patient measures fluid intake and output; records are reviewed to ensure accuracy.
- Patient returns to normal, appropriate diet.

DOCUMENTATION

- Observations of physical findings
- Intake and output
- Weight (recorded daily)
- Drainage from indwelling tubes and catheters, including amount, color, and consistency
- Skin turgor, mucous membranes, vital signs, and other physical findings
- Urine specific gravity and other laboratory values
- Amount, color, and odor of drainage on dressings
- Patient teaching about fluid intake and diet
- Patient's response to interventions
- Evaluations for expected outcomes

REFERENCES

Li, J. S. C., Chan, J. Y. H., Tai, M. M. Y., Wong, S. M., Pang, S. M., Lam, F. Y. F., … Chak, W. L. (2018). Hydration and nutritional status in patients on home-dialysis—A single centre study. *Journal of Renal Care, 44*(3), 142–151.

Paulis, S. J. C., Everink, I. H. J., Halfens, R. J. G., Lohrmann, C., & Schols, J. M. G. A. (2018). Prevalence and risk factors of dehydration among nursing home residents: A systematic review. *Journal of the American Medical Directors Association, 19*(8), 646–657.

Shells, R., & Morrell-Scott, N. (2018). Prevention of dehydration in hospital patients. *British Journal of Nursing, 27*(10), 565–569.

Suminski, R. R., Poston, W. S. C., Day, R. S., Jitnarin, N., Haddock, C. K., Jahnke, S. A., & Dominick, G. M. (2019). Steady state hydration levels of career firefighters in a large, population-based sample. *Journal of Occupational & Environmental Medicine, 61*(1), 47–50.

Excess Fluid Volume

DEFINITION

Surplus retention of fluid

RELATED FACTORS (R/T)

- Excessive fluid intake
- Excessive sodium intake
- Ineffective medication self-management

ASSOCIATED CONDITIONS

- Deviations affecting fluid elimination
- Pharmaceutical preparations

ASSESSMENT

- Neurologic status, including level of consciousness, orientation, and mental status
- Cardiovascular status, including skin color, temperature, and turgor; jugular venous pressure; central venous pressure and pulmonary artery pressure (if available); heart rate and rhythm; blood pressure; heart sounds, electrocardiogram (ECG) results; and hemoglobin (Hb) level and hematocrit (HCT)
- Respiratory status, including rate, depth, and pattern of respiration; breath sounds; chest x-ray; and arterial blood gas levels
- Renal status, including intake and output, urine specific gravity, weight, serum electrolyte and serum and urine osmolality levels, and blood urea nitrogen (BUN), urine and serum creatinine, and serum protein levels
- Endocrine status, including general appearance, size and body proportions, skin color and condition, and distribution of body hair

DEFINING CHARACTERISTICS

- Adventitious breath sounds
- Altered blood pressure
- Altered mental status
- Altered pulmonary artery pressure
- Altered respiratory pattern
- Altered urine specific gravity
- Anxiety
- Azotemia
- Decreased serum hematocrit levels
- Decreased serum hemoglobin level
- Edema
- Hepatomegaly
- Increased central venous pressure
- Intake exceeds output
- Jugular vein distension
- Oliguria
- Pleural effusion
- Positive hepatojugular reflex
- Presence of S3 heart sound
- Psychomotor agitation
- Pulmonary congestion
- Weight gain over short period of time

EXPECTED OUTCOMES

- Patient's blood pressure and vital signs will be within normal limits.
- Patient will demonstrate no signs of hyperkalemia on ECG.
- Patient's urine specific gravity will remain within normal limits.
- Patient's HCT will be within normal limits.
- Patient's BUN, creatinine, sodium, and potassium levels will stay within acceptable range.
- Patient will plan 24-hour fluid intake, as prescribed.
- Patient will tolerate restricted intake with no physical or emotional discomfort.
- Patient will assist with activities of daily living without undue fatigue.

▤ Patient will demonstrate skill in selecting permitted foods, such as those low in sodium and potassium.
▤ Patient will describe signs and symptoms that require medical treatment.
▤ Patient will return to baseline weight.
▤ Patient will have unlabored respirations.
▤ Patient will have elastic skin turgor.

Suggested NOC Outcomes

Electrolyte & Acid–Base Balance; Fluid Balance; Fluid Overload Severity; Hydration; Kidney Function; Knowledge: Disease Process; Knowledge: Treatment Regimen; Nutritional Status: Food & Fluid Intake; Urinary Elimination; Vital Signs; Weight: Body Mass

INTERVENTIONS AND RATIONALES

S ▤ Monitor blood pressure, pulse rate, heart rhythm, temperature, and breath sounds at least every 4 hours; record and report changes. *Changed parameters may indicate altered fluid or electrolyte status.*

▤ Carefully monitor intake, output, and urine specific gravity at least every 4 hours. *Intake greater than output and change in specific gravity may indicate fluid retention or overload.*

S ▤ Monitor BUN, creatinine, electrolyte, and Hb levels and HCT. *BUN and creatinine levels indicate renal function; electrolyte and Hb levels and HCT help indicate fluid status.*

▤ Administer diuretics *to promote fluid excretion.* Record effects.

▤ Assess patient daily for edema, including ascites and dependent or sacral edema. *Fluid overload or decreased osmotic pressure may result in edema, especially in dependent areas.*

▤ Weigh patient daily before breakfast, as ordered, *to provide consistent readings.* Check for signs of fluid retention, such as dependent edema, sacral edema, and ascites.

▤ Give fluids, as ordered. Monitor IV flow rate carefully *because excess IV fluids can worsen patient's condition.*

▤ If oral fluids are allowed, help patient make a schedule for fluid intake. *Patient involvement encourages compliance.*

EBP ▤ Explain reasons for fluid and dietary restrictions *to enhance patient's understanding and compliance.*

PCC ▤ Learn patient's food preferences and plan accordingly within prescribed dietary restrictions *to enhance compliance.*

▤ Provide mouth care every 4 hours. Keep mucous membranes moist with water-soluble lubricant *to prevent them from dehydrating.*

EBP ▤ Provide sour hard candy *to decrease thirst and improve taste.*

PCC ▤ Support patient with positive feedback about adherence to restrictions *to encourage compliance.*

▤ Give skin care every 4 hours. Change patient's position at least every 2 hours. Elevate edematous extremities. *These measures enhance venous return, reduce edema, and prevent skin breakdown.*

▤ Alternate periods of rest and activity *to avoid worsening fatigue caused by electrolyte imbalance.*

▤ Increase patient's activity level, as tolerated; for example, ambulate and increase self-care measures performed by patient. *Gradually increasing activity helps body adjust to increased tissue oxygen demand and possible increased venous return.*

S ▦ Help patient into a position that aids breathing, such as Fowler's position or semi-Fowler's position, *to increase chest expansion and improve ventilation.*

S ▦ Administer oxygen, as ordered, *to enhance arterial blood oxygenation.*

S ▦ Apply antiembolism stockings or intermittent pneumatic compression stockings *to increase venous return.* Remove for 1 hour and inspect skin every 8 hours or according to facility policy.

▦ Assess skin turgor *to monitor for edema.*

▦ Measure abdominal girth every shift and report changes *to monitor for ascites.*

T&C ▦ Have dietitian see patient *to teach or reinforce dietary restrictions.*

EBP ▦ Educate patient regarding
  ▦ environmental safety measures
  ▦ fluid restriction and diet
  ▦ signs and symptoms requiring immediate medical treatment
  ▦ medications (name, dosage, frequency, therapeutic effects, and adverse effects)
  ▦ activity level
  ▦ ways to prevent infection

These measures encourage patient and family members to participate more fully in care.

Suggested NIC Interventions

Acid–Base Management; Electrolyte Management; Fluid Management; Fluid Monitoring; Medication Management; Nutrition Management; Urinary Elimination Management; Vital Signs Monitoring; Weight Management

EVALUATIONS FOR EXPECTED OUTCOMES

▦ Patient's vital signs remain within established limits.

▦ Patient indicates, verbally and through behavior, ability to breathe comfortably.

▦ Signs of hyperkalemia (peaked or elevated T waves, prolonged PR intervals, widened QRS complexes, or depressed ST segments) don't appear on ECG.

▦ Patient's fluid intake and output remain within established limits.

▦ Patient's urine specific gravity remains within established limits.

▦ Patient's HCT remains above specified level.

▦ Patient's electrolyte levels remain within established limits.

▦ Patient plans 24-hour fluid intake.

▦ Patient doesn't indicate discomfort with restricted fluid intake, either verbally or through behavior.

▦ Patient plans own menu and selects foods low in sodium and potassium. Patient follows other dietary restrictions (specify).

▦ Patient expresses understanding of health problem.

▦ Patient demonstrates skill in health-related behaviors, such as maintaining weight and monitoring intake and output.

▦ Patient and caregiver list signs and symptoms that require medical attention.

DOCUMENTATION

▦ Expression of patient's needs, desires, or perceptions of situation

▦ Specific changes in patient's physical status

▦ Observations about patient's response to treatment

▦ Observations about how patient appears to be coping with fluid and dietary restrictions

- Condition of skin and mucous membranes
- Interventions performed to alleviate or resolve diagnosis
- Interventions to correct fluid volume excess
- Patient's demonstration of skills
- Evaluations for expected outcomes

REFERENCES

Cheuvront, S. N., Kenefick, R. W., Charkoudian, N., Mitchell, K. M., Luippold, A. J., Bradbury, K. E., & Vidyasagar, S. (2018). Efficacy of glucose or amino acid-based commercial beverages in meeting oral rehydration therapy goals after acute hypertonic and isotonic dehydration. *JPEN Journal of Parenteral & Enteral Nutrition, 42*(7), 1185–1193.

Evans, G. H., Miller, J., Whiteley, S., & James, L. J. (2017). A sodium drink enhances fluid retention during 3 hours of post-exercise recovery when ingested with a standard meal. *International Journal of Sport Nutrition & Exercise Metabolism, 27*(4), 344–350.

Lucena, A. D. F., Magro, C. Z., da Costa Proença, M. C., Bertoldo Pires, A. U., Monteiro Moraes, V., & Badin Aliti, G. (2017). Validation of the nursing interventions and activities for patients on hemodialytic therapy. *Revista Gaucha de Enfermagem, 38*(3), 1–9.

Risk for Imbalanced Fluid Volume

DEFINITION

Susceptible to a decrease, increase, or rapid shift from one to the other of intravascular, interstitial, and/or intracellular fluid, which may compromise health

ASSESSMENT

- Cardiovascular status including heart rate and rhythm, blood pressure, peripheral pulses
- Fluid and electrolyte status, weight, intake and output, urine specific gravity, skin turgor, mucous membranes, jugular vein distention
- Results of laboratory studies including serum electrolytes, blood urea nitrogen, hemoglobin, hematocrit
- History of cardiovascular, renal, gastrointestinal dysfunction

RISK FACTORS

- Altered fluid intake
- Difficulty accessing water
- Excessive sodium intake
- Inadequate knowledge about fluid needs
- Ineffective medication self-management
- Insufficient muscle mass
- Malnutrition

ASSOCIATED CONDITIONS

- Active fluid volume loss
- Deviations affecting fluid absorption
- Deviations affecting fluid elimination

- Deviations affecting fluid intake
- Deviations affecting vascular permeability
- Excessive fluid loss through normal route
- Fluid loss through abnormal route
- Pharmaceutical preparations
- Treatment regimen

EXPECTED OUTCOMES

- Patient will remain hemodynamically stable.
- Patient will not experience electrolyte imbalance.
- Patient will maintain adequate urine output.
- Patient will identify risk factors contributing to possible imbalanced fluid volume.

Suggested NOC Outcomes

Client Satisfaction: Fluid Balance; Hydration; Vital Signs

INTERVENTIONS AND RATIONALES

PCC ▪ Assess for conditions that may contribute to imbalanced fluid volume. *Prompt treatment of underlying cause may prevent serious complications of fluid imbalance.*

S ▪ Monitor vital signs and other assessment parameters frequently. *Changes in heart rate and rhythm, blood pressure, and breath sounds may indicate altered fluid status.*

▪ Collect and evaluate urine output frequently. Measure urine specific gravity as indicated. *Decreased urine volume and elevated urine specific gravity indicate hypovolemia.*

▪ Collect and evaluate serum electrolyte levels. *Fluid alterations may affect electrolyte levels.*

▪ Administer intravenous fluids as indicated. *Proactive fluid management may prevent serious imbalances.*

EBP ▪ Educate patient and family regarding fluid restrictions or need for increased fluids, depending on the underlying condition. *Knowledge will enhance feeling of participation and sense of control.*

PCC ▪ Provide encouragement and support for cooperation with prescribed treatment regimen. *Positive reinforcement will promote compliance.*

T&C ▪ Coordinate care with other members of the health care team *to effectively manage underlying medical condition and prevent any alteration in fluid balance.*

Suggested NIC Interventions

Fluid Management; Fluid Monitoring; Intravenous (IV) Therapy

EVALUATIONS FOR EXPECTED OUTCOMES

- Patient remains hemodynamically stable.
- Electrolytes remain within acceptable limits.
- Patient has no electrolyte imbalances as a result of altered fluid status.
- Patient has adequate urine output.
- Patient states risk factors contributing to altered fluid status.

▩ Patient's intake and output measurements
▩ Patient's vital signs and physical assessment findings
▩ Relevant lab results
▩ Patient's understanding of behaviors that promote fluid balance
▩ Evaluations for expected outcomes

REFERENCES

Davies, H., Leslie, G. D., & Morgan, D. (2017). A retrospective review of fluid balance control in CRRT. *Australian Critical Care, 30*(6), 314–319.
Li, C., Wang, H., Liu, N., Jia, M., Hou, X., Zhang, H., & Xi, X. (2018). Early negative fluid balance is associated with lower mortality after cardiovascular surgery. *Perfusion, 33*(8), 630–637.
Samransamruajkit, R., Saelim, K., Hantragool, S., Deerojanawong, J., Sritippayawan, S., & Prapphal, N. (2017). A comparison of NSS vs balanced salt solution as a fluid resuscitation and impact of fluid balance on clinical outcomes in pediatric septic shock. *Critical Care & Shock, 20*(3), 68–75.
Van Regenmortel, N., Verbrugghe, W., Roelant, E., Van den Wyngaert, T., & Jorens, P. G. (2018). Maintenance fluid therapy and fluid creep impose more significant fluid, sodium, and chloride burdens than resuscitation fluids in critically ill patients: A retrospective study in a tertiary mixed ICU population. *Intensive Care Medicine, 44*(4), 409–417.

Frail Elderly Syndrome

Dynamic state of unstable equilibrium that affects the older individual experiencing deterioration in one or more domain of health (physical, functional, psychological, or social) and leads to increased susceptibility to adverse health effects, in particular disability

▩ Activity intolerance
▩ Anxiety
▩ Average daily physical activity is less than recommended for gender and age
▩ Decrease in energy
▩ Decrease in muscle strength
▩ Depression
▩ Exhaustion
▩ Fear of falling
▩ Immobility
▩ Impaired balance
▩ Impaired mobility
▩ Insufficient social support
▩ Malnutrition
▩ Muscle weakness
▩ Obesity
▩ Sadness
▩ Sedentary lifestyle
▩ Social isolation

ASSOCIATED CONDITIONS

- Alteration in cognitive functioning
- Altered clotting process
- Anorexia
- Chronic illness
- Decrease in serum 25-hydroxyvitamin D concentration
- Endocrine regulatory dysfunction
- Psychiatric disorder
- Sarcopenia
- Sarcopenic obesity
- Sensory deficit
- Suppressed inflammatory response
- Unintentional loss of 25% of body weight over one year
- Unintentional weight loss > 10 pounds (>4.5 kg) in one year
- Walking 15 feet requires >6 seconds (4 m > 5 seconds)

ASSESSMENT

- Ability to complete activities of daily living
- Cognitive level
- Level of physical activity
- Nutritional status
- Oxygenation status
- Presence of depression
- Self-report of exhaustion
- Slowness
- Weakness
- Weight

DEFINING CHARACTERISTICS

- Activity intolerance
- Bathing self-care deficit
- Decreased cardiac output
- Dressing self-care deficit
- Fatigue
- Feeding self-care deficit
- Hopelessness
- Imbalanced nutrition: Less than body requirements
- Impaired memory
- Impaired physical mobility
- Impaired walking
- Social isolation
- Toileting self-care deficit

EXPECTED OUTCOMES

- Patient will have improved physical function.
- Patient will have improved psychological function.
- Patient will have improved social function.

Suggested NOC Outcomes

Physical Aging; Psychosocial Adjustment: Life Change; Client Satisfaction: Functional Assistance

INTERVENTIONS AND RATIONALES

- **S** ■ Conduct environmental assessment. *Can identify risks for falls and ability to manage care outside the hospital.*
- **EBP** ■ Educate on importance of regular exercise. *Can improve mobility, improve gait, decrease incidence of falls, increase muscle strength.*
- **T&C** ■ Implement interdisciplinary treatment plan. *Can improve physical and psychological function, improve patient satisfaction, decrease need for hospitalization.*
- ■ Provide antidepressants as ordered. *Delay of treatment may accelerate decline of patient status.*
- ■ Provide appetite-stimulating medications as ordered *to possibly increase appetite.*
- **PCC** ■ Provide patient with ample time to complete activities of daily living (ADLs) *to increase ability to complete ADLs.*
- **T&C** ■ Provide physical and occupational therapy as needed *to improve functional impairment.*
- **PCC** ■ Provide socialization opportunities. *Isolation can exacerbate depression.*
- ■ Provide stimulating activities *to keep cognitive mind engaged.*
- ■ Provide supplemental nutritional drinks *to provide extra calories and energy intake.*

Suggested NIC Interventions

Physical Exercise; Strength Training; Balance Training

EVALUATIONS FOR EXPECTED OUTCOMES

- ■ Patient has no deterioration of physical function.
- ■ Patient has no deterioration of psychological function.
- ■ Patient has no deterioration of social function.

DOCUMENTATION

- ■ Ability to complete ADLs
- ■ Body weight
- ■ Cognitive level
- ■ Mental status
- ■ Mobility status
- ■ Vital signs

REFERENCES

Ljungbeck, B., & Sjögren Forss, K. (2017). Advanced nurse practitioners in municipal healthcare as a way to meet the growing healthcare needs of the frail elderly: A qualitative interview study with managers, doctors and specialist nurses. *BMC Nursing, 16,* 1–9.

Longstaff, S., Rees, J., Good, E., & Kirby, E. (2018). Case study of home care for isolated and frail elderly patients by general practice nurses. *Journal of Integrated Care, 26*(3), 211–218.

Lopez, P., Pinto, R. S., Radaelli, R., Rech, A., Grazioli, R., Izquierdo, M., & Cadore, E. L. (2018). Benefits of resistance training in physically frail elderly: A systematic review. *Aging Clinical & Experimental Research, 30*(8), 889–899.

Oliveira Crossetti, M. D. G., Antunes, M., Ferreira Waldman, B., Rubin Unicovsky, M. A., Henrique de Rosso, L., & Dalla Lana, L. (2018). Factors that contribute to a NANDA nursing diagnosis of risk for frail elderly syndrome. *Revista Gaucha de Enfermagem, 39*(1), 1–17.

Risk for Frail Elderly Syndrome

DEFINITION

Susceptible to a dynamic state of unstable equilibrium that affects the older individual experiencing deterioration in one or more domain of health (physical, functional, psychological, or social) and leads to increased susceptibility to adverse health effects, in particular disability

RISK FACTORS

- Activity intolerance
- Anxiety
- Average daily physical activity is less than recommended for gender and age
- Decrease in energy
- Decrease in muscle strength
- Depression
- Exhaustion
- Fear of falling
- Immobility
- Impaired balance
- Impaired mobility
- Insufficient knowledge of modifiable factors
- Insufficient social support
- Malnutrition
- Muscle weakness
- Obesity
- Sadness
- Sedentary lifestyle
- Social isolation

ASSOCIATED CONDITIONS

- Alteration in cognitive functioning
- Altered clotting process
- Anorexia
- Chronic illness
- Decrease in serum 25-hydroxyvitamin D concentration
- Endocrine regulatory dysfunction
- Psychiatric disorder
- Sarcopenia
- Sarcopenic obesity
- Sensory deficit
- Suppressed inflammatory response

- Unintentional loss of 25% of body weight over one year
- Unintentional weight loss >10 lb (>4.5 kg) in one year
- Walking 15 feet requires >6 seconds (4 m > 5 seconds)

ASSESSMENT

- Ability to complete activities of daily living (ADLs)
- Cognitive level
- Fall risk
- Level of physical activity
- Muscle strength
- Nutritional status
- Oxygenation status
- Presence of depression
- Self-report of exhaustion
- Slowness
- Weakness
- Weight

EXPECTED OUTCOMES

- Patient will not experience deterioration in physical domain.
- Patient will not experience deterioration in functional domain.
- Patient will not experience deterioration in psychological domain.
- Patient will not experience deterioration in social domain.
- Patient will not be susceptible to adverse health effects.

Suggested NOC Outcomes

Physical Aging; Psychosocial Adjustment: Life Change; Client Satisfaction: Functional Assistance

INTERVENTIONS AND RATIONALES

- **S** Conduct environmental assessment. *Patient should be able to identify risks for falls and ability to manage care outside the hospital.*
- **EBP** Educate on importance of regular exercise, which *can improve mobility, improve gait, decrease incidence of falls, increase muscle strength.*
- **T&C** Implement interdisciplinary treatment plan, which *can improve physical and psychological function, improve patient satisfaction, decrease need for hospitalization.*
- **PCC** Provide patient with ample time to complete ADLs *to increase ability to complete ADLs.*
- **T&C** Provide physical and occupational therapy as needed *to improve functional impairment.*
- **PCC** Provide socialization opportunities. *Isolation can exacerbate depression.*
- Provide stimulating activities *to keep cognitive mind engaged.*
- Provide supplemental nutritional drinks *to provide extra calories and energy intake.*

Suggested NIC Interventions

Physical Exercise; Strength Training; Balance Training

EVALUATIONS FOR EXPECTED OUTCOMES

- Patient has no deterioration in physical domain.
- Patient has no deterioration in psychological domain.
- Patient has no deterioration in functional domain.
- Patient has no deterioration in social domain.
- Patient is not susceptible to adverse health effects.

DOCUMENTATION

- Ability to complete ADLs
- Body weight
- Cognitive level
- Fall risk
- Mental status
- Mobility status
- Vital signs

REFERENCES

Gale, C. R., Westbury, L., & Cooper, C. (2018). Social isolation and loneliness as risk factors for the progression of frailty: The English Longitudinal Study of Ageing. *Age & Ageing, 47*(3), 392–397.

Ørum, M., Gregersen, M., Jensen, K., Meldgaard, P., & Damsgaard, E. M. S. (2018). Frailty status but not age predicts complications in elderly cancer patients: A follow-up study. *Acta Oncologica, 57*(11), 1458–1466.

Rodríguez-Sánchez, I., García-Esquinas, E., Mesas, A. E., Martín-Moreno, J. M., Rodríguez-Mañas, L., & Rodríguez-Artalejo, F. (2019). Frequency, intensity and localization of pain as risk factors for frailty in older adults. *Age & Ageing, 48*(1), 74–80.

Romão Preto, L. S., Dias da Conceição, M. D. C., Soeiro Amaral, S. I., Martins Figueiredo, T., & Barreira Preto, P. M. (2018). Frailty and associated risk factors in independent older people living in rural areas. *Revista de Enfermagem Referência, 4*(16), 73–82.

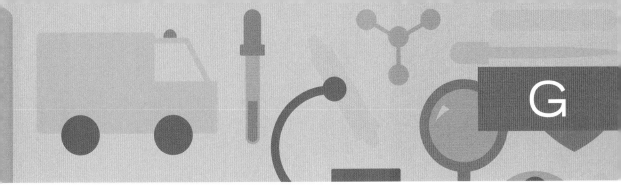

Impaired Gas Exchange

Excess or deficit in oxygenation and/or carbon dioxide elimination

- Ineffective airway clearance
- Ineffective breathing pattern
- Pain

- Alveolar-capillary membrane changes
- Asthma
- General anesthesia
- Heart diseases
- Ventilation-perfusion imbalance

- Age
- Gender
- Smoking history
- Neurologic status, including level of consciousness, orientation, and mental status
- Respiratory status, including respiratory rate and depth, symmetry of chest expansion, use of accessory muscles, cough, sputum, palpation for fremitus, percussion of lung fields, auscultation of breath sounds, arterial blood gas (ABG) levels, and pulmonary function studies
- Cardiovascular status, including skin color and temperature, heart rate and rhythm, blood pressure, and complete blood count
- Activity status, including such functional capabilities as range of motion and muscle strength, activities of daily living (ADLs), and occupation

- Abnormal arterial pH
- Abnormal skin color
- Altered respiratory depth
- Altered respiratory rhythm
- Bradypnea

- Confusion
- Decreased carbon dioxide level
- Diaphoresis
- Headache upon awakening
- Hypercapnia
- Hypoxemia
- Hypoxia
- Irritable mood
- Nasal flaring
- Psychomotor agitation
- Somnolence
- Tachycardia
- Tachypnea
- Visual disturbance

EXPECTED OUTCOMES

- Patient will maintain respiratory rate within five breaths of predetermined baseline.
- Patient will sustain sufficient fluid intake to prevent dehydration: ___ mL/24 hours.
- Patient will exercise and perform ADLs without experiencing dyspnea or excessive fatigue.
- Patient will maintain adequate ventilation and have clear breath sounds on auscultation.
- Patient or family members will state understanding of causes for impaired gas exchange and behaviors to prevent it.
- Patient will have normal breath sounds.
- Patient's ABG levels will return to baselines: ___ pH; ____ partial pressure of arterial oxygen (Pao_2); ____ partial pressure of arterial carbon dioxide ($Paco_2$).
- Patient will perform relaxation techniques every 4 hours.
- Patient will use correct bronchial hygiene.

Suggested NOC Outcomes

Cognition; Electrolyte & Acid–Base Balance; Respiratory Status: Gas Exchange; Respiratory Status: Ventilation; Tissue Perfusion: Pulmonary; Vital Signs

INTERVENTIONS AND RATIONALES

- Establish baseline values for respiratory assessment *to distinguish age-related changes that may mimic disease states from disease. Older adults take shorter breaths. This decreases maximum breathing capacity, vital capacity, residual volume, and functional capacity.*
- **S** Assess and record pulmonary status every 4 hours or more frequently if patient's condition is unstable. *Poor pulmonary status may result in hypoxemia.*
- Monitor vital signs and heart rhythm at least every 4 hours *to detect tachycardia and tachypnea, which could indicate hypoxemia.*
- Place patient in position that best facilitates chest expansion *to enhance gas exchange.*
- **S** Change patient's position at least every 2 hours *to mobilize secretions and allow aeration of all lung fields.*
- Perform bronchial hygiene, as ordered, including coughing, percussion, postural drainage, and suctioning. *These measures promote drainage and keep airways clear.*

▨ Give medications, as ordered, *to improve oxygenation*. Monitor and record efficacy and adverse reactions *to guide treatment*.

S ▨ Administer and monitor oxygen therapy, as ordered, *to enhance oxygenation and detect signs of decompensation. Older patients have a high incidence of chronic cardiac and chronic pulmonary disorders. Detecting early changes in condition allows for early intervention.*

▨ Record intake and output *to monitor patient's fluid status*.

▨ Report signs of dehydration or fluid overload immediately. *Dehydration may hinder tissue perfusion and secretion mobilization; fluid overload may cause pulmonary edema.*

PCC ▨ Assist patient with ADLs *to decrease tissue oxygen demand*.

EBP ▨ Encourage patient to alternate periods of rest and activity. *Activity increases tissue oxygen demand; rest enhances tissue oxygen perfusion.*

S ▨ Monitor ABG levels and notify physician immediately if PaO_2 or arterial oxygen saturation drops or $PaCO_2$ rises. Administer endotracheal intubation and mechanical ventilation if needed. *This helps increase ventilation and gas exchange.*

EBP ▨ Have patient turn, cough, and deep breathe every 4 hours *to prevent atelectasis or fluid buildup in lungs and to enhance blood oxygen level*.

EBP ▨ Teach patient relaxation techniques *to reduce tissue oxygen demand*.

▨ Have patient perform relaxation techniques every 4 hours *to establish routine and reduce oxygen demand.*

Suggested NIC Interventions

Acid-Base Management; Airway Management; Airway Suctioning; Anxiety Reduction; Energy Management; Mechanical Ventilation; Oxygen Therapy; Positioning; Respiratory Monitoring

EVALUATIONS FOR EXPECTED OUTCOMES

▨ Patient's respiratory rate remains within established limits.

▨ Patient doesn't experience dyspnea.

▨ Patient's fluid intake remains sufficient to prevent dehydration.

▨ Patient performs ADLs without exhibiting dyspnea or other signs of abnormal ABG levels.

▨ Patient has normal breath sounds.

▨ Patient's pH, PaO_2, and $PaCO_2$ return to and remain within established limits.

▨ Patient performs relaxation techniques every 4 hours.

▨ Patient uses correct bronchial hygiene.

DOCUMENTATION

▨ Patient's complaints of dyspnea, headache, and restlessness

▨ Patient's expression of well-being

▨ Observations of physical findings

▨ Effectiveness of medications

▨ Teaching provided and patient's response

▨ Patient response to interventions

▨ Other treatments performed by nurse

▨ Evaluations for expected outcomes

REFERENCES

Gilpin, R. (2017). Understanding the gas exchange process. *EMS World, 46*(4), 50–56.

Johnson, N. J., Luks, A. M., & Glenny, R. W. (2017). Gas exchange in the prone posture. *Respiratory Care, 62*(8), 1097–1110.

Marinus, N., Bervoets, L., Massa, G., Verboven, K., Stevens, A., Takken, T., & Hansen, D. (2017). Altered gas-exchange at peak exercise in obese adolescents: Implications for verification of effort during cardiopulmonary exercise testing. *Journal of Sports Medicine and Physical Fitness, 57*(12), 1687–1694.

Oribabor, C., Gulkarov, I., Khusid, F., Fischer, E., Esan, A., Rizzuto, N., … Kenney, B. (2018). The use of high-frequency percussive ventilation after cardiac surgery significantly improves gas exchange without impairment of hemodynamics. *Canadian Journal of Respiratory Therapy, 54*(3), 58–61.

Dysfunctional Gastrointestinal Motility

DEFINITION

Increased, decreased, ineffective, or lack of peristaltic activity within the gastrointestinal system

RELATED FACTORS (R/T)

- Anxiety
- Change in water source
- Eating habit change
- Immobility
- Malnutrition
- Sedentary lifestyle
- Stressors
- Unsanitary food preparation

ASSOCIATED CONDITIONS

- Decrease in gastrointestinal circulation
- Diabetes mellitus
- Enteral feedings
- Food intolerance
- Gastroesophageal reflux disease
- Infection
- Pharmaceutical agent
- Treatment regimen

ASSESSMENT

- Health status, educational level, cultural status, requests for information; demonstrated understanding of material
- Diet
- Recent travel
- Recent surgical procedures
- Fluid and electrolyte status, including blood urea nitrogen level, creatinine level, intake and output, mucous membranes, serum electrolyte levels, and skin turgor
- Nutritional status, including dietary patterns, laboratory tests, and serum protein level
- Neurologic status, including level of consciousness, mental status, motor function, and sensory pattern
- Gastrointestinal (GI) status, including nausea and vomiting, bowel habits, stool characteristics, history of GI problems, disease, or surgery; bowel sounds

DEFINING CHARACTERISTICS

- Abdominal cramping
- Abdominal pain
- Absence of flatus
- Acceleration of gastric emptying
- Bile-colored gastric residual
- Change in bowel sounds
- Diarrhea
- Difficulty with defecation
- Distended abdomen
- Hard, formed stool
- Increased gastric residual
- Nausea
- Regurgitation
- Vomiting

EXPECTED OUTCOMES

- Patient will not experience gastrointestinal cramping/pain.
- Patient will not have gastrointestinal distention.
- Patient will have bowel movements every 1 to 3 days.
- Patient will have normoactive bowel sounds.
- Patient will verbalize strategies to promote healthy bowel function.
- Patient will acknowledge the importance of seeking medical help for persistent alteration in GI motility.
- Patient will not experience any fluid and electrolyte imbalance as a result of altered motility.
- Patient will understand the need for early ambulation following abdominal surgery.

Suggested NOC Outcomes

Bowel Elimination; Electrolyte and Acid–Base Balance; Gastrointestinal Function

INTERVENTIONS AND RATIONALES

- **S** Assess abdomen including auscultation in all four quadrants noting character and frequency *to determine increased or decreased motility*.
- Assess current manifestations of altered GI motility *to help identify cause of alteration and guide development of nursing interventions*.
- Monitor intake and output *to identify need for restoration of fluid balance*.
- Assess for nausea, vomiting, bloating, and pain *as these are signs of decreased gastric motility*.
- Collect and evaluate laboratory electrolyte specimens. *Some altered motility states may require electrolyte replacement therapy*.
- **S** Insert nasogastric tube as prescribed for patients with absent bowel sounds *to relieve the pressures caused by accumulation of air and fluid*.
- **EBP** Educate patient regarding importance of maintaining diet high in natural fiber and adequate fluid intake. *Fiber increases stool bulk and softens the stool. Fluid will promote normal bowel elimination pattern*.

▦ Encourage activities such as walking as tolerated for patients with decreased GI motility. *Increased activity will stimulate peristalsis and facilitate elimination.*

 ▦ Collaborate with dietitian and other health care professionals as needed *to meet the unique needs of each individual patient.*

Suggested NIC Interventions

Fluid/Electrolyte Management; Gastrointestinal Intubation; Tube Care: Gastrointestinal

EVALUATIONS FOR EXPECTED OUTCOMES

▦ Patient does not experience bowel/abdominal cramping.
▦ Patient does not exhibit signs of abdominal distention.
▦ Patient has a bowel movement every 1 to 3 days.
▦ Patient verbalizes strategies to promote healthy bowel function.
▦ Patient states plan to seek medical assistance for GI problems.
▦ Patient maintains normal electrolyte balance.
▦ Patient ambulates according to schedule.

DOCUMENTATION

▦ Patient's laboratory results and bowel characteristics
▦ Observations of physiologic and behavioral manifestations of decreased GI motility
▦ Interventions performed for management of nasogastric tube
▦ Teaching provided and patient's response
▦ Patient's response to interventions
▦ Evaluations for expected outcomes

REFERENCES

Eastwick, E., Leise, J., Sabo, J., Clute, L., & Stoj, P. (2017). Effect of gum chewing on bowel motility following elective colon resection. *MEDSURG Nursing, 26*(3), 185–189.

Frazer, C., Hussey, L., & Bemker, M. (2018). Gastrointestinal motility problems in critically ill patients. *Critical Care Nursing Clinics of North America, 30*(1), 109–121.

Kashima, H., Sugimura, K., Taniyawa, K., Kondo, R., Endo, M. Y., Tanimoto, S., ... Fukuba, Y. (2018). Timing of post-resistance exercise nutrient ingestion: Effects on gastric emptying and glucose and amino acid responses in humans. *British Journal of Nutrition, 120*(9), 995–1005.

Madsen, J. L., Damgaard, M., Fuglsang, S., Dirksen, C., Holst, J. J., & Graff, J. (2019). Gastrointestinal motility, gut hormone secretion, and energy intake after oral loads of free fatty acid or triglyceride in older and middle-aged men. *Appetite, 132*, 18–24.

Risk for Dysfunctional Gastrointestinal Motility

DEFINITION

Susceptible to increased, decreased, ineffective, or lack of peristaltic activity within the gastro-intestinal system, which may compromise health

RISK FACTORS

▦ Anxiety
▦ Change in water source

- Eating habit change
- Immobility
- Malnutrition
- Sedentary lifestyle
- Stressors
- Unsanitary food preparation

ASSOCIATED CONDITIONS

- Decrease in gastrointestinal circulation
- Diabetes mellitus
- Enteral feedings
- Food intolerance
- Gastroesophageal reflux disease
- Infection
- Pharmaceutical agent
- Treatment regimen

ASSESSMENT

- Diet
- Recent travel
- Recent surgical procedures
- Health status, educational level, cultural status, requests for information; demonstrated understanding of material
- Fluid and electrolyte status, including blood urea nitrogen level, creatinine level, intake and output, mucous membranes, serum electrolyte levels, and skin turgor
- Nutritional status, including dietary patterns, laboratory tests, and serum protein level
- Neurologic status, including level of consciousness, mental status, motor function, and sensory pattern
- Gastrointestinal (GI) status, including nausea and vomiting, bowel habits, stool characteristics, history of GI problems, disease, or surgery; bowel sounds

EXPECTED OUTCOMES

- Patient will not experience gastrointestinal cramping/pain.
- Patient will not have gastrointestinal distention.
- Patient will identify diet selections and lifestyle changes that would promote healthy GI function.
- Patient will verbalize strategies to promote healthy bowel function.
- Patient will acknowledge the importance of seeking medical help for persistent alteration in GI motility.
- Patient will not experience altered GI motility related to prescribed medications.
- Patient will recognize chronic conditions that may contribute to altered GI motility, for example, diabetes, gastroesophageal reflux disease.

Suggested NOC Outcomes

Electrolyte and Acid–Base Balance; Fluid Balance; Bowel Elimination

INTERVENTIONS AND RATIONALES

S ▦ Assess patient for signs of fluid or electrolyte imbalance related to increased or decreased GI motility. *Fluid and electrolyte alterations can result from either increased or decreased GI motility.*

▦ Assess patient for positive risk factors for altered GI motility. *This will allow for timely interventions to prevent complications associated with GI dysfunction.*

S ▦ Assist patient taking prescribed medications that affect motility with strategies to avoid GI complications. *Awareness of preventive measures will decrease GI complications.*

EBP ▦ Encourage early ambulation for postoperative patients receiving opioids for pain control. *Early ambulation will reduce the risk of narcotic-related constipation.*

EBP ▦ Educate patient regarding the risk factors related to altered GI motility, including certain food choices, fluid intake, medications, travel, and activity. *Promotion of healthy lifestyle choices will contribute to positive patient outcomes.*

PCC ▦ Provide encouragement and support for behaviors that enhance GI health. *Positive reinforcement results in improved confidence in self-management of health behaviors.*

T&C ▦ Coordinate care with other disciplines as needed *to reinforce positive behaviors or to assist with complex situations.*

Suggested NIC Interventions

Diarrhea Management; Electrolyte Monitoring; Fluid Management; Nutrition Management

EVALUATIONS FOR EXPECTED OUTCOMES

▦ Patient does not report gastrointestinal cramping/pain.
▦ Patient makes dietary and fluid selections to maintain a healthy GI system.
▦ Patient seeks medical help for persistent alteration in GI motility.
▦ Patient has no adverse reaction to medications.
▦ Patient verbalizes the relationship of chronic conditions to GI motility.

DOCUMENTATION

▦ Patient's expressions of concern about adverse reaction and symptoms of altered GI motility
▦ Observations of physiologic and behavioral manifestations of decreased GI motility
▦ Interventions performed to allay adverse GI reactions to medications
▦ Teaching provided and patient's response
▦ Patient's response to interventions
▦ Evaluations for expected outcomes

REFERENCES

Jacob, L. (2017). Auscultation of bowel sounds in critical care: The role of the nurse. *British Journal of Nursing, 26*(17), 962–963. doi:10.12968/bjon.2017.26.17.962

Lovén Wickman, U., Yngman-Uhlin, P., Hjortswang, H., Wenemark, M., Stjernman, H., Riegel, B., & Hollman Frisman, G. (2019). Development of a self-care questionnaire for clinical assessment of self-care in patients with inflammatory bowel disease: A psychometric evaluation. *International Journal of Nursing Studies, 89,* 1–7.

Stoner, P. L., Kamel, A., Ayoub, F., Tan, S., Iqbal, A., Glover, S. C., & Zimmermann, E. M. (2018). Perioperative care of patients with inflammatory bowel disease: Focus on nutritional support. *Gastroenterology Research and Practice, 2018,* 1–13.

Thompson, J. (2017). Improving clinical care for patients with irritable bowel syndrome. *British Journal of Nursing, 26*(2), 76–80. doi:10.12968/bjon.2017.26.2.76

Maladaptive Grieving

DEFINITION

A disorder that occurs after the death of a significant other, in which the experience of distress accompanying bereavement fails to follow sociocultural expectations

RELATED FACTORS (R/T)

- Difficulty dealing with concurrent crises
- Excessive emotional disturbance
- High attachment anxiety
- Inadequate social support
- Low attachment avoidance

ASSOCIATED CONDITIONS

- Anxiety disorders
- Depression

ASSESSMENT

- History of loss
- Length of grief process
- Pattern of coping (grief delayed or avoided)
- Self-destructive behaviors
- Sleep assessment
- Nutritional assessment
- Changes in presentation of self
- Social or spiritual support
- Ability to maintain roles at occupation and within family

DEFINING CHARACTERISTICS

- Anxiety
- Decreased life role performance
- Depressive symptoms
- Diminished intimacy levels
- Disbelief
- Excessive stress
- Experiencing symptoms the deceased experienced
- Expresses anger
- Expresses being overwhelmed
- Expresses distress about the deceased person
- Expresses feeling detached from others
- Expresses feeling of emptiness
- Expresses feeling stunned
- Expresses shock
- Fatigue
- Gastrointestinal symptoms
- Grief avoidance
- Increased morbidity

- Longing for the deceased person
- Mistrust of others
- Nonacceptance of a death
- Persistent painful memories
- Preoccupation with thoughts about a deceased person
- Rumination about deceased person
- Searching for a deceased person
- Self-blame

EXPECTED OUTCOMES

- Patient will express appropriate feelings of loss, guilt, fear, anger, or sadness.
- Patient will identify the loss and describe what it means to him or her.
- Patient will appropriately move through stages of grief.
- Patient will maintain healthy patterns of sleep, activity, and eating.
- Patient will verbalize understanding that grief is normal.
- Patient will use healthy coping mechanisms and social support systems.
- Patient will seek fulfillment through preferred spiritual practices.
- Patient will begin planning for future.

Suggested NOC Outcomes

Coping; Family Coping; Grief Resolution; Life Change; Psychosocial Adjustment

INTERVENTIONS AND RATIONALES

- **PCC** Encourage patient to express grief and feelings of anger, guilt, and sadness. *Inability to express these feelings may result in maladaptive behaviors.*
- **PCC** Encourage journaling to express grief and loss. *Writing and exploring feelings is an active process that may assist in grieving.*
- **PCC** Help patient identify an area of hope in life. *Focusing on a life purpose may decrease anger and feelings of frustration.*
- **T&C** Refer patient to community support systems *to help patient deal with bereavement and grief process.*
- **T&C** Contact patient's preferred spiritual leader if patient desires; *this may provide relief from spiritual distress.*
- **PCC** Help patient focus realistically on changes the loss has brought about. *This will assist patient in forming plans for the future and improving social relationships.*
- **PCC** Encourage patient and family to engage in reminiscing; *this will give purpose and meaning to the loss and assist in maintenance of self-esteem.*
- **PCC** Help patient formulate goals for the future; *this helps patient place loss in perspective and move on to new situations and relationships.*
- **PCC** Identify previous losses and assess for depression; *in the elderly, losses frequently occur without adequate recovery time before the next loss.*

Suggested NIC Interventions

Calming Technique; Coping Enhancement; Counseling; Emotional Support; Family Therapy; Grief Facilitation Work

- Patient expresses feelings, which may include grief, guilt, anger, or sadness.
- Patient verbalizes feelings and behaviors related to the grieving process and applies these behaviors and feelings to daily life.
- Patient appropriately moves through stages of grief.
- Patient maintains healthy patterns of sleep, activity, and eating.
- Patient communicates understanding that grieving is an appropriate response to loss and comes to terms with own grief response.
- Patient uses coping mechanisms and discusses loss with others, including support group and family.
- Patient experiences satisfaction and support from chosen religious practices.
- Patient begins planning for future.

- Patient's verbal expression of grief
- Observations of emotional responses, attempts at coping, and interactions with family and staff
- Interventions to assist coping with loss
- Patient's response to nursing interventions
- Evaluations for expected outcomes

REFERENCES

Fields, S. A., Johnson, W. M., Mears, J., & Johnson, W. M. (2018). How to treat complicated grief. *Journal of Family Practice, 67*(10), 637–640.

Glickman, K., Shear, M. K., & Wall, M. M. (2018). Therapeutic alliance and outcome in complicated grief treatment. *International Journal of Cognitive Therapy, 11*(2), 222–233. doi:10.1007/s41811-018-0018-9

Maccallum, F., & Bryant, R. A. (2019). Symptoms of prolonged grief and posttraumatic stress following loss: A latent class analysis. *Australian and New Zealand Journal of Psychiatry, 53*(1), 59–67. doi:10.1177/0004867418768429

Tal, I., Mauro, C., Reynolds, C. F., III, Shear, M. K., Simon, N., Lebowitz, B., … Zisook, S. (2017). Complicated grief after suicide bereavement and other causes of death. *Death Studies, 41*(5), 267–275. doi:10.1080/07481187.2016.1265028

Risk for Maladaptive Grieving

Susceptible to a disorder that occurs after the death of a significant other, in which the experience of distress accompanying bereavement fails to follow sociocultural expectations, which may compromise health

- Difficulty dealing with concurrent crises
- Excessive emotional disturbance
- High attachment anxiety
- Inadequate social support
- Low attachment avoidance

- Anxiety disorders
- Depression

- History of loss
- Length of grief process
- Pattern of coping (grief delayed or avoided)
- Self-destructive behaviors
- Sleep assessment
- Nutritional assessment
- Changes in presentation of self
- Social or spiritual support
- Ability to maintain roles at occupation and within family
- Behavioral status, understanding of health problem and treatment plan, past history with health care providers, participation in health care planning and decision-making; recognition and realization of potential growth, health, and autonomy

- Patient will express appropriate feelings of loss, guilt, fear, anger, or sadness.
- Patient will identify loss and describe meaning of loss.
- Patient will appropriately move through stages of grieving.
- Patient will maintain healthy patterns of sleep, activity, and eating.
- Patient will list personal strengths.
- Patient will use healthy coping mechanisms and social support systems.
- Patient will seek fulfillment through preferred spiritual practices.
- Patient will begin planning for future.

Suggested NOC Outcomes

Grief Resolution; Life Change Adjustment

- **PCC** Identify areas of hope in patient's life *to help decrease anger and feelings of frustration.*
- Identify previous losses and assess for depression *to establish a baseline.*
- **EBP** Perform interventions to promote sleep such as giving snacks, pillows, backrubs, or showers *to enhance rest.*
- **EBP** Teach patient relaxation techniques such as guided imagery, meditation, or progressive muscle relaxation *to promote feelings of comfort.*
- **PCC** Encourage patient to express grief and feelings of anger, guilt, and sadness. *Inability to express these feelings may result in maladaptive behaviors.*
- **PCC** Encourage patient to express feelings in a way the patient is most comfortable with, for example, crying, talking, writing, and/or drawing. *Dysfunctional grieving may result from an inability to express feelings freely.*

PCC ▪ Encourage patient to keep a journal to express feelings of grief and loss. The act of writing about feelings may aid in the grieving process. *Help patient form goals for the future to place the loss in perspective and to move on to new situations and relationships.*

T&C ▪ Refer patient to community support systems to assist with grieving process. Contact patient's preferred spiritual leader if patient desires. *This may provide relief from spiritual distress.*

Suggested NIC Interventions

Coping Enhancement; Counseling; Emotional Support; Family Therapy; Grief Facilitation Work

EVALUATIONS FOR EXPECTED OUTCOMES

▪ Patient expresses feelings of loss and grief.
▪ Patient describes the impact of the loss.
▪ Patient articulates movement through stages of grief.
▪ Patient's personal strengths are sufficient for normal functioning.
▪ Patient uses healthy coping strategies and social support systems.
▪ Patient states plan for future and uses spiritual practices satisfactorily.

DOCUMENTATION

▪ Patient's expressions of grief and loss
▪ Observations of physiologic and behavioral manifestations of grief
▪ Interventions performed to allay sleeping problems
▪ Patient's use of journal
▪ Patient's response to interventions
▪ Evaluations for expected outcomes

REFERENCES

McSpedden, M., Mullan, B., Sharpe, L., Breen, L. J., & Lobb, E. A. (2017). The presence and predictors of complicated grief symptoms in perinatally bereaved mothers from a bereavement support organization. *Death Studies, 41*(2), 112–117. doi:10.1080/07481187.2016.1210696

Perng, A., & Renz, S. (2018). Identifying and treating complicated grief in older adults. *Journal for Nurse Practitioners, 14*(4), 289–295. doi:10.1016/j.nurpra.2017.12.001

Thimm, J. C., & Holland, J. M. (2017). Early maladaptive schemas, meaning making, and complicated grief symptoms after bereavement. *International Journal of Stress Management, 24*(4), 347–367. doi:10.1037/str0000042

Tofthagen, C. S., Kip, K., Witt, A., & McMillan, S. C. (2017). Complicated grief: Risk factors, interventions, and resources for oncology nurses. *Clinical Journal of Oncology Nursing, 21*(3), 331–337. doi:10.1188/17.CJON.331-337

Readiness for Enhanced Grieving

DEFINITION

A pattern of integration of a new functional reality that arises after an actual, anticipated, or perceived significant loss, which can be strengthened

ASSESSMENT

▪ Age, gender, developmental stage
▪ Patient's perceived value of loss

- Emotional status, including evidence of anger, apathy, depression, or hostility
- Support systems, including family members, significant other, friends, and clergy
- Spiritual practices, including religious affiliation and use of spiritual support systems
- Customs and beliefs related to illness, death, and suffering

DEFINING CHARACTERISTICS

- Expresses desire to carry on legacy of the deceased
- Expresses desire to engage in previous activities
- Expresses desire to enhance coping with pain
- Expresses desire to enhance forgiveness
- Expresses desire to enhance hope
- Expresses desire to enhance personal growth
- Expresses desire to enhance sleep–wake cycle
- Expresses desire to integrate feelings of anger
- Expresses desire to integrate feelings of despair
- Expresses desire to integrate feelings of guilt
- Expresses desire to integrate feelings of remorse
- Expresses desire to integrate positive feelings
- Expresses desire to integrate positive memories of deceased
- Expresses desire to integrate possibilities for a joyful life
- Expresses desire to integrate possibilities for a meaningful life
- Expresses desire to integrate possibilities for a purposeful life
- Expresses desire to integrate possibilities for a satisfactory life
- Expresses desire to integrate the loss
- Expresses desire to invest energy in new interpersonal relations

EXPECTED OUTCOMES

- Patient will carry on legacy of the deceased.
- Patient will engage in previous activities.
- Patient will enhance coping with pain.
- Patient will enhance forgiveness.
- Patient will enhance hope.
- Patient will enhance personal growth.
- Patient will enhance sleep–wake cycle.
- Patient will integrate feelings of anger.
- Patient will integrate feelings of despair.
- Patient will integrate feelings of guilt.
- Patient will integrate feelings of remorse.
- Patient will integrate positive feelings.
- Patient will integrate positive memories of deceased.
- Patient will integrate possibilities for a joyful life.
- Patient will integrate possibilities for a meaningful life.
- Patient will integrate possibilities for a purposeful life.
- Patient will integrate possibilities for a satisfactory life.
- Patient will integrate the loss.
- Patient will invest energy in new interpersonal relations.

Suggested NOC Outcomes

Coping; Depression Level; Family Coping; Grief Resolution; Life Change; Psychosocial Adjustment

PCC ▪ Assist patient in identifying the meaning of the loss. *Identifying the nature of the attachment is the first step in developing a grieving strategy.*

EBP ▪ Encourage patient to express feelings about the loss. *Identifying and expressing feelings enhances coping with the loss.*

PCC ▪ Assist patient to understand grieving process and accept feelings; *this enhances patient's understanding and ability to cope.*

PCC ▪ Monitor patient progress through the psychological stages associated with grief, including shock and denial, anger, bargaining, depression, and acceptance, *foster anticipation of the patient's psychological needs. Keep in mind, however, that not all grieving patients go through each stage.*

PCC ▪ Reassure the patient that it is all right to be angry or sad. Assess whether the patient feels responsible for the loss, and clear up misconceptions *to help alleviate guilt feelings.*

PCC ▪ Reassure the patient that grief is a normal reaction to loss; explain the stages of the grieving process and normal responses. Reinforce that the patient's feelings and sadness are normal in the grieving process. *Understanding the grieving process will enhance the patient's ability to cope.*

T&C ▪ Offer the option of referral to a spiritual counselor or clergy member. *Spiritual beliefs often become stronger and occupy a more important place in the life of the patient during times of grieving.*

PCC ▪ Encourage the patient to express feelings through drawing or hobbies *to provide a safe outlet for pent-up emotions.*

T&C ▪ Encourage expression of grief in a support group; *comfort is received in knowing that the pain from grief is normal.*

T&C ▪ Involve an interdisciplinary team (psychologist, nurse, patient, nutritionist, physician, physical therapist, and chaplain) in providing care for a dying patient. *Each team member offers unique expertise to meet the patient's needs.*

PCC ▪ Help patient make a specific plan for coping to enable patient *to integrate the loss and adjust to new lifestyle.*

Suggested NIC Interventions

Active Listening; Anticipatory Guidance; Coping Enhancement; Emotional Support; Family Support; Grief Work Facilitation; Presence; Touch; Spiritual Support

▪ Patient reminisces and shares memories of the deceased.
▪ Patient maintains previous activities.
▪ Patient resolves feelings about loss.
▪ Patient maintains living environment, personal grooming and hygiene, nutrition, sleep, and sexual desire.
▪ Patient describes the meaning of the loss.
▪ Patient expresses spiritual beliefs and feelings about loss and death.
▪ Patient seek social support.
▪ Patient invest in building new interpersonal relationships.

▪ Patient's perception of loss
▪ Patient statements that indicate understanding of the grieving process, coping techniques, and necessary self-care skills

- Patient's response to interventions and teaching
- Literature provided to patient about loss and grief
- Observations of patient's demonstrations of health literacy techniques
- Evaluations for expected outcomes

REFERENCES

Hone, L. (2020). Resilient grieving: Positive psychology-based healthy adaptation to loss. *AI Practitioner, 22*(2), 36–41.

LeRoy, A. S., Robles, B., Kilpela, L. S., & Garcini, L. M. (2020). Dying in the face of the COVID-19 pandemic: Contextual considerations and clinical recommendations. *Psychological Trauma: Theory, Research, Practice, and Policy, 12*, S98–S99. doi:10.1037/tra0000818

Schellekens, M. P., van den Hurk, D. G., Jansen, E. T., van der Lee, M. L., Prins, J. B., van der Drift, M. A., & Speckens, A. E. (2021). Perspectives of bereaved partners of lung cancer patients on the role of mindfulness in dying and grieving: A qualitative study. *Palliative Medicine, 35*(1), 200–208.

Valliani, K., & Mughal, F. B. (2021). Human emotions during COVID-19: A lens through Kubler-Ross grief theory. *Psychological Trauma: Theory, Research, Practice, and Policy.* doi:10.1037/tra0001064

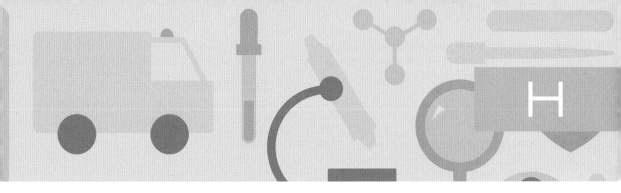

Deficient Community Health

Presence of one or more health problems or factors that deter wellness or increase the risk of health problems experienced by an aggregate

- Inadequate consumer satisfaction with program
- Inadequate program budget
- Inadequate program evaluation plan
- Inadequate program outcome data
- Inadequate social support for program
- Insufficient access to health care provider
- Insufficient community experts
- Insufficient resources
- Program incompletely addresses health problem

- Community demographics, including age and sex distribution, ethnic and racial groups, education, and income levels
- Prevalence of health problems in community, availability of health care services, and use of health care services
- Psychosocial status of community members, including cognitive abilities, access to transportation, physical disabilities, communication problems, environmental factors, financial resources, support systems, and beliefs and practices regarding health

- Health problem experienced by groups or populations
- Program unavailable to eliminate health problem(s) of group or population
- Program unavailable to enhance wellness of a group or population
- Program unavailable to prevent health problem(s) of a group or population
- Program unavailable to reduce health problem(s) of a group or population
- Risk of hospitalization experienced by groups or populations
- Risk of physiologic states experienced by groups or populations
- Risk of psychological states experienced by groups or populations

EXPECTED OUTCOMES

- Community members will conduct a formal comprehensive survey assessing the parameters of the community that impact its health.
- Community members will develop a plan to secure professional, governmental, social, and financial/economic resources that sustain a community's health.
- Community members will develop processes that enable individuals, organizations, and agencies to work together to accomplish the community's health goals.
- Community members will implement systems that meet the community's health needs.

Suggested NOC Outcomes

> Health-Promoting Behavior; Health-Seeking Behavior; Knowledge: Health Behavior; Knowledge: Health Resources; Community Health Status

INTERVENTIONS AND RATIONALES

T&C ■ Select a qualified leader/coordinator to establish and direct community resources to assess the health care needs of the residents. *A leader is necessary to coordinate the efforts of individuals working to improve the structures supporting community health.*

PCC ■ Communicate widely and through multiple media outlets the need for participation in surveys and assessments to determine deficiencies in community health. *Understanding proposed actions and expectations reduces anxiety and suspicion; it increases cooperation among the community residents.*

■ Assess community demographics. *An understanding of who has health needs to be addressed provides efficiency and effectiveness in delivering care.*

QI ■ Evaluate prevalence of health problems and risk behaviors. *Understanding the medical conditions and nursing needs are essential components of providing professional services to meet the community's needs.*

QI ■ Establish scope of need and the reality of resources available to meet the needs. *Integrating the knowledge gained about community deficit enables community leaders to identify scope of need, scope of work, and means to accomplish it.*

T&C ■ Create opportunities for community resources to begin services to the community residents in need. *Volunteers and concerned individuals can provide local services to meet the needs of "their neighbors" and promote goodwill.*

PCC ■ Foster relationships at all levels (local, regional, and national) that secure resources to enable policy, funding, and actions plans that correct deficiencies in community health. *In communities of any size, working together for common goals creates synergy and moves the agenda forward.*

QI ■ Plan for resident (community)-centered, safe, equitable, effective, efficient, quality, and timely delivery of health care. *These aims from the Institute for Medicine provide guidance in the outcomes desired for the community health care delivery.*

EBP ■ Teach the community members about their roles in self-care, disease management, and community care. *This facilitates autonomy to improve health and promote community-centered care.*

EBP ■ Educate students about their responsibilities, self-care, health maintenance, and health protection. *Positive health habits, positive self-esteem, disease avoidance, pregnancy avoidance, and successful completion of high school coupled with plans for a vocation or higher education reduce the current and future burden on the community's health.*

PCC ■ Support and encourage the community as it moves forward. *Barriers and challenges to initiatives may develop and can be surmounted with professional guidance.*

T&C ■ Encourage groups, agencies, and residents to find common ground and goals to work on together to identify solutions to meet the needs of the community. *In finding common ground, a commitment to the group process and the outcomes goal evolve into a solution.*

T&C ▪ Solicit a cadre of individuals with expertise to enhance the assessment, planning, and implementation phases of the community health plan. *Advanced knowledge of the community health assessment and promotion process enables local leaders and residents to move steadily toward positive health outcomes.*

QI ▪ Engage local educators and community leaders to provide insight and recommendations for implementing the health plan. *Local experts can be translational leaders in bringing the right residents forward to benefit from the ideas and resources made available through the community health initiatives.*

Suggested NIC Interventions

Community Health Development; Program Development; Environmental Management: Community; Health Screening; Community Disease Management

EVALUATIONS FOR EXPECTED OUTCOMES

▪ Community members complete health surveys and assessments.
▪ Community members develop health care plan.
▪ Community members participate in health care planning, implementation, and evaluation.
▪ Community resources are adequate to meet health care needs.

DOCUMENTATION

▪ Results of surveys and assessments done
▪ Minutes of meetings held
▪ Public relations announcements
▪ Educational materials produced
▪ Evaluations for expected outcomes

REFERENCES

Caffrey, A., Pointer, C., Steward, D., & Vohra, S. (2018). The role of community health needs assessments in medicalizing poverty. *Journal of Law, Medicine & Ethics, 46*(3), 615–621. doi:10.1177/1073110518804212

Carlton, E. L., & Singh, S. R. (2018). Joint community health needs assessments as a path for coordinating community-wide health improvement efforts between hospitals and local health departments. *American Journal of Public Health, 108*(5), 676–682. doi:10.2105/AJPH.2018.304339

Shah, G. H. (2018). Local health departments' role in nonprofit hospitals' community health needs assessment. *American Journal of Public Health, 108*(5), 595–597. doi:10.2105/AJPH.2018.304382

Van Gelderen, S. A., Krumwiede, K. A., Krumwiede, N. K., & Fenske, C. (2018). Trialing the community-based collaborative action research framework: Supporting rural health through a community health needs assessment. *Health Promotion Practice, 19*(5), 673–683. doi:10.1177/1524839917754043

Risk-Prone Health Behavior

DEFINITION

Impaired ability to modify lifestyle and/or actions in a manner that improves the level of wellness

RELATED FACTORS (R/T)

▪ Inadequate comprehension
▪ Insufficient social support

- Low self-efficacy
- Negative perception of health care provider
- Negative perception of recommended health care strategy
- Social anxiety
- Stressors

ASSESSMENT

- Nature and impact of medical diagnosis
- Behavioral responses, including verbal or nonverbal, engagement or disengagement, interest or apathy, acceptance or denial, and independence or dependence
- Knowledge of health condition
- Past experiences with family, friends, and media
- Psychosocial factors, such as age, gender, ethnic and cultural background, religious preference and beliefs, values, occupation, family support, and coping style
- Nutritional status, including modifications in diet and weight changes

DEFINING CHARACTERISTICS

- Failure to achieve optimal sense of control
- Failure to take action that prevents health problems
- Minimizes health status change
- Nonacceptance of health status change
- Smoking
- Substance misuse

EXPECTED OUTCOMES

- Patient will identify inability to cope and will adjust adequately.
- Patient will express understanding of the illness or disease.
- Patient will participate in health care regimen and will plan care-related activities.
- Patient will demonstrate ability to manage health problem.
- Patient will show ability to accept and adapt to a new health status and integrate learning.
- Patient will demonstrate new coping strategies.

Suggested NOC Outcomes

Acceptance: Health Status; Adaptation to Physical Disability; Coping; Health Seeking Behavior; Participation in Health Care Decisions; Psychosocial Adjustment: Life Change; Social Support; Treatment Behavior: Illness or Injury

INTERVENTIONS AND RATIONALES

- **PCC** Encourage patient to express feelings in a safe, private environment. *This allows patient to gain insight into and rationally define fears, goals, and potential problems.*
- Allow patient to grieve. Grieving is a normal and essential aspect with any kind of negative change in health status. *After working through denial and isolation, anger, bargaining, and depression, patient will progress toward acceptance.*
- **PCC** Provide reassurance that patient's feelings, under these circumstances, are normal. *By realizing that it's acceptable to grieve, the patient will be ready to look for positive ways of coping.*

EBP ▪ Begin teaching patient and caregivers the skills needed to adequately manage care. This will *encourage compliance and adjustment to optimum wellness.*

PCC ▪ Spend time listening to patient's feelings. *This helps reassure patient you're interested and care.*

PCC ▪ Help patient identify areas where it's possible to maintain control. *This prevents feelings of powerlessness and allows the patient to feel part of a team effort.*

PCC ▪ Encourage patient to plan for care activities, such as time of treatment, personal hygiene, and rest periods. *Doing this offers patient an opportunity to control facets of care and increases feelings of self-determination.*

T&C ▪ Arrange for others who have suffered similar health problems to speak with patient and family. *This exposes patient to suitable role models and may allow a trusting, supportive relationship to develop.*

PCC ▪ Discuss health problems and implications with family members *to enable them to participate in patient's care and to foster a trusting relationship.*

T&C ▪ Obtain a consultation with a mental health specialist if patient develops severe depression or other psychiatric problems. *Although trauma or illness commonly causes some depression, consultation with a mental health professional may help minimize it.*

Suggested NIC Interventions

Anxiety Reduction; Behavior Modification; Coping Enhancement; Counseling; Knowledge; Decision-Making Support; Emotional Support; Mutual Goal Setting; Role Enhancement; Simple Relaxation Therapy; Support System Enhancement

EVALUATIONS FOR EXPECTED OUTCOMES

▪ Patient recognizes necessity of learning to live with impairment.
▪ Patient understands that grieving is a normal response to impairment.
▪ Patient meets learning objectives before discharge.
▪ Patient identifies and contacts sources of continued psychological support if needed.
▪ Patient identifies two areas in which he or she can maintain control despite altered health status.
▪ Patient meets with individual who has similar health problem and reports results of meeting.

DOCUMENTATION

▪ Patient's verbalizations of specific behaviors that cause impairment of health
▪ Patient's nonverbal behaviors
▪ Patient's verbal expressions of denial, anger, or guilt because of the illness or disease process
▪ Patient's ability or inability to participate in care
▪ Evaluations for expected outcomes

REFERENCES

James, S., Donnelly, L., Brooks-Gunn, J., & McLanahan, S. (2018). Links between childhood exposure to violent contexts and risky adolescent health behaviors. *Journal of Adolescent Health, 63*(1), 94–101. doi:10.1016/j.jadohealth.2018.01.013

Kim, J.-N., Oh, Y. W., & Krishna, A. (2018). Justificatory information forefending in digital age: Self-sealing informational conviction of risky health behavior. *Health Communication, 33*(1), 85–93. doi:10.1080/10410236.2016.1242040

Nelson, K., Carey, K., Scott-Sheldon, L., Eckert, T., Park, A., Vanable, P., ... Carey, M. P. (2017). Gender differences in relations among perceived family characteristics and risky health behaviors in urban adolescents. *Annals of Behavioral Medicine, 51*(3), 416–422. doi:10.1007/s12160-016-9865-x

Vahedi, Z., Sibalis, A., & Sutherland, J. E. (2018). Are media literacy interventions effective at changing attitudes and intentions towards risky health behaviors in adolescents? A meta-analytic review. *Journal of Adolescence, 67*, 140–152. doi:10.1016/j.adolescence.2018.06.007

Readiness for Enhanced Health Literacy

DEFINITION

A pattern of using and developing a set of skills and competencies (literacy, knowledge, motivation, culture and language) to find, comprehend, evaluate and use health information and concepts to make daily health decisions to promote and maintain health, decrease health risks and improve overall quality of life, which can be strengthened

ASSESSMENT

- Age
- Developmental stage
- Education level and reading level
- Usual sources of health care information
- Readiness to participate in plan of care
- Need and use of assistance reading hospital materials
- Confidence level for filling out medical forms
- Problems learning about medical condition
- Difficulty understanding written information

DEFINING CHARACTERISTICS

- Expresses desire to enhance ability to read, write, speak, and interpret numbers for everyday health needs
- Expresses desire to enhance awareness of civic and/or government processes that impact public health
- Expresses desire to enhance health communication with health care providers
- Expresses desire to enhance knowledge of current determinants of health on social and physical environments
- Expresses desire to enhance personal health care decision-making
- Expresses desire to enhance social support for health
- Expresses desire to enhance understanding of customs and beliefs to make health care decisions
- Expresses desire to enhance understanding of health information to make health care choices
- Expresses desire to obtain sufficient information to navigate the health care system

EXPECTED OUTCOMES

- Patient will express desire to interpret personal health information.
- Patient will express desire to comprehend government processes that impact personal and public health.

- Patient will have meaningful communication with health care providers.
- Patient will express confidence in personal health care decision-making.
- Patient will identify sources of social support for health.
- Patient will have sufficient information to navigate the health care system.

Suggested NOC Outcomes

Client Satisfaction; Client Satisfaction: Access to Care Resources; Client Satisfaction: Communication; Client Satisfaction: Functional Assistance; Client Satisfaction: Protection of Rights; Decision-Making; Health Beliefs: Perceived Control; Knowledge: Health Promotion; Knowledge: Health Resources

INTERVENTIONS AND RATIONALES

- **PCC** Provide privacy when discussing health care matters. *Patients may be reluctant to discuss personal issues and health problems where others may hear or see.*
- **PCC** Write instructions in clear and simple language *to promote understanding and provide ease in reading.*
- **PCC** Use common, non medical terms when discussing care. *Individuals outside of the health care field do not always know and understand medical terminology.*
- **PCC** Use clear language and include pictures, graphs, and diagrams to clarify written materials and instructions. *Visuals and graphics clarify material.*
- **PCC** If needed, assist patient with forms and documents. *Allows patient to see examples of process.*
- **PCC** Review instructions with patient. Verify understanding of information and instructions by having patient repeat back using their own words. *Verifies that patient fully understands instructions.*
- **T&C** Refer patient to agencies that can provide additional information and services. *Allows patient to seek appropriate information from reputable sources.*
- **PCC** Provide copies of test results and/or reports. Highlight important information. *Helps patient keep a record of health information.*
- **PCC** Clarify any questions patient may have regarding care.

Suggested NIC Interventions

Active Listening; Decision-Making Support; Health Education; Health Literacy Enhancement; Health Policy Monitoring; Health System Guidance; Learning Facilitation; Learning Readiness Enhancement; Self-Efficacy Enhancement

EVALUATIONS FOR EXPECTED OUTCOMES

- Patient seeks information regarding personal health.
- Patient monitors government processes that impact personal and public health and asks questions for understanding.
- Patient communicates openly with health care providers.
- Patient makes personal health care decisions using resources and by consulting providers.
- Patient identifies sources of social support for health.
- Patient navigates the health care system.

- Patient's perception of health issues
- Patient statements that indicate understanding of disease, health-promoting activities, management techniques during exercise and illness, and necessary self-care skills
- Patient's response to interventions and teaching
- Literature provided to patient about managing the disorder
- Observations of patient's demonstrations of health literacy techniques
- Evaluations for expected outcomes

REFERENCES

Alberti, T. L., & Morris, N. J. (2017). Health literacy in the urgent care setting: What factors impact consumer comprehension of health information? *Journal of the American Association of Nurse Practitioners, 29*(5), 242–247. doi:10.1002/2327-6924.12452

Fernβndez, G. M., Bas, S. P., Albar, M. M. J., Paloma, C. O., & Romero, S. J. M. (2018). Health literacy interventions for immigrant populations: A systematic review. *International Nursing Review, 65*(1), 54–64. doi:10.1111/inr.12373

Harbour, P., & Grealish, L. (2018). Health literacy of the baby boomer generation and the implications for nursing. *Journal of Clinical Nursing, 27*(19/20), 3472–3481. doi:10.1111/jocn.14549

Huhta, A.-M., Hirvonen, N., & Huotari, M.-L. (2018). Health literacy in web-based health information environments: Systematic review of concepts, definitions, and operationalization for measurement. *Journal of Medical Internet Research, 20*(12), 16. doi:10.2196/10273

Peralta, L., Rowling, L., Samdal, O., Hipkins, R., & Dudley, D. (2017). Conceptualising a new approach to adolescent health literacy. *Health Education Journal, 76*(7), 787–801. doi:10.1177/0017896917714812

Ineffective Health Maintenance Behaviors

Management of health knowledge, attitudes, and practices underlying health actions that are unsatisfactory for maintaining or improving well-being or preventing illness and injury

- Cognitive dysfunction
- Competing demands
- Competing lifestyle preferences
- Conflict between health behaviors and social norms
- Conflicts between spiritual beliefs and health practices
- Depressive symptoms
- Difficulty accessing community resources
- Difficulty navigating complex health care systems
- Difficulty with decision-making
- Inadequate health resources
- Inadequate social support
- Inadequate trust in health care professional
- Individuals with limited decision-making experience
- Ineffective communication skills
- Ineffective coping strategies
- Ineffective family coping
- Low self-efficacy
- Maladaptive grieving

- Neurobehavioral manifestations
- Perceived prejudice
- Spiritual distress

ASSOCIATED CONDITIONS

- Chronic disease
- Developmental disabilities
- Mental disorders
- Motor skills disorders

ASSESSMENT

- Age
- Gender
- Developmental stage, including cognitive ability and physical maturity
- Level of knowledge about routine health practices, preventive needs and safety measures, and treatment and follow-up
- Level of motivation to perform self-care
- Current health status, including height, weight, recent illnesses, and patient's perception of personal health status
- Social status, including lifestyle, activity level, sports, interests, and socioeconomic status
- Family health history
- Community demographics, including age and sex distribution, ethnic and racial groups, education, and income levels
- Prevalence of health problems in community, availability of health care services, and use of health care services
- Psychosocial status of community members, including access to transportation, communication problems, environmental factors, financial resources, support systems, and beliefs and practices regarding health

DEFINING CHARACTERISTICS

- Failure to take action that prevents health problem
- Failure to take action that reduces risk factor
- Inadequate commitment to a plan of action
- Inadequate health literacy
- Inadequate interest in improving health
- Inadequate knowledge about basic health practices
- Ineffective choices in daily living for meeting health goal
- Pattern of lack of health-seeking behavior

EXPECTED OUTCOMES

- Patient will express confidence in disease self-management.
- Patient will adapt to environmental changes.
- Patient will express desire to improve health behaviors.
- Patient will describe proper techniques for managing signs and symptoms of disease.
- Patient will demonstrate ability to perform self-care activities, such as properly administering medications and choosing appropriate foods.
- Patient will express desire to learn about available resources.
- Patient will seek support from health care professionals.

Suggested NOC Outcomes

Health Beliefs: Perceived Resources; Health-Promoting Behavior; Health-Seeking Behavior; Knowledge: Health Behavior; Knowledge: Health Resources; Knowledge: Treatment Regimen; Risk Detection; Symptom Control

INTERVENTIONS AND RATIONALES

PCC ▪ Evaluate patient's understanding of disease and attitude about the need to manage it. *This assists in determining which teaching interventions to use.*

PCC ▪ Correct any misconceptions about disease and the therapeutic regimen *to increase knowledge and instill confidence in management ability.*

PCC ▪ Observe as patient performs self-care activities *to assess skills and overall progress.*

EBP ▪ Teach patient how to interpret test results and correlate these values with the degree of disease control *to increase autonomy and decision-making skills.*

PCC ▪ Provide written materials that cover each teaching topic. *These materials help reinforce learning and can refresh patient's memory later.*

T&C ▪ Describe resources available to help patient manage the disorder. Consider arranging a visit with the other members of the health care team *to reinforce teaching.*

PCC ▪ Work with patient to develop an exercise plan *to promote health.* The plan should identify a support person capable of assisting during an emergency. *This ensures patient's safety while allowing participation in activities.*

EBP ▪ Discuss how to manage health during an illness. Explain the importance of following prescribed regimen. *These measures help provide a sense of control, ensure safety, and prevent complications.*

EBP ▪ Teach patient to recognize signs and symptoms that must be reported to health care provider *to improve management skills and ensure safety.*

EBP ▪ Discuss possible complications. *Understanding possible major complications may encourage patient to adhere to the prescribed regimen.*

T&C ▪ Encourage patient to contact a support group *to provide peer support.*

T&C ▪ Help patient identify specific neighborhood resources. For example, a senior citizen may need nutrition support services, whereas young families may need information about immunizations and child safety. *Targeting resources that meet specific health needs increases chances that they'll be used.*

T&C ▪ Assist patient in learning about community and resources available, such as the American Heart Association, Agency on Aging, American Cancer Society, Meals on Wheels, and Alzheimer Disease support group, *to help empower patient.*

Suggested NIC Interventions

Health Education; Patient Contracting; Self-Modification Assistance; Self-Responsibility Facilitation; Support System Enhancement; Teaching: Disease Process

EVALUATIONS FOR EXPECTED OUTCOMES

▪ Patient expresses confidence in disease self-management.
▪ Patient adapts to environmental changes with no complications.
▪ Patient expresses desire to improve health behaviors.
▪ Patient describes proper techniques for managing signs and symptoms of disease.

- Patient performs self-care activities, such as properly administering medications and choosing appropriate foods.
- Patient lists available resources.
- Patient seeks support from health care professionals.

DOCUMENTATION

- Patient's perception of health issues
- Patient statements that indicate understanding of disease, health-promoting activities, management techniques during exercise and illness, and necessary self-care skills
- Patient's response to interventions and teaching
- Literature provided to patient about managing the disorder
- Observations of patient's demonstrations of self-care techniques
- Referrals to community resources or hospital services
- Evaluations for expected outcomes

REFERENCES

Adongo, W. B., & Asaarik, M. J. A. (2018). Health seeking behaviors and utilization of healthcare services among rural dwellers in under-resourced communities in Ghana. *International Journal of Caring Sciences, 11*(2), 840–850.

Basch, C. H., MacLean, S. A., Romero, R.-A., & Ethan, D. (2018). Health information seeking behavior among college students. *Journal of Community Health, 43*(6), 1094–1099. doi:10.1007/s10900-018-0526-9

Park, A. R., So, H. S., & Song, C. E. (2017). Impact of risk factors, autonomy support and health behavior compliance on the relapse in patients with coronary artery disease. *Korean Journal of Adult Nursing, 29*(1), 32–40. doi:10.7475/kjan.2017.29.1.32

Van de Ven, K., Memedovic, S., Maher, L., Wand, H., Iversen, J., & Jackson, E. (2018). Health risk and health seeking behaviours among people who inject performance and image enhancing drugs who access needle syringe programs in Australia. *Drug and Alcohol Review, 37*(7), 837–846. doi:10.1111/dar.12831

Ineffective Health Self-Management

DEFINITION

Unsatisfactory management of symptoms; treatment regimen; physical, psychosocial, and spiritual consequences; and lifestyle changes inherent in living with a chronic condition

RELATED FACTORS (R/T)

- Cognitive dysfunction
- Competing demands
- Competing lifestyle preferences
- Conflict between cultural beliefs and health practices
- Conflict between health behaviors and social norms
- Conflict between spiritual beliefs and treatment regimen
- Decreased perceived quality of life
- Depressive symptoms
- Difficulty accessing community resources
- Difficulty managing complex treatment regimen
- Difficulty with decision-making

- Inadequate commitment to a plan of action
- Inadequate health literacy
- Inadequate knowledge of treatment regimen
- Inadequate number of cues to action
- Inadequate role models
- Inadequate social support
- Individuals with limited decision-making experience
- Limited ability to perform aspects of treatment regimen
- Low self-efficacy
- Negative feelings toward treatment regimen
- Neurobehavioral manifestations
- Nonacceptance of condition
- Perceived barrier to treatment regimen
- Perceived social stigma associated with condition
- Substance misuse
- Unrealistic perception of seriousness of condition
- Unrealistic perception of susceptibility to sequelae
- Unrealistic perception of treatment benefit

ASSOCIATED CONDITIONS

- Asymptomatic disease
- Developmental disabilities
- High acuity illness
- Neurocognitive disorders
- Polypharmacy
- Significant comorbidity

ASSESSMENT

- Age
- Current health status
- History of neurologic, sensory, or psychological impairment
- Neurologic status, including level of consciousness, orientation, cognition (memory, insight, and judgment), sensory ability, and motor ability
- Knowledge of health practices, including body maintenance, preventive health care needs, health care team follow-up, and safety measures
- Learning ability including demonstrated skills in managing health problems
- Recognition and realization of potential growth, health, and autonomy
- Personal habits, such as smoking and alcohol consumption
- Psychosocial support, including lifestyle, communication status (verbal, nonverbal, phone, and written), family members, and finances

DEFINING CHARACTERISTICS

- Exacerbation of disease signs
- Exacerbation of disease symptoms
- Exhibits dissatisfaction with quality of life
- Failure to attend appointments with health care provider
- Failure to include treatment regimen into daily living
- Failure to take action that reduces risk factor
- Inattentive to disease signs
- Inattentive to disease symptoms
- Ineffective choices in daily living for meeting health goal

EXPECTED OUTCOMES

- Patient will identify necessary health activities.
- Patient will perform daily health maintenance activities (specify) to level of ability.
- Patient will acknowledge responsibility to manage own health condition.
- Patient will identify any barriers to optimal self-health management and determine plan to address them.
- Patient will increase self-efficacy, the confidence that one can carry out a behavior necessary to reach a desired goal.
- Patient will identify community and social resources available to help with health maintenance.

Suggested NOC Outcomes

Adherence Behavior; Compliance Behavior; Decision-Making; Health Beliefs: Perceived Resources; Health Promoting Behavior; Health Seeking Behaviors; Health Status; Knowledge: Health Behavior; Knowledge: Health Promotion; Motivation; Personal Health Status; Self-Care Status; Social Support; Spiritual Health

INTERVENTIONS AND RATIONALES

PCC ▪ Discuss health maintenance needs with patient while carrying out routine activities *to reinforce their importance.*

PCC ▪ Involve patient in decision-making by allowing choices in determining where, when, and how activities are to be carried out. Ask, for example, "Would you like a bath or shower in the morning or evening?" *Participation in decision-making increases feelings of independence.*

PCC ▪ Monitor patient's self-efficacy and use of problem-solving skills as patient manages own health. *These concepts reflect a new paradigm in health management that acknowledges that patients need many skills and confidence to carry out plan of care.*

PCC ▪ Help patient perform health maintenance activities, such as daily skin inspection and weekly catheterization for residual urine. *Encouraging skill development in patient promotes continued use of those skills after discharge.*

EBP ▪ Instruct patient in specific skills needed in monitoring health status *to prompt participation in self-care.* Allow patient to perform skills *to encourage independence.*

PCC ▪ Assist patient in setting goals and making informed choices. *This patient–nurse collaborative relationship helps patient and nurse identify barriers to optimal health management and overcome them.*

EBP ▪ Teach patient about disease states and regimens but, more importantly, teach problem-solving skills *to ensure active participation in self-health management despite any possible setbacks.*

PCC ▪ Provide encouragement to help motivate patient to maximize healthy behaviors. *This highlights that behavior is best changed by internal motivation rather than by external motivation.*

T&C ▪ Consult with social services or other health care team members to identify health care resources (e.g., Meals on Wheels or homemaker services) and help patient contact and arrange for follow-up. *These resources can help patient maintain independence after discharge.*

PCC ▪ Encourage patient and family members to verbalize feelings and concerns related to health maintenance *to help them develop greater understanding and better manage their health.*

PCC ▪ Help family members develop coping skills necessary to deal with patient. *If patient's illness is prolonged, family members could develop maladaptive coping strategies.*

▪ Make referrals, as appropriate, to psychiatric liaison nurse and social services *to help prevent burnout among family members.*

 ▪ Coordinate care with social services and colleagues in other disciplines *to ensure that family, economic, and social barriers to optimal self-health management have been addressed.*

Suggested NIC Interventions

Anticipatory Guidance; Behavior Modification; Complex Relationship Building; Decision-Making Support; Health Education; Health System Guidance; Learning Facilitation; Mutual Goal Setting; Referral; Support System Enhancement; Self-Awareness Enhancement; Teaching: Disease Process

EVALUATIONS FOR EXPECTED OUTCOMES

▪ Patient identifies health maintenance activities.
▪ Patient communicates understanding of importance of monitoring health status.
▪ Patient identifies and contacts community resources to assist with health maintenance, if needed.
▪ Patient acknowledges responsibility for management of own health.
▪ Patient identifies barriers to self-health management and strategies to address them.
▪ Patient begins to develop confidence in managing own health and achieving goals.

DOCUMENTATION

▪ Patient's identified health needs and perceptions and limitations in achieving them
▪ Patient's willingness to make decisions and participate in health maintenance activities
▪ Patient's statement of responsibility for self-health management
▪ Patient's identified barriers to self-health management and planned strategies
▪ Observations of motor abilities, level of skill performance, and health status
▪ Patient's response to nursing interventions
▪ Evaluations for expected outcomes

REFERENCES

Cohen-Mansfield, J., & Sommerstein, M. (2019). Motivating inactive seniors to participate in physical activity: A pilot RCT. *American Journal of Health Behavior, 43*(1), 195–206. doi:10.5993/AJHB.43.1.16

Montiel, L. A., Núñez, M. A. J., Martín, A. E., García, D. F., Toro, T. M. C., González, C. J. A., & Polipresact. (2018). Prevalence and related factors of ineffective self-health management in polymedicated patients over the age of 65 years. *International Journal of Nursing Knowledge, 29*(2), 133–142. doi:10.1111/2047-3095.12155

Sevinc, S., & Argon, G. (2018). Application of Pender's health promotion model to post-myocard infarction patients in Turkey. *International Journal of Caring Sciences, 11*, 409–418.

Worawong, C., Borden, M. J., Cooper, K. M., Pérez, O. A., & Lauver, D. (2018). Evaluation of a person-centered, theory-based intervention to promote health behaviors. *Nursing Research, 67*(1), 6–15. doi:10.1097/NNR.0000000000000254

Readiness for Enhanced Health Self-Management

DEFINITION

A pattern of satisfactory management of symptoms; treatment regimen; physical, psychosocial, and spiritual consequences; and lifestyle changes inherent in living with a chronic condition, which can be strengthened

DEFINING CHARACTERISTICS

- Expresses desire to enhance acceptance of the condition
- Expresses desire to enhance choices of daily living for meeting health goals
- Expresses desire to enhance commitment to follow-up care
- Expresses desire to enhance decision-making
- Expresses desire to enhance inclusion of treatment regimen into daily living
- Expresses desire to enhance management of risk factors
- Expresses desire to enhance management of signs
- Expresses desire to enhance management of symptoms
- Expresses desire to enhance recognition of disease signs
- Expresses desire to enhance recognition of disease symptoms
- Expresses desire to enhance satisfaction with quality of life

ASSESSMENT

- Age
- Current health status
- History of neurologic, sensory, or psychological impairment
- Neurologic status, including level of consciousness, orientation, cognition (memory, insight, and judgment), sensory ability, and motor ability
- Knowledge of health practices, including body maintenance, preventive health care needs, health care team follow-up, and safety measures
- Learning ability including demonstrated skills in managing health problems
- Recognition and realization of potential growth, health, and autonomy
- Personal habits, such as smoking and alcohol consumption
- Psychosocial support, including lifestyle, communication status (verbal, nonverbal, phone, and written), family members, and finances

EXPECTED OUTCOMES

- The patient will acknowledge responsibility to manage own health condition.
- The patient will identify any barriers to optimal self-health management and determine plan to address them.
- The patient will refine problem-solving skills over time.
- The patient will increase self-efficacy, the confidence that one can carry out a behavior necessary to reach a desired goal.

Suggested NOC Outcomes

Adherence Behavior; Compliance Behavior; Decision-Making; Health Orientation; Health Promoting Behavior; Personal Health Status; Self-Direction of Care; Knowledge: Health Promotion

INTERVENTIONS AND RATIONALES

PCC ▪ Monitor patient's self-efficacy and use of problem-solving skills as patient manages own health. *These concepts reflect a new paradigm in health management that acknowledges that patients need many skills and confidence to carry out plan of care.*

PCC ▪ Assist patient in setting goals and making informed choices. *This patient–nurse collaborative relationship helps patient and nurse identify barriers to optimal health management and overcome them.*

EBP ▪ Teach patients about their disease states and regimens, but more importantly, teach patients problem-solving skills *to ensure that they actively participate in their self-health management despite any setbacks that they might experience.*

PCC ▪ Provide encouragement to help motivate patient to maximize healthy behaviors. *This high-lights that behavior is best changed by internal motivation rather than by external motivation.*

T&C ▪ Coordinate with social services and colleagues in other disciplines *to ensure that family, economic, and social barriers to optimal self-health management have been addressed.*

Suggested NIC Interventions

Behavior Modification; Complex Relationship Building; Decision-Making Support; Health Education; Learning Facilitation; Mutual Goal-Setting; Self-Awareness Enhancement

EVALUATIONS FOR EXPECTED OUTCOMES

▪ The patient accepts responsibility to manage and improve own health condition.
▪ The patient identifies any barriers to optimal self-health management and determines plan to address them.
▪ The patient works to refine problem-solving skills.
▪ The patient increases self-efficacy and the confidence to carry out behaviors necessary to reach desired goals.

DOCUMENTATION

▪ Patient's identified health needs and desire in improving them
▪ Patient's willingness to make decisions and participate in health maintenance activities
▪ Patient's statement of responsibility for self-health management
▪ Patient's identified barriers to self-health management and planned strategies to overcome them
▪ Patient's response to nursing interventions
▪ Evaluations for expected outcomes

REFERENCES

Fu, Y., Yu, G., McNichol, E., Marczewski, K., & Closs, S. J. (2018). The association between patient-professional partnerships and self-management of chronic back pain: A mixed methods study. *European Journal of Pain, 22*(7), 1229–1244. doi:10.1002/ejp.1210

Jacobson, A. F., Sumodi, V., Albert, N. M., Butler, R. S., DeJohn, L., Walker, D., … Ross, D. M. (2018). Patient activation, knowledge, and health literacy association with self-management behaviors in persons with heart failure. *Heart & Lung, 47*(5), 447–451. doi:10.1016/j.hrtlng.2018.05.021

Jeddi, F., Nabovati, E., & Amirazodi, S. (2017). Features and effects of information technology-based interventions to improve self-management in chronic kidney disease patients: A systematic review of the literature. *Journal of Medical Systems, 41*(11), 170. doi:10.1007/s10916-017-0820-6

Roberts, S., Marshall, A., & Chaboyer, W. (2017). Hospital staffs' perceptions of an electronic program to engage patients in nutrition care at the bedside: A qualitative study. *BMC Medical Informatics and Decision Making, 17*, 105. doi:10.1186/s12911-017-0495-4

Ineffective Family Health Self-Management

DEFINITION

Unsatisfactory management of symptoms; treatment regimen; physical, psychosocial, and spiritual consequences; and lifestyle changes inherent in living with one or more family members' chronic condition

- Cognitive dysfunction
- Cognitive dysfunction of one or more caregivers
- Competing demands on family unit
- Competing lifestyle preferences within family unit
- Conflict between health behaviors and social norms
- Conflict between spiritual beliefs and treatment regimen
- Difficulty accessing community resources
- Difficulty dealing with role changes associated with condition
- Difficulty managing complex treatment regimen
- Difficulty navigating complex health care systems
- Difficulty with decision-making
- Family conflict
- Inadequate commitment to a plan of action
- Inadequate health literacy of caregiver
- Inadequate knowledge of treatment regimen
- Inadequate number of cues to action
- Inadequate social support
- Ineffective communication skills
- Ineffective coping skills
- Limited ability to perform aspects of treatment regimen
- Low self-efficacy
- Negative feelings toward treatment regimen
- Nonacceptance of condition
- Perceived barrier to treatment regimen
- Perceived social stigma associated with condition
- Substance misuse
- Unrealistic perception of seriousness of condition
- Unrealistic perception of susceptibility to sequelae
- Unrealistic perception of treatment benefit
- Unsupportive family relations

ASSOCIATED CONDITIONS

- Chronic disease
- Mental disorders
- Neurocognitive disorders
- Terminal illness

ASSESSMENT

- Family status, including marital status, family composition, communication patterns, coping skills, drug or alcohol abuse, psychiatric history, and beliefs and attitudes about health and illness
- Health status, including chronic or terminal illness and severely disabling physical conditions
- Socioeconomic factors, including financial status, insurance, accessibility of health care, availability of health care providers, and transportation system
- Social status, including communication skills, size of social network, degree of trust in others, self-esteem, and ability to function in social and occupational roles
- Spiritual status, including religious or church affiliation and description of faith and religious practices

DEFINING CHARACTERISTICS

- Caregiver strain
- Decrease in attention to illness in one or more family members
- Depressive symptoms of caregiver
- Exacerbation of disease signs of one or more family members
- Exacerbation of disease symptoms of one or more family members
- Failure to take action to reduce risk factor in one or more family members
- Ineffective choices in daily living for meeting health goal of family unit
- One or more family members report dissatisfaction with quality of life.

EXPECTED OUTCOMES

- Family members will identify behaviors that lead to conflict.
- Family members will participate in family therapy sessions and openly express feelings about illness of family member.
- Family members will express desire to have help in resolving conflicts.
- Family members will describe coping mechanisms that help reduce conflicts.
- Family members will cooperate in finding ways to incorporate therapeutic regimen into their lifestyle.
- Family members will express desire to carry out therapeutic regimen.
- Family members will plan for future course of illness.

Suggested NOC Outcomes

Compliance Behavior; Family Coping; Family Functioning; Family Normalization; Family Participation in Professional Care; Knowledge: Treatment Regimen; Risk Control; Symptom Control

INTERVENTIONS AND RATIONALES

- **PCC** Spend time with family, get to know each family member individually, and establish a trusting relationship with each family member *to help identify measures that will increase family cohesiveness.*
- **PCC** Encourage family members to attend and participate in family therapy sessions *to strengthen family unit and promote resolution of conflict.*
- **PCC** Help family members describe feelings associated with the illness of a relative to bring family conflict into the open. *Unresolved family conflicts may prevent family members from fully implementing therapeutic regimen.*
- **PCC** Elicit family members' personal beliefs about the illness and review relevant information *to establish their support for improving management of therapeutic regimen.*
- **EBP** Educate family members about the pathophysiology of illness and explain relationship between the pathophysiology and the therapeutic regimen. *If family members know reasons for specific behaviors, they may be more willing to adjust lifestyle.*
- **PCC** Work with family members to identify behaviors that have contributed to family conflict and help them identify alternative behaviors *to promote resolution of the conflict.*
- **PCC** Encourage family members to address individual needs assertively *to promote healthy interactions within family.*
- **PCC** Help family members clarify values associated with their lifestyle *to enhance understanding of conflicts between lifestyle and demands of therapeutic regimen.*
- **PCC** Work with family members to develop a daily routine for managing the therapeutic regimen that fits with lifestyle. *Collaboration with family members makes it possible to incorporate lifestyle factors, such as culture, family dynamics, and finances, into a plan for managing the illness.*

EBP ▪ Assist family members in modifying factors (such as lack of supportive behaviors among family members) that interfere with treatment management *to enhance level of care.*

PCC ▪ Work with family in establishing goals for coping with conflicts *to focus their energy on achievable objectives and to foster hope.*

EBP ▪ Refer family members to appropriate agencies, if needed. This can ensure continued family support and help reduce conflicts.

PCC ▪ Help family members plan for a future course of the illness. *Planning enhances family members' abilities to develop an appropriate strategy to manage the therapeutic regimen.*

Suggested NIC Interventions

Case Management; Coping Enhancement; Decision-Making Support; Family Involvement Promotion; Family Process Maintenance; Family Therapy

EVALUATIONS FOR EXPECTED OUTCOMES

- Family members identify unresolved conflicts.
- Family members attend and participate in family therapy sessions.
- Family members express a desire to resolve conflicts.
- Family members describe coping mechanisms that can reduce conflicts.
- Family members successfully incorporate components of therapeutic regimen into daily activities.
- Family members carry out therapeutic regimen.
- Family members establish a plan for coping with future course of illness.

DOCUMENTATION

- Description of each family member's understanding of patient's illness
- Family members' expressions of feelings regarding patient's illness
- Compliance with participation in family therapy sessions
- Evaluations for expected outcomes

REFERENCES

Aarthun, A., Øymar, K. A., & Akerjordet, K. (2018). How health professionals facilitate parents' involvement in decision-making at the hospital: A parental perspective. *Journal of Child Health Care*, 22(1), 108–121. doi:10.1177/1367493517744279

Koren, D., Laidsaar-Powell, R., Tilden, W., Latt, M., & Butow, P. (2018). Health care providers' perceptions of family caregivers' involvement in consultations within a geriatric hospital setting. *Geriatric Nursing*, 39(4), 419–427. doi:10.1016/j.gerinurse.2017.12.013

Whiston, L., Barry, J. M., & Darker, C. D. (2017). Participation of patients and family members in healthcare services at the service and national levels: A lesson learned in Dublin, Ireland. *Patient Education and Counseling*, 100(3), 583–591. doi:10.1016/j.pec.2016.10.025

Ineffective Home Maintenance Behaviors

DEFINITION

An unsatisfactory pattern of knowledge and activities for the safe upkeep of one's residence

RELATED FACTORS (R/T)

- Cognitive dysfunction
- Competing demands

- Depressive symptoms
- Difficulty with decision-making
- Environmental constraints
- Impaired physical mobility
- Impaired postural balance
- Inadequate knowledge of home maintenance
- Inadequate knowledge of social resources
- Inadequate organizing skills
- Inadequate role models
- Inadequate social support
- Insufficient physical endurance
- Neurobehavioral manifestations
- Powerlessness
- Psychological distress

ASSOCIATED CONDITIONS

- Depression
- Mental disorders
- Neoplasms
- Neurocognitive disorders
- Sensation disorders
- Vascular diseases

ASSESSMENT

- Age and gender of occupants at home
- Home environment
- Financial resources
- Patient's and family's knowledge of care requirements
- Patient's and family's psychological status, including perception of reality, communication patterns, assignment of responsibilities, degree of awareness and concern, and history of psychiatric illness
- Drug or alcohol abuse
- Support systems, including close friends, organizations with which patient is affiliated, and community resources

DEFINING CHARACTERISTICS

- Cluttered environment
- Difficulty maintaining a comfortable environment
- Failure to request assistance with home maintenance
- Home task-related anxiety
- Home task-related stress
- Impaired ability to regulate finances
- Negative affect toward home maintenance
- Neglected laundry
- Pattern of hygiene-related diseases
- Trash accumulation
- Unsafe cooking equipment
- Unsanitary environment

- Patient/family members will maintain a healthy home environment.
- Patient/family members develop a plan to correct health and safety hazards at home.
- Patient/family members will utilize community resources available to help maintain home.

Suggested NOC Outcomes

Family Functioning; Role Performance; Self-Care: Instrumental Activities of Daily Living (IADLs)

PCC ◾ Help patient/family identify strengths and weaknesses in current home maintenance practices *to provide a focus for interventions.*

PCC ◾ Discuss with patient/family obstacles to meeting home maintenance needs *to provide the basis for a program to meet health and safety requirements.*

PCC ◾ Determine patient/family ability and motivation to achieve a higher level of home maintenance. *Self-motivation is necessary to ensure change.*

PCC ◾ Discuss obstacles to effective home maintenance management with patient and family *to develop understanding of potential and actual health and safety hazards.*

PCC ◾ Help family members assign responsibilities for household care and establish appropriate expectations *to aid communication and help set realistic goals.*

PCC ◾ Help family members establish daily and weekly home maintenance activities and assignments *to impose structure on family's routine and set standards for measuring progress.*

S ◾ Conduct a home visit or evaluate patient's description of own home *to assess safety needs and make recommendations for structural alterations. For example, the patient may benefit from installing ramps, enlarging doorways, or moving a second-floor bedroom to the first-floor family room.*

S ◾ Based on assessment of patient's health and home environment, determine the need for assistive devices, including: *Using assistive devices improves safe environment.*
  - Telephones for hearing impaired
  - Telephone dial covers with large numbers
  - Telephones with programmed dialing
  - Amplifiers for phone receivers
  - Clocks that chime or recite time
  - Handrails
  - Safety bars for toilet and bath
  - Automatic chair lifts
  - Commode chairs
  - Shower chairs

S ◾ Discuss alternative housing opportunities with patient and caregiver, such as moving patient to a life-care community, *to provide necessary information to make appropriate decisions regarding patient's future.*

EBP ◾ Provide family with written information on medications and various aspects of patient's treatment. *The more competent family members feel, the greater the possibility patient will progress without difficulty.*

PCC ◾ Encourage weekly discussions about progress in maintaining home maintenance *schedule to develop family unity and allow members to address problems before they become overwhelming.*

T&C ▥ Assist patient and family members in exploring available resources *to help with home and safety needs.*

T&C ▥ Help family members contact community resources that can assist them in their efforts to improve home maintenance management, such as self-help groups, cleaning services, and exterminators. *Community resources can lessen family's burden while members learn to function independently.*

Suggested NIC Interventions

Caregiver Support; Counseling; Emotional Support; Environmental Management; Family Support; Family Integrity Promotion; Family Support; Home Maintenance Assistance; Role Enhancement; Support System Enhancement

EVALUATIONS FOR EXPECTED OUTCOMES

▥ Patient and family members establish and follow daily and weekly schedule for home maintenance.

▥ Patient and family members describe changes needed to promote maximum health and safety at home.

▥ Patient and family members list agencies that can assist with home care.

▥ Patient and family members contact community resources.

▥ Patient and family members identify individuals or organizations that may provide assistance.

DOCUMENTATION

▥ Patient's and family members' expressions of difficulty in maintaining household

▥ Patient's and family members' perception of problem

▥ Patient's and family members' mental status

▥ Presence of health hazards, such as filth, rodents, and waste matter

▥ Presence of safety hazards, such as faulty wiring

▥ Presence of offensive odors

▥ Patient's and family members' understanding of home maintenance management and resources

▥ Interventions to improve home maintenance skills

▥ Patient's and family members' responses to nursing interventions

▥ Evaluations for expected outcomes

REFERENCES

Gutman, S., Berg, J., Amarantos, K., Chen, E., Schlugar, Z., & Peters, R. (2017). Assessing home safety fall and accident risk in the prematurely aging, formerly homeless population. *American Journal of Occupational Therapy, 71*, 21. doi:10.5014/ajot.2017.71S1-PO6127

Polletta, V. L., Reid, M., Barros, E., Duarte, C., Donaher, K., Wensley, H., & Wolff, L. (2017). Role of landlords in creating healthy homes: Section 8 landlord perspectives on healthy housing practices. *American Journal of Health Promotion, 31*(6), 511–514. doi:10.1177/0890117116671081

Rostad, W., McFry, E., Self-Brown, S., Damashek, A., & Whitaker, D. (2017). Reducing safety hazards in the home through the use of an evidence-based parenting program. *Journal of Child and Family Studies, 26*(9), 2602–2609. doi:10.1007/s10826-017-0756-y

Woodruff, R. C., Haardörfer, R., Kegler, M. C., Gazmararian, J. A., Ballard, D., Addison, A. R., … Tucker, R. B. (2019). Home environment-focused intervention improves dietary quality: A secondary analysis from the healthy homes/healthy families randomized trial. *Journal of Nutrition Education and Behavior, 51*(1), 96–100. doi:10.1016/j.jneb.2018.06.007

Risk for Ineffective Home Maintenance Behaviors

DEFINITION

Susceptible to an unsatisfactory pattern of knowledge and activities for the safe upkeep of one's residence, which may compromise health

RISK FACTORS

- Cognitive dysfunction
- Competing demands
- Depressive symptoms
- Difficulty with decision-making
- Environmental constraints
- Impaired physical mobility
- Impaired postural balance
- Inadequate knowledge of home maintenance
- Inadequate knowledge of social resources
- Inadequate organizing skills
- Inadequate role models
- Inadequate social support
- Insufficient physical endurance
- Neurobehavioral manifestations
- Powerlessness
- Psychological distress

ASSOCIATED CONDITIONS

- Depression
- Mental disorders
- Neoplasms
- Neurocognitive disorders
- Sensation disorders
- Vascular diseases

ASSESSMENT

- Age and gender of occupants of home
- Home environment
- Financial resources
- Patient's and family's knowledge of home maintenance requirements
- Patient's and family's psychological status including perception of reality, communication patterns, assignment of responsibilities, degree of awareness and concern, and history of psychiatric illness
- Drug or alcohol abuse
- Support systems, including close friends, organizations with which patient is affiliated, and community resources

EXPECTED OUTCOMES

- Patient/family members will maintain a healthy home environment.

- Patient/family members will identify health and safety risks in home.
- Patient/family members will utilize community resources available to help maintain home.

Suggested NOC Outcomes

Family Functioning; Knowledge: Healthy Lifestyle; Role Performance; Self-Care: Instrumental Activities of Daily Living (IADLs)

INTERVENTIONS AND RATIONALES

PCC — Assist family in determining home maintenance requirements. *Having a list of requirements allows for best planning of time and resources.*

PCC — Help the patient/family identify the strengths and weaknesses in current home maintenance practices *to provide a focus for interventions.*

S — Discuss with the patient/family obstacles to meeting home maintenance needs *to provide the basis for a program to meet health and safety requirements.*

PCC — Determine the patient/family ability and motivation to achieve a higher level of home maintenance. *Self-motivation is necessary to ensure change.*

PCC — Discuss obstacles to effective home maintenance management with patient and family *to develop understanding of potential and actual health and safety hazards.*

PCC — Help family members assign responsibilities for household care and establish appropriate expectations *to aid communication and help set realistic goals.*

PCC — Help family members establish daily and weekly home maintenance activities and assignments *to impose structure on family's routine and set standards for measuring progress.*

PCC — Encourage weekly discussions about progress in maintaining home maintenance *schedule to develop family unity and allow members to address problems before they become overwhelming.*

T&C — Assist patient and family members to explore available resources *to help with home and safety needs.*

T&C — Help family members contact community resources that can assist them in their efforts to improve home maintenance management, such as self-help groups, cleaning services, and exterminators. *Community resources can lessen family's burden while members learn to function independently.*

Suggested NIC Interventions

Caregiver Support; Counseling; Emotional Support; Environmental Management; Family Support; Family Integrity Promotion; Family Support; Home Maintenance Assistance; Role Enhancement; Support System Enhancement

EVALUATIONS FOR EXPECTED OUTCOMES

- Patient and family members establish and follow daily and weekly schedule for home maintenance.
- Patient and family members describe changes needed to promote maximum health and safety at home.
- Patient and family members list agencies that can assist with home care.
- Patient and family members contact community resources.
- Patient and family members identify individuals or organizations that may provide assistance.

DOCUMENTATION

- Patient's and family members' expressions of difficulty in maintaining household
- Patient's and family members' perception of problem
- Patient's and family members' mental status
- Presence of health hazards such as filth, rodents, and waste matter
- Presence of safety hazards such as faulty wiring
- Presence of offensive odors
- Patient's and family members' understanding of home maintenance management and resources
- Interventions to improve home maintenance skills
- Patient's and family members' responses to nursing interventions
- Evaluations for expected outcomes

REFERENCES

Bleske-Rechek, A., & Gunseor, M. M. (2021). Gendered perspectives on sharing the load: Men's and women's attitudes toward family roles and household and childcare tasks. *Evolutionary Behavioral Sciences.* doi:10.1037/ebs0000257

Giovannetti, T., Mis, R., Hackett, K., Simone, S. M., & Ungrady, M. B. (2021). The goal-control model: An integrated neuropsychological framework to explain impaired performance of everyday activities. *Neuropsychology, 35*(1), 3–18. doi:10.1037/neu0000714

Hou, W. K., Lai, F. T. T., Hougen, C., Hall, B. J., & Hobfoll, S. E. (2019). Measuring everyday processes and mechanisms of stress resilience: Development and initial validation of the sustainability of living inventory (SOLI). *Psychological Assessment, 31*(6), 715–729. doi:10.1037/pas0000692

Rende, R. (2021). Chores: Why they still matter and how to engage youth. *Brown University Child & Adolescent Behavior Letter, 37*(6), 1–4.

Readiness for Enhanced Home Maintenance Behaviors

DEFINITION

A pattern of knowledge and activities for the safe upkeep of one's residence, which can be strengthened

ASSESSMENT

- Family's perception and knowledge of home maintenance requirements
- Financial resources
- Cultural status, including affiliation with racial, ethnic, or religious groups
- Support systems, including close friends, organizations with which patient is affiliated, and community resources

DEFINING CHARACTERISTICS

- Expresses desire to enhance affect toward home tasks
- Expresses desire to enhance attitude toward home maintenance
- Expresses desire to enhance comfort of the environment
- Expresses desire to enhance home safety
- Expresses desire to enhance household hygiene
- Expresses desire to enhance laundry management skills
- Expresses desire to enhance organizational skills
- Expresses desire to enhance regulation of finances
- Expresses desire to enhance trash management

EXPECTED OUTCOMES

- Patient/family will maintain a positive attitude toward home maintenance.
- Patient/family will enhance the comfort of the environment.
- Patient/family will enhance home safety.
- Patient/family will enhance household hygiene.
- Patient/family will enhance laundry management skills.
- Patient/family will enhance organizational skills.
- Patient/family will enhance regulation of finances.
- Patient/family will enhance trash management.

Suggested NOC Outcomes

Family Functioning; Knowledge: Healthy Lifestyle; Role Performance; Self-Care: Instrumental Activities of Daily Living (IADLs)

INTERVENTIONS AND RATIONALES

- **PCC**   Determine the patient/family's ability and motivation to achieve a higher level of home maintenance. *Self-motivation is necessary to ensure change.*
- **PCC**   Help the patient/family identify the strengths and weaknesses in current home maintenance practices *to provide a focus for interventions.*
- **PCC**   Help family members assign responsibilities for household care and establish appropriate expectations *to aid communication and help set realistic goals.*
- **PCC**   Encourage weekly discussions about progress in maintaining home maintenance *schedule to develop family unity and allow members to address problems before they become overwhelming.*
- **T&C**   Assist patient and family members explore available resources *to help with home and safety needs.*
- **T&C**   Help family members contact community resources that can assist them in their efforts to improve home maintenance management, such as self-help groups, cleaning services, and exterminators. *Community resources can lessen family's burden while members learn to function independently.*

Suggested NIC Interventions

Caregiver Support; Counseling; Emotional Support; Environmental Management; Family Support; Family Integrity Promotion; Family Support; Home Maintenance Assistance; Role Enhancement; Support System Enhancement

EVALUATIONS FOR EXPECTED OUTCOMES

- Patient and family members express a positive attitude toward home maintenance.
- Patient and family members express their perception of the comfort of the environment.
- Patient and family members maintain regular home safety practices.
- Patient and family members participate in household hygiene activities.
- Patient and family members develop a laundry routine that meets all members' needs.
- Patient and family members develop a plan to organize household items. Patient and family members seek education for budgeting and regulation of finances.
- Patient and family members develop a waste removal plan.
- Patient and family members identify individuals or organizations that may provide assistance.

DOCUMENTATION

- Patient's and family members' expressions of desire to maintain a safe and healthy household
- Patient's and family members' understanding of home maintenance management and resources
- Interventions to build or enhance home maintenance skills
- Patient's and family members' responses to nursing interventions
- Evaluations for expected outcomes

REFERENCES

Bleske-Rechek, A., & Gunseor, M. M. (2021). Gendered perspectives on sharing the load: Men's and women's attitudes toward family roles and household and childcare tasks. *Evolutionary Behavioral Sciences.* doi:10.1037/ebs0000257

Giovannetti, T., Mis, R., Hackett, K., Simone, S. M., & Ungrady, M. B. (2021). The goal-control model: An integrated neuropsychological framework to explain impaired performance of everyday activities. *Neuropsychology, 35*(1), 3–18. doi:10.1037/neu0000714

Hou, W. K., Lai, F. T. T., Hougen, C., Hall, B. J., & Hobfoll, S. E. (2019). Measuring everyday processes and mechanisms of stress resilience: Development and initial validation of the sustainability of living inventory (SOLI). *Psychological Assessment, 31*(6), 715–729. doi:10.1037/pas0000692

Rende, R. (2021). Chores: Why they still matter and how to engage youth. *Brown University Child & Adolescent Behavior Letter, 37*(6), 1–4.

Readiness for Enhanced Hope

DEFINITION

A pattern of expectations and desires for mobilizing energy to achieve positive outcomes, or avoid a potentially threatening or negative situation, which can be strengthened

ASSESSMENT

- Patient's expression of desire to build on possibilities for the future
- Patient's ability to align desires and expectations
- Patient's expression of hope regarding health situation
- Patient's desire to maintain and enhance relationships with others
- Patient's problem-solving approach to health situation
- Patient's expressed need for increased spiritual connection

DEFINING CHARACTERISTICS

- Expresses desire to enhance ability to set achievable goals
- Expresses desire to enhance belief in possibilities
- Expresses desire to enhance congruency of expectation with goal
- Expresses desire to enhance deep inner strength
- Expresses desire to enhance giving and receiving of care
- Expresses desire to enhance giving and receiving of love
- Expresses desire to enhance initiative
- Expresses desire to enhance involvement with self-care
- Expresses desire to enhance positive outlook on life
- Expresses desire to enhance problem-solving to meet goal
- Expresses desire to enhance sense of meaning in life
- Expresses desire to enhance spirituality

- Patient will express desire for positive health outcomes.
- Patient will share personal goals to increase autonomy and personal satisfaction.
- Patient will discuss measures to increase quality of life.
- Patient will share strategies to live a meaningful life.
- Patient will express awareness of the need for developing and maintaining a positive attitude of hope.
- Patient will share need for emotional support.
- Patient will maintain a sense of humor and positive sense of self.
- Patient will seek spiritual support as needed.

Suggested NOC Outcomes

Hope; Personal Well-Being; Quality of Life; Will to Live

PCC ▪ Assist patient in adapting to stressor *to promote acceptance and understanding of physical condition, thereby improving management of therapeutic regimen.*

PCC ▪ Assess patient's adaptation to current health status; *baseline assessment is needed to develop care plan.*

PCC ▪ Implement a plan to build on patient's optimal role performance; *establish a plan with patient that promotes clear mutual expectations.*

PCC ▪ Facilitate opportunities for spiritual nourishment and growth *to address patient's holistic needs for maximal therapeutic environment.*

PCC ▪ Assist patient in building and maintaining meaningful interpersonal relationships *to maintain highest level of well-being.*

PCC ▪ Discuss the issue of hope with patient's family. Encourage patient to allow including family in discussions about hope. *It is important to understand what the differences and similarities are in their expectations.*

Suggested NIC Interventions

Emotional Support; Hope Instillation; Self-Esteem Enhancement; Spiritual Growth Facilitation; Support Systems

- Patient expresses desire for positive health outcomes.
- Patient shares personal goals to increase autonomy and personal satisfaction.
- Patient discusses measures utilized to increase quality of life.
- Patient shares own strategies for living a meaningful life.
- Patient demonstrates awareness of the need for developing and maintaining a positive attitude of hope.
- Patient shares the need for emotional support.
- Patient maintains a sense of humor and positive sense of self.
- Patient seeks spiritual support as needed.

- Patient's assessment of situation and hopeful resolution of problems
- Community resources to support patient's positive outcomes

▥ Future plans to maximize patient's preferred outcomes
▥ Evaluations for expected outcomes

REFERENCES

Bjørnnes, A. K., Parry, M., Lie, I., Falk, R., Leegaard, M., & Rustøen, T. (2018). The association between hope, marital status, depression and persistent pain in men and women following cardiac surgery. *BMC Women's Health, 18*, 2. doi:10.1186/s12905-017-0501-0

Elsegood, K. J., Anderson, L., & Newton, R. (2018). Introducing the recovery inspiration group: Promoting hope for recovery with inspirational recovery stories. *Advances in Dual Diagnosis, 11*(4), 137–146. doi:10.1108/ADD-03-2018-0004

Sheikhpourkhani, M., Abbaszadeh, A., Borhani, F., & Rassouli, M. (2018). Hope-promoting strategies: Perspectives of Iranian women with breast cancer about the role of social support. *International Journal of Cancer Management, 11*(11), e83317. doi:10.5812/ijcm.83317

Thomas, S. P. (2017). Maintaining hope in a time of hatred. *Issues in Mental Health Nursing, 38*(6), 463. doi:10.1080/01612840.2017.1319167

Hopelessness

DEFINITION

The feeling that one will not experience positive emotions or an improvement in one's condition

RELATED FACTORS (R/T)

▥ Chronic stress
▥ Fear
▥ Inadequate social support
▥ Loss of belief in spiritual power
▥ Loss of belief in transcendent values
▥ Low self-efficacy
▥ Prolonged immobility
▥ Social isolation
▥ Unaddressed violence
▥ Uncontrolled severe disease symptoms

ASSOCIATED CONDITIONS

▥ Critical illness
▥ Depression
▥ Deterioration in physiological condition
▥ Feeding and eating disorders
▥ Mental disorders
▥ Neoplasms
▥ Terminal illness

ASSESSMENT

▥ Psychological status, including changes in appetite, energy level, motivation, and personal hygiene
▥ Mental status, including cognitive functioning, affect, and mood
▥ Communication, including verbal (speech content, quality, and quantity), nonverbal (body positioning, eye contact, and facial expression), and quality of interactions with others

- Family status, including family composition, level of education of family members, family member's occupations, ability of family to meet patient's physical and emotional needs, coping patterns, and evidence of abuse
- Nutritional status, including alteration in appetite or body weight
- Motivation level, including personal hygiene, therapies (physical and occupational), use of diversional activities, and sense of control over current life situation
- Developmental stage, including age and role in family
- Disruption in usual roles and activities and losses (real and perceived)
- Number and types of stressors
- Coping mechanisms and decision-making ability
- Support systems, including clergy, family, and friends
- Spiritual values or religious beliefs

DEFINING CHARACTERISTICS

- Anorexia
- Avoidance behaviors
- Decreased affective display
- Decreased initiative
- Decreased response to stimuli
- Decreased verbalization
- Depressive symptoms
- Expresses despondency
- Expresses diminished hope
- Expresses feeling of uncertain future
- Expresses inadequate motivation for the future
- Expresses negative expectations about self
- Expresses negative expectations about the future
- Expresses sense of incompetency in meeting goals
- Inadequate involvement with self-care
- Overestimates the likelihood of unfortunate events
- Passivity
- Reports altered sleep-wake cycle
- Suicidal behaviors
- Unable to imagine life in the future
- Underestimates the occurrence of positive events

EXPECTED OUTCOMES

- Patient will identify feelings of hopelessness and seek help when they're overwhelming.
- Patient will identify ways to deal with stress.
- Patient will develop coping mechanisms to deal with feelings of hopelessness.
- Patient will begin making positive statements about self and others.
- Patient will seek positive social interactions.
- Patient will participate in self-care activities and in decisions regarding care planning.
- Patient will resume and maintain as many former roles as possible.
- Patient will regain and maintain self-esteem.
- Patient will begin to develop feelings of hope.

Suggested NOC Outcomes

Comfort Level; Coping; Decision-Making; Depression Control; Depression Level; Depression Self-Control; Hope; Mood Equilibrium; Quality of Life; Will to Live; Spiritual Health

S ■ Assess for evidence of self-destructive behavior. *Assessment for suicide potential in a depressed patient is a nursing care priority.*

PCC ■ If possible, assign a primary nurse to patient to encourage establishment *of a therapeutic relationship between patient and nurse.*

PCC ■ Allow for specific amount of uninterrupted, non–care-related time each shift to talk with patient. Encourage verbal response with open-ended statements and questions. If patient chooses not to talk, spend time in silence. *This establishes rapport with depressed patient even if patient talks little.*

PCC ■ Provide for appropriate physical outlets for expression of feelings (punching bag, walking) *to help patient release hostilities, thereby decreasing tension and anxiety.*

PCC ■ Convey belief in patient's ability to develop and use coping skills *to increase patient's self-esteem and reduce feelings of dependence.*

PCC ■ Acknowledge patient's pain. Encourage patient to express feelings of depression, anger, guilt, and sadness. Convey to patient that all these feelings are appropriate. *This will help patient work through stages of coming to terms with chronic illness.*

PCC ■ Identify patient's strengths and encourage putting strengths to use *to maintain optimal functioning.*

PCC ■ Encourage patient's participation in self-care to fullest extent possible *to reduce feelings of helplessness.*

PCC ■ Help patient to participate in usual activities as strength, energy, and time permit *to maintain a sense of being connected to others.*

PCC ■ Encourage patient to identify enjoyable diversions and to participate in them *to decrease negative thinking and enhance self-esteem.*

PCC ■ Encourage positive thinking. Convey a sense of confidence in patient's ability to cope with illness *to promote an optimistic outlook.*

PCC ■ Provide positive reinforcement for patient's efforts to participate in self-care activities *to encourage patient to participate in self-care.* Encourage patient to establish self-care schedule *to enhance feelings of usefulness and control.*

PCC ■ Assist patient with hygiene and grooming needs *to help enhance patient's self-esteem.*

PCC ■ Offer patient and family a realistic assessment of situation and communicate hope for immediate future. *This facilitates acceptance, helps promote patient safety and security, and allows planning of future health care.*

PCC ■ Encourage patient to identify spiritual needs and facilitate fulfillment of those needs *to help patient come to terms with chronic illness and its limitations.*

PCC ■ Involve patient and family members in care planning and allow patient to choose degree of self-involvement on a continuing basis. Begin by offering patient a choice between two alternatives. Increase alternatives as initiative improves. *Cognitive disturbances associated with anxiety or depression usually prevent patient from making healthy decisions.*

EBP ■ Teach patient and family members how to manage illness, prevent complications, and control factors in the environment that affect patient's health. *Education enables family members to become resources in patient's care.*

T&C ■ Refer patient and family members to other caregivers (such as dietitian, social worker, clergyman, and mental health clinical nurse specialist) or support groups, as necessary. *Referrals to outside specialists ensure continuity of care. Support groups give patient chance to discuss illness with others similarly affected.*

Suggested NIC Interventions

Coping Enhancement; Counseling; Decision-Making Support; Energy Management; Family Mobilization; Family Support; Hope Instillation; Mood Management; Spiritual Growth Facilitation

EVALUATIONS FOR EXPECTED OUTCOMES

- Patient discusses negative feelings
- Patient asks for help when unable to cope with feelings.
- Patient demonstrates positive coping mechanisms.
- Patient demonstrates positive methods of dealing with stress.
- Patient interacts with others and regains involvement in life experiences.
- Patient states that feelings of hopelessness are less frequent and expresses feelings of hope.
- Patient attempts to make positive statements about self and others.

DOCUMENTATION

- Patient's responses to treatment regimen
- Patient's mental and emotional status (baseline and ongoing)
- Patient education, counseling, and precautions taken to maintain or enhance patient's level of functioning
- Interventions to help patient deal with daily stressors
- Interventions to protect patient from self-harm
- Patient's response to nursing interventions
- Evaluations for expected outcomes

REFERENCES

Brenner, L. A., Forster, J. E., Hoffberg, A. S., Matarazzo, B. B., Hostetter, T. A., Signoracci, G., & Simpson, G. K. (2018). Window to hope: A randomized controlled trial of a psychological intervention for the treatment of hopelessness among veterans with moderate to severe traumatic brain injury. *Journal of Head Trauma Rehabilitation, 33*(2), E64–E73. doi:10.1097/HTR.0000000000000351

Gum, A. M., Shiovitz-Ezra, S., & Ayalon, L. (2017). Longitudinal associations of hopelessness and loneliness in older adults: Results from the US health and retirement study. *International Psychogeriatrics, 29*(9), 1451–1459. doi:10.1017/S1041610217000904

Lan, X., Xiao, H., & Chen, Y. (2017). Effects of life review interventions on psychosocial outcomes among older adults: A systematic review and meta-analysis. *Geriatrics & Gerontology International, 17*(10), 1344–1357. doi:10.1111/ggi.12947

Ribeiro, J. D., Huang, X., Fox, K. R., & Franklin, J. C. (2018). Depression and hopelessness as risk factors for suicide ideation, attempts and death: Meta-analysis of longitudinal studies. *British Journal of Psychiatry, 212*(5), 279–286. doi:10.1192/bjp.2018.27

Risk for Compromised Human Dignity

DEFINITION

Susceptible for perceived loss of respect and honor, which may compromise health

RISK FACTORS

- Cultural incongruence
- Dehumanizing treatment
- Disclosure of confidential information
- Exposure of the body
- Humiliation
- Insufficient comprehension of health information
- Intrusion by clinician
- Invasion of privacy

- Limited decision-making experience
- Loss of control of body functions
- Stigmatization

ASSESSMENT

- Patient's perception of present health problem and problem-solving techniques used
- Patient health status; attitude toward and use of health care services; and beliefs, values, and attitudes about illness
- Family status, including family composition; responsibilities assumed in caring for family members (including patient); and ability of family to meet their physical, social, emotional, and economic needs
- Support systems, including family members, friends, and clergy
- Health history, including medical or mental illness, self-care abilities, and disabilities and deformities
- Legal status, including patient's authority to give consent for treatments or procedures
- Attitude of health care providers toward the patient
- Welfare and health care system and reliance on welfare for support

EXPECTED OUTCOMES

- Patient and family will express satisfaction with level of respect received.
- Patient will express reduced feelings of powerlessness and vulnerability and increased feelings of autonomy.
- Patient and family will develop and implement plans to protect privacy and confidentiality of patient.
- Patient and family will report a reduction or elimination of compromised human dignity.

Suggested NOC Outcomes

Client Satisfaction: Protection of Rights; Coping; Personal Autonomy; Self-Esteem

INTERVENTIONS AND RATIONALES

PCC ■ Assess patient's satisfaction with health care environment *to determine the extent of positive perception of the nursing staff's concern for patient.*

PCC ■ Work with patient to develop a plan to increase autonomy *to promote feelings of control and independence in making life decisions.*

PCC ■ Include patient or patient's representative in all decision-making. *This demonstrates a sense of respect for patient's right to make decisions that affect personal well-being.*

T&C ■ Work closely with patient and health professionals *to promote the positive perception of protection of a patient's legal and moral rights provided by nursing and other staff.*

PCC ■ Implement a program to promote patient dignity that involves staff, family, and community *to assist patient in coping to manage the stressors that tax personal resources.*

T&C ■ Work with various health professionals, families, educators, and students *to determine the extent of the problem of protecting human dignity in the delivery of health care.*

T&C ■ Encourage health professional groups and religious and social service organizations to feature guest speakers *to provide information on aspects of bioethics and human dignity in the care of patients.*

EBP ■ Provide education on the legal and ethical rights of patients to human dignity and have current information available at community and senior centers. *Access to information provides patients and their families with appropriate resources to seek help.*

PCC ▦ Encourage patient and family to participate in support networks that allow them to discuss caregiving and illness pressures and other issues related to the provision of human dignity. *This gives patient and family a chance to express their feelings openly and obtain support.*

T&C ▦ Develop a referral list for patient and family that includes resources that promote human dignity, including charities, clinics, support groups, and senior centers *to promote family involvement in decision-making and delivery and evaluation of care.*

Suggested NIC Interventions

Body Image Enhancement; Presence; Self-Awareness Enhancement; Self-Esteem Enhancement

EVALUATIONS FOR EXPECTED OUTCOMES

▦ Patient and family express satisfaction with level of respect for the patient.
▦ Patient and family articulate plan to reduce feelings of powerlessness and vulnerability and increase feelings of patient autonomy.
▦ Patient and family develop and implement plan to protect patient privacy and confidentiality.
▦ Patient and family report success of plan to protect patient privacy and confidentiality.
▦ Patient and family report a reduction or elimination of compromised human dignity.

DOCUMENTATION

▦ Patient and family perception of understanding of the need for human dignity
▦ Community resources that exist to promote human dignity
▦ Patient and family plans to promote human dignity
▦ Nursing interventions to promote and protect human dignity of patient
▦ Patient response to nursing interventions
▦ Evaluations for expected outcomes

REFERENCES

Bentwich, M. E., Dickman, N., & Oberman, A. (2018). Human dignity and autonomy in the care for patients with dementia: Differences among formal caretakers from various cultural backgrounds. *Ethnicity & Health, 23*(2), 121–141. doi:10.1080/13557858.2016.1246519

Hubbard, R. E., Bak, M., Watts, J., Shum, D., Lynch, A., & Peel, N. M. (2018). Enhancing dignity for older inpatients: The photograph-next-to-the-bed study. *Clinical Gerontologist, 41*(5), 468–473. doi:10.1080/07317115.2017.1398796

Kirchhoffer, D. G. (2017). Human dignity and human enhancement: A multidimensional approach. *Bioethics, 31*(5), 375–383. doi:10.1111/bioe.12343

Nyholm, L., & Koskinen, C. A.-L. (2017). Understanding and safeguarding patient dignity in intensive care. *Nursing Ethics, 24*(4), 408–418. doi:10.1177/0969733015605669

Neonatal Hyperbilirubinemia

DEFINITION

The accumulation of unconjugated bilirubin in the circulation (less than 15 mL/dL) that occurs after 24 hours of life

RELATED FACTORS (R/T)

▦ Deficient feeding pattern
▦ Delay in meconium passage
▦ Infants with inadequate nutrition

ASSOCIATED CONDITIONS

- Bacterial infection
- Infant with liver malfunction
- Infant with enzyme deficiency
- Internal bleeding
- Prenatal infection
- Sepsis
- Viral infection

ASSESSMENT

- Infant weight gain patterns and trends
- Laboratory studies including bilirubin level
- Labor and delivery history
- Maternal risk factors (Rh, ABO)
- Infant fluid and electrolyte status
- Infant bowel elimination, stool characteristics

DEFINING CHARACTERISTICS

- Abnormal blood profile
- Bruised skin
- Yellow mucous membranes
- Yellow sclera
- Yellow-orange skin color

EXPECTED OUTCOMES

- Neonate will establish effective feeding pattern (breast or bottle) that enhances stooling.
- Neonate will not experience injury as a result of increasing bilirubin levels.
- Neonate will receive bilirubin assessment and screening within first week of life to detect increasing levels of serum bilirubin.
- Neonate will receive appropriate therapy to enhance bilirubin excretion.
- Neonate will receive nursing assessment to determine risk for severity of jaundice.

Suggested NOC Outcomes

Bowel Elimination; Breastfeeding Establishment; Infant; Nutritional Status; Risk Control; Risk Detection

INTERVENTIONS AND RATIONALES

- Evaluate maternal and delivery history for risk factors for neonatal jaundice (Rh, ABO, glucose-6-phosphate dehydrogenase deficiency, direct Coombs, prolonged labor, maternal viral illness, medications) *to anticipate which neonates are at highest risk for jaundice.*
- **S** Collect and evaluate laboratory blood specimens as ordered or per unit protocol *to permit accurate and timely diagnosis and treatment of neonatal jaundice.*
- **EBP** Educate parents regarding newborn care at home in relation to appearance of jaundice in association with any of the following: no stool in 48 hours, lethargy with refusal to nurse or bottle-feed, less than one wet diaper in 12 hours, abnormal infant behavior. *Parent*

education is crucial for the time after neonate is discharged from the hospital. Parents are the major decision-makers concerning whether and when to bring neonate back for medical and nursing assessments after being discharged from the hospital.

PCC ▪ Provide caring support to family if a breastfed neonate must receive supplementation. *It can be upsetting and result in feelings of inadequacy to a breastfeeding mother for her neonate to require supplementation.*

T&C ▪ Coordinate care and facilitate communication between family, nursing staff, pediatrician, and lactation specialist. *A multidisciplinary approach that includes family enhances communication and improves outcomes.*

Suggested NIC Interventions

Attachment Promotion; Kangaroo Care; Newborn Monitoring; Vital Signs Monitoring; Infant Care; Breastfeeding Assistance; Bottle-Feeding; Teaching: Infant Nutrition; Capillary Blood Sample; Surveillance; Risk Identification: Childbearing Family; Bowel Management; Discharge Planning

EVALUATIONS FOR EXPECTED OUTCOMES

▪ An effective feeding pattern has been achieved for the neonate that enhanced stooling.
▪ Neonate did not experience any injury as a result of increased bilirubin levels.
▪ Bilirubin assessment and screening was completed within first week of life.
▪ Neonate received the appropriate therapy to enhance bilirubin excretion.

DOCUMENTATION

▪ Neonate's feeding pattern
▪ Neonate will receive appropriate therapy to enhance bilirubin excretion
▪ Record of completed assessments
▪ Therapy used to promote bilirubin excretion
▪ Evaluations for expected outcomes

REFERENCES

Donneborg, M. L., Vandborg, P. K., Hansen, B. M., Rodrigo-Domingo, M., & Ebbesen, F. (2018). Double versus single intensive phototherapy with LEDs in treatment of neonatal hyperbilirubinemia. *Journal of Perinatology, 38*(2), 154–158. doi:10.1038/jp.2017.167

Garg, B. D., Kabra, N. S., & Balasubramanian, H. (2019). Role of massage therapy on reduction of neonatal hyperbilirubinemia in term and preterm neonates: A review of clinical trials. *Journal of Maternal-Fetal & Neonatal Medicine, 32*(1), 301–309. doi:10.1080/14767058.2017.1376316

Goyal, P., Mehta, A., Kaur, J., Jain, S., Guglani, V., & Chawla, D. (2018). Fluid supplementation in management of neonatal hyperbilirubinemia: A randomized controlled trial. *Journal of Maternal-Fetal & Neonatal Medicine, 31*(20), 2678–2684. doi:10.1080/14767058.2017.1351535

Özdemir, R., Olukman, Ö., Karadeniz, C., Çelik, K., Katipoğlu, N., Muhtar Yılmazer, M., … Arslanoğlu, S. (2018). Effect of unconjugated hyperbilirubinemia on neonatal autonomic functions: Evaluation by heart rate variability. *Journal of Maternal-Fetal & Neonatal Medicine, 31*(20), 2763–2769. doi:10.1080/14767058.2017.1355901

Risk for Neonatal Hyperbilirubinemia

DEFINITION

Susceptible to the accumulation of unconjugated bilirubin in the circulation (15 mL/dL) that occurs after 24 hours of life which may compromise health

- Deficient feeding pattern
- Delay in meconium passage
- Infants with inadequate nutrition

- Bacterial infection
- Infant with liver malfunction
- Infant with enzyme deficiency
- Internal bleeding
- Prenatal infection
- Sepsis
- Viral infection

- Infant weight gain patterns and trends
- Laboratory studies, including bilirubin level
- Maternal risk factors (e.g., Rh, ABO)
- Labor and delivery history
- Infant fluid and electrolyte status
- Infant bowel elimination, stool characteristics

- Parents will identify factors that place infant at risk for neonatal jaundice.
- Parents will identify potential signs of neonatal jaundice in infant.
- Neonate will establish effective feeding pattern (breast or bottle) that enhances stooling.
- Neonate will not experience injury as a result of increasing bilirubin levels.
- Neonate will receive bilirubin assessment and screening within first week of life to detect increasing levels of serum bilirubin.

Suggested NOC Outcomes

Bowel Elimination; Breastfeeding Establishment; Infant; Nutritional Status; Risk Control; Risk Detection

- Review history of mother and prior obstetrical and medical histories in determining risk factors leading to neonatal jaundice. *Utilizing knowledge about maternal factors and blood type incompatibilities that can lead to neonatal jaundice aids provider team in preparations.*
- **S** At birth, assess neonate for gestational age. *Neonates less than 38 weeks are at higher risk for jaundice.*
- **S** At birth, assess neonate for birthing trauma such as excessive bruising. *Bruising is indicative of increased bleeding, which results in hemolysis and leads to increased bilirubin.*
- **S** At birth, place neonate to the breast for initial feeding. *This stimulates the production of milk, initiating the process to produce sufficient milk for infant over the next days.*
- **S** Inject vitamin K (phylloquinone) into vastus lateralis muscle of neonate as prescribed. *Neonates lack vitamin K and cannot produce sufficient amounts for several weeks; injecting vitamin K provides a primary chemical for the clotting factors.*

S ▦ Examine skin and head of the neonate carefully to determine bruising or the presence of cephalohematoma. *Presence of bruising/hematoma indicates bleeding and increases the risk for jaundice as the red blood cells are reabsorbed.*

▦ Rely on laboratory analysis for total serum bilirubin (TSB) or calibrated transcutaneous bilirubin (TcB) graphed on the Bhutani nomogram. *Accurate clinical observations of neonate's skin color for jaundice is difficult in varying lighting settings and varying skin tone pigmentation. Laboratory and calibrated cutaneous readings provide consistent accurate measures and are interpreted using the nomogram.*

EBP ▦ Adhere to nursery protocol on time intervals to obtain readings/heel stick blood. *Clinical protocols are critical for assessment and treatment of hyperbilirubinemia since there are specific time–rate increase factors. This differentiates "normal physiologic" hyperbilirubinemia from more serious hemolytic forms.*

EBP ▦ If the neonate is less than 38 weeks, at 12 hours postpartum, obtain a heel stick blood sample for TSB; graph results to the Bhutani nomogram; continue every 12 hours per protocol or provider orders. *At-risk premature neonates have elevated TSB in comparison with 38-week neonates.*

▦ Maintain nursery protocol on assessing vital signs, bilirubin, weight, intake, diaper output, and other parameters. *Close vigilance by the caregivers will inform the providers of progress in the neonate's health status and hydration status.*

▦ Institute the treatment plan—aggressive breastfeeding and/or phototherapy. *Sufficient breast milk intake by the neonate prevents dehydration and assists in the elimination of bilirubin; exposure to therapeutic photo light converts insoluble bilirubin to a water-soluble form that is easily eliminated.*

EBP ▦ Provide information to mother/family unit of the identified factors that may lead to neonatal jaundice. *Understanding information and expectations reduces anxiety.*

EBP ▦ Breastfeeding eight to 12 times a day (every 2 to 3 hours), beginning immediately at birth, with adequate amounts of milk, decreases the incidence of hyperbilirubinemia. *Understanding information and expectations allows the mother to participate in the care of her newborn.*

EBP ▦ Provide detailed information to family unit regarding the interventions to prevent bleeding and increased bilirubin, assessment findings, the lab values, and treatments for neonate. *Understanding expectations improves confidence and reduces anxiety.*

PCC ▦ Support family when they receive the knowledge that risk factors exist. *Understanding information and expectations reduces anxiety and allows family to prepare for their participation in treatment plan.*

PCC ▦ Encourage mother to breastfeed her newborn. *This allows the mother to be the active agent intervening for her newborn by breastfeeding.*

PCC ▦ Support bonding of neonate and mother/family unit if neonate receives phototherapy. *Understanding information and expectations of how neonate will appear during therapy reduces anxiety and reduces barriers to bonding.*

T&C ▦ Refer to lactation consultant to manage breastfeeding and methods to enhance milk production. *Expertise and support provide the confidence to achieve success in breastfeeding.*

S ▦ Emphasize the importance of follow-up at discharge for any level of hyperbilirubinemia; adhere to the clinical protocols and clinical pathways. *Neonates are frequently discharged after 24 hours and need to have professional evaluation to ensure that the bilirubin levels follow a predicted decrease.*

Suggested NIC Interventions

Attachment Promotion; Kangaroo Care; Newborn Monitoring; Vital Signs Monitoring; Infant Care; Breastfeeding Assistance; Bottle-Feeding; Teaching: Infant Nutrition; Capillary Blood Sample; Surveillance; Risk Identification: Childbearing Family; Bowel Management; Discharge Planning

EVALUATIONS FOR EXPECTED OUTCOMES

▪ Parents identify risk factors for neonatal jaundice.
▪ Parents identify potential signs of neonatal jaundice.
▪ Neonate establishes effective feeding pattern.
▪ Neonate has no injuries related to elevated bilirubin.
▪ Neonate's bilirubin is within normal limits.

DOCUMENTATION

▪ Results of risk assessment
▪ Parents' expression of knowledge of signs of neonatal jaundice
▪ Results of blood test, weight, urine, and stool
▪ Nursing interventions and mother's/infant's response to them
▪ Evaluations for expected outcomes

REFERENCES

Chang, P. W., Kuzniewicz, M. W., McCulloch, C. E., & Newman, T. B. (2017). A clinical prediction rule for rebound hyperbilirubinemia following inpatient phototherapy. *Pediatrics, 139*(3), e20162896. doi:10.1542/peds.2016-2896
Golden, W. C. (2017). The African-American neonate at risk for extreme hyperbilirubinemia: A better management strategy is needed. *Journal of Perinatology, 37*(4), 321–322. doi:10.1038/jp.2017.1
Jones, K. D. J., Grossman, S. E., Kumaranayakam, D., Rao, A., Fegan, G., & Aladangady, N. (2017). Umbilical cord bilirubin as a predictor of neonatal jaundice: A retrospective cohort study. *BMC Pediatrics, 17*, 186. doi:10.1186/s12887-017-0938-1

Hyperthermia

DEFINITION

Core body temperature above the normal diurnal range due to failure of thermoregulation

RELATED FACTORS (R/T)

▪ Dehydration
▪ Inappropriate clothing
▪ Increase in metabolic rate
▪ Vigorous activity

ASSOCIATED CONDITIONS

▪ Decrease in sweat response
▪ Illness
▪ Ischemia
▪ Pharmaceutical agent
▪ Sepsis
▪ Trauma

ASSESSMENT

▪ Age
▪ History of present illness
▪ History of exposure to communicable disease

- Health history, including chronic disease or disability, pathologic conditions known to cause dehydration, recent traumatic event, exposure to sources of infection, exposure to communicable diseases, and other related events
- Medications
- Physiologic manifestations of fever, including vital signs and skin temperature and color
- Fluid and electrolyte status, including skin turgor, intake and output, mucous membranes, serum electrolyte levels, and urine specific gravity
- Laboratory studies, including white blood cell count and culture and sensitivity findings
- Neurologic status, including level of consciousness (LOC) and orientation
- Skin integrity, including open lesions and rashes

DEFINING CHARACTERISTICS

- Abnormal posturing
- Apnea
- Coma
- Flushed skin
- Hypotension
- Infant does not maintain suck
- Irritability
- Lethargy
- Seizure
- Skin warm to touch
- Stupor
- Tachycardia
- Tachypnea
- Vasodilation

EXPECTED OUTCOMES

- Patient will remain afebrile.
- Patient will maintain adequate hydration, with balanced intake and output within normal limits for age, urine specific gravity between 1.010 and 1.015, moist mucous membranes, and skin turgor within normal limits.
- Patient will remain alert and responsive and won't show evidence of seizure activity or decreased LOC.
- Patient will identify appropriate measures to reduce fever and prevent dehydration.

Suggested NOC Outcomes

Comfort Level; Hydration; Infection Severity; Thermoregulation; Vital Signs

INTERVENTIONS AND RATIONALES

S — Take temperature every 1 to 4 hours *to obtain an accurate core temperature.* Identify route and record measurements. Use the same method each time temperature is taken *to track accurate trends of temperature and maintain accuracy of results.*

S — Administer antipyretics as prescribed and record effectiveness. *Antipyretics act on hypothalamus to regulate temperature.*

EBP — Use nonpharmacologic measures to reduce excessive fever, such as removing sheets, blankets, and most clothing; placing ice bags on axillae and groin; and sponging with tepid water. Explain these measures to patient. *Nonpharmacologic measures lower body* temperature and promote comfort. *Sponging reduces body temperature by increasing evaporation from skin. Tepid water is used because cold water increases shivering, thereby increasing metabolic rate and causing temperature to rise.*

EBP ▪ Use a hypothermia blanket if patient's temperature rises above 103°F (39.4°C). Monitor vital signs every 15 minutes for 1 hour and then as indicated. *Temperatures that exceed 103°F cannot be controlled with antipyretics alone.*

EBP ▪ Turn hypothermia blanket off if shivering occurs. *Shivering increases metabolic rate, increasing temperature.*

S ▪ Monitor heart rate and rhythm, blood pressure, respiratory rate, LOC and level of responsiveness, and capillary refill time every 1 to 4 hours *to evaluate effectiveness of interventions and monitor for complications.*

PCC ▪ Determine patient's preferences for oral fluids and encourage patient to drink as much as possible, unless contraindicated. Monitor and record intake and output, and administer IV fluids, if indicated. *Because insensible fluid loss increases by 10% for every 1.8°F (1°C) increase in temperature, patient must increase fluid intake to prevent dehydration.*

Suggested NIC Interventions

Environmental Management; Fever Treatment; Fluid Management; Temperature Regulation: Vital Signs Monitoring

EVALUATIONS FOR EXPECTED OUTCOMES

▪ Patient remains afebrile.
▪ Patient maintains adequate hydration:
  ▪ Intake and output are balanced and within normal limit for age.
  ▪ Urine specific gravity ranges from 1.005 to 1.015.
▪ Patient exhibits moist mucous membranes.
▪ Patient exhibits good skin turgor.
▪ Patient remains alert and responsive.
▪ Patient identifies appropriate measures to reduce fever and prevent dehydration.

DOCUMENTATION

▪ Observations of physical assessment findings
▪ Nursing interventions and patient's response to interventions
▪ Administration of medication, such as antipyretics
▪ Patient's response (behavioral, cognitive, and physiologic) to interventions, including administration of antipyretics
▪ Evaluations for expected outcomes

REFERENCES

Butts, C. L., Spisla, D. L., Smith, C. R., Paulsen, K. M., Caldwell, A. R., Ganio, M. S., ... Adams, J. D. (2017). Effectiveness of ice-sheet cooling following exertional hyperthermia. *Military Medicine, 182*(9), e1951–e1957. doi:10.7205/MILMED-D-17-00057

Chiappini, E., Cangelosi, A. M., Becherucci, P., Pierattelli, M., Galli, L., & de Martino, M. (2018). Knowledge, attitudes and misconceptions of Italian healthcare professionals regarding fever management in children. *BMC Pediatrics, 18*(1), 194. doi:10.1186/s12887-018-1173-0

Hekmatpou, D., & Karimi Kia, M. (2018). Investigation of fever control in febrile patients: A narrative review. *Medical-Surgical Nursing Journal, 7*(2), e85154. doi:10.5812/msnj.85154

O'Mara, S. K. (2017). Management of postoperative fever in adult cardiac surgical patients. *Dimensions of Critical Care Nursing, 36*(3), 182–192. doi:10.1097/DCC.0000000000000248

Hypothermia

DEFINITION

Core body temperature below the normal diurnal range in individuals >28 days of life

RELATED FACTORS (R/T)

- Alcohol consumption
- Excessive conductive heat transfer
- Excessive convective heat transfer
- Excessive evaporative heat transfer
- Excessive radiative heat transfer
- Inactivity
- Inadequate caregiver knowledge of hypothermia prevention
- Inadequate clothing
- Low environmental temperature
- Malnutrition

ASSOCIATED CONDITIONS

- Damage to hypothalamus
- Decreased metabolic rate
- Pharmaceutical preparations
- Radiotherapy
- Trauma

ASSESSMENT

- History of present illness
- Exposure to cold
- Circumstances surrounding development of hypothermia
- Age
- Medication history
- Neurologic status, including level of consciousness, mental status, motor status, and sensory status
- Cardiovascular status, including blood pressure, capillary refill time, electrocardiogram results, heart rate and rhythm, pulses (apical, peripheral), and temperature
- Respiratory status, including arterial blood gas analysis; breath sounds; and rate, depth, and character of respirations
- Integumentary status, including color, temperature, and turgor
- Nutritional status, including current (and normal) weight and dietary pattern
- Fluid and electrolyte status, including blood urea nitrogen level, intake and output, serum electrolyte levels, and urine specific gravity
- Psychosocial status, including behavior, financial resources, mood, and occupation

DEFINING CHARACTERISTICS

- Acrocyanosis
- Bradycardia
- Cyanotic nail beds
- Decreased blood glucose level

- Decreased ventilation
- Hypertension
- Hypoglycemia
- Hypoxia
- Increased metabolic rate
- Increased oxygen consumption
- Peripheral vasoconstriction
- Piloerection
- Shivering
- Skin cool to touch
- Slow capillary refill
- Tachycardia

Neonates

- Infant with insufficient energy to maintain sucking
- Infant with insufficient weight gain (<30 g/day)
- Irritability
- Jaundice
- Metabolic acidosis
- Pallor
- Respiratory distress

EXPECTED OUTCOMES

- Patient will exhibit body temperature within normal limits.
- Patient's skin will feel warm and dry.
- Patient's heart rate and blood pressure will remain within normal range.
- Patient won't shiver.
- Patient will express feelings of comfort.
- Patient will show no complications associated with hypothermia, such as soft tissue injury, fracture, dehydration, and hypovolemic shock, if warmed too quickly.
- Patient will verbalize how hypothermia develops and will state measures to prevent recurrence of hypothermia.

Suggested NOC Outcomes

Comfort Level; Neurological Status: Autonomic; Thermoregulation; Vital Signs

INTERVENTIONS AND RATIONALES

- **S** Monitor body temperature at least every 4 hours or more frequently, if indicated, *to evaluate effectiveness of interventions*. Record temperature and route *to allow accurate data comparison*. Baseline temperatures vary, depending on route used. If temperature drops below 95°F (35°C), use a low-reading thermometer *to obtain accurate reading*.
- **S** Monitor and record neurologic status at least every 4 hours. *Falling body temperature and metabolic rate reduce pulse rate and blood pressure, which reduces blood perfusion to brain, resulting in disorientation, confusion, and unconsciousness.*
- **S** Monitor and record heart rate and rhythm, blood pressure, and respiratory rate at least every 4 hours. Blood pressure and pulse decrease in hypothermia. *During rewarming, patient may develop hypovolemic shock. During warming, ventricular fibrillation and cardiac arrest may occur, possibly signaled by irregular pulse.*

EBP ▦ Provide supportive measures, such as placing patient in warm bed and covering with warm blankets, removing wet or constrictive clothing, and covering metal or plastic surfaces that contact patient's body. *These measures protect patient from heat loss.*

EBP ▦ Follow prescribed treatment regimen for hypothermia:
  - ▦ As ordered, administer medications *to prevent shivering to avoid overheating.* Monitor and record effectiveness.
  - ▦ As ordered, administer analgesic *to relieve pain associated with warming.* Monitor and record effectiveness.
  - ▦ Use hyperthermia blanket to *warm patient* if temperature drops below 95°F (35°C). Warm patient to 97°F (36.1°C).
  - ▦ As appropriate, administer fluids during rewarming *to prevent hypovolemic shock.* If administering large volumes of IV fluids, consider using a fluid warmer *to avoid heat loss.*

PCC ▦ Discuss precipitating factors with patient, if indicated. *Patient may require community outreach assistance with certain precipitating factors, including inadequate living conditions, insufficient finances, and abuse of medications (such as sedatives and alcohol).*

EBP ▦ Instruct patient in precautionary measures to avoid hypothermia, such as dressing warmly even when indoors, eating proper diet, and remaining as active as possible. *Precautions help to prevent accidental hypothermia.*

Suggested NIC Interventions

Circulatory Precautions; Comfort Level; Environmental Management; Fluid Management; Hypothermia Treatment; Temperature Regulation; Vital Signs Monitoring

EVALUATIONS FOR EXPECTED OUTCOMES

- ▦ Patient's temperature returns to normal limits.
- ▦ Patient's skin is warm and dry.
- ▦ Patient's heart rate and blood pressure return to within normal limits.
- ▦ Patient doesn't shiver.
- ▦ Patient voices feelings of comfort.
- ▦ Patient doesn't develop complications associated with hypothermia.
- ▦ Patient describes measures to prevent further episodes of hypothermia.

DOCUMENTATION

- ▦ Patient's shivering and complaints of coldness
- ▦ Observations of physical findings
- ▦ Nursing interventions and patient's response to interventions, including physiologic, behavioral, and cognitive
- ▦ Evaluations for expected outcomes

REFERENCES

Purnamasari, M. D., Rustina, Y., & Waluyanti, F. T. (2017). Heat loss prevention education aids nurses' knowledge in prevention of hypothermia in newborns. *Comprehensive Child and Adolescent Nursing, 40*, 37–44. doi:10.1080/24694193.2017.1386969

Saqe-Rockoff, A., Schubert, F. D., Ciardiello, A., & Douglas, E. (2018). Improving thermoregulation for trauma patients in the emergency department : An evidence-based practice project. *Journal of Trauma Nursing, 25*(1), 14–20. doi:10.1097/JTN.0000000000000336

Shabeer, M. P., Abiramalatha, T., Devakirubai, D., Rebekah, G., & Thomas, N. (2018). Standard care with plastic bag or portable thermal nest to prevent hypothermia at birth: A three-armed randomized controlled trial. *Journal of Perinatology, 38*(10), 1324–1330. doi:10.1038/s41372-018-0169-9

Steelman, V. M. (2017). Conductive skin warming and hypothermia: An observational study. *AANA Journal, 85*(6), 461–468.

Svendsen, Ø. S., Grong, K., & Husby, P. (2018). Neuroprotective treatment strategies after rewarming from accidental hypothermia. *Resuscitation, 122,* e9–e10. doi:10.1016/j.resuscitation.2017.10.017

Risk for Hypothermia

DEFINITION

Susceptible to a failure of thermoregulation that may result in a core body temperature below the normal diurnal range in individuals >28 days of life, which may compromise health

RISK FACTORS

- Alcohol consumption
- Excessive conductive heat transfer
- Excessive convective heat transfer
- Excessive evaporative heat transfer
- Excessive radiative heat transfer
- Inactivity
- Inadequate caregiver knowledge of hypothermia prevention
- Inadequate clothing
- Low environmental temperature
- Malnutrition

Neonates

- Decrease in metabolic rate
- Delay in breastfeeding
- Early bathing of newborn
- Increase in oxygen demand

ASSOCIATED CONDITIONS

- Damage to hypothalamus
- Decreased metabolic rate
- Pharmaceutical preparations
- Radiotherapy
- Trauma

ASSESSMENT

- History of present illness
- Exposure to cold
- Circumstances surrounding development of hypothermia
- Age
- Medication history
- Neurologic status, including level of consciousness, mental status, motor status, and sensory status
- Cardiovascular status, including blood pressure, capillary refill time, electrocardiogram results, heart rate and rhythm, pulses (apical, peripheral), and temperature
- Respiratory status, including arterial blood gas analysis; breath sounds; and rate, depth, and character of respirations

- Integumentary status, including color, temperature, and turgor
- Nutritional status, including current (and normal) weight and dietary pattern
- Fluid and electrolyte status, including blood urea nitrogen level, intake and output, serum electrolyte levels, and urine specific gravity
- Psychosocial status, including behavior, financial resources, mood, and occupation

EXPECTED OUTCOMES

- Patient will exhibit body temperature within normal limits.
- Patient's skin will feel warm and dry.
- Patient's heart rate and blood pressure will remain within normal range.
- Patient won't shiver.
- Patient will express feelings of comfort.
- Patient will show no complications associated with hypothermia, such as soft tissue injury, fracture, dehydration, and hypovolemic shock, if warmed too quickly.
- Patient will verbalize how hypothermia develops and will state measures to prevent recurrent hypothermia.

Suggested NOC Outcomes

Neurological Status: Autonomic; Thermoregulation; Vital Signs; Risk Control: Hypothermia

INTERVENTIONS AND RATIONALES

- **S** Monitor body temperature every 1 to 3 hours by axillary or inguinal route. Record temperature and route. *Monitoring body temperature helps detect developing complications.*
- **S** Monitor and record neurologic status every 1 to 4 hours. *Falling body temperature and slowed metabolic rate may cause decreased LOC.*
- **S** Monitor and record vital signs every 1 to 4 hours. As ordered, initiate and maintain continuous electronic cardiorespiratory monitoring. *These measures help avert metabolic acidosis and respiratory arrest.*
- **S** Maintain appropriate room temperature. *Environmental temperature assists in preventing hypothermic episodes.*
- **PCC** Discuss precipitating factors with patient *to help prevent occurrence.*
- **EBP** Instruct patient in preventive measures, such as dressing appropriately and adequate nutrition. *These precautions may prevent a cold stress episode.*
- **EBP** Provide education about dressing in layers and wearing synthetic fabrics when outdoors in cold temperatures. *Synthetic fabrics help to wick away moisture and keep the body warm even when wet.*
- **EBP** Provide education to patient for outdoor activity, to frequently replace wet layers of clothing with dry layers. *Wet clothing contributes to heat loss.*
- **EBP** Provide education to patient when outdoors, to exercise or work in small or short bursts *to generate heat and prevent fatigue.*

Suggested NIC Interventions

Comfort Level; Fluid Management; Hypothermia Treatment; Temperature Regulation; Vital Signs Monitoring

EVALUATIONS FOR EXPECTED OUTCOMES

- Patient's temperature returns to normal limits.
- Patient's skin is warm and dry.

- Patient's heart rate and blood pressure return to within normal limits.
- Patient doesn't shiver.
- Patient voices feelings of comfort.
- Patient doesn't develop complications associated with hypothermia.
- Patient describes measures to prevent further episodes of hypothermia.

DOCUMENTATION

- Patient's shivering and complaints of coldness
- Observations of physical findings
- Nursing interventions and patient's response to interventions, including physiologic, behavioral, and cognitive
- Patient teaching and response
- Evaluations for expected outcomes

REFERENCES

Higginson, R. (2018). Causes of hypothermia and the use of patient-rewarming techniques. *British Journal of Nursing, 27*(21), 1222–1224. doi:10.12968/bjon.2018.27.21.1222

Procter, E., Brugger, H., & Burtscher, M. (2018). Accidental hypothermia in recreational activities in the mountains: A narrative review. *Scandinavian Journal of Medicine & Science in Sports, 28*(12), 2464–2472. doi:10.1111/sms.13294

Spruce, L. (2018). Back to basics: Unplanned patient hypothermia. *AORN Journal, 108*(5), 533–541. doi:10.1002/aorn.12389

Trevisanuto, D., Testoni, D., & de Almeida, M. F. B. (2018). Maintaining normothermia: Why and how? *Seminars in Fetal & Neonatal Medicine, 23*(5), 333–339. doi:10.1016/j.siny.2018.03.009

Watson, J. (2018). Inadvertent postoperative hypothermia prevention: Passive versus active warming methods. *ACORN: The Journal of Perioperative Nursing in Australia, 31*(1), 43–46.

Neonatal Hypothermia

DEFINITION

Core body temperature of an infant below the normal diurnal range

RELATED FACTORS (R/T)

- Delayed breastfeeding
- Early bathing of newborn
- Excessive conductive heat transfer
- Excessive convective heat transfer
- Excessive evaporative heat transfer
- Excessive radiative heat transfer
- Inadequate caregiver knowledge of hypothermia prevention
- Inadequate clothing
- Malnutrition

ASSOCIATED CONDITIONS

- Damage to hypothalamus
- Immature stratum corneum
- Increased pulmonary vascular resistance
- Ineffective vascular control
- Inefficient nonshivering thermogenesis
- Low appearance, pulse, grimace, activity, and respiration (APGAR) scores
- Pharmaceutical preparations

ASSESSMENT

▦ Core temperature
▦ Weight
▦ Cardiovascular status, including heart rate and rhythm
▦ Respiratory status, including oxygen saturation and respirations
▦ Neurologic status, including muscle tone, neonatal reflexes, excessive crying, lethargy, irritability, seizures, tremors, and assessments such as appearance, pulse, grimace, activity, and respiration (APGAR) scores
▦ Blood glucose
▦ Sensory status, including responsiveness to visual, tactile, and auditory stimuli and experience with pain

DEFINING CHARACTERISTICS

▦ Acrocyanosis
▦ Bradycardia
▦ Decreased blood glucose level
▦ Decreased metabolic rate
▦ Decreased peripheral perfusion
▦ Decreased ventilation
▦ Hypertension
▦ Hypoglycemia
▦ Hypoxia
▦ Increased oxygen demand
▦ Insufficient energy to maintain sucking
▦ Irritability
▦ Metabolic acidosis
▦ Pallor
▦ Peripheral vasoconstriction
▦ Respiratory distress
▦ Skin cool to touch
▦ Slow capillary refill
▦ Tachycardia
▦ Weight gain less than 30 g/day

EXPECTED OUTCOMES

▦ Infant will exhibit adequate perfusion (HR, skin color, capillary refill—WNL)
▦ Infant will have core temperature of greater than 36.5°C (97.7°F)

Suggested NOC Outcomes

Knowledge: Infant Care; Knowledge: Preterm Infant Care; Newborn Adaptation; Thermoregulation: Newborn

INTERVENTIONS AND RATIONALES

EBP ▦ Warm neonate in an incubator or under a radiant warmer. *Hypothermia is treated by warming in an incubator or under a radiant warmer.*

EBP ▦ Monitor and treat hypoglycemia, hypoxemia, and apnea. *Treat underlying conditions that may cause complications.*

EBP ▦ Keep room temperature warm at 23 to 25°C (74 to 77°F) *to prevent radiant heat loss on surfaces.*

EBP ▓ The temperature of birthing room should be at least 25°C, free from the drafts from open windows, doors, or fans, to *prevent cooling of surfaces and radiant heat loss. Temperature of the birthing room should not be determined by adult comfort.*

EBP ▓ Supplies needed to keep the newborn warm should be prepared ahead of time *to prevent surface cooling.*

EBP ▓ Dry and swaddle neonate (including the head) in a warm blanket *to prevent evaporative, conductive, and convective losses.*

EBP ▓ While drying newborn, place on mother's or partner's chest or abdomen (skin-to-skin contact) *to prevent heat loss.* Uncover neonate as little as possible during assessments and interventions *to prevent heat loss.*

EBP ▓ Initiate breastfeeding preferably within 1 hour of birth, which *helps to maintain the skin-to-skin contact and encourages sucking reflexes.*

EBP ▓ Place a cap on neonate's head *to prevent radiant heat loss.*

S ▓ If neonate must be transported, cover with loose clothing and wrap in blanket to *prevent heat loss due to air temperature.*

EBP ▓ Teach parents and families about the risks of hypothermia and hyperthermia *to prevent unnecessary exposure of neonate.*

Suggested NIC Interventions

Hypothermia Treatment; Infant Care: Newborn; Infant Care: Preterm; Temperature Regulation

EVALUATIONS FOR EXPECTED OUTCOMES

▓ Infant's heart rate, skin color, and capillary refill are within the defined limits.
▓ Infant's core temperature remains greater than 36.5°C (97.7°F).

DOCUMENTATION

▓ Assessment of factors that affect infant's temperature
▓ Parents' expression of feelings about caring for infant
▓ Nursing interventions and infant's response to them
▓ Evaluations for expected outcomes

REFERENCES

Beletew, B., Mengesha, A., Wudu, M., & Abate, M. (2020). Prevalence of neonatal hypothermia and its associated factors in East Africa: A systematic review and meta-analysis. *BMC Pediatrics, 20*, 1–14. doi:10.1186/s12887-020-02024-w

Chen, K.-Y., Wei, T.-Y., Huang, H.-Y., & Hsu, Y.-H. (2019). Project to decrease the incidence of neonatal hypothermia in the newborn center. *Journal of Nursing, 66*(4), 71–78.

Nebiyu, S., Berhanu, M., & Liyew, B. (2021). Magnitude and factors associated with neonatal hypothermia among neonates admitted in neonatal intensive care units: Multicenter cross-sectional study. *Journal of Neonatal Nursing, 27*(2), 111–117.

Vilinsky-Redmond, A., Brenner, M., Nugent, L., & McCann, M. (2020). Active warming after caesarean section to prevent neonatal hypothermia: A systematic review. *British Journal of Midwifery, 28*(12), 829–837.

Risk for Neonatal Hypothermia

DEFINITION

Susceptibility of an infant to a core body temperature below the normal diurnal range, which may compromise health

RISK FACTORS

- Delayed breastfeeding
- Early bathing of newborn
- Excessive conductive heat transfer
- Excessive convective heat transfer
- Excessive evaporative heat transfer
- Excessive radiative heat transfer
- Inadequate caregiver knowledge of hypothermia prevention
- Inadequate clothing
- Malnutrition

ASSOCIATED CONDITIONS

- Damage to hypothalamus
- Immature stratum corneum
- Increased pulmonary vascular resistance
- Ineffective vascular control
- Inefficient nonshivering thermogenesis
- Low appearance, pulse, grimace, activity, and respiration (APGAR) scores
- Pharmaceutical preparations

ASSESSMENT

- Core temperature
- Weight
- Cardiovascular status, including heart rate and rhythm
- Respiratory status, including oxygen saturation and respirations
- Neurologic status, including muscle tone, neonatal reflexes, excessive crying, lethargy, irritability, seizures, tremors, and assessments such as appearance, pulse, grimace, activity, and respiration (APGAR) scores
- Blood glucose
- Sensory status, including responsiveness to visual, tactile, and auditory stimuli and experience with pain

EXPECTED OUTCOMES

- Infant will exhibit adequate perfusion (HR, skin color, capillary refill—WNL).
- Infant will have core temperature of greater than 36.5°C (97.7°F).

Suggested NOC Outcomes

Knowledge: Infant Care; Knowledge: Preterm Infant Care; Newborn Adaptation; Thermoregulation: Newborn

INTERVENTIONS AND RATIONALES

EBP ■ Warm neonate in an incubator or under a radiant warmer. *Hypothermia is treated by warming in an incubator or under a radiant warmer.*

EBP ■ Monitor and treat hypoglycemia, hypoxemia, and apnea. *Treat underlying conditions that may cause complications.*

EBP ▦ Keep room temperature warm at 23 to 25°C (74 to 77°F) *to prevent radiant heat loss on surfaces.*

EBP ▦ The temperature of birthing room should be at least 25°C, free from the drafts from open windows, doors, or fans, to *prevent cooling of surfaces and radiant heat loss. Temperature of the birthing room should not be determined by adult comfort.*

EBP ▦ Supplies needed to keep the newborn warm should be prepared ahead of time *to prevent surface cooling.*

EBP ▦ Dry and swaddle neonate (including the head) in a warm blanket *to prevent evaporative, conductive, and convective losses.*

EBP **PCC** ▦ While drying newborn, place on mother's or partner's chest or abdomen (skin-to-skin contact) *to prevent heat loss.*

EBP ▦ Uncover neonate as little as possible during assessments and interventions *to prevent heat loss.*

EBP **PCC** ▦ Initiate breastfeeding preferably within 1 hour of birth, which *helps to maintain the skin-to-skin contact and encourages sucking reflexes.*

EBP ▦ Place a cap on neonate's head *to prevent radiant heat loss.*

S ▦ If neonate must be transported, cover with loose clothing and wrap in blanket to *prevent heat loss due to air temperature.*

EBP ▦ Teach parents and families about the risks of hypothermia and hyperthermia *to prevent unnecessary exposure of neonate.*

Suggested NIC Interventions

Hypothermia Treatment; Infant Care: Newborn; Infant Care: Preterm; Temperature Regulation

EVALUATIONS FOR EXPECTED OUTCOMES

▦ Infant's heart rate, skin color, and capillary refill are within the defined limits.
▦ Infant's core temperature remains greater than 36.5°C (97.7°F).

DOCUMENTATION

▦ Assessment of factors that affect infant's temperature
▦ Parents' expression of feelings about caring for infant
▦ Nursing interventions and infant's response to them
▦ Evaluations for expected outcomes

REFERENCES

Beletew, B., Mengesha, A., Wudu, M., & Abate, M. (2020). Prevalence of neonatal hypothermia and its associated factors in East Africa: A systematic review and meta-analysis. *BMC Pediatrics, 20*, 1–14. doi:10.1186/s12887-020-02024-w
Chen, K.-Y., Wei, T.-Y., Huang, H.-Y., & Hsu, Y.-H. (2019). Project to decrease the incidence of neonatal hypothermia in the newborn center. *Journal of Nursing, 66*(4), 71–78.
Nebiyu, S., Berhanu, M., & Liyew, B. (2021). Magnitude and factors associated with neonatal hypothermia among neonates admitted in neonatal intensive care units: Multicenter cross-sectional study. *Journal of Neonatal Nursing, 27*(2), 111–117.
Vilinsky-Redmond, A., Brenner, M., Nugent, L., & McCann, M. (2020). Active warming after caesarean section to prevent neonatal hypothermia: A systematic review. *British Journal of Midwifery, 28*(12), 829–837.

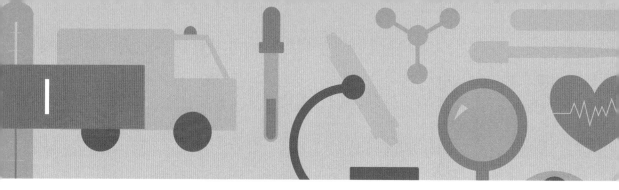

Risk for Complicated Immigration Transition

Susceptible to experiencing negative feelings (loneliness, fear, anxiety) in response to unsatisfactory consequences and cultural barriers to one's immigration transition, which may compromise health

RISK FACTORS

- Available work below educational preparation
- Cultural barriers in host county
- Unsanitary housing
- Insufficient knowledge about the process to access resources in the host county
- Insufficient social support in host country
- Language barriers in host country
- Multiple nonrelated persons within household
- Overcrowded housing
- Overt discrimination
- Parent–child conflicts related to enculturation in the host country
- Abusive landlord

ASSESSMENT

- Age and developmental stage
- Education
- Primary language and other languages spoken
- Migration reason and immigration status
- Employment status, working conditions, and any specialized training
- Livings conditions and housing status including number of residents and relationships in same household
- Availability of family and/or friends
- Expectations of immigration
- Coping mechanisms and decision-making ability
- Psychosocial support, including lifestyle, communication status (verbal, nonverbal, phone, and written), family members, and finances

EXPECTED OUTCOMES

- Patient will not experience complications from immigration transition.
- Patient will adapt to culture of host country.
- Patient will not experience isolation during transition.

344

- Patient will not experience feelings of fear.
- Patient will not experience feelings of anxiety.
- Patient will identify healthy coping strategies for stress.
- Patient will have sanitary housing.
- Patient will have effective communication in host country.
- Patient will identify sources of support in host country.

Suggested NOC Outcomes

Community Competence; Community Program Effectiveness; Decision-Making; Family Social Climate; Knowledge: Health Resources; Personal Safety Behavior

INTERVENTIONS AND RATIONALES

PCC — Provide a nonthreatening environment. *A safe environment facilitates communication.*

S — Discuss specific situation or individuals that threaten the patient or family. *Identifying threats guides service needs.*

PCC — Establish communication methods with patient. *Adequate communication must be implemented to effectively work with the patient.*

PCC — Provide instructions in formats that patient can understand. *Use of appropriate language, pictures, and graphs assists comprehension.*

PCC — Assist patient in clarifying values and expectation *to make informed decisions about the situation.*

PCC — Respect patient's right to receive or not to receive information and assistance. *Patient may need time to ingest and process the current situation.*

— Determine status of basic living needs. *Identifies needed support systems.*

EBP — Educate patient about the different types of health care facilities available. *The many types of services can be overwhelming.*

T&C — Facilitate care between patient and other health care providers. *Acting as the patient's advocate will help navigation through the health care system.*

T&C — Educate patient about community resources and contact persons. *Knowing where to find assistance encourages appropriate use.*

T&C — Refer patient to support as needed: legal aid, support groups, social services. *Each support entity has specialized knowledge to guide patient through transition process.*

Suggested NIC Interventions

Coping Enhancement; Counseling; Crisis Intervention; Decision-Making Support; Health Literacy Enhancement; Health System Guidance; Risk Identification

EVALUATIONS FOR EXPECTED OUTCOMES

- Patient does not experience complications from immigration transition.
- Patient adapts to culture of host country.
- Patient does not experience feelings of fear.
- Patient does not experience feelings of anxiety.
- Patient identifies healthy coping strategies for stress.
- Patient obtains sanitary housing.
- Patient has effective communication in host country.
- Patient identifies sources of support in host country.

DOCUMENTATION

- Patient's perception of issues
- Patient statements that indicate understanding of health-promoting activities, health care systems, support agencies, and necessary self-care skills
- Patient's response to interventions and teaching
- Literature provided to patient
- Evaluations for expected outcomes

REFERENCES

Cadenas, G. A., Bernstein, B. L., & Tracey, T. J. G. (2018). Critical consciousness and intent to persist through college in DACA and U.S. citizen students: The role of immigration status, race, and ethnicity. *Cultural Diversity & Ethnic Minority Psychology, 24*(4), 564–575. doi:10.1037/cdp0000200

Philbin, M. M., Flake, M., Hatzenbuehler, M. L., & Hirsch, J. S. (2018). State-level immigration and immigrant-focused policies as drivers of Latino health disparities in the United States. *Social Science & Medicine, 199*, 29–38. doi:10.1016/j.socscimed.2017.04.007

Roche, K. M., Vaquera, E., White, R. M. B., & Rivera, M. I. (2018). Impacts of immigration actions and news and the psychological distress of U.S. Latino parents raising adolescents. *Journal of Adolescent Health, 62*(5), 525–531. doi:10.1016/j.jadohealth.2018.01.004

Vargas, E., & Ybarra, V. (2017). U.S. citizen children of undocumented parents: The link between state immigration policy and the health of Latino children. *Journal of Immigrant & Minority Health, 19*(4), 913–920. doi:10.1007/s10903-016-0463-6

Ineffective Impulse Control

DEFINITION

A pattern of performing rapid, unplanned reactions to internal or external stimuli without regard for the negative consequences of these reactions to the impulsive individual or to others

RELATED FACTORS (R/T)

- Hopelessness
- Mood disorder
- Smoking
- Substance misuse

ASSOCIATED CONDITIONS

- Alteration in cognitive functioning
- Alteration in development
- Organic brain disorder
- Personality disorder

ASSESSMENT

- History or current presence of stress reactions in response to internal or external forces expressed by such physical findings as choking sensation, hyperventilation, dizziness, increased heart rate and/or blood pressure, perspiration, pupillary dilation, polyuria, and elevated blood glucose, cholesterol, and free fatty acid levels
- History or current presence of stress reactions in response to internal or external forces expressed by such behavioral cues as insomnia, restlessness, "scattered" thoughts, disorganized speech, restlessness, irritability, and altered concentration

- Physical stressors, including extreme heat or cold, malnutrition, disease, infection, and pain
- Psychological stressors, including fear, sense of failure, change in company or home location, success, holiday, vacation, or promotion
- Level of stress, positive coping mechanisms, realistic thought patterns, behaviors, or energy level
- Medication history, including use of drugs, caffeine, tobacco, or alcohol, which stimulate the sympathetic nervous system
- Sleep patterns or changes in daily activities that could be perceived as stressful, including too many or too few activities
- Sociologic factors, including job satisfaction, presence of support systems, family coping mechanisms, or hobbies

DEFINING CHARACTERISTICS

- Acting without thinking
- Asking personal questions despite discomfort of others
- Gambling addiction
- Inability to save money or regulate finances
- Inappropriate sharing of personal details
- Irritability
- Overly familiar with strangers
- Sensation seeking
- Sexual promiscuity
- Temper outburst
- Violent behavior

EXPECTED OUTCOMES

- Patient will identify triggers that lead to self-destructive actions.
- Patient will identify appropriate coping mechanisms to prevent self-harm and minimize engaging in impulsive behaviors.
- Patient will identify strategies that will aid in maintaining positive relationships.
- Patient will report to staff any thoughts of harming self or others.
- Patient will work with staff in planning ongoing treatment.

Suggested NOC Outcomes

Aggression Control; Anxiety Control; Coping; Impulse Control; Self-Esteem; Self-Mutilation Restraint; Social Interaction Skills

INTERVENTIONS AND RATIONALES

- Assess patient for thoughts of suicide, homicide, or self-mutilation. *Findings may require immediate safety precautions and psychological support.*
- **S** Assess for history of previous or current medical conditions and any pharmacologic side effects that may be contributing to current symptoms, *as brain trauma, organic brain disorders, or medications can present with impulse control symptoms.*
- **PCC** Decrease environmental stimuli if the patient is feeling unsafe. *A quiet and nonstimulating environment will assist in decreasing level of anxiety.*
- Assist patient in identifying stressors that lead to inappropriate or harmful impulsive behaviors *as patient is usually unaware of impulsive behaviors and will require assistance in identifying them.*

T&C ▪ Encourage patient to attend milieu therapies. *Milieu therapies will offer patient an opportunity to share feelings and learn/practice new coping and social skills with peers.*

▪ Educate patient regarding cognitive therapies that can be used *to reinforce appropriate coping and social skills.*

PCC ▪ Dedicate quality time to patient in a therapeutic and consistent manner *in order to help patient feel safe and allow an open and trusting relationship to develop.*

▪ Refer patient for treatment, which may include but is not limited to medication management, individual therapy sessions, peer support groups, and crisis center contacts *to ensure continuation of treatment.*

Suggested NIC Interventions

Anger Control Assistance; Anxiety Reduction; Cognitive Restructuring; Coping Enhancement; Impulse Control Training; Support Group

EVALUATIONS FOR EXPECTED OUTCOMES

▪ Patient shows no physical or mental signs of self-destructive actions.
▪ Patient uses appropriate coping mechanisms.
▪ Patient can manage own impulsive behavior.
▪ Patient reports no harm to self or others.
▪ Patient states plan for continuing therapy.

DOCUMENTATION

▪ Results of assessment for suicidal ideation, thoughts of homicide, or self-mutilation
▪ Response to decreased environmental stimuli
▪ Milieu therapies attended and response to treatment
▪ Response to nursing interventions
▪ External agencies suggested
▪ Evaluations for expected outcomes

REFERENCES

Davis, J., Dumas, T., Berey, B., Merrin, G., Cimpian, J. R., & Roberts, B. (2017). Effect of victimization on impulse control and binge drinking among serious juvenile offenders from adolescence to young adulthood. *Journal of Youth & Adolescence, 46*(7), 1515–1532. doi:10.1007/s10964-017-0676-6

Guillaume, S., Gay, A., Jaussent, I., Sigaud, T., Billard, S., Attal, J., … Courtet, P. (2018). Improving decision-making and cognitive impulse control in bulimia nervosa by rTMS: An ancillary randomized controlled study. *International Journal of Eating Disorders, 51*(9), 1103–1106. doi:10.1002/eat.22942

Rose, M. H., Nadler, E. P., & Mackey, E. R. (2018). Impulse control in negative mood states, emotional eating, and food addiction are associated with lower quality of life in adolescents with severe obesity. *Journal of Pediatric Psychology, 43*(4), 443–451. doi:10.1093/jpepsy/jsx127

Weintraub, D., & Mamikonyan, E. (2019). Impulse control disorders in Parkinson's disease. *American Journal of Psychiatry, 176*(1), 5–11. doi:10.1176/appi.ajp.2018.18040465

Disability-Associated Urinary Incontinence

DEFINITION

Involuntary loss of urine not associated with any pathology or problem related to the urinary system

RELATED FACTORS (R/T)

- Avoidance of nonhygienic toilet use
- Caregiver inappropriately implements bladder training techniques.
- Cognitive dysfunction
- Difficulty finding the bathroom
- Difficulty obtaining timely assistance to bathroom
- Embarrassment regarding toilet use in social situations
- Environmental constraints that interfere with continence
- Habitually suppresses urge to urinate
- Impaired physical mobility
- Impaired postural balance
- Inadequate motivation to maintain continence
- Increased fluid intake
- Neurobehavioral manifestations
- Pelvic floor disorders

ASSOCIATED CONDITIONS

- Heart diseases
- Impaired coordination
- Impaired hand dexterity
- Intellectual disability
- Neuromuscular diseases
- Osteoarticular diseases
- Pharmaceutical preparations
- Psychological disorder
- Vision disorders

ASSESSMENT

- Age
- Gender
- Vital signs
- History of mental illness
- Genitourinary status, including frequency and voiding pattern
- Fluid and electrolyte status, including blood urea nitrogen level, creatinine level, intake and output, mucous membranes, serum electrolyte levels, and skin turgor
- Neuromuscular status, including activities of daily living, mental status, mobility, and sensory ability to perceive bladder fullness
- Psychosocial status, including behavior before and after voiding, support from family members, impact of incontinence on self and others, and stressors (family, job, and change in environment)

DEFINING CHARACTERISTICS

- Adaptive behaviors to avoid others' recognition of urinary incontinence
- Mapping routes to public bathrooms prior to leaving home
- Time required to reach toilet is too long after sensation of urge.
- Use of techniques to prevent urination
- Voiding prior to reaching toilet

EXPECTED OUTCOMES

- Patient will void at appropriate intervals.
- Patient will not have an incontinent occurrence.
- Patient will have minimal, if any, complications.
- Patient and family members will demonstrate skill in managing incontinence.
- Patient will discuss impact of incontinence on self and family members.
- Patient and family members will identify resources to assist with care following discharge.

Suggested NOC Outcomes

Coordinated Movement; Self-Care: Toileting; Symptom Control; Urinary Continence; Urinary Elimination

INTERVENTIONS AND RATIONALES

- Monitor and record patient's voiding patterns *to ensure correct fluid replacement therapy*.
- Assist with specific bladder elimination procedures, such as the following:
  - Bladder training. Place patient on commode or toilet every 2 hours while awake and once during night. *Successful bladder training revolves around adequate fluid intake, muscle-strengthening exercises, and carefully scheduled voiding times.*
  - Rigid toilet regimen. Place patient on toilet at specific intervals (every 2 hours or after meals). Note whether patient was wet or dry and whether voiding occurred at each interval. *This helps patient adapt to routine physiologic function.*
  - Behavior modification. Reward continence or voiding in lavatory. Don't punish unwanted behavior such as voiding in wrong place. Reinforce behavior consistently, using social or material rewards. *This helps patient learn alternatives to maladaptive behaviors.*
  - Use of external catheter. Apply according to established procedure and maintain patency. Observe condition of perineal skin and clean with soap and water at least twice daily. *This ensures effective therapy and prevents infection and skin breakdown.*
  - Application of protective pads and garments. Use only when interventions have failed to prevent infection and skin breakdown and promote social acceptance. Allow at least 4 to 6 weeks for trial period. *Establishing continence requires prolonged effort.*
- **PCC** Maintain continence based on patient's voiding patterns and limitations.
  - Use reminders. *Reminders help limit amount of information patient must retain in memory.*
  - Orient patient to toileting environment: time, place, and activity. *A structured environment offers security and helps patient with elimination problems.*
  - Stimulate patient's voiding reflexes (give patient water to drink while on toilet, stroke area over bladder, or pour water over perineum). *External stimulation triggers bladder's spastic reflex.*
  - Provide hyperactive patient with distraction, such as a magazine, to occupy attention while on toilet. *This reduces anxiety and eases voiding.*
  - Provide privacy and adequate time *to void to allow patient to void easily without anxiety.*
  - Praise successful performance *to give patient a sense of control and to encourage compliance.*
  - Change wet clothes to accustom patient *to dry clothes.*
  - Teach family members and support personnel to assist, *thus reducing anxiety that results from noninvolvement and increasing chances for successful treatment.*

- Respond to patient's call light promptly *to avoid delays in voiding routine.*
- Choose patient's clothing to promote easy dressing and undressing (e.g., use Velcro fasteners and gowns instead of pajamas). *This reduces patient's frustration with voiding routine.*

PCC ▪ Schedule patient's fluid intake to encourage voiding at convenient times. Maintain adequate hydration up to 3,000 mL daily, unless contraindicated. *Scheduling fluid intake promotes regular bladder distention and optimal time intervals between voidings.* Limit fluid intake to 150 mL after dinner *to reduce need to void at night.*

EBP ▪ Instruct patient and family members in continence techniques to use at home *to increase chances of successful bladder retraining.*

PCC ▪ Encourage patient and family members to share feelings related to incontinence. *This allows specific problems to be identified and resolved. Attentive listening conveys recognition and respect.*

T&C ▪ Refer patient and family members to psychiatric liaison nurse, home health care agency, or support group *to provide access to additional community resources.*

Suggested NIC Interventions

Environmental Management; Pelvic Muscle Exercise; Prompted Voiding; Self-Care Assistance; Urinary Elimination Management; Urinary Habit Training

EVALUATIONS FOR EXPECTED OUTCOMES

- Patient voids at appropriate intervals, with minimal episodes of incontinence.
- Patient recognizes urge to void, undresses without assistance, and uses toilet.
- Patient doesn't experience urinary tract infection, skin breakdown, or other complications related to incontinence.
- Patient and family members demonstrate proper procedures for managing incontinence.
- Patient expresses feelings about condition and its effect on family. Patient and family members are neither overwhelmed nor excessively optimistic about patient's condition.
- Patient and family members contact support group or home health care agency, if needed.

DOCUMENTATION

- Observations of incontinence and response to treatment regimen
- Interventions to provide supportive care and patient's response to supportive care
- Instructions given to patient and family members; return demonstration of knowledge and skills needed to carry out continence management techniques
- Patient's expression of concern about incontinence and motivation to participate in self-care
- Evaluations for expected outcomes

REFERENCES

Lai, C. K. Y., & Wan, X. (2017). Using prompted voiding to manage urinary incontinence in nursing homes: Can it be sustained? *Journal of the American Medical Directors Association, 18*(6), 509–514. doi:10.1016/j.jamda.2016.12.084

Payne, D. (2018). Managing urinary incontinence in patients living with dementia. *British Journal of Community Nursing, 23*(1), 24–28. doi:10.12968/bjcn.2018.23.1.24

Prud'homme, G., Alexander, L., & Orme, S. (2018). Management of urinary incontinence in frail elderly women. *Obstetrics, Gynaecology & Reproductive Medicine, 28*(2), 39–45. doi:10.1016/j.ogrm.2017.11.004

Mixed Urinary Incontinence

DEFINITION

Involuntary loss of urine in combination with or following a strong sensation or urgency to void and also with activities that increase intra-abdominal pressure

RELATED FACTORS (R/T)

- Incompetence of the bladder neck
- Incompetence of the urethral sphincter
- Overweight
- Pelvic organ prolapse
- Skeletal muscular atrophy
- Smoking
- Weak anterior wall of the vagina

ASSOCIATED CONDITIONS

- Diabetes mellitus
- Estrogen deficiency
- Motor disorders
- Pelvic floor disorders
- Prolonged urinary incontinence
- Surgery for stress urinary incontinence
- Urethral sphincter injury

ASSESSMENT

- History of sensory or neuromuscular impairment
- History of urinary tract disease, trauma, surgery, or infection
- Genitourinary status, including bladder palpation, residual urine volume after voiding, urinalysis, urine characteristics, urine culture and sensitivity, and voiding patterns
- Neuromuscular status, including anal sphincter tone, motor ability to start and stop urine stream, neuromuscular function, sensory ability to perceive bladder fullness and voiding, and involuntary voiding after stimulation of skin on abdomen, thighs, or genitals
- Fluid and electrolyte status, including blood urea nitrogen level, creatinine level, intake and output, medication history, mucous membranes, serum electrolyte levels, skin turgor, and urine specific gravity
- Sexuality status, including capability, concerns, and habits
- Psychosocial status, including coping skills, self-concept, and perception of problem by patient and family members

DEFINING CHARACTERISTICS

- Expresses incomplete bladder emptying
- Involuntary loss of urine upon coughing
- Involuntary loss of urine upon effort
- Involuntary loss of urine upon laughing
- Involuntary loss of urine upon physical exertion
- Involuntary loss of urine upon sneezing
- Nocturia
- Urinary urgency

EXPECTED OUTCOMES

- Patient will completely empty bladder upon urination.
- Patient will have postvoid residual of <50 mL.
- Patient will have reduction in urinary incontinence episodes or complete absence of urinary incontinence.
- Patient and family members will demonstrate skill in managing urinary incontinence.
- Patient will express understanding of condition and activities to prevent/reduce overflow incontinence.

Suggested NOC Outcomes

Coordinated Movement; Self-Care: Toileting; Symptom Control; Urinary Continence; Urinary Elimination

INTERVENTIONS AND RATIONALES

- **PCC** Monitor and record patient's voiding patterns *to determine existence and extent of incontinence.*
- **PCC** Ask patient to keep a bladder diary of continent and incontinent voids to promote understanding of the extent of the problem of overflow incontinence. Discuss voiding and fluid intake patterns. *Accurate understanding of patient's pattern provides a baseline for introducing new activities.*
- **PCC** Provide privacy and adequate time to void *to decrease anxiety and promote relaxation of sphincter.*
- **PCC** Assist patient to assume usual position for voiding. *Some patients are unable to void while lying in bed and may develop urinary retention and overflow incontinence.*
- **EBP** Massage (credé) the bladder area during urination to increase pressure in the pelvic area *to encourage drainage of urine from the bladder.*
- **PCC** Assist with application of pads and protective garments (used only as a last resort) *to prevent skin breakdown and odor and to promote social acceptance.*
- **EBP** Teach patient and/or family to catheterize patient with chronic overflow incontinence related to urinary retention using clean technique *to manage long-term overflow incontinence.*
- **EBP** Teach stress management and relaxation techniques. *Stress and anxiety interfere with sphincter relaxation, causing urinary retention and overflow incontinence.*
- **PCC** Encourage patient to share feelings related to incontinence *to reduce anxiety.*
- **EBP** Encourage patient to drink six to eight glasses of noncaffeinated, nonalcoholic, and noncarbonated liquid, preferably water, per day (unless contraindicated). *1,500 to 2,000 mL/day promotes optimal renal function and flushes bacteria and solutes from the urinary tract. Caffeine and alcohol promote diuresis and may contribute to excess fluid loss and irritation of the bladder wall.*
- **PCC** Encourage patient to respond to the urge to void in a timely manner. *Ignoring the urge to urinate may cause incontinence.*
- **EBP** Encourage patient to participate in regular exercise, including walking and modified sit-ups (unless contraindicated). *Weak abdominal and perineal muscles weaken bladder and sphincter control.*
- **EBP** Encourage patient to avoid anticholinergics, opioids, psychotropics, α-adrenergic agonists, β-adrenergic agonists, and calcium-channel blockers (unless contraindicated), *which inhibit relaxation of the urinary sphincter and cause urinary retention.*
- **T&C** Provide referrals for physical therapy or psychological counseling as necessary *to enhance success.*

Suggested NIC Interventions

Pelvic Muscle Exercise; Urinary Bladder Training; Urinary Elimination Management; Urinary Incontinence Care

EVALUATIONS FOR EXPECTED OUTCOMES

- Patient successfully demonstrates chosen technique for bladder control.
- Patient voids at appropriate intervals, with minimal episodes of incontinence.
- Patient recognizes urge to void.

DOCUMENTATION

- Observations of incontinence and response to treatment regimen
- Interventions to provide supportive care and patient's response to supportive care
- Instructions given to patient; return demonstration of knowledge and skills needed to carry out continence management techniques.
- Patient's expression of concern about incontinence and motivation to participate in self-care
- Evaluations for expected outcomes

REFERENCES

Barzegari, M., Vahidi, B., Safarinejad, M. R., & Ebad, M. (2020). A computational analysis of the effect of supporting organs on predicted vesical pressure in stress urinary incontinence. *Medical & Biological Engineering & Computing, 58*(5), 1079–1089.

Le Berre, M., Morin, M., Corriveau, H., Hamel, M., Nadeau, S., Filiatrault, J., & Dumoulin, C. (2019). Characteristics of lower limb muscle strength, balance, mobility, and function in older women with urge and mixed urinary incontinence: An observational pilot study. *Physiotherapy Canada, 71*(3), 250–260.

Legendre, G., Fritel, X., Panjo, H., Zins, M., & Ringa, V. (2020). Incidence and remission of stress, urge, and mixed urinary incontinence in midlife and older women: A longitudinal cohort study. *Neurourology and Urodynamics, 39*(2), 650–657. doi:10.1002/nau.24237

Nygaard, I. E. (2019). Evidence-based treatment for mixed urinary incontinence. *The Journal of the American Medical Association, 322*(11), 1049. doi:10.1001/jama.2019.12659

Stress Urinary Incontinence

DEFINITION

Involuntary loss of urine with activities that increase intra-abdominal pressure, which is not associated with urgency to void

RELATED FACTORS (R/T)

- Overweight
- Pelvic floor disorders
- Pelvic organ prolapse

ASSOCIATED CONDITIONS

- Damaged pelvic floor muscles
- Degenerative changes in pelvic floor muscles
- Intrinsic urethral sphincter deficiency

- Nervous system diseases
- Prostatectomy
- Urethral sphincter injury

ASSESSMENT

- Age
- Gender
- Vital signs
- Mobility status
- Current medication regimen
- History of incontinence symptoms, including onset and pattern
- History of long-term use of tranquilizers, multiple pregnancies, prolonged or difficult labor, surgery, trauma, and vaginal infections
- Genitourinary status, including inspection of abdomen for scars from previous surgeries, rectal examination, vaginal examination, voiding pattern, and leakage of urine during sneezing, laughing, vomiting, coughing, defecating, physical exertion, or change from prone to upright position
- Fluid and electrolyte status, including creatinine level, blood urea nitrogen level, estrogen levels, intake and output, mucous membranes, serum electrolyte levels, and skin turgor
- Nutritional status, including appetite, dietary habits, and present weight
- Neuromuscular status, including degree of neuromuscular function, motor ability to start or stop urine stream, and sensory ability to perceive fullness
- Physical observations, including personal and perineal hygiene and complete bladder assessment
- Sexuality status, including capability, concerns, habits, and patterns
- Psychosocial status, including coping skills, self-concept, stressors (such as finances, family, and job), and perception of problem by family members

DEFINING CHARACTERISTICS

- Involuntary loss of urine in the absence of detrusor contraction
- Involuntary loss of urine in the absence of overdistended bladder
- Involuntary loss of urine upon coughing
- Involuntary loss of urine upon effort
- Involuntary loss of urine upon laughing
- Involuntary loss of urine upon physical exertion
- Involuntary loss of urine upon sneezing

EXPECTED OUTCOMES

- Patient will maintain continence.
- Patient will understand causes of stress incontinence.
- Patient will establish plan compatible with lifestyle to manage symptoms.
- Patient will maintain continence with the aid of incontinence pads or frequent toileting.
- Patient will perform Kegel exercises.
- Patient will state understanding of treatment.
- Patient and family members will identify resources to assist with care following discharge.

Suggested NOC Outcomes

Comfort Level; Referral; Tissue Integrity: Skin & Mucous Membranes; Urinary Continence; Urinary Elimination

INTERVENTIONS AND RATIONALES

- Observe patient's voiding patterns, time of voiding, amount voided, and whether voiding is provoked by stimuli. *Accurate, thorough assessment forms the basis of an effective treatment plan.*

PCC Discuss stress incontinence and associated social stigma with patient in a nonjudgmental manner. Tell patient that many people experience incontinence. *Patient may be reluctant to discuss incontinence, which can have a negative effect on self-image. A nonjudgmental approach may help ease embarrassment and encourage open discussion of the problem.*

PCC Assist patient in obtaining appropriate evaluation and care for the underlying causes of stress incontinence *to ensure prompt diagnosis and treatment.*

PCC Develop an individualized toileting schedule, increasing intervals by 30 minutes until the patient achieves a 2- to 3-hour pattern. *Bladder retraining may help alleviate symptoms.*

EBP Teach patient to do Kegel exercises to strengthen pelvic floor muscles. Instruct patient to tighten muscles of pelvic floor to stop flow of urine while urinating and then to release muscles to restart flow *to strengthen the urinary sphincter muscle and restore control.*

EBP Help patient reduce intra-abdominal pressure by losing weight, avoiding heavy lifting, avoiding chairs or beds that are too high or too low. *These measures reduce intra-abdominal pressure and bladder pressure.*

EBP Promote patient's awareness of condition through education *to help patient understand illness as well as treatment.*

PCC Provide supportive measures:
  - Respond to call bell quickly, assign patient to bed next to bathroom, put night-light in bathroom, and have patient wear easily removable clothing (gown rather than pajamas, and Velcro fasteners rather than buttons or zippers). *Early recognition of problems promotes continence; easily removed clothing reduces patient frustration and helps achieve continence.*
  - Provide privacy during toileting *to reduce anxiety and promote elimination.*
  - Have patient empty bladder before meals, at bedtime, and before leaving accessible bathroom area *to promote elimination, avoid accidents, and help relieve intra-abdominal pressure.*
  - Encourage high fluid intake, unless contraindicated, *to moisten mucous membranes and maintain hydration.*
  - Suggest patient eat increased amount of salty food before going on a long trip (unless contraindicated). *Increased sodium decreases urine production.*
  - Make protective pads available for patient's undergarments, if needed, *to absorb urine, protect skin, and control odors.*

- If surgery is scheduled, give attentive, appropriate preoperative and postoperative instructions and care *to reduce patient's anxiety and build trust in caregivers.*

PCC Encourage patient to express feelings and concerns about urologic problems. *This helps patient focus on specific problem.*

PCC Review the current medication regimen for drugs that can contribute to stress incontinence, including diuretics, central nervous system depressants, and anticholinergics. Discuss with the physician the possibility of changing medications or the medication schedule *to relieve symptoms.*

T&C Refer patient and family members to psychiatric liaison nurse, support group, or other resources, as appropriate. *Community resources typically provide health care not available from other health agencies.*

EBP Alert patient and family members about need for toilet schedule. Prepare for discharge according to individual needs *to ensure that patient will receive proper care.*

Suggested NIC Interventions

Pelvic Muscle Exercise; Teaching: Individual; Urinary Elimination Management; Urinary Habit Training; Urinary Incontinence Care

EVALUATIONS FOR EXPECTED OUTCOMES

- Patient maintains continence.
- Patient expresses, without embarrassment, understanding of causes of stress incontinence.
- Patient manages symptoms successfully.
- Patient maintains continence with aid of incontinence pads or frequent toileting.
- Patient performs Kegel exercises.
- Patient expresses satisfaction with progress in overcoming stress incontinence.
- Patient expresses understanding of techniques to reduce intra-abdominal pressure and other supportive measures.
- Patient and family members contact appropriate community resources.

DOCUMENTATION

- Patient's symptoms of stress incontinence, including onset and pattern
- Patient teaching, including Kegel exercises, use of incontinence pads, and other control strategies
- Patient's response to nursing interventions
- Observations of urologic condition and patient's response to treatment regimen
- Interventions to provide supportive care and patient's response to interventions
- Instructions given to patient and family members on patient's urologic problem, their response to instructions, and demonstrated ability to carry out self-care management
- Patient's expression of concern about urologic problem and its impact on body image and lifestyle
- Patient's motivation to participate in self-care
- Evaluations for expected outcomes

REFERENCES

Capobianco, G., Madonia, M., Morelli, S., Dessole, F., De Vita, D., Cherchi, P. L., & Dessole, S. (2018). Management of female stress urinary incontinence: A care pathway and update. *Maturitas, 109*, 32–38. doi:10.1016/j.maturitas.2017.12.008

Lasak, A. M., Jean-Michel, M., Le, P. U., Durgam, R., & Harroche, J. (2018). The role of pelvic floor muscle training in the conservative and surgical management of female stress urinary incontinence: Does the strength of the pelvic floor muscles matter? *PM & R: Journal of Injury, Function & Rehabilitation, 10*(11), 1198–1210. doi:10.1016/j.pmrj.2018.03.023

MacDonald, S., Colaco, M., & Terlecki, R. (2017). Waves of change: National trends in surgical management of male stress incontinence. *Urology, 108*(1), 175–179. doi:10.1016/j.urology.2017.04.055

Sjöström, M., Lindholm, L., & Samuelsson, E. (2017). Mobile app for treatment of stress urinary incontinence: A cost-effectiveness analysis. *Journal of Medical Internet Research, 19*(5), 1. doi:10.2196/jmir.7383

Urge Urinary Incontinence

DEFINITION

Involuntary loss of urine in combination with or following a strong sensation or urgency to void

RELATED FACTORS (R/T)

- Alcohol consumption
- Anxiety
- Caffeine consumption
- Carbonated beverage consumption
- Fecal impaction
- Ineffective toileting habits
- Involuntary sphincter relaxation
- Overweight
- Pelvic floor disorders
- Pelvic organ prolapse

ASSOCIATED CONDITIONS

- Atrophic vaginitis
- Bladder outlet obstruction
- Depression
- Diabetes mellitus
- Nervous system diseases
- Nervous system trauma
- Overactive pelvic floor
- Pharmaceutical preparations
- Treatment regimen
- Urologic diseases

ASSESSMENT

- History of stroke, urinary tract disease, spinal cord injury, surgery, or infection
- Medication history
- Vital signs
- Genitourinary status, including cystometrogram, pain or discomfort, urinalysis, urine specific gravity, use of urinary assistive devices, and voiding pattern
- Fluid and electrolyte status, including blood urea nitrogen level, creatinine level, intake and output, mucous membranes, postvoiding residual volume, skin turgor, and serum electrolyte levels
- Neuromuscular status, including ambulation ability, degree of neuromuscular function, dexterity, and sensory ability to perceive fullness
- Sexuality status, including capability, concerns, habits, and sexual partner
- Psychosocial status, including coping skills, self-concept, stressors (such as finances, family, and job), and perception of health problem by patient and family members

DEFINING CHARACTERISTICS

- Decreased bladder capacity
- Feeling of urgency with triggered stimulus
- Increased urinary frequency
- Involuntary loss of urine before reaching toilet
- Involuntary loss of urine with bladder contractions
- Involuntary loss of urine with bladder spasms
- Involuntary loss of varying volumes of urine between voids, with urgency
- Nocturia

- Patient will not have episode of incontinence.
- Patient will state understanding of treatment.
- Patient will have minimal, if any, complications.
- Patient will discuss impact of disorder on self and family members.
- Patient and family members will demonstrate skill in managing incontinence.

Suggested NOC Outcomes

Knowledge: Treatment Regimen; Self-Esteem; Tissue Integrity: Skin & Mucous Membranes; Treatment Behavior: Illness or Injury; Urinary Continence; Urinary Elimination

- Observe voiding pattern; document intake and output. *This ensures correct fluid replacement therapy and provides information about patient's ability to void adequately.*
- **EBP** Provide appropriate care for patient's urologic condition, monitor progress, and report patient's responses to treatment. *Patient should receive adequate care and take part in decisions about care as much as possible.*
- **EBP** Provide supportive measures:
  - Administer pain medication and monitor effectiveness. *Patient's knowledge that pain can be alleviated reduces tension and anxiety.*
  - Prepare pleasant toilet environment that's warm, clean, and free from odors *to promote continence.*
  - Place commode next to bed, or assign patient bed next to bathroom. *A bedside commode or convenient bathroom requires less energy expenditure than bedpan.*
  - Keep bed and commode at same level *to facilitate patient's movements.*
  - Provide good lighting from bed to bathroom *to reduce sensory misinterpretation.*
  - Remove all obstacles between bed and bathroom *to reduce chance of falling.*
  - Provide clock *to help patient maintain voiding schedule through self-monitoring.*
  - Unless contraindicated, maintain fluids to 3,000 mL daily *to moisten mucous membranes and ensure hydration*; limit patient to 150 mL after dinner *to reduce need to void at night.*
  - Have patient wear easily removable clothes (gown instead of pajamas and Velcro fasteners instead of buttons or zippers) *to reduce frustration and delay in voiding routine.*
  - If patient loses control on way to bathroom, instruct patient to stop and take a deep breath. *Anxiety and rushing may strengthen bladder contractions.*
- **PCC** Assist with specific bladder elimination procedures, such as the following:
  - Bladder training. Place patient on commode every 2 hours while awake and once during night. Provide privacy. Gradually increase intervals between toileting. *These measures aim to restore a regular voiding pattern.*
  - Rigid toilet regimen. Place patient on toilet at specific times. *This aids adaptation to routine physiologic function.* Keep baseline micturition record for 3 to 7 days *to monitor toileting effectiveness.*
- **PCC** Encourage patient to express feelings and concerns about the urologic problem *to identify patient's fears.*
- **EBP** Explain urologic condition to patient and family members; include instructions on preventive measures and established bladder schedule. *Patient education begins with*

educational assessment and depends on establishing a therapeutic relationship with patient and family. Prepare patient for discharge according to individual needs *to allow patient to practice under supervision.*

EBP ▪ Instruct patient and family members in continence techniques for home use. *This reduces fear and anxiety resulting from lack of knowledge of patient's condition, and reassures patient of continuing care.*

T&C ▪ Refer patient and family members to psychiatric liaison nurse, support group, or other resources, as appropriate. *Community resources typically provide health care not available from other health agencies.*

Suggested NIC Interventions

Bathing; Environmental Management; Fluid Monitoring; Perineal Care; Self-Care Assistance: Toileting; Urinary Elimination Management; Urinary Habit Training; Urinary Incontinence Care

EVALUATIONS FOR EXPECTED OUTCOMES

▪ Patient maintains continence.
▪ Patient expresses understanding of treatment.
▪ Patient doesn't experience incontinence or other complications.
▪ Patient expresses feelings about condition.
▪ Patient and family members discuss treatment of urologic condition and home bladder schedule; they also demonstrate necessary skills.

DOCUMENTATION

▪ Observations of urologic condition and patient's response to treatment regimen
▪ Interventions to provide supportive care
▪ Patient's response to nursing interventions
▪ Instructions given to patient and family members on urologic problem, their response to instructions, and their demonstrated ability to carry out self-care management
▪ Patient's expression of concern about urologic problem and its impact on body image and lifestyle; patient's motivation to participate in self-care
▪ Evaluations for expected outcomes

REFERENCES

Chung, E., Katz, D. J., & Love, C. (2017). Adult male stress and urge urinary incontinence—A review of pathophysiology and treatment strategies for voiding dysfunction in men. *Australian Family Physician, 46*(9), 661–666.

Kuzina, I., Prokofyeva, A., Kosilov, K., Loparev, S., Kosilova, L., & Ivanovskaya, M. (2018). Effectiveness of a new tool for self-evaluation of adherence to antimuscarinic drug treatment in older patients of both sexes with urge incontinence. *Geriatrics & Gerontology International, 18*(1), 115–122. doi:10.1111/ggi.13150

Lukacz, E. S., Santiago-Lastra, Y., Albo, M. E., & Brubaker, L. (2017). Urinary incontinence in women: A review. *JAMA: Journal of the American Medical Association, 318*(16), 1592–1604. doi:10.1001/jama.2017.12137

Risk for Urge Urinary Incontinence

DEFINITION

Susceptible to involuntary passage of urine occurring soon after a strong sensation of urgency to void, which may compromise health

- Alcohol consumption
- Anxiety
- Caffeine consumption
- Carbonated beverage consumption
- Fecal impaction
- Ineffective toileting habits
- Involuntary sphincter relaxation
- Overweight
- Pelvic floor disorders
- Pelvic organ prolapse

- Atrophic vaginitis
- Bladder outlet obstruction
- Depression
- Diabetes mellitus
- Nervous system diseases
- Nervous system trauma
- Overactive pelvic floor
- Pharmaceutical preparations
- Treatment regimen
- Urologic diseases

- Age and gender
- Vital signs
- Drug history
- History of illness that may cause neuromuscular dysfunction, including stroke, spinal cord injury, head injury, urinary tract disease, and infection
- Genitourinary status, including pain or discomfort, urinalysis, urine specific gravity, use of urinary assistive devices, voiding pattern, and cystometrogram results
- Fluid and electrolyte status, including intake and output, mucous membranes, postvoiding residual volume, skin turgor, and serum electrolyte, blood urea nitrogen, and creatinine levels
- Neuromuscular status, including ambulation ability, cognitive status, sensory ability, and degree of neuromuscular function
- Sexuality status, including patient's or partner's expressions of concern
- Psychosocial status, including coping skills, self-concept, stressors (finances, family, job), patient's and family members' perceptions of health problem, and patient's motivation to meet self-care needs

- Patient will state possibility of anticipating when episodes of incontinence are likely to occur.
- Patient will state understanding of potential causes of urge incontinence and its treatment.
- Patient will avoid complications of urge incontinence or such complications will be minimized.
- Patient will discuss potential effects of urologic dysfunction on self and family members.
- Patient or family members will demonstrate skill in managing incontinence.
- Patient and family members will identify community resources to help them cope with alterations in urinary status.

Suggested NOC Outcomes

Knowledge: Treatment Regimen; Urinary Continence; Urinary Elimination

INTERVENTIONS AND RATIONALES

- Observe patient's voiding pattern and document intake and output *to ensure correct fluid replacement therapy and provide information about patient's ability to void adequately.*
- Determine patient's premorbid elimination status *to ensure that interventions are realistic and based on patient's health status and goals.*
- **T&C** Use an interdisciplinary approach to management of incontinence. Incorporate recommendations from a urologist, urology nurse specialist, other health care providers, and patient. Monitor progress and report patient's response to interventions. *An interdisciplinary approach helps to ensure that patient receives adequate care. Encouraging patient participation on the team will help foster motivation.*
- **PCC** Assess patient's ability to sense and communicate elimination needs *to maximize self-care.*
- **PCC** Make sure patient's toilet environment is warm, clean, and free from odor *to promote continence.*
- **S** Place a commode beside the bed if impaired mobility is an issue. *A bedside commode requires less energy expenditure than using a bedpan or ambulating to a bathroom.*
- **S** Keep the bed and commode at same level *to facilitate easy access.*
- **S** Provide good lighting from bed to bathroom *to reduce confusion and risk of falls.*
- **S** Remove all obstacles between bed and bathroom *to reduce risk of falls.*
- **EBP** Unless contraindicated, provide 2.5 to 3 L of fluid daily *to moisten mucous membranes and ensure adequate hydration.* Space out fluid intake through the day and limit it to 150 mL after supper *to reduce the need to void at night.*
- **PCC** Have patient wear easily removable articles of clothing (a gown instead of pajamas, Velcro fasteners instead of buttons or zippers) *to facilitate faster removal of clothing and foster independence.*
- **EBP** Instruct patient to stop and take a deep breath if experiencing an intense urge to urinate before reaching a bathroom. *Anxiety and rushing may increase bladder contraction.*
- **PCC** Have patient keep a diary recording episodes of incontinence. Use the information from the diary as a basis for planning interventions. Possible bladder training interventions may include voiding every 2 hours, avoiding high fluid intake, maintaining proper hygiene, or notifying a health care professional if urge incontinence occurs frequently. *Individualized interventions help promote self-care, foster motivation, and avoid incontinence.*
- **PCC** Incorporate patient's suggestions for managing incontinent episodes into a care plan *to foster motivation.*
- **PCC** Encourage patient to express feelings regarding incontinence *to provide emotional support and identify areas for further patient teaching.*
- **EBP** Explain urge incontinence to patient and family members, especially preventive measures and potential underlying causes, *to foster compliance.*
- Note if patient expresses concern about the effect of incontinence on sexuality. If appropriate, refer him to a sex therapist *to promote sexual health.*
- Refer patient and family members to community resources such as support groups, as appropriate, *to help ensure continuity of care.*

Suggested NIC Interventions

Fluid Monitoring; Urinary Elimination Management; Urinary Habit Training; Urinary Incontinence Care

EVALUATIONS FOR EXPECTED OUTCOMES

- Patient states the possibility of anticipating when episodes of incontinence are likely to occur.
- Patient states understanding of potential causes of urge incontinence and its treatment.
- Patient avoids complications of urge incontinence or complications are minimized.
- Patient discusses potential effects of urologic dysfunction on self and family members.
- Patient or family members demonstrate skill in managing incontinence.
- Patient and family members identify community resources to help them cope with alterations in urinary status.

DOCUMENTATION

- Patient's urologic status
- Episodes of urge incontinence
- Nursing interventions and patient's response
- Instruction given to patient and family and their responses
- Demonstrated ability to meet self-care needs
- Patient's expression of concern about potential changes in urologic status and its impact on body image and lifestyle
- Patient's statements indicating motivation to meet self-care needs
- Evaluations for expected outcomes

REFERENCES

Alvarenga-Martins, N., Pinto, P. F., Arreguy-Sena, C., Campos Paschoalin, H., Alves de Moura, D. C., & Vasconcelos Teixeira, C. (2017). Urinary incontinence: An analysis in the perspective of aging policies. *Journal of Nursing UFPE/Revista de Enfermagem UFPE, 11*(3), 1189–1199. doi:10.5205/reuol.10544-93905-1-RV.1103201709

Wiers, S. G., & Keilman, L. J. (2017). Improving care for women with urinary incontinence in primary care. *Journal for Nurse Practitioners, 13*(10), 675–680. doi:10.1016/j.nurpra.2017.08.010

Yates, A. (2017). Incontinence and associated complications: Is it avoidable? *Nurse Prescribing, 15*(6), 288–295. doi:10.12968/npre.2017.15.6.288

Yates, A. (2017). Urinary continence care for older people in the acute setting. *British Journal of Nursing, 26*(9), S28–S30. doi:10.12968/bjon.2017.26.9.S28

Risk for Infection

DEFINITION

Susceptible to invasion and multiplication of pathogenic organisms, which may compromise health

RISK FACTORS

- Difficulty managing long-term invasive devices
- Difficulty managing wound care

- Dysfunctional gastrointestinal motility
- Exclusive formula feeding
- Impaired skin integrity
- Inadequate access to individual protective equipment
- Inadequate adherence to public health recommendations
- Inadequate environmental hygiene
- Inadequate health literacy
- Inadequate hygiene
- Inadequate knowledge to avoid exposure to pathogens
- Inadequate oral hygiene habits
- Inadequate vaccination
- Malnutrition
- Mixed breastfeeding
- Obesity
- Smoking
- Stasis of body fluid

ASSOCIATED CONDITIONS

- Altered pH of secretion
- Anemia
- Chronic illness
- Decreased ciliary action
- Immunosuppression
- Invasive procedure
- Leukopenia
- Premature rupture of amniotic membrane
- Prolonged rupture of amniotic membrane
- Suppressed inflammatory response

ASSESSMENT

- Age, gender, weight
- Current health status, including vital signs, nutritional status, and integumentary status (including any wounds)
- Health history, including accidents, allergies, falls, hyperthermia, hypothermia, poisoning, seizures, trauma, and exposure to pollutants
- Presence of medical conditions such as diabetes mellitus that may increase incidence of infection
- Current medical treatments, including radiation therapy, chemotherapy, antibiotic or antifungal therapy, steroid treatment, anticoagulant or thrombolytic therapy, and immunosuppressive therapy
- Presence of invasive devices, including indwelling urinary catheter, endotracheal tube, tracheostomy tube, IV lines, central venous and arterial lines, drains, and gastric feeding tubes
- Sensory or perceptual changes (auditory, gustatory, kinesthetic, olfactory, tactile, and visual)
- Circumstances of present situation that could lead to infection
- Neurologic status, including level of consciousness, mental status, and orientation

- Laboratory studies, including clotting factors, hemoglobin (Hb) level, hematocrit, platelet count, serum albumin level, white blood cell (WBC) count, and cultures of blood, body fluid, sputum, urine, and wound drainage
- Home environment, including structural barriers, availability of soap and water for hand washing, clean preparation area, access to telephone, and need for special equipment

EXPECTED OUTCOMES

- Patient will remain free from signs and symptoms of infection.
- Patient's vital signs will remain within normal range.
- Patient's WBC count and differential will stay within normal range.
- Patient's cultures won't show evidence of pathogens.
- Patient's respiratory secretions will be clear and odorless.
- Patient's urine will remain clear, yellow, odorless, and free from sediment.
- Patient's wounds and incisions will appear clean, pink, and free from purulent drainage.
- Patient's IV sites won't show signs of inflammation.
- Patient will state infection risk factors.
- Patient will identify signs and symptoms of infection.

Suggested NOC Outcomes

> Immune Status; Infection Severity; Infection Status; Knowledge: Infection Control; Knowledge: Treatment Procedure(s); Nutritional Status; Risk Control; Risk Detection; Wound Healing: Primary Intention; Wound Healing: Secondary Intention

INTERVENTIONS AND RATIONALES

EBP ▪ Minimize patient's risk of infection by:
- washing hands before and after providing care. *Hand washing is the single best way to avoid spreading pathogens.*
- wearing gloves to maintain asepsis when providing direct care. *Gloves offer protection when handling wound dressings or carrying out various treatments.*

EBP ▪ Identify risk factors predisposing patient to infection. *A complete nursing assessment allows development of an individualized care plan.*

S ▪ Follow the facility's infection control policy *to minimize the risk of nosocomial infection.*

S ▪ Maintain standard precautions. Wear gloves if you might come into contact with the patient's blood and body secretions. *Standard precautions protect you and the patient from the transfer of microorganisms.*

S ▪ Monitor temperature at least every 4 hours, and record on graph paper. Report elevations immediately. *Sustained temperature elevation after surgery may signal onset of pulmonary complications, wound infection or dehiscence, urinary tract infection, or thrombophlebitis.*

S ▪ Monitor WBC count, as ordered. Report elevations or depressions. Elevated total WBC count indicates infection. *Markedly decreased WBC count may indicate decreased production resulting from extreme debilitation or severe lack of vitamins and amino acids. Any damage to bone marrow may suppress WBC formation.*

S ▪ Culture urine, respiratory secretions, wound drainage, or blood according to facility policy and physician's order. *This identifies pathogens and guides antibiotic therapy.*

S ▪ Help patient wash hands before and after meals and after using bathroom, bedpan, or urinal. *Hand washing prevents spread of pathogens to other objects and food.*

PCC ▪ Assist patient when necessary to ensure that perianal area is clean after elimination. *Cleaning perineal area by wiping from area of least contamination (urinary meatus) to area of most contamination (anus) helps prevent genitourinary infections.*

PCC ▪ Instruct patient to report incidents of loose stools or diarrhea. Inform physician immediately. *Diarrhea or loose stools may indicate need to discontinue or change antibiotic therapy. It may also indicate need to test for* Clostridium difficile.

S ▪ Offer oral hygiene to patient every 4 hours to prevent colonization of bacteria and reduce risk of descending infection. *Disease and malnutrition may reduce moisture in mucous membranes of mouth and lips.*

S ▪ Use strict sterile technique when performing invasive procedures, such as urinary catheterization or IV line insertion, *to minimize the risk of introducing pathogens into the body.*

S ▪ Use strict sterile technique when suctioning lower airway, inserting indwelling urinary catheters, inserting IV catheters, and providing wound care *to avoid spreading pathogens.*

S ▪ Change IV tubing, and give site care every 24 to 48 hours or as facility policy dictates *to help keep pathogens from entering body.*

S ▪ Rotate IV sites every 48 to 72 hours or as facility policy dictates *to reduce chances of infection at individual sites.*

S ▪ Have patient cough and deep breathe every 4 hours after surgery *to help remove secretions and prevent pulmonary complications.*

▪ Provide tissues and disposal bags for expectorated sputum. *Convenient disposal encourages expectoration; sanitary disposal reduces spread of infection.*

S ▪ Help patient turn every 2 hours. Provide skin care, particularly over bony prominences, *to help prevent venous stasis and skin breakdown.*

S ▪ Use sterile water for humidification or nebulization of oxygen. *This prevents drying and irritation of respiratory mucosa, impaired ciliary action, and thickening of secretions within respiratory tract.*

S ▪ Encourage fluid intake of 3,000 to 4,000 mL daily unless contraindicated *to help thin mucus secretions.*

EBP ▪ Ensure adequate nutritional intake. Offer high-protein supplements unless contraindicated. *This helps stabilize weight, improves muscle tone and mass, and aids wound healing.*

S ▪ Arrange for protective isolation if patient has compromised immune system. Monitor flow and number of visitors. *These measures protect patient from pathogens in environment.*

▪ Administer topical, oral, and parenteral antibiotics as ordered *to eradicate pathogenic organisms.*

EBP ▪ Teach patient about:
- Good hand washing technique.
- Factors that increase infection risk.
- Signs and symptoms of infection. *These measures allow patient to participate in care and help patient modify lifestyle to maintain optimum health.*

Suggested NIC Interventions

Incision Site Care; Infection Control; Infection Protection; Teaching: Nutrition Therapy; Procedure/Treatment; Wound Care

EVALUATIONS FOR EXPECTED OUTCOMES

▪ Patient's vital signs remain within normal limits.
▪ Patient's WBC count and differential remain within normal range.

- Patient's cultures don't exhibit pathogen growth.
- Patient demonstrates appropriate personal and oral hygiene.
- Patient's respiratory secretions remain clear and odorless.
- Patient's urine remains clear, yellow, odorless, and free from sediment.
- Patient's bowel patterns remain normal.
- Patient's incisions or wounds remain clear, pink, and free from purulent drainage.
- Patient's IV sites don't show signs of inflammation.
- Patient's skin doesn't exhibit signs of breakdown.
- Patient's fluid and protein intake remains at specified levels.
- Patient does not experience signs and symptoms of infection.

DOCUMENTATION

- Patient's activity level
- Temperature
- Dates, times, and sites of all cultures
- Dates, times, and sites of all catheter insertions
- Appearance of all invasive catheter sites, tube sites, and wounds
- Interventions performed to reduce infection risk
- Patient's response to nursing interventions
- Evaluations for expected outcomes

REFERENCES

Burden, M., & Thornton, M. (2018). Reducing the risks of surgical site infection: The importance of the multidisciplinary team. *British Journal of Nursing, 27*(17), 976–979. doi:10.12968/bjon.2018.27.17.976

Kee, K. K., Nair, H. K. R., & Yuen, N. P. (2019). Risk factor analysis on the healing time and infection rate of diabetic foot ulcers in a referral wound care clinic. *Journal of Wound Care, 28,* S4–S13. doi:10.12968/jowc.2019.28.Sup1.S4

Palmer, S., & Dixon, R. (2019). Reducing catheter-associated urinary tract infections through best practice: Sherwood Forest Hospitals' experience. *British Journal of Nursing, 28*(1), 11–15. doi:10.12968/bjon.2019.28.1.11

Wood, D. (2019). Infection prevention in care homes: The role of community nurses. *British Journal of Community Nursing, 24*(1), 16–19. doi:10.12968/bjcn.2019.24.1.16

Risk for Injury

DEFINITION

Susceptible to physical damage due to environmental conditions interacting with the individual's adaptive and defense resources, which may compromise health

RISK FACTORS

- Compromised nutritional source
- Exposure to pathogen
- Exposure to toxic chemical
- Immunization level within community
- Insufficient knowledge of modifiable factors
- Malnutrition
- Nosocomial agent
- Physical barrier
- Unsafe mode of transport

- Abnormal blood profile
- Alteration in cognitive functioning
- Alteration in psychomotor functioning
- Alteration in sensation
- Autoimmune dysfunction
- Biochemical dysfunction
- Effector dysfunction
- Immune dysfunction
- Sensory integration dysfunction
- Tissue hypoxia

- Age
- Gender
- Physical head-to-toe examination
- Patient's health status, including presence of acute or chronic illness and changes or deterioration in mental or physical functioning
- Developmental status, including cognitive abilities (language and reasoning), sensory perception, response to stimuli (pain, touch, and warmth), level of independence, and motor skills
- Health history, including accidents, falls, and exposure to environmental hazards
- Environmental factors, including household layout, electrical wiring, lighting, utilities, fire precautions, presence of toxic or noxious substances, medications, special safety needs, and childproofing
- Mental status, including mood, affect, thought processes, thought content, orientation, judgment, and ability to perform activities of daily living
- Knowledge level, including understanding of household safety precautions and automobile safety
- Participation in recreational activities, such as swimming, diving, motorcycling, bicycling, and contact sports
- Family status, including caregiver relationship to patient; time and resources available for caregiving; willingness and ability to meet patient's physical, social, and psychological needs; feelings of frustration; and history of abuse of any family member

- Patient will remain free from physical injury.
- Patient and family will follow safety precautions in and out of home.
- Patient and family members will develop strategy to maintain safety.

Suggested NOC Outcomes

Immune Status; Risk Control; Safety Behavior: Home Physical Environment; Risk Detection; Safe Home Environment; Safety Behavior: Personal; Safety Status: Physical Injury

 ■ Assist patient and family to identify situations and hazards that can cause accidents *to increase patient's awareness of potential dangers.*

PCC ■ Assess and document any motor, mental, or sensory deficits *to identify specific safety needs.*

- Assess patient for evidence of physical or mental abuse or neglect. Observe for bruises or abrasions, body odor, or a dirty, unkempt appearance *to ensure safety and well-being.*

PCC - Question patient privately about findings *to encourage trust and promote open communication.*

S - Encourage patient to make repairs and remove potential safety hazards from environment *to decrease possibility of injury.*

S - Encourage adults to discuss safety rules with children. For example:
  - Don't play with matches.
  - Use electrical equipment carefully.
  - Know location of fire escape route.
  - Don't speak to strangers.
  - Dial 911 in an emergency.
  Teaching by parents fosters household safety.

S - Improve environmental safety, as needed:
  - Orient patient to environment.
  - Assess patient's ability to use call bell, side rails, and bed positioning controls.
  - Keep bed at lowest level, and conduct close night watch. *These measures will help patient cope with unfamiliar surroundings.*
  - Teach patient and family about need for safe illumination.
  - Advise patient to wear sunglasses to reduce glare.
  - Advise using contrasting colors in household furnishings. *These measures will enhance visual discrimination.*
  - Test heating pads and bath water before using; assess extremities daily for injury *to assist patient with decreased tactile sensitivity.*
  - For patient with hearing loss, encourage use of hearing aid *to minimize deficit.*
  - Teach patient with unstable gait correct use of adaptive devices *to decrease potential for injury.*

S - Promote electrical safety. Apply electrical outlet covers to all unused outlets. Inspect all electrical appliances brought from home and have them approved by a safety officer before use. Don't place liquids, jellies, or creams on electrical appliances. Finally, test all electrical equipment before using on a patient. *Electrical appliances pose potential hazards for patient and staff members.*

EBP - Provide additional patient teaching as needed. Possible topics may include household, automobile, and pedestrian safety. Refer patient to appropriate resources (police, fire, and home health care agency) for more information. *Health education can help patient take steps to prevent injury.*

EBP - Instruct the child and family members in standard safety practices, including
  - wiping up spills immediately.
  - providing nonslip surfaces in hallways, on stairs, and in bathtubs and shower stalls.
  - draining all water from bathtubs immediately after a bath.
  - placing toxic substances in locked cabinets or out of reach of the child. *Teaching promotes household safety.*

S - Immediately report malfunctioning equipment to appropriate personnel for replacement or repair *to help prevent accidents.*

T&C - Refer patient to appropriate community resources for more information about identifying and removing safety hazards. *This enables patient and family to alter environment to achieve optimal safety level.*

Suggested NIC Interventions

Environmental Management; Fall Prevention; Health Education; Risk Identification; Surveillance: Safety; Home Maintenance Assistance

EVALUATIONS FOR EXPECTED OUTCOMES

▦ Patient remains free from physical injury.
▦ Patient and family identify and eliminate safety hazards in their surroundings.
▦ Patient and family members demonstrate prevention and safety precautions.
▦ Children describe safety measures they have learned.
▦ Patient and family point out evidence of childproofing measures in home.
▦ Patient increases self-care activities within limits posed by sensorimotor limitations.

DOCUMENTATION

▦ Patient's statements about situations that cause accidents and injuries
▦ Patient's lack of awareness of, or disregard for, safety hazards
▦ Assessment of home environment
▦ Observation of physical findings
▦ Patient's and family members' knowledge of safety practices
▦ Patient's cognitive deficits that inhibit learning or attention to safety hazards
▦ Interventions to help patient recognize and eliminate safety hazards
▦ Patient's or family's response to nursing interventions
▦ Evaluations for expected outcomes

REFERENCES

Ambutas, S. (2017). Continuous quality improvement. Fall reduction and injury prevention toolkit: Implementation on two medical-surgical units. *MEDSURG Nursing, 26*(3), 175–197.

Kahriman, I. L., & Karadeniz, H. (2018). Effects of a safety-awareness-promoting program targeting mothers of children aged 0–6 years to prevent pediatric injuries in the home environment: Implications for nurses. *Journal of Trauma Nursing, 25*(5), 327–335. doi:10.1097/JTN.0000000000000384

Marshall, M., Cruickshank, L., Shand, J., Perry, S., Anderson, J., Parker, D., & de Silva, D. (2017). Assessing the safety culture of care homes: A multimethod evaluation of the adaptation, face validity and feasibility of the Manchester Patient Safety Framework. *BMJ Quality & Safety, 26*(9), 751–759. doi:10.1136/bmjqs-2016-006028

Ruiz-Millo, O., Climente-Martí, M., & Navarro-Sanz, J. R. (2018). Patient and health professional satisfaction with an interdisciplinary patient safety program. *International Journal of Clinical Pharmacy, 40*(3), 635–641. doi:10.1007/s11096-018-0627-7

Risk for Corneal Injury

DEFINITION

Susceptible to infection of inflammatory lesion in the corneal tissue that can affect superficial or deep layers, which may compromise health

RISK FACTORS

▦ Exposure of the eyeball
▦ Insufficient knowledge of modifiable factors

ASSOCIATED CONDITIONS

▦ Blinking <5 times/minute
▦ Glasgow Coma Scale score <7

- Intubation
- Mechanical ventilation
- Oxygen therapy
- Periorbital edema
- Pharmaceutical agent
- Tracheostomy

ASSESSMENT

- Neurologic status, including level of consciousness, orientation, motor activity, and strength in all extremities
- Glasgow Coma Scale score
- Detailed eye assessment, including blinking rate, amount of moisture in the eye, quality of the eye moisture, ability or inability to maintain eyelid closure

EXPECTED OUTCOMES

- Patient will not develop dry eyes.
- Patient's eyes will not become infected.
- Patient will not develop corneal abrasion or injury.

Suggested NOC Outcomes

Risk Control; Risk Detection; Tissue Integrity: Skin/Mucous Membranes; Knowledge: Health Behavior

INTERVENTIONS AND RATIONALES

- Assess eyes with each head-to-toe assessment *to identify any changes as soon as they occur.*
- **S** Complete hand hygiene prior to performing eye care. *This reduces the potential for infection.*
- **EBP** Perform eye care as indicated by hospital policy or protocol *to keep eyes clean.*
- **EBP** When performing eye care, wipe eye from nasal edge and outward *to avoid wiping discharge into the lacrimal duct.*
- **EBP** When performing eye care, use a new sterile gauze for the second eye *to reduce the risk for infection.*
- **EBP** Implement prescribed treatments to protect the eyes such as prescribed eye drops or hydrogel dressings *to maintain the moisture in the eyes.*
- **EBP** Educate patient on prescribed eye care regimen *to alleviate fears.*

Suggested NIC Interventions

Risk Management; Risk Identification; Behavior Management

EVALUATIONS FOR EXPECTED OUTCOMES

- Moisture maintained in patient's eyes.
- Patient shows no signs of infection in eyes.
- Patient's corneas are free from injury.

DOCUMENTATION

- Observations of the eye, including blink rate, moisture, and ability to maintain eye lid closure
- Interventions performed
- Patient response to interventions
- Evaluations for expected outcomes

REFERENCES

Carniciu, A. L., Fazzari, M. J., Tabibian, P., Batta, P., Gentile, R. C., Grendell, J. H., ... Barzideh, N. (2017). Corneal abrasion following anaesthesia for non-ocular surgical procedures: A case-controlled study. *Journal of Perioperative Practice, 27*(11), 246–253. doi:10.1177/175045891702701102

Chatterjee, S., & Agrawal, D. (2017). Primary prevention of ocular injury in agricultural workers with safety eyewear. *Indian Journal of Ophthalmology, 65*(9), 859–864. doi:10.4103/ijo.IJO_334_17

Kroll, M. W., Ritter, M. B., Kennedy, E. A., Silverman, N. K., Shinder, R., Brave, M. A., & Williams, H. E. (2018). Eye injuries from electrical weapon probes: Incidents, prevalence, and legal implications. *Journal of Forensic & Legal Medicine, 55*, 52–57. doi:10.1016/j.jflm.2018.02.013

Miller, K. N., Collins, C. L., Chounthirath, T., & Smith, G. A. (2018). Pediatric sports- and recreation-related eye injuries treated in US emergency departments. *Pediatrics, 141*(2), 1–9. doi:10.1542/peds.2017-3083

Risk for Thermal Injury

DEFINITION

Susceptible to extreme temperature damage to skin and mucous membranes, which may compromise health

RISK FACTORS

- Fatigue
- Inadequate protective clothing
- Inadequate supervision
- Inattentiveness
- Insufficient caregiver knowledge of safety precautions
- Insufficient knowledge of safety precautions
- Smoking
- Unsafe environment

ASSOCIATED CONDITIONS

- Alcohol intoxication
- Drug intoxication
- Alteration in cognitive functioning
- Neuromuscular impairment
- Neuropathy
- Treatment regimen

ASSESSMENT

- Cardiovascular status, including blood pressure, capillary refill time, electrocardiogram results, heart rate and rhythm, pulses (apical, peripheral), and temperature

- Health history, including past episodes of allergy; food, pollen, or drug allergy; multiple surgical history; spina bifida; and asthma
- Current health status, including temperature, blood pressure, respiratory status, and other vital signs
- Knowledge level, including patient's current understanding of physical condition and physical, mental, and emotional readiness to learn
- Self-care abilities, including knowledge and use of adaptive equipment, preparation of equipment and supplies, and technical or mechanical skills

EXPECTED OUTCOMES

- Patient will not experience thermal injury.
- Patient will acknowledge presence of environmental hazards in home.
- Patient will take safety precautions to prevent injury.

Suggested NOC Outcomes

Risk Control; Risk Detection; Safe Home Environment; Knowledge: Personal Safety

INTERVENTIONS AND RATIONALES

- **S** Assess environment for potential risks for thermal injury *to prevent accidents.*
- **S** Assess patient for any cognitive impairment *that would increase risk for thermal injury.*
- **S** Assess knowledge of fire safety and emergency response *to ensure rapid notification of emergency personnel.*
- **S** Remove dangerous or potentially dangerous items from the environment *to avoid injury.*
- **S** Suggest a decrease in the maximum water temperature *to decrease potential scalding.*
- **S** Ensure proper functioning of all fire/smoke alarms *to provide quick intervention in case of fire.*
- **S** Encourage adults/family member to discuss fire safety measures with children and elderly family members *to promote household safety.*
- **S** Encourage use of flame-retardant sleepwear *to minimize injury in the event of a fire.*
- **S** Encourage patient/family to report any potential safety hazards *to decrease chance of thermal accident.*
- **T&C** Refer patient/family to community resources for fire safety to ensure all possible precautions have been identified and implemented.
- **T&C** Refer at-risk patients who are living alone to home health services *for follow-up home safety evaluation.*

Suggested NIC Interventions

Environmental Management: Safety; Fire Setting Precautions; Risk Identification; Surveillance: Safety

EVALUATIONS FOR EXPECTED OUTCOMES

- Patient has no incidents of thermal injury.
- Patient removes environmental hazards from home.
- Patient uses appropriate safety measures.

- Patient's expressions of concern about risk for thermal injury
- Observations of measures taken to minimize environmental hazards
- Interventions performed to allay thermal injury risk
- Patient's response to interventions
- Evaluations for expected outcomes

REFERENCES

Ashman, H. (2018). Cooling of thermal burn injuries: A literature review. *Journal of Paramedic Practice,* *10*(5), 200–204. doi:10.12968/jpar.2018.10.5.200

Prasad, V., West, J., Sayal, K., & Kendrick, D. (2018). Injury among children and young people with and without attention-deficit hyperactivity disorder in the community: The risk of fractures, thermal injuries, and poisonings. *Child: Care, Health & Development, 44*(6), 871–878. doi:10.1111/cch.12591

Price, C. (2018). Nutrition: Reducing the hypermetabolic response to thermal injury. *British Journal of Nursing, 27*(12), 661–670. doi:10.12968/bjon.2018.27.12.661

Risk for Urinary Tract Injury

Susceptible to damage of the urinary tract structures from use of catheters, which may compromise health

- Cognitive dysfunction
- Confusion
- Inadequate caregiver knowledge regarding urinary catheter care
- Inadequate knowledge regarding urinary catheter care
- Neurobehavioral manifestations
- Obesity

- Anatomical variation in the pelvic organs
- Condition preventing ability to secure catheter
- Detrusor sphincter dyssynergia
- Latex allergy
- Long-term use of urinary catheter
- Medullary injury
- Prostatic hyperplasia
- Repetitive catheterizations
- Retention balloon inflated to ≥30 mL
- Use of large caliber urinary catheter

- History of urinary tract disease, trauma, surgery, or previous urethral infection
- Age
- Gender
- Vital signs

▓ Genitourinary status, including characteristics of urine, excretory urography, pain or discomfort, palpation of bladder, urinalysis, and voiding patterns
▓ Catheter placement, including securing devices
▓ Psychosocial status, including coping skills, patient's perception of health problem, self-concept (body image), family members, and stressors

EXPECTED OUTCOMES

▓ Patient will not experience injury from urinary catheter.
▓ Patient will voice no discomfort with catheter placement.
▓ Patient will voice understanding of treatment.
▓ Patient will have few, if any, complications.
▓ Patient will discuss impact of urologic disorder on self and family members.
▓ Patient will demonstrate skill in managing urinary elimination problem.

Suggested NOC Outcomes

Hydration; Mobility; Physical Aging; Self-Care Toileting; Urinary Elimination

INTERVENTIONS AND RATIONALES

PCC ▓ Administer appropriate catheter care and monitoring of secure device. *Appropriate care prevents complications and alerts health care team to developing problems.*

S ▓ Monitor patency of indwelling urinary catheter. Keep tubing free from kinks and keep drainage bag below the level of the bladder *to avoid urine reflux.*

S ▓ Clean the urinary meatus according to the established policy and maintain a closed drainage system *to prevent skin irritation and bacteriuria.*

S ▓ Secure the catheter to patient's leg (female) or abdomen (male); avoid tension on the sphincter. *Anchoring the catheter avoids straining the trigone muscle of the bladder and prevents friction leading to inflammation.*

EBP ▓ Only use urinary catheters as necessary. Discontinue catheter if patient is able to void spontaneously. *Decreased time of use prevents injury and infection.*

S ▓ Do not overfill retention balloon of indwelling catheters. *Overfilling can lead to pressure on the bladder floor.*

S ▓ For intermittent catheterization, catheterize patient using clean or sterile technique. *These measures prevent infection and help maintain integrity of ureterovesical function.*

S ▓ For intermittent catheterization, consider using bladder scan. *Determines if catheterization is necessary.*

Suggested NIC Interventions

Fluid Management; Perineal Care; Self-Care Assistance: Toileting; Urinary Elimination Management

EVALUATIONS FOR EXPECTED OUTCOMES

▓ Patient does not experience injury from urinary catheter.
▓ Patient reports no discomfort with catheter placement.
▓ Patient reports understanding of treatment and self-catheterization.

▣ Patient has no complications.
▣ Patient is able to discuss impact of urologic disorder on self and family members.
▣ Patient demonstrates skill in managing urinary elimination problem.

DOCUMENTATION

▣ Observations of urologic condition and response to treatment regimen
▣ Catheter placement and patency of securing devices
▣ Need for continued use of catheter
▣ Interventions to provide supportive care and patient's response
▣ Instructions given to patient and family members on urologic problem, response to instructions, and demonstrated ability to manage patient's urinary elimination needs
▣ Patient's expression of concern about urologic problem and its impact on body image and lifestyle; patient's motivation to participate in self-care
▣ Evaluations for expected outcomes

REFERENCES

Davis, N. F., Cunnane, E. M., Mooney, R. O., Forde, J. C., & Walsh, M. T. (2018). Clinical evaluation of a safety-device to prevent urinary catheter inflation related injuries. *Urology, 115*(1), 179–183. doi:10.1016/j.urology.2018.02.026

Greenberg, J. A., Grazul-Bilska, A. T., Webb, B. T., Sun, X., & Vonnahme, K. A. (2017). A preliminary evaluation of ovine bladder mucosal damage associated with 2 different indwelling urinary catheters. *Urology, 110*(1), 248–252. doi:10.1016/j.urology.2017.08.020

Matsuo, K., Hom, M. S., Machida, H., Shabalova, A., Mostofizadeh, S., Takiuchi, T., & Muderspach, L. I. (2017). Incidence of urinary tract injury and utility of routine cystoscopy during total laparoscopic hysterectomy for endometrial cancer. *European Journal of Obstetrics & Gynecology & Reproductive Biology, 213*, 141–142. doi:10.1016/j.ejogrb.2017.03.027

Wong, J. M. K., Bortoletto, P., Tolentino, J., Jung, M. J., & Milad, M. P. (2018). Urinary tract injury in gynecologic laparoscopy for benign indication: A systematic review. *Obstetrics & Gynecology, 131*(1), 100–108. doi:10.1097/AOG.0000000000002414

Insomnia

DEFINITION

Inability to initiate or maintain sleep, which impairs functioning

RELATED FACTORS (R/T)

▣ Anxiety
▣ Average daily physical activity is less than recommended for age and gender.
▣ Caffeine consumption
▣ Caregiver role strain
▣ Consumption of sugar-sweetened beverages
▣ Depressive symptoms
▣ Discomfort
▣ Dysfunctional sleep beliefs
▣ Environmental disturbances
▣ Fear
▣ Frequent naps during the day
▣ Inadequate sleep hygiene
▣ Lifestyle incongruent with normal circadian rhythms

- Low psychological resilience
- Obesity
- Stressors
- Substance misuse
- Use of interactive electronic devices

ASSOCIATED CONDITIONS

- Chronic disease
- Hormonal change
- Pharmaceutical preparations

ASSESSMENT

- Age
- Daytime activity and work patterns
- Normal bedtime
- Travel history
- Detailed sleep history, including number of hours of sleep required
- Problems associated with sleep, including early morning awakening, difficulty falling and staying asleep, nightmares, and sleepwalking
- Quality of sleep
- Sleeping environment
- Activities associated with sleep, including bath, drink, food, and medication
- Personal beliefs about sleep
- Chemical ingestion, including alcohol, caffeine, hypnotics, and nicotine
- Use of herbal or dietary products used to facilitate sleep
- Any illness or injury related to lack of sleep

DEFINING CHARACTERISTICS

- Altered affect
- Altered attention
- Altered mood
- Early awakening
- Expresses dissatisfaction with quality of life
- Expresses dissatisfaction with sleep
- Expresses forgetfulness
- Expresses need for frequent naps during the day
- Impaired health status
- Increased absenteeism
- Increased accidents
- Insufficient physical endurance
- Nonrestorative sleep-wake cycle

EXPECTED OUTCOMES

- Patient will identify factors that prevent or disrupt sleep.
- Patient will sleep ___ hours a night.
- Patient will express feeling of being well rested.

- Patient won't show physical signs of sleep deprivation.
- Patient won't exhibit sleep-related behavioral symptoms, such as restlessness, irritability, lethargy, and disorientation.
- Patient will perform relaxation exercises at bedtime.

Suggested NOC Outcomes

Anxiety Level; Anxiety Self-Control; Fear Level; Medication Response; Personal Well-Being; Rest; Sleep; Stress Level

INTERVENTIONS AND RATIONALES

PCC ▦ Assess environmental factors that may inhibit patient's sleep. *Sleeping in strange or new environment tends to influence both rapid eye movement (REM) and non-REM sleep.*

EBP ▦ Explore sleep promoting techniques with patient *to allow patient to take an active role in treatment.*

PCC ▦ Make a detailed plan to provide patient with a set number of hours of uninterrupted sleep, if possible. *This allows consistent nursing care and gives patient uninterrupted sleep time.*

PCC ▦ Allow patient to discuss any concerns that may be preventing sleep. *Active listening helps determine causes of difficulty with sleep.*

EBP ▦ Provide patient with usual sleep aids, such as pillows, bath before sleep, food or drink, and reading materials. Milk and some high-protein snacks, such as cheese and nuts, contain L-tryptophan, a sleep promoter. *Personal hygiene and pre-bedtime rituals precede and promote sleep in many patients.*

PCC ▦ Create quiet environment conducive to sleep; for example, close curtains, adjust lighting, and close door. *These measures promote rest and sleep.*

▦ Administer medications that promote normal sleep patterns, as ordered. Monitor and record adverse effects and effectiveness. *Hypnotic agents induce sleep; tranquilizers reduce anxiety.*

EBP ▦ Promote involvement in diversional activities or exercise program during day. Discuss and relate exercise and activity to improved sleep. Discourage excessive napping. *Activity and exercise promote sleep by increasing fatigue and relaxation.*

PCC ▦ Ask patient to keep a sleep log describing sleep disturbances and the impact on daytime functioning, such as with cognition, mood, coping skills, and physical complaints. *This allows increased awareness of potential sleep disturbances.*

PCC ▦ Ask patient to describe in specific terms each morning the quality of sleep during the previous night. *This helps detect sleep-related behavioral symptoms.*

EBP ▦ Educate patient about such relaxation and stress-reducing techniques as guided imagery, progressive muscle relaxation, aromatherapy, relaxation music, and meditation. *Purposeful relaxation efforts usually help promote sleep.*

EBP ▦ Instruct patient to eliminate or reduce caffeine and alcohol intake and avoid foods that interfere with sleep (e.g., spicy foods). *Foods and beverages containing caffeine consumed fewer than 4 hours before bedtime may interfere with sleep. Alcohol disrupts normal sleep, especially when ingested immediately before retiring.*

Suggested NIC Interventions

Calming Technique; Coping Enhancement; Energy Management; Medication Management; Positioning; Simple Relaxation Therapy; Sleep Enhancement

- Patient identifies factors that prevent or disrupt sleep.
- Patient sleeps specified number of hours nightly.
- Patient expresses feeling well rested.
- Patient doesn't exhibit signs of sleep deprivation.
- Patient doesn't exhibit sleep-related behavioral symptoms.
- Patient reports changing diet habits and making lifestyle changes to promote sleep.
- Patient performs relaxation exercises at bedtime.

- Patient's complaints about sleep disturbances
- Patient's report of improvement in sleep patterns
- Observations of physical and behavioral sleep-related disturbances
- Interventions to alleviate sleep disturbances
- Patient's response to nursing interventions
- Evaluations for expected outcomes

REFERENCES

Duman, M., & Taşhan, S. T. (2018). The effect of sleep hygiene education and relaxation exercises on insomnia among postmenopausal women: A randomized clinical trial. *International Journal of Nursing Practice, 24*(4), 1–8. doi:10.1111/ijn.12650

Maurer, L. F., Espie, C. A., & Kyle, S. D. (2018). How does sleep restriction therapy for insomnia work? A systematic review of mechanistic evidence and the introduction of the Triple-R model. *Sleep Medicine Reviews, 42*, 127–138. doi:10.1016/j.smrv.2018.07.005

Miner, B., Gill, T. M., Yaggi, H. K., Redeker, N. S., Van Ness, P. H., Han, L., & Fragoso, C. A. V. (2018). Insomnia in community-living persons with advanced age. *Journal of the American Geriatrics Society, 66*(8), 1592–1597. doi:10.1111/jgs.15414

Reynolds, M. E., & Cone, P. H. (2018). Managing adult insomnia confidently. *Journal for Nurse Practitioners, 14*(10), 718–724. doi:10.1016/j.nurpra.2018.08.019

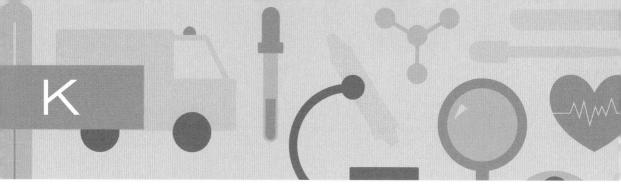

K

Deficient Knowledge

DEFINITION

Absence of cognitive information related to a specific topic, or its acquisition

RELATED FACTORS (R/T)

- Anxiety
- Cognitive dysfunction
- Depressive symptoms
- Inadequate access to resources
- Inadequate awareness of resources
- Inadequate commitment to learning
- Inadequate information
- Inadequate interest in learning
- Inadequate knowledge of resources
- Inadequate participation in care planning
- Inadequate trust in health care professional
- Low self-efficacy
- Misinformation
- Neurobehavioral manifestations

ASSOCIATED CONDITIONS

- Depression
- Developmental disabilities
- Neurocognitive disorders

ASSESSMENT

- Psychosocial status, including age; learning ability (affective, cognitive, and psychomotor domains); decision-making ability; developmental stage; financial resources; interest in learning, knowledge and skills related to current health problem; obstacles to learning, support systems (willingness and ability of others to help patient), and usual coping pattern
- Neurologic status, including level of consciousness, memory, mental status, and orientation

DEFINING CHARACTERISTICS

- Inaccurate follow-through of instruction
- Inaccurate performance on a test
- Inaccurate statements about a topic
- Inappropriate behavior

- Patient will be motivated to learn.
- Patient will communicate need to gain knowledge and establish learning goals.
- Patient will state or demonstrate understanding of what has been taught.
- Patient will demonstrate ability to perform new health-related behaviors as they're taught and will list specific skills and realistic target dates for each.
- Patient will set realistic learning goals.
- Patient will state intention to make needed changes in lifestyle, including seeking help from health professional, when needed.

Suggested NOC Outcomes

Client Satisfaction: Teaching; Cognition; Concentration; Information Processing; Knowledge: Disease Process; Knowledge: Health Behaviors; Knowledge: Health Resources; Knowledge: Illness Care; Motivation; Stress Level

PCC ▦ Find a quiet, private environment for teaching *patient and support person. Freed from distractions, patient and support person will learn more effectively.*

PCC ▦ Establish environment of mutual trust and respect to enhance learning. *Comfort with growing self-awareness, ability to share this awareness with others, receptiveness to new experiences, and consistency between actions and words form the basis of trusting relationship.*

PCC ▦ Communicate openly and honestly with patient and encourage parents and others to visit regularly *to enhance child's feelings of trust in the staff and comfort within the hospital environment.*

PCC ▦ Assess patient's level of knowledge *to determine whether patient requires the basic information or reinforcement of previous learning.*

PCC ▦ Identify patient's level of cognitive, physical, linguistic, and perceptual development *to establish appropriate learning goals.*

PCC ▦ Negotiate with patient to develop goals for learning. *Involving patient in planning meaningful goals encourages follow-through.*

EBP ▦ Select teaching strategies (such as discussion, demonstration, role-playing, and visual materials) appropriate for patient's individual learning style (specify) *to enhance teaching effectiveness.*

PCC ▦ Consider patient's life experiences when developing a teaching plan. *New information is easier to assimilate if it's built on existing knowledge.*

EBP ▦ Provide written materials explaining skills patient is trying to develop and facts patient must remember. *Words and pictures will reinforce things the patient must learn to care for self.*

EBP ▦ Encourage patient to use memory aids, such as preset alarms on a watch, a calendar for noting scheduled appointments, and a small notepad for recording questions or symptoms, *to help compensate for memory lapses.*

EBP ▦ Limit the length of each teaching session *to avoid information overload.*

PCC ▦ Don't place unrealistic demands on patient *to avoid exacerbating feelings of inadequacy and anxiety.*

PCC ▦ Have patient incorporate learned skills into daily routine during hospitalization (specify skills). *This allows patient to practice new skills and receive feedback.*

▦ Answer questions in terms patient can understand. If patient can't understand, refer patient to the physician *to ensure patient's right to informed consent is protected.*

EBP ▦ Provide all equipment needed for each self-care measure patient must learn. *This reduces frustration, aids learning, and minimizes dependence by promoting self-care.*

PCC ▦ When teaching self-care measures, go slowly and repeat frequently. Offer small amounts of information, and present it in various ways. *By building cognition, patient will be better able to complete self-care measures.*

- Have patient practice each task. Provide positive reinforcement each time patient performs task correctly. *This encourages desired behavior.*

PCC ■ Encourage family members to participate in patient's learning process *to help create an encouraging, therapeutic climate after discharge.*

EBP ■ Have patient give return demonstration of any skills taught. *This provides hands-on experience with equipment, builds confidence, and encourages compliance.*

PCC ■ Regularly discuss progress toward goal achievement with the child and family members. Make changes in the care plan as necessary. *Evaluation helps to reinforce effective learning techniques and identify ineffective techniques. It allows analysis of progress and redirection of activities as necessary.*

T&C ■ Provide patient with names and telephone numbers of resource people or organizations *to provide continuity of care and follow-up after discharge.*

T&C ■ As needed, arrange for interpreter. *Patient who doesn't speak English may understand health-related behaviors, but may need interpreter to express them.*

T&C ■ Refer family members to outside agencies, such as a home health care organization, for assistance after patient's discharge. *This ensures continuity of care and assistance with follow-up after discharge.*

Suggested NIC Interventions

Behavior Management; Behavior Modification; Decision-Making Support; Energy Management; Discharge Planning; Health Education; Family Support; Health Education; Learning Facilitation; Learning Readiness Enhancement; Support System Enhancement

EVALUATIONS FOR EXPECTED OUTCOMES

- Patient expresses motivation to learn.
- Patient expresses desire to overcome lack of knowledge.
- Patient states understanding of all that has been learned.
- Patient demonstrates newly learned health-related behaviors.
- Patient develops realistic learning goals and performs new skills by target date.
- Patient identifies specific changes in lifestyle needed to promote optimal health.

DOCUMENTATION

- Progress made by patient in learning each specific task
- Patient's statements of information and skills that patient knows and doesn't know
- Expressions of need to know and motivation to learn
- Learning objectives
- Methods used to teach patient
- Information imparted
- Skills demonstrated
- Patient's responses to teaching
- Family members' participation in learning process
- Referrals to outside agencies
- Evaluations for expected outcomes

REFERENCES

Crawford, T., Roger, P., & Candlin, S. (2018). Supporting patient education using schema theory: A discourse analysis. *Collegian, 25*(5), 501–507. doi:10.1016/j.colegn.2017.12.004

Day, D. M., & Edson, W. N. (2017). Postpartum patient teaching success. *JOGNN: Journal of Obstetric, Gynecologic & Neonatal Nursing, 46*, S48–S49. doi:10.1016/j.jogn.2017.04.094

Docherty, A., Warkentin, P., Borgen, J., Garthe, K., Fischer, K. L., & Najjar, R. H. (2018). Enhancing student engagement: Innovative strategies for intentional learning. *Journal of Professional Nursing, 34*(6), 470–474. doi:/10.1016/j.profnurs.2018.05.001

Klingbeil, C., & Gibson, C. (2018). The teach back project: A system-wide evidence based practice implementation. *Journal of Pediatric Nursing, 42*, 81–85. doi:10.1016/j.pedn.2018.06.002

Readiness for Enhanced Knowledge

DEFINITION

A pattern of cognitive information related to a specific topic, or its acquisition, which can be strengthened

ASSESSMENT

- Age and gender
- Psychosocial status, including age; learning ability (affective, cognitive, and psychomotor domains); decision-making ability; developmental stage; financial resources; interest in learning; knowledge and skills related to current health problem; obstacles to learning; support systems (willingness and ability of others to help patient); and usual coping pattern
- Neurologic status, including level of consciousness, memory, mental status, and orientation
- Health problems, restrictions, and limitations
- Roles in family and community
- Socioeconomic factors
- Cultural background

DEFINING CHARACTERISTICS

Expresses a desire to enhance learning

EXPECTED OUTCOMES

- Patient will identify new sources for enhancing knowledge in the topic of interest.
- Patient will make use of all relevant resources to enhance knowledge.
- Patient will ask questions where new information needs clarification.
- Patient will begin practicing new behaviors gleaned from enhanced knowledge.

Suggested NOC Outcomes

Knowledge: Health Promotion

INTERVENTIONS AND RATIONALES

PCC ▪ Determine exactly what patient knows and to what level patient wishes to and can enhance knowledge and understanding. *This information will assist the nurse in planning with the patient.*

EBP ▪ Assist patient in acquiring knowledge necessary for positive decision-making. *Making positive decisions that produce benefits will reinforce health-seeking behaviors.*

EBP   ▪ Provide books and videos that will help patient's quest for enhanced knowledge. *Supplying some materials directly may motivate patient to want to search further.*

T&C   ▪ Direct patient to use other sources for information, such as libraries, the internet, or professional organizations. *An independent search results in patient developing confidence in own ability to go much deeper into the area of interest.*

PCC   ▪ Be available to answer questions and correct misconceptions for patient *in order to enhance the effectiveness of what patient is learning.*

PCC   ▪ Provide feedback to patient for incorporating new knowledge into lifestyle. *This reinforces behaviors resulting from enhanced knowledge.*

PCC   ▪ Work with patient to help develop a plan that takes into account the resources identified as being helpful to the patient in attaining an optimal level of self-care. *This will help patient maintain control of own decision-making about health while using the input of others whom the patient trusts.*

Suggested NIC Interventions

Learning Facilitation; Learning Readiness Enhancement

EVALUATIONS FOR EXPECTED OUTCOMES

▪ Patient expresses motivation for enhanced knowledge.
▪ Patient expresses desire to increase knowledge.
▪ Patient states understanding of all that has been learned.
▪ Patient uses various resources to achieve success.
▪ Patient questions things that aren't clearly understood.
▪ Patient practices skills derived from enhanced knowledge.

DOCUMENTATION

▪ Patient's current level of knowledge and skill
▪ Patient's expressions of motivation to enhance knowledge
▪ Resources used to enhance knowledge
▪ Patient's response to learning resources
▪ Evaluations for expected outcomes

REFERENCES

Chung, L. M. Y., & Fong, S. S. M. (2018). Role of behavioural feedback in nutrition education for enhancing nutrition knowledge and improving nutritional behaviour among adolescents. *Asia Pacific Journal of Clinical Nutrition, 27*(2), 466–472. doi:/10.6133/apjcn.042017.03

Crawford, T., Roger, P., & Candlin, S. (2018). Supporting patient education using schema theory: A discourse analysis. *Collegian, 25*(5), 501–507. doi:10.1016/j.colegn.2017.12.004

Walsh, J. C. (2017). A nurse led clinic's contribution to patient education and promoting self-care in heart failure patients: A systematic review. *International Journal of Integrated Care (IJIC), 17*, 1–2. doi:10.5334/ijic.3812

Wigg, J. (2017). Enhancing lymphoedema patients' learning through education. *British Journal of Nursing, 26*(4), 204–206. doi:10.12968/bjon.2017.26.4.204

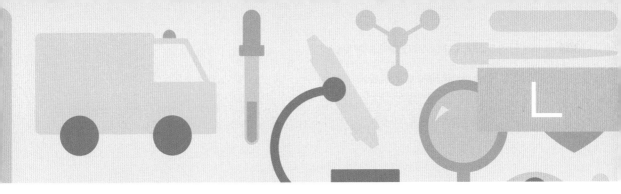

Risk for Latex Allergy Reaction

Susceptible to a hypersensitive reaction to natural latex rubber products or latex reactive foods, which may compromise health

- Inadequate knowledge about avoidance of relevant allergens
- Inattentive to potential environmental latex exposure
- Inattentive to potential exposure to latex reactive foods

- Asthma
- Atopy
- Food allergy
- Hypersensitivity to natural latex rubber protein
- Multiple surgical procedures
- Poinsettia plant allergy
- Urinary bladder diseases

- Age, gender, and weight
- Occupation
- Current health status, including vital signs, respiratory status, and integumentary status
- Health history, including drug, food, or pollen allergies; surgical history; chronic disease such as spina bifida; and previous local or systemic allergic reactions
- Laboratory studies, such as immunoglobulin E level, complete blood count, radioallergosorbent test, and scratch test

- Patient's vital signs, especially respirations, will remain within normal limits.
- Patient's skin will remain free from erythema, edema, urticaria, and breakdown.
- Patient's nasal passages and laryngeal area will remain clear and free from edema and secretions.
- Patient and family members will express understanding of risk of latex allergy.
- Patient and family members will state intention to take precautions to avoid contact with latex products.

Suggested NOC Outcomes

Allergy Response: Localized; Immune Hypersensitivity Response; Knowledge: Health Behavior; Risk Control; Risk Detection

INTERVENTIONS AND RATIONALES

S ▪ Conduct a nursing assessment to identify factors in patient's life that set up a risk for allergy to latex products. *There may be occupational exposure or consumption of certain foods that patient has not thought to attribute to the symptoms he or she is experiencing.*

S ▪ Remove all products containing latex from patient's room *to reduce risk of allergic reaction.*

S ▪ Use only nonlatex products when caring for patient *to reduce risk of latex allergy reaction in patient.*

T&C ▪ Make sure all personnel are aware of the risk of latex allergy and refrain from using latex products during diagnostic procedures. *Communication with other health care personnel allows for continuity of care and reduces the risk of latex allergy reaction.*

EBP ▪ Educate patient and family about the risk of latex allergy *to prevent allergic reaction due to contact with latex products.*

EBP ▪ Explain that although some reactions to latex are relatively minor (such as sneezing and runny nose), others are life-threatening. *This will foster awareness of the serious nature of risk.*

EBP ▪ Educate patient and family about the symptoms of allergic reaction and the need for quick treatment if symptoms appear. *Rapid response to allergic reaction may help prevent complications, such as skin infection (with local reaction) and respiratory failure (with systemic reaction).*

EBP ▪ Give patient and family a list of household items containing latex and emphasize the importance of avoiding these. Tell them about nonlatex product substitutes. *Prevention is the foundation of treatment of latex allergy.*

T&C ▪ Emphasize the need to inform all health care providers—including emergency medical service—about patient's latex sensitivity. Stress the importance of wearing a medical identification bracelet that specifies latex sensitivity *to prevent future contact and allergic reactions.*

PCC ▪ Provide emotional support to help patient cope with stress. *Fear of latex exposure can cause a high level of stress in a latex-sensitive patient. Some patients are afraid to seek medical help for fear of latex exposure.*

Suggested NIC Interventions

Allergy Management; Environmental Management; Health System Guidance; Latex Precautions; Risk Identification; Teaching: Individual

EVALUATIONS FOR EXPECTED OUTCOMES

▪ Patient's vital signs, especially respirations, remain within normal limits.
▪ Patient's skin remains free from erythema, edema, urticaria, and breakdown.
▪ Patient's nasal passages and laryngeal area remain clear and free from edema and secretions.
▪ Patient and family members express understanding of risk of latex allergy.
▪ Patient and family members state intention to take precautions to avoid contact with latex products.

- Results of nursing assessment
- Presence of risk factors
- Communication of risk factors to health care personnel involved in care or diagnostic studies of patient
- Teaching provided to patient and family members about risk factors and symptoms of allergic reactions
- Patient's and family members' statements indicating understanding of risk factors and symptoms of allergic reactions
- Evaluations for expected outcomes

REFERENCES

Carstensen, C. (2018). When a child is diagnosed with severe allergies: An autoethnographic account. *Nursing Praxis in New Zealand*, *34*(2), 6–16.

Hohler, S. E. (2017). Keeping children with latex allergies safe. *Nursing*, *47*(10), 1–5. doi:10.1097/01. NURSE.0000524760.51000.bd

Iio, M., Hamaguchi, M., Nagata, M., & Yoshida, K. (2018). Stressors of school-age children with allergic diseases: A qualitative study. *Journal of Pediatric Nursing*, *42*, e73–e78. doi:10.1016/j. pedn.2018.04.009

Liberatore, K. (2019). Protecting patients with latex allergies. *AJN American Journal of Nursing*, *119*(1), 60–63. doi:10.1097/01.NAJ.0000552616.96652.72

McBride, D. L. (2019). Life-threatening allergic reactions increasing among children. *Journal of Pediatric Nursing*, *44*, 127–129. doi:10.1016/j.pedn.2018.05.013

Sedentary Lifestyle

DEFINITION

An acquired mode of behavior that is characterized by waking hour activities that require low energy expenditure

RELATED FACTORS (R/T)

- Conflict between cultural beliefs and health practices
- Decreased activity tolerance
- Difficulty adapting areas for physical activity
- Exceeds screen time recommendations for age
- Impaired physical mobility
- Inadequate interest in physical activity
- Inadequate knowledge of consequences of sedentarism
- Inadequate knowledge of health benefits associated with physical activity
- Inadequate motivation for physical activity
- Inadequate resources for physical activity
- Inadequate role models
- Inadequate social support
- Inadequate time management skills
- Inadequate training for physical exercise
- Low self-efficacy
- Low self-esteem
- Negative affect toward physical activity
- Pain

- Parenting practices that inhibit child's physical activity
- Perceived physical disability
- Perceived safety risk

ASSESSMENT

- Age, gender, and cognitive status
- Daytime activity and work patterns
- Possible precipitating factors
- Height, weight, body mass index (BMI), and muscle and weight-bearing
- Underlying conditions or medications
- Overall quality and duration of sleep
- Situational daily stressors
- Nutritional status and opportunity for exercise and social interaction
- Convenience of exercise facilities and safety of environment
- Recent changes in health status or lifestyle
- Dietary and medication history
- Culturally determined expectations of body image or dietary intake
- Risk assessment for substance abuse, smoking, and high-risk behaviors
- Disabilities

DEFINING CHARACTERISTICS

- Average daily physical activity is less than recommended for age and gender
- Chooses a daily routine lacking physical exercise
- Does not exercise during leisure time
- Expresses preference for low physical activity
- Performs majority of tasks in a reclining posture
- Performs majority of tasks in a sitting posture
- Physical deconditioning

EXPECTED OUTCOMES

- Older adults will maintain independent living status with reduced risk for falling.
- Patient will identify barriers to increasing physical activity level.
- Patient will identify health benefits to increasing physical activity level.
- Patient will increase physical activity and limit inactive forms of diversion, such as television and computer games.
- Patient will seek professional consultation to develop an appropriate plan to increase physical activity.
- Patient will identify factors that enhance readiness for sleep.
- Patient will demonstrate readiness for enhanced sleep through the use of appropriate sleep hygiene measures.
- Patient's amount of sleep and rapid eye movement (REM) sleep will be congruent with developmental needs.
- Patient will express a feeling of being rested after sleep.
- Patient will increase lean muscle and bone strength and decrease body fat.
- Patient will demonstrate weight control and, if appropriate, weight loss.
- Patient will demonstrate enhanced psychological well-being and reduced risk of depression.
- Patient will have reduced depression and anxiety and an improved mood.
- Patient with certain chronic, disabling conditions will have increased ability to perform activities of daily living (ADLs).

Suggested NOC Outcomes

Activity Intolerance; Adherent Behavior; Client Satisfaction: Teaching; Endurance; Energy Conservation; Health-Promoting Behavior; Immobility Consequences: Physiological; Immobility Consequences: Psycho-cognitive; Knowledge: Diet; Knowledge: Rest; Knowledge: Risk Control; Knowledge: Sleep

INTERVENTIONS AND RATIONALES

PCC ▪ Provide counseling tailored to patient's risk factors, needs, preferences, and abilities *to enhance emotional well-being and motivation for physical activity.*

EBP ▪ Discuss behavioral risk factors in lack of motivation to increase physical activity, such as ingestion of carbohydrates, caffeine, nicotine, alcohol, sedatives, and hypnotics and fluid intake, *to focus behavior on positive outcomes of increased physical activity.*

PCC ▪ Instruct patient to keep a daily activity and dietary log *to help obtain a more objective view of patient's behavior.*

PCC ▪ Identify barriers and enhancers to increasing physical activity, including time management, access to facilities, and safe environments in which to be active. *Breaking down barriers and building opportunities for activity increase the probability of consistent physical activity.*

EBP ▪ Educate patient about how sedentary lifestyle increases cardiovascular risk factors (such as hypertension, dyslipidemia, hyperinsulinemia, insulin resistance) *to motivate patient to be more active.*

▪ Discuss the need for activity that will improve psychosocial well-being.

PCC ▪ Develop a behavior modification plan based on patient's condition, history, and precipitating factors *to maximize physical activity and compliance.*

EBP ▪ Provide education about community resources available to increase physical activity *to decrease barriers to activity.*

EBP ▪ Teach exercises for increasing strength and endurance *to maintain mobility and prevent musculoskeletal degeneration.*

EBP ▪ Educate patient about using the bedroom only for sleep or sexual activity and avoiding other activities such as watching television, reading, and eating *to increase sleep efficiency.*

Suggested NIC Interventions

Activity Therapy; Body Mechanics Promotion; Energy Management; Risk Identification; Sleep Enhancement; Teaching: Prescribed Activity/Exercise

EVALUATIONS FOR EXPECTED OUTCOMES

▪ Patient seeks professional consultation to develop a plan to increase physical activity and limit inactive forms of diversion, such as watching television.

▪ Patient's BMI is appropriate for patient's height and weight.

▪ Patient verbalizes how sedentary lifestyle impacts morbidity and mortality.

▪ Patient reduces high-risk behaviors.

▪ Patient demonstrates increased ability to perform ADLs and, if appropriate, to maintain independent living status.

▪ Patient demonstrates motivation to increase physical activity.

▪ Patient demonstrates readiness for enhanced sleep through the use of appropriate sleep hygiene measures.

▪ Patient's amount of sleep and REM sleep matches developmental needs.

▨ Patient demonstrates behaviors of psychological well-being and reduced risk for developing depression.
▨ Patient experiences reduced depression and anxiety and improved mood.
▨ Change in sedentary lifestyle is congruent with cultural expectations.
▨ Facility policies and staff behaviors reflect opportunities to provide physical activity for patients and limit inactive forms of diversion, such as television watching and computer games.

DOCUMENTATION

▨ Daytime activity and work patterns
▨ Behavioral modification plan
▨ Dietary and drug history
▨ Height, weight, and BMI
▨ High-risk behavior assessment
▨ Sleep hygiene behaviors
▨ Culturally determined expectations
▨ Nursing interventions to increase patient's physical activity
▨ Response to nursing interventions
▨ Evaluations for expected outcomes

REFERENCES

Bramante, C. T., King, M. M., Story, M., Whitt-Glover, M. C., & Barr-Anderson, D. J. (2018). Worksite physical activity breaks: Perspectives on feasibility of implementation. *Work, 59*(4), 491–499. doi:10.3233/WOR-182704

Donaldson-Feilder, E., Lewis, R., Pavey, L., Jones, B., Green, M., & Webster, A. (2017). Perceived barriers and facilitators of exercise and healthy dietary choices: A study of employees and managers within a large transport organisation. *Health Education Journal, 76*(6), 661–675. doi:10.1177/0017896917712296

Giusti Rossi, P., Carnaz, L., Bertollo, W. L., & de Medeiros Takahashi, A. C. (2018). Causes of drop out from a physical exercise supervised program specific to older adults. *Fisioterapia Em Movimento, 31*(1), 1–11. doi:10.1590/1980-5918.031.AO33

Said, M. A., Abdelmoneem, M., Almaqhawi, A., Kotob, A. A. H., Alibrahim, M. C., & Bougmiza, I. (2018). Multidisciplinary approach to obesity: Aerobic or resistance physical exercise? *Journal of Exercise Science & Fitness, 16*(3), 118–123. doi:10.1016/j.jesf.2018.11.001

Risk for Impaired Liver Function

DEFINITION

Susceptible to a decrease in liver function, which may compromise health

RISK FACTORS

Substance misuse

ASSOCIATED CONDITIONS

▨ Human immunodeficiency virus (HIV) coinfection
▨ Pharmaceutical agent
▨ Viral infection

- Risk management
- Pharmacologic function
- Fluid and electrolyte status, including blood urea nitrogen level, creatinine level, intake and output, mucous membranes, serum electrolyte levels, and skin turgor

- Patient will state effects of environmental and ingested chemicals and substances on health and liver function.
- Patient will work with industry managers and with public health officials to lower or eliminate the presence of environmental chemicals and substances in work or living environment.
- Patient will have liver function indicators within normal limits.
- Patient will modify lifestyle and behaviors to avoid risk of hepatic dysfunction and inflammation.
- Patient will manage concurrent disease processes that impact hepatic function.
- Patient will acknowledge the impact of medications on hepatic function.
- Patient will observe measures to avoid the spread of infection to self and to others.
- Patient will maintain long-term follow-up for chronic illness with health care provider.
- Patient will optimize nutritional intake for needs.

Suggested NOC Outcomes

Health-Promoting Behavior; Risk Control—Alcohol; Risk Control—Drug Use; Safe Home Environment; Substance Addiction Consequences

S - Assist patient and family in assessing workplace and home environments for potential hepatotoxic substances *to increase patient's awareness of hazards in the environment and to lower potential for hepatic injury.*

S - Monitor for clinical manifestations of hepatic inflammation and dysfunction *to notify physician in order to initiate treatment if liver function is compromised.* Clinical manifestations may include fatigue, depression or mood changes, anorexia, right upper quadrant tenderness, pruritus, jaundice, bruising, or nontraumatic bleeding.

S - Monitor customary clinical laboratory tests *to alert the health care provider of the status of the immune/inflammatory response, the degree of hepatic metabolic dysfunction, and the impact of concurrent disorders on liver function.* Clinical laboratory tests include complete blood cell count: lower red blood cell count, elevated WBC (increased immunocyte and inflammatory responses); basic metabolic panel: altered electrolyte balance, elevated glucose, elevated blood urea nitrogen and creatinine level, elevated HbA_{1c}; hepatic plasma markers: elevated liver enzymes (alanine aminotransferase, aspartate aminotransferase, and γ-glutamyltranspeptidase); positive immunoassays *for pathogen and viral antigens*; elevated ammonia; elevated bilirubin; low coagulation factors; low total protein/albumin; elevated lipid panel.

- Carry out postprocedure measures as ordered *to identify and/or minimize complications.*

EBP - Teach patient about the following: perform hand hygiene before and after personal hygiene and care; cover draining and nonhealing wounds; report to care provider;

inform others of infectious condition *so that each observes barrier precautions*; adhere to prescribed plan of care and treatment with immune system modifiers (antibiotics, antivirals, interferon, others); maintain a balanced nutritional diet intake. *These measures minimize patient's risk for self-infection and spread of infection and allow patient to help modify lifestyle to maintain optimum health level for self and for others.*

T&C ▥ Along with health care team, prepare patient for and later evaluate the results of liver biopsy, and provide explanation to patient and family. *Patient and family need understanding of purpose for and implications of results obtained from a liver biopsy. This support and education help patient understand rationale for plan of treatment and genetic counseling for genetically linked hepatic disorders.*

PCC ▥ Provide a nonjudgmental attitude toward patient's lifestyle choices *to promote feelings of self-worth.*

T&C ▥ Refer patient to counseling and therapy to address lifestyle choices and risk behaviors. *Modification of behaviors will provide risk avoidance for drug and alcohol abuse and exposure to body substance pathogen infection.*

Suggested NIC Interventions

Behavioral Modification; Environment Risk Protection; Infection Protection; Risk Identification; Risk Identification—Genetic; Self-Modification Assistance; Sports Injury Prevention; Surveillance

EVALUATIONS FOR EXPECTED OUTCOMES

▥ Patient verbalizes impact of contaminants and exposure to chemicals on health.
▥ Patient follows prescribed treatment plan.
▥ Patient expresses feelings about condition and its effect on family.
▥ Patient describes response to procedures.

DOCUMENTATION

▥ Liver function tests
▥ Interventions to provide supportive care and patient's response to supportive care
▥ Instructions given to patient and family members; return demonstration of knowledge and skills needed to carry out postprocedure regimen
▥ Patient's expression of concern about hepatic function and motivation to participate in self-care
▥ Evaluations for expected outcomes

REFERENCES

Assi, N., Gunter, M. J., Thomas, D. C., Leitzmann, M., Stepien, M., Chajès, V., ... Jenab, M. (2018). Metabolic signature of healthy lifestyle and its relation with risk of hepatocellular carcinoma in a large European cohort. *American Journal of Clinical Nutrition, 108*(1), 117–126. doi:10.1093/ajcn/nqy074

Greenslade, L. (2017). Providing high-quality care for patients with liver disease. *British Journal of Nursing, 26*(13), 739. doi:10.12968/bjon.2017.26.13.739

Melendez-Rosado, J., Alsaad, A., Stancampiano, F. F., & Palmer, W. C. (2018). Abnormal liver enzymes. *Gastroenterology Nursing, 41*(6), 487–507. doi:10.1097/SGA.0000000000000346

Presky, J., Webzell, I., Murrells, T., Heaton, N., & Lau-Walker, M. (2018). Understanding alcohol-related liver disease patients' illness beliefs and views about their medicine. *British Journal of Nursing, 27*(13), 730–736. doi:10.12968/bjon.2018.27.13.730

Risk for Loneliness

DEFINITION

Susceptible to experiencing discomfort associated with a desire or need for more contact with others, which may compromise health

RISK FACTORS

- Affectional deprivation
- Emotional deprivation
- Physical isolation
- Social isolation

ASSESSMENT

- Family status, including family composition, presence of a spouse, ability of family to meet patient's physical and emotional needs, conflicts between patient's needs and family's ability to meet them, and family member's feelings of self-worth
- Psychological status, including changes in appetite, behavior, energy level, mood, motivation, self-image, self-esteem, or sleep patterns; alcohol and drug consumption; recent death, job loss, loss of loved one, or relocation; and psychiatric history
- Social status, including interpersonal skills, size of social network, quality of relationships, degree of trust in others, level of self-esteem, and ability to function in social and occupational roles
- Health history, including medical illness, disabilities, and deformities
- Spiritual status, including religious or church affiliation, description of faith and religious practices, and support network (family, clergy, and friends)

EXPECTED OUTCOMES

- Patient will identify feelings of loneliness and will express desire to socialize more.
- Patient will identify behaviors that lead to loneliness.
- Patient will identify people whose support and acceptance are most likely.
- Patient will spend time with others.
- Patient will be comfortable in social settings, will interact with peers, and will receive support from others.
- Patient will make specific plans to continue involvement with others, such as through recreational activities or social interaction groups.

Suggested NOC Outcomes

Grief Resolution; Loneliness Severity; Risk Control; Social Involvement; Social Support

INTERVENTIONS AND RATIONALES

- **PCC** Spend sufficient time with patient to allow self-expression of feelings of loneliness *to establish trusting relationship.*
- **PCC** Inform patient that you'll help with expression of feelings of loneliness and identify ways to increase social activity *to bring issue into open and help patient understand that you want to be of help.*

PCC ▦ Work with patient to identify factors and behaviors that have contributed to loneliness *to begin changing behaviors that may have alienated others.*

PCC ▦ Help patient identify feelings associated with loneliness *to lessen their impact and mobilize energy to counteract them.*

PCC ▦ Help patient curb feelings of loneliness by encouraging one-on-one interaction with others whose acceptance is likely—for example, church members or patients with similar health problems—*to promote feelings of acceptance and support.*

PCC ▦ Encourage patient to address personal needs assertively. *By being assertive, patient assumes responsibility for meeting personal needs, without anger or guilt.*

PCC ▦ As patient's comfort level improves, encourage patient to attend group activities and social functions *to promote use of social skills.*

PCC ▦ Help patient identify social activities that patient can initiate, such as becoming active in a support group or volunteer organization, *to foster feelings of control and increase social contacts.*

PCC ▦ Help patient come to terms with being viewed differently by others because of patient's illness, and explore ways of coping with their reactions *to help patient learn to cope with stigma associated with the illness.*

PCC ▦ Work with patient to establish goals for reducing feelings of loneliness after patient leaves health care setting *to focus energy on specific objectives.*

T&C ▦ Refer patient and family to social service agencies, mental health center, and appropriate support groups *to ensure continued care and maintain social involvement.*

Suggested NIC Interventions

Activity Therapy; Anxiety Reduction; Counseling; Emotional Support; Energy Management; Socialization Enhancement; Spiritual Support; Visitation Facilitation

EVALUATIONS FOR EXPECTED OUTCOMES

▦ Patient expresses feelings of loneliness.
▦ Patient describes behaviors that lead to loneliness.
▦ Patient lists at least _____ (specify) people whose support and acceptance are most likely.
▦ Patient initiates conversations with peers.
▦ Patient participates in group activities.
▦ Patient describes plans to continue involvement with others.

DOCUMENTATION

▦ Patient's statements of loneliness
▦ Observations of patient's behaviors and problems associated with loneliness
▦ Patient's choice of activities to end isolation
▦ Teaching of new coping methods
▦ Goals established by patient
▦ Evidence of efforts to use new coping mechanisms
▦ Referral
▦ Evaluations for expected outcomes

REFERENCES

Chang, E. C., Chang, O. D., Lucas, A. G., Li, M., Beavan, C. B., Eisner, R. S., ... Hirsch, J. K. (2019). Depression, loneliness, and suicide risk among Latino college students: A Test of a Psychosocial Interaction Model. *Social Work, 64*(1), 51–60. doi:10.1093/sw/swy052

Cheung, J. C. S., Chan, K. H. W., Lui, Y. W., Tsui, M. S., & Chan, C. (2018). Psychological well-being and adolescents' internet addiction: A school-based cross-sectional study in Hong Kong. *Child & Adolescent Social Work Journal, 35*(5), 477–487. doi:10.1007/s10560-018-0543-7

Kovaleva, M., Spangler, S., Clevenger, C., & Hepburn, K. (2018). Chronic stress, social isolation, and perceived loneliness in dementia caregivers. *Journal of Psychosocial Nursing & Mental Health Services, 56*(10), 36–43. doi:10.3928/02793695-20180329-04

Nyatanga, B. (2017). Being lonely and isolated: Challenges for palliative care. *British Journal of Community Nursing, 22*(7), 360. doi:10.12968/bjcn.2017.22.7.360

Paque, K., Bastiaens, H., Van Bogaert, P., & Dilles, T. (2018). Living in a nursing home: A phenomenological study exploring residents' loneliness and other feelings. *Scandinavian Journal of Caring Sciences, 32*(4), 1477–1484. doi:10.1111/scs.12599

Ineffective Lymphedema Self-Management

DEFINITION

Unsatisfactory management of symptoms, treatment regimen, physical, psychosocial, and spiritual consequences and lifestyle changes inherent in living with edema related to obstruction or disorders of lymph vessels or nodes

RELATED FACTORS (R/T)

- Cognitive dysfunction
- Competing demands
- Competing lifestyle preferences
- Conflict between health behaviors and social norms
- Decreased perceived quality of life
- Difficulty accessing community resources
- Difficulty managing complex treatment regimen
- Difficulty navigating complex health care systems
- Difficulty with decision-making
- Inadequate commitment to a plan of action
- Inadequate health literacy
- Inadequate knowledge of treatment regimen
- Inadequate number of cues to action
- Inadequate role models
- Inadequate social support
- Limited ability to perform aspects of treatment regimen
- Low self-efficacy
- Negative feelings toward treatment regimen
- Neurobehavioral manifestations
- Nonacceptance of condition
- Perceived barrier to treatment regimen
- Perceived social stigma associated with condition
- Unrealistic perception of seriousness of condition
- Unrealistic perception of susceptibility to sequelae
- Unrealistic perception of treatment benefit

ASSOCIATED CONDITIONS

- Chemotherapy
- Chronic venous insufficiency

- Developmental disabilities
- Infections
- Invasive procedure
- Major surgery
- Neoplasms
- Obesity
- Radiotherapy
- Removal of lymph nodes
- Trauma

ASSESSMENT

- Age
- Weight
- Symptoms of affected limb; fibrosis, infection, edema, swelling
- Physical activity, range of motion, and level of discomfort
- Patient's perception of problem, coping mechanisms, problem-solving ability, decision-making competencies
- Patient's desire to perform self-management behaviors (skin care, massage, compression, exercise)
- Neurologic status, including level of consciousness; orientation; and mental, sensory, and motor status

DEFINING CHARACTERISTICS

Lymphedema Signs

- Fibrosis in affected limb
- Recurring infections
- Swelling in affected limb

Lymphedema Symptoms

- Expresses dissatisfaction with quality of life
- Reports feeling of discomfort in affected limb
- Reports feeling of heaviness in affected limb
- Reports feeling of tightness in affected limb

Behaviors

- Average daily physical activity is less than recommended for age and gender
- Inadequate manual lymph drainage
- Inadequate protection of affected area
- Inappropriate application of night-time bandaging
- Inappropriate diet
- Inappropriate skin care
- Inappropriate use of compression garments
- Inattentive to carrying heavy objects
- Inattentive to extreme temperatures
- Inattentive to lymphedema signs
- Inattentive to lymphedema symptoms
- Inattentive to sunlight exposure

- Reduced range of motion of affected limb
- Refuses to apply night-time bandages
- Refuses to use compression garments

EXPECTED OUTCOMES

- Patient will demonstrate function of affected limb.
- Patient will verbalize diminished fear and anxiety concerning task planning and execution.
- Patient will demonstrate improved physical activity.
- Patient will be free of infection.

Suggested NOC Outcomes

Comfort Status: Physical; Health Beliefs: Perceived Ability to Perform; Knowledge: Lymphedema Management; Lymphedema Severity; Self-Management: Lymphedema

INTERVENTIONS AND RATIONALES

- **EBP** Educate patient about self-management strategies: self-massage, skin care, compression garments, and exercise *provides tools to successfully manage lymphedema.*
- **EBP** Educate patient about complete decongestive therapy (CDT) performed by a certified lymphedema therapist—24-hour multilayer compression, daily manual lymphatic drainage, exercises, and skin care *to allow patient to plan for treatment and ask questions.*
- **EBP** Educate patient about maintenance compression therapy of bandages for day and night-time *to allow patient to plan for treatment and ask questions.*
- **PCC** Facilitate an exercise plan for deep breathing, general aerobic, and resistance exercises *to improve drainage and perfusion.*
- **S** Instruct patient not to lift heavy objects, wear constrictive clothing, or obtain new tattoos *to prevent trauma, injury, and infection.*
- **EBP** Educate how to perform daily massage and/or Manual Lymphatic Drainage (MLD) *to facilitate drainage.*
- **S** Assess skin daily for cracks, wounds, and signs of infection. *Prevents complications of infection.*
- **PCC** Educate patient about use low-pH moisturizer *to protect skin and prevent breakdown.*
- **PCC** Teach patient how to measure the circumference of the limb *to monitor edema.*
- **S** Refer patient to lymphedema program specialists *to provide support and disease focus.*

Suggested NIC Interventions

Anxiety Reduction; Behavior Management; Body Image Enhancement; Comfort; Protection from Infection; Self-efficacy Enhancement; Skin Surveillance

EVALUATIONS FOR EXPECTED OUTCOMES

- Patient exhibits functionality of affected limb.
- Patient verbalizes diminished fear and anxiety concerning task planning and execution.
- Patient demonstrates improved physical activity.
- Patient does not exhibit signs or symptoms of infection.
- Patient has reduced edema.

DOCUMENTATION

▦ Patient's edema, limb circumference, weight
▦ Patient's range of motion of affected limb
▦ Condition of patient's skin
▦ Patient's statements of improved self-confidence in self-management techniques
▦ Patient's stated goals for lymphedema management
▦ Evaluations for expected outcomes

REFERENCES

Bowman, C., Devesh, O., Radke, L., Francis, G. J., & Carlson, L. E. (2021). Living with leg lymphedema: Developing a novel model of quality lymphedema care for cancer survivors. *Journal of Cancer Survivorship, 15*(1), 140–150. doi:10.1007/s11764-020-00919-2

Huihui, Z., Wu, Y., Chunlan, Z., Li, W., Li, X., & Chen, L. (2021). Breast cancer-related lymphedema patient and healthcare professional experiences in lymphedema self-management: A qualitative study. *Supportive Care in Cancer, 29*(12), 8027–8044. doi:10.1007/s00520-021-06390-8

Jaimala, V. S., Jain, A. S., Sheral, T. K., & Ekta, N. P. (2021). A model for self-management of chronic filarial lymphoedema with acute dermato-lymphangio-adenitis. *BMJ Case Reports, 14*(11). doi:10.1136/bcr-2021-244721

McLaughlin, T. M., Broadhurst, J. J., Harris, C. J., McGarry, S., & Keesing, S. L. (2020). A randomized pilot study on self-management in head and neck lymphedema. *Laryngoscope Investigative Otolaryngology, 5*(5), 879–889. doi:10.1002/lio2.455

Risk for Ineffective Lymphedema Self-Management

DEFINITION

Susceptible to unsatisfactory management of symptoms, treatment regimen, physical, psychosocial and spiritual consequences and lifestyle changes inherent in living with edema related to obstruction or disorders of lymph vessels or nodes, which may compromise health

RISK FACTORS

▦ Cognitive dysfunction
▦ Competing demands
▦ Competing lifestyle preferences
▦ Conflict between health behaviors and social norms
▦ Decreased perceived quality of life
▦ Difficulty accessing community resources
▦ Difficulty managing complex treatment regimen
▦ Difficulty navigating complex health care systems
▦ Difficulty with decision-making
▦ Inadequate commitment to a plan of action
▦ Inadequate health literacy
▦ Inadequate knowledge of treatment regimen
▦ Inadequate number of cues to action
▦ Inadequate role models
▦ Inadequate social support
▦ Limited ability to perform aspects of treatment regimen
▦ Low self-efficacy
▦ Negative feelings toward treatment regimen
▦ Neurobehavioral manifestations
▦ Nonacceptance of condition
▦ Perceived barrier to treatment regimen
▦ Perceived social stigma associated with condition

- Unrealistic perception of seriousness of condition
- Unrealistic perception of susceptibility to sequelae
- Unrealistic perception of treatment benefit

ASSOCIATED CONDITIONS

- Chemotherapy
- Chronic venous insufficiency
- Developmental disabilities
- Infections
- Invasive procedure
- Major surgery
- Neoplasms
- Obesity
- Radiotherapy
- Removal of lymph nodes
- Trauma

ASSESSMENT

- Age, weight
- History of present illness
- Symptoms of affected limb; fibrosis, infection, edema, swelling
- Physical activity, range of motion, and level of discomfort
- Patient's perception of problem, coping mechanisms, problem-solving ability, decision-making competencies
- Patient's desire to perform self-management behaviors (skin care, massage, compression, exercise)
- Neurologic status, including level of consciousness; orientation; and mental, sensory, and motor status
- Sources of support: health care, social, financial, and emotional

EXPECTED OUTCOMES

- Patient will maintain function of affected limb.
- Patient will verbalize risk factors associate with lymphedema and present condition.
- Patient will verbalize realistic seriousness of condition.
- Patient will verbalize realistic perception of susceptibility to sequelae.
- Patient will verbalize realistic perception of treatment benefit.
- Patient will maintain physical activity.
- Patient will be free of infection.

Suggested NOC Outcomes

Comfort Status: Physical; Health Beliefs: Perceived Ability to Perform; Knowledge: Lymphedema Management; Lymphedema Severity; Self-Management: Lymphedema

INTERVENTIONS AND RATIONALES

`PCC` - Provide support to patient about self-management strategies: self-massage, skin care, compression garments, and exercise *provides tools to successfully manage lymphedema.*

`PCC` - Monitor need for complete decongestive therapy (CDT) performed by a certified lymphedema therapist—24-hour multilayer compression, daily manual lymphatic drainage, exercises, and skin care *to allow patient to plan for treatment and ask questions.*

EBP ▦ Educate patient about maintenance compression therapy of bandages for day and night-time *to allow patient to plan for treatment and ask questions.*

PCC ▦ Facilitate an exercise plan for deep breathing, general aerobic, and resistance exercises *to improve drainage and perfusion.*

S ▦ Instruct patient not to lift heavy objects, wear constrictive clothing, or obtain new tattoos *to prevent trauma, injury, and infection.*

EBP ▦ Educate how to perform daily massage and/or Manual Lymphatic Drainage (MLD) *to facilitate drainage.*

S ▦ Assess skin daily for cracks, wounds, and signs of infection. *Prevents complications of infection.*

PCC ▦ Educate patient about use low-pH moisturizer *to protect skin and prevent breakdown.*

PCC ▦ Teach patient how to measure the circumference of the limb *to monitor edema.*

T&C ▦ Refer patient to lymphedema program specialists *to provide support and disease focus.*

Suggested NIC Interventions

Anxiety Reduction; Behavior Management; Body Image Enhancement; Comfort; Protection from Infection; Self-efficacy Enhancement; Skin Surveillance

EVALUATIONS FOR EXPECTED OUTCOMES

▦ Patient verbalizes realistic seriousness of condition.

▦ Patient verbalizes realistic perception of susceptibility to sequelae.

▦ Patient verbalizes realistic perception of treatment benefit.

▦ Patient verbalizes diminished fear and anxiety concerning task planning and execution.

▦ Patient does not exhibit signs or symptoms of infection.

▦ Patient has reduced edema.

DOCUMENTATION

▦ Activities and management performed by patient

▦ Patient's edema, limb circumference, weight

▦ Patient's range of motion of affected limb

▦ Condition of patient's skin

▦ Patient's statements of improved self-confidence in self-management techniques

▦ Patient's stated goals for lymphedema management

▦ Evaluations for expected outcomes

REFERENCES

Bowman, C., Devesh, O., Radke, L., Francis, G. J., & Carlson, L. E. (2021). Living with leg lymphedema: Developing a novel model of quality lymphedema care for cancer survivors. *Journal of Cancer Survivorship, 15*(1), 140–150. doi:10.1007/s11764-020-00919-2

Huihui, Z., Wu, Y., Chunlan, Z., Li, W., Li, X., & Chen, L. (2021). Breast cancer-related lymphedema patient and healthcare professional experiences in lymphedema self-management: A qualitative study. *Supportive Care in Cancer, 29*(12), 8027–8044. doi:10.1007/s00520-021-06390-8

Jaimala, V. S., Jain, A. S., Sheral, T. K., & Ekta, N. P. (2021). A model for self-management of chronic filarial lymphoedema with acute dermato-lymphangio-adenitis. *BMJ Case Reports, 14*(11). doi:10.1136/bcr-2021-244721

McLaughlin, T. M., Broadhurst, J. J., Harris, C. J., McGarry, S., & Keesing, S. L. (2020). A randomized pilot study on self-management in head and neck lymphedema. *Laryngoscope Investigative Otolaryngology, 5*(5), 879–889. doi:10.1002/lio2.455

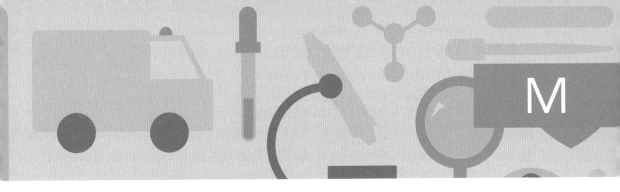

Risk for Disturbed Maternal–Fetal Dyad

DEFINITION

Susceptible to disruption of the symbiotic maternal–fetal dyad relationship as a result of co-morbid or pregnancy-related conditions, which may compromise health

RISK FACTORS

■ Inadequate prenatal care
■ Presence of abuse
■ Substance misuse

ASSOCIATED CONDITIONS

■ Alteration in glucose metabolism
■ Compromised fetal oxygen transport
■ Pregnancy complication
■ Treatment regimen

ASSESSMENT

■ Patient's understanding of health condition and treatment plan, past participation in health care planning, and decision-making
■ Patient's recognition and realization of potential growth, health, and autonomy
■ Support systems, expressed concerns regarding maternal role
■ Family status, including roles of family members
■ Cultural status, including affiliation with racial, ethnic, or religious groups

EXPECTED OUTCOMES

■ Patient will be compliant with recommendations for self-care activities to minimize prenatal complications and optimize maternal/fetal health.
■ Patient will verbalize fears and uncertainty related to prenatal conditions.
■ Patient will actively involve significant other/support systems with pregnancy expectations and plan of care.
■ Patient will demonstrate the "maternal tasks of pregnancy," culminating in an unconditional acceptance of the fetus before delivery.

Suggested NOC Outcomes

Prenatal Health Behavior; Knowledge: Pregnancy; Role Performance; Family Integrity

PCC ▪ Assess physical condition, psychosocial well-being, and cultural beliefs at each prenatal visit *to be able to counsel and/or refer as needed.*

PCC ▪ Encourage support/involvement of significant other(s) during the course of pregnancy *to enhance maternal role adaptation.*

PCC ▪ Incorporate the cultural beliefs, rites, and rituals of childbearing family into the plan of care *to foster feelings of normalcy with pregnancy.*

EBP ▪ Educate patient/significant other on role transition and maternal tasks of pregnancy *to provide anticipatory guidance on expected psychosocial changes.*

EBP ▪ Teach trimester-specific risk/danger signs and emphasize importance of self-monitoring *to empower the patient and reduce potential for adverse fetal effects.*

PCC ▪ Encourage patient to express disappointments/concerns related to relationships, physical condition, and fetal well-being *to promote therapeutic communication.*

T&C ▪ Refer to community resources as needed (e.g., prenatal classes, psychological counseling, pastoral care, social services) *to facilitate appropriate role adaptation.*

Suggested NIC Interventions

Anticipatory Guidance; Childbirth Preparation; Coping Enhancement; Role Enhancement

▪ Patient's physical and psychosocial well-being remained stable.
▪ Patient's maternal role adaptation was enhanced by support from significant other.
▪ Patient's cultural beliefs regarding childbearing were incorporated into the plan of care.
▪ Patient understood the trimester-specific risks and dangers and the importance of self-monitoring.
▪ Patient was able to express concerns related to relationships, physical condition, and fetal well-being.
▪ Patient was aware of appropriate resources to use to help with role adaptation.

▪ Patient's prenatal record of physical and psychosocial condition
▪ Plan of care, including cultural beliefs related to childbearing
▪ Patient's understanding of trimester-specific risks and dangers and self-monitoring abilities
▪ Evaluations for expected outcomes

REFERENCES

Farré-Sender, B., Torres, A., Gelabert, E., Andrés, S., Roca, A., Lasheras, G., ... Garcia-Esteve, L. (2018). Mother-infant bonding in the postpartum period: Assessment of the impact of pre-delivery factors in a clinical sample. *Archives of Women's Mental Health, 21*(3), 287–297. doi:10.1007/s00737-017-0785-y

Lind, J. N., Interrante, J. D., Ailes, E. C., Gilboa, S. M., Khan, S., Frey, M. T., ... Broussard, C. S. (2017). Maternal use of opioids during pregnancy and congenital malformations: A systematic review. *Pediatrics, 139*(6), 1–25. doi:10.1542/peds.2016-4131

Scott, C. (2017). Resolving perceived maternal–fetal conflicts through active patient–physician collaboration. *American Journal of Bioethics, 17*(1), 100–102. doi:10.1080/15265161.2016.1251636

Sebastiani, G., Borrás-Novell, C., Alsina Casanova, M., Pascual Tutusaus, M., Ferrero Martínez, S., Gómez Roig, M. D., & García-Algar, O. (2018). The effects of alcohol and drugs of abuse on maternal nutritional profile during pregnancy. *Nutrients, 10*(8), 1008. doi:10.3390/nu10081008

Impaired Memory

DEFINITION

Persistent inability to remember or recall bits of information or skills, while maintaining the capacity to independently perform activities of daily living

RELATED FACTORS (R/T)

Depressive symptoms
Inadequate intellectual stimulation
Inadequate motivation
Inadequate social support
Social isolation
Water–electrolyte imbalance

ASSOCIATED CONDITIONS

- Anemia
- Brain hypoxia
- Cognition disorders

ASSESSMENT

- Age, gender, level of education, occupation, and living arrangements
- Cardiovascular status, including vital signs, apical pulse, pulse rate and rhythm, and heart sounds; color of skin, lips, and nails; fatigue on exertion, dyspnea, and dizziness; history of hypertension, chest pain, or anoxia; and complete blood count and differential, thyroid studies, electrocardiography, and echocardiography
- Family status, including household composition and marital status (presence of a spouse, length of marriage, divorce, or death of spouse)
- Neurologic status, including mental status (abstract thinking, insight about present situation, judgment, long- and short-term memory, cognition, and orientation to time, place, and person); level of consciousness; sensory ability; fine and gross motor functioning; history of neurologic disorder, head injury, or psychiatric illness; medication use; and computed tomography scan, magnetic resonance imaging, cerebral angiography, electroencephalography, toxicology studies, thyroid function, and serotonin levels
- Psychological status, including changes in appetite, behavior, energy level, mood, motivation, self-image, self-esteem, and sleep patterns; alcohol and drug consumption; recent divorce, separation, death, job loss, loss of loved one, relocation, or physical or emotional trauma; and psychiatric history
- Self-care status, including ability to carry out voluntary activities and use of adaptive equipment

DEFINING CHARACTERISTICS

- Consistently forgets to perform a behavior at the scheduled time
- Difficulty acquiring a new skill
- Difficulty acquiring new information
- Difficulty recalling events
- Difficulty recalling factual information
- Difficulty recalling familiar names
- Difficulty recalling familiar objects

- Difficulty recalling familiar words
- Difficulty recalling if a behavior was performed
- Difficulty retaining a new skill
- Difficulty retaining new information

EXPECTED OUTCOMES

- Patient will express feelings about memory impairment.
- Patient will acknowledge need to take measures to cope with memory impairment.
- Patient will identify coping skills to deal with memory impairment.
- Patient and family members will state specific plans to modify lifestyle.
- Patient and family members will establish realistic goals to deal with further memory loss.

Suggested NOC Outcomes

Cognition; Cognitive Orientation; Concentration; Depression Level; Memory; Neurological Status

INTERVENTIONS AND RATIONALES

S — Observe patient's thought processes during every shift. Document and report any changes. *Changes may indicate progressive improvement or a decline in patient's underlying condition.*

S — Implement appropriate safety measures to protect patient from injury. *Patient may be unable to provide for own safety needs.*

PCC — Call patient by name and mention your name. Provide background information (place, time, and date) frequently throughout the day *to provide reality orientation.* Use a reality orientation board *to visually reinforce reality orientation.*

PCC — Spend sufficient time with patient to allow him or her to become comfortable discussing memory loss *to establish a trusting relationship.*

PCC — Inform patient that you're aware of patient's memory loss and that you'll provide help in coping with the condition *to bring the issue into the open and help patient understand that your goal is to be supportive.*

EBP — Be clear, concise, and direct in establishing goals *so that patient can maximize the use of remaining cognitive skills.*

EBP — Offer short, simple explanations to patient each time you carry out any medical or nursing procedure *to avoid confusion.*

S — Label patient's personal possessions and photos, keeping them in the same place as much as possible *to reduce confusion and create a secure environment.*

PCC — Encourage patient to develop a consistent routine for performing activities of daily living *to enhance patient's self-esteem and increase self-awareness and awareness of patient's environment.*

EBP — Teach patient ways to cope with memory loss—for example, using an alarm to remind patient when to eat or take medications, using a pillbox organized by days of the week, keeping lists in notebooks or a pocket calendar, and having family members or friends provide reminders of important tasks. *Reminders help limit the amount of information patient must maintain in memory.*

- Encourage patient to interact with others *to increase social involvement, which may decline with memory loss.*

PCC — Encourage patient to express the feelings associated with impaired memory *to reduce the impact of memory impairment on patient's self-image and lessen anxiety.*

PCC — Help patient and family members establish goals for coping with memory loss. Discuss with family members the need to maintain the least restrictive environment possible.

Instruct them on how to maintain a safe home environment for patient. *This helps ensure that patient's needs are met and promotes independence.*

S ▦ Demonstrate reorientation techniques to family members and provide time for supervised return demonstrations *to prepare them to cope with the patient with memory impairment.*

T&C ▦ Help family members identify appropriate community support groups, mental health services, and social service agencies *to assist in coping with the effects of patient's illness or injury.*

Suggested NIC Interventions

Anxiety Reduction; Calming Technique; Cerebral Perfusion Promotion; Dementia Management; Fluid/Electrolyte Management; Memory Training; Neurologic Monitoring; Reality Orientation

EVALUATIONS FOR EXPECTED OUTCOMES

▦ Patient expresses feelings about memory impairment.
▦ Patient acknowledges need to take measures to cope with memory impairment.
▦ Patient describes mechanisms for coping with memory loss.
▦ Patient and family members describe plans to modify lifestyle.
▦ Patient and family members set realistic goals to cope with further memory loss.

DOCUMENTATION

▦ Description of patient's mental status, including documentation of changes from shift to shift
▦ Outline of goals for helping patient cope with memory loss
▦ Response of family members to techniques for keeping patient functioning at maximal level
▦ Referrals to community support groups
▦ Evaluations for expected outcomes

REFERENCES

Jonsdottir, I. H., Nordlund, A., Ellbin, S., Ljung, T., Glise, K., Währborg, P., ... Wallin, A. (2017). Working memory and attention are still impaired after three years in patients with stress-related exhaustion. *Scandinavian Journal of Psychology, 58*(6), 504–509. doi:10.1111/sjop.12394

Koeritzer, M. A., Rogers, C. S., Van Engen, K. J., & Peelle, J. E. (2018). The impact of age, background noise, semantic ambiguity, and hearing loss on recognition memory for spoken sentences. *Journal of Speech, Language & Hearing Research, 61*(3), 740–751. doi:10.1044/2017_JSLHR-H-17-0077

Smirni, D., Smirni, P., Di Martino, G., Fontana, M. L., Cipolotti, L., Oliveri, M., & Turriziani, P. (2019). Early detection of memory impairments in older adults: Standardization of a short version of the verbal and nonverbal Recognition Memory Test. *Neurological Sciences, 40*(1), 97–103. doi:10.1007/s10072-018-3587-8

Stein, K. F., Morys-Carter, W. L., Hinkley, L., & Fredman Stein, K. (2018). Rumination and impaired prospective memory. *Journal of General Psychology, 145*(3), 266–279. doi:10.1080/00221309.2018.1469464

Risk for Metabolic Syndrome

DEFINITION

Susceptible to developing a cluster of symptoms that increase risk of cardiovascular disease and type 2 diabetes mellitus, which may compromise health

RISK FACTORS

- Absence of interest in improving health behaviors
- Average daily physical activity is less than recommended for age and gender
- Body mass index above normal range for age and gender
- Excessive accumulation of fat for age and gender
- Excessive alcohol intake
- Excessive stress
- Inadequate dietary habits
- Inadequate knowledge of modifiable factors
- Inattentive to second-hand smoke
- Smoking

ASSOCIATED CONDITIONS

- Hyperuricemia
- Insulin resistance
- Polycystic ovary syndrome

ASSESSMENT

- Biologic factors, including age, gender, height, weight, and body mass index
- Weight fluctuations over past 10 years
- Vital signs and trends from last year
- Underlying conditions or medications
- Laboratory results: chemistry panel including albumin, blood glucose, uric acid; include result for HbA1c
- Nutritional status, including change in type of food tolerated, financial resources, meal preparation, serum albumin level, sociocultural influences, and usual dietary pattern
- History of eating disorders
- Sociocultural factors, including moral or health concerns about food and eating, financial status, and cultural background influence on food choices
- Activity level for work and leisure time
- History of smoking, alcoholic beverages, recreational drug use
- Situational daily stressors, current stress level, and coping behaviors

EXPECTED OUTCOMES

- Patient will adapt life routine for optimal health.
- Patient will seek information to improve health status.
- Patient will participate in plan of care to decrease risk for metabolic syndrome.
- Patient will take self-initiated actions to promote optimal wellness.
- Patient will take action to comply with health care provider–recommended daily physical activity plan.
- Patient will take action to comply with health care provider–recommended diet.
- Patient will maintain blood pressure within normal limits.
- Patient will maintain blood glucose level within normal limits.

Suggested NOC Outcomes

Adherence Behavior; Compliance Behavior: Prescribed Activity; Compliance Behavior: Prescribed Diet; Hyperglycemia Severity; Hypertension Severity; Knowledge: Chronic Disease Management; Knowledge: Healthy Diet; Knowledge: Healthy Lifestyle; Risk Control: Hypertension; Self-management: Lipid Disorder

INTERVENTIONS AND RATIONALES

EBP ▪ Assess hemodynamic status, including blood pressure, heart rate, oxygen saturation, and respiratory rate, for any abnormalities *that may be early indicators of high or low blood pressure.*

S ▪ Treat episodes of high or low blood pressure promptly. *Perfusion is decreased if blood pressure is not within normal limits.*

S ▪ Monitor serum levels of electrolytes, albumin, total protein, and blood glucose. *Identifying negative results quickly limits potential complications.*

PCC ▪ Discuss with patient the need to lose weight. *Even a 10% decrease in body weight yields health benefits.*

PCC ▪ Determine patient's motivation to change. *Motivation leads to positive action.*

PCC ▪ Help patient set realistic goals for losing weight. *This aids positive reinforcement and reduces frustration.*

PCC ▪ Support and encourage healthy patient behavior. *Creates positive relationship and reinforces healthy behaviors.*

PCC ▪ Weigh patient in a private, nonthreatening setting. *Builds trust with care team and prevents embarrassment.*

EBP ▪ Assess for health comorbidities, such as diabetes, skin breakdown, and hypertension. *Obesity is linked to other health concerns, which can be exacerbated by weight fluctuations.*

T&C ▪ Encourage attendance in support groups. *Support groups offer a place to share ideas and offer emotional support.*

PCC ▪ Evaluate for depression and anxiety. *Eating disorders can be linked to emotion.*

PCC ▪ Assist patient in identifying strengths and reinforce those. *Maintaining a positive outlook fosters participation in prescribed plan of care.*

PCC ▪ Assist patient in identifying small successes. *Identifying positive steps toward goal helps to motivate more positive actions.*

PCC ▪ Discuss patient's normal food preferences *to evaluate eating habits and include preferred foods (if nutritious) in patient's diet.*

T&C ▪ Evaluate nutritional status and refer to registered dietitian as needed. *Obese patients may be malnourished because of improper diet habits.*

EBP ▪ Discuss with patient the need for activity. *Lack of activity causes physical deconditioning and may also have a negative impact on psychological well-being.*

PCC ▪ Help patient select an exercise program (such as walking, jogging, aerobics, or swimming) appropriate to patient's age and physical condition. *Besides aiding weight loss, such activities offer an alternative to eating to alleviate stress.*

S **PCC** ▪ Teach patient exercises for increasing strength and endurance *to improve breathing and promote general physical reconditioning.*

PCC ▪ Instruct patient and family on risk factor modification (smoking cessation, diet, and exercise) *to lower modifiable risks.*

S **PCC** ▪ Support and encourage activity to patient's level of tolerance *to help foster patient's independence.*

EBP ▪ Provide patient with information regarding modifiable risk factors. *Knowledge of risk factors will contribute to informed decisions about lifestyle changes.*

T&C ▪ Collaborate with other members of the health care team to ensure that all underlying medical conditions are being managed effectively. *This will minimize the possibility of high and low blood pressure complications.*

Suggested NIC Interventions

Behavior Modification; Nutrition Therapy; Risk Identification; Teaching: Prescribed Diet; Teaching: Prescribed Exercise; Weight Reduction Assistance

EVALUATIONS FOR EXPECTED OUTCOMES

- Patient makes changes in life routine to achieve optimal health.
- Patient seeks information to improve health status.
- Patient participates in plan of care to decrease risk for metabolic syndrome.
- Patient takes self-initiated actions to promote optimal wellness.
- Patient complies with health care provider–recommended daily physical activity plan.
- Patient complies with health care provider–recommended diet.
- Patient makes necessary changes to maintain blood pressure within normal limits.
- Patient makes necessary changes to maintain blood glucose level within normal limits.

DOCUMENTATION

- Patient's vital signs
- Patient's concerns or perceptions of circumstances; willingness to accept and participate in treatment
- Assessment of body systems at risk for deterioration
- Observations of patient's behaviors
- Interventions to provide preventive or supportive care and prescribed treatment
- Treatment given to patient and patient's understanding and demonstrated ability to carry out instructions
- Patient's response to nursing interventions
- Evaluations for expected outcomes

REFERENCES

Crowther, M. R., Ford, C. D., Vinson, L. D., Huang, C. H., Wayde, E., & Guin, S. (2018). Assessment of metabolic syndrome risk factors among rural-dwelling older adults requires innovation: Partnerships and a mobile unit can help. *Quality in Ageing & Older Adults, 19*(4), 251–260. doi:10.1108/QAOA-12-2017-0052

Kim, J., Lee, I., & Lim, S. (2017). Overweight or obesity in children aged 0 to 6 and the risk of adult metabolic syndrome: A systematic review and meta-analysis. *Journal of Clinical Nursing, 26*(23–24), 3869–3880. doi:10.1111/jocn.13802

Kim J. Y., Yang Y., & Sim Y. J. (2018). Effects of smoking and aerobic exercise on male college students' metabolic syndrome risk factors. *Journal of Physical Therapy Science, 30*(4), 595–600.

Ochoa Sangrador, C., & Ochoa, B. J. (2018). Waist-to-height ratio as a risk marker for metabolic syndrome in childhood. A meta-analysis. *Pediatric Obesity, 13*(7), 421–432. doi:10.1111/ijpo.12285

Impaired Bed Mobility

DEFINITION

Limitation in independent movement from one bed position to another

RELATED FACTORS (R/T)

- Cognitive dysfunction
- Decreased flexibility
- Environmental constraints
- Impaired postural balance
- Inadequate angle of headboard

- Inadequate knowledge of mobility strategies
- Insufficient muscle strength
- Obesity
- Pain
- Physical deconditioning

ASSOCIATED CONDITIONS

- Artificial respiration
- Critical illness
- Dementia
- Drain tubes
- Musculoskeletal impairment
- Neurodegenerative disorders
- Neuromuscular diseases
- Parkinson's disease
- Pharmaceutical preparations
- Sedation

ASSESSMENT

- Age and gender
- Vital signs
- History of neuromuscular disorder or dysfunction
- Drug history
- Musculoskeletal status, including coordination, muscle size and strength, muscle tone, range of motion (ROM), and functional mobility as follows:
  0 = completely independent
  1 = requires use of equipment or device
  2 = requires help, supervision, or teaching from another person
  3 = requires help from another person and use of equipment or device
  4 = dependent; doesn't participate in activity
- Neurologic status, including level of consciousness, motor ability, and sensory ability

DEFINING CHARACTERISTICS

- Difficulty moving between long sitting and supine positions
- Difficulty moving between prone and supine positions
- Difficulty moving between sitting and supine positions
- Difficulty reaching objects on the bed
- Difficulty repositioning self in bed
- Difficulty returning to the bed
- Difficulty rolling on the bed
- Difficulty sitting on edge of bed
- Difficulty turning from side to side

EXPECTED OUTCOMES

- Patient won't exhibit complications associated with impaired bed mobility, such as altered skin integrity, contractures, venous stasis, thrombus formation, depression, altered health maintenance, and falls.
- Patient will maintain or improve muscle strength and joint ROM.

- Patient will achieve highest level of bed mobility possible (independence, independence with device, verbalization of needs for assistance with bed mobility, requires assistance of one person, requires assistance of two people).
- Patient will maintain safety while in bed.
- Patient will demonstrate ability to use equipment or devices to assist with moving about in bed safely.
- Patient will adapt to alteration in ability to move about in bed.
- Patient will participate in social, physical, and occupational activities to the extent possible.

Suggested NOC Outcomes

Body Positioning: Self-initiated; Immobility Consequences: Physiological; Immobility Consequences: Psycho-cognitive; Mobility

INTERVENTIONS AND RATIONALES

S
- Perform ROM exercises to affected joints, unless contraindicated, at least once per shift. Progress from passive to active ROM as tolerated *to prevent joint contractures and muscle atrophy*.

- Assist patient in maintaining anatomically correct and functional body positioning. Encourage repositioning every 2 hours while in bed. Establish a turning schedule for immobile patients. *Proper positioning relieves pressure, thereby preventing skin breakdown, and helps prevent fluid accumulation in dependent extremities*.

PCC
- Identify patient's level of independence using the functional mobility scale. Communicate your findings to staff *to provide continuity of care and preserve the documented level of independence*.

S
- Monitor and record daily evidence of complications related to impaired bed mobility (contractures, venous stasis, skin breakdown, thrombus formation, depression, altered health maintenance or self-care skills, falls). *Patients with neuromuscular dysfunction are at risk for complications*.

S
- Perform prescribed medical regimen to manage or prevent complications (e.g., administer prophylactic heparin for venous stasis) *to promote patient's health and well-being*.

S
- Assess patient's skin every 2 hours *to maintain skin integrity*.

- Help patient move about in bed. Encourage progressive mobility up to the limits imposed by patient's condition *to maintain muscle tone, prevent complications associated with immobility, and promote self-care*.

T&C
- Refer patient to a physical therapist for development of a program to improve bed mobility *to assist with rehabilitation of musculoskeletal deficits*.

T&C
- Refer the patient to an occupational therapist for development of a program to maximize self-care *to promote restoration of self-care skills*.

T&C
- Encourage patient to participate in physical and occupational therapy sessions. Incorporate equipment, devices, and techniques used by therapists into your care. Request written instructions from patient's therapists to use as a reference *to help ensure continuity of care and reinforce learned skills*.

S
- If you're uncertain about your ability to move patient, request help from colleagues *to maintain safety*.

EBP ▦ Instruct patient and family members in techniques to improve bed mobility and ways to prevent complications *to help prepare the patient and family members for discharge.*

EBP ▦ Demonstrate patient's bed mobility regimen and note the date. Have patient and family members perform a return demonstration *to ensure continuity of care and use of proper technique.*

T&C ▦ Assist patient in identifying and contacting resources for social and spiritual support *to promote patient's reintegration into the community and help him/her maintain psychosocial health.*

Suggested NIC Interventions

Bed Rest Care; Body Mechanics Promotion; Circulatory Precautions; Exercise Promotion: Strength Training; Exercise Therapy: Joint Mobility; Fall Prevention; Positioning; Skin Surveillance

EVALUATIONS FOR EXPECTED OUTCOMES

▦ Patient doesn't exhibit complications associated with impaired bed mobility, such as altered skin integrity, contractures, venous stasis, thrombus formation, depression, altered health maintenance, and falls.

▦ Patient maintains or improves muscle strength and joint ROM.

▦ Patient achieves highest level of bed mobility possible (independence, independence with device, verbalization of needs for assistance with bed mobility, requires assistance of one person, requires assistance of two people).

▦ Patient maintains safety while in bed.

▦ Patient demonstrates ability to use equipment or devices to assist with moving about in bed safely.

▦ Patient adapts to alteration in ability to move about in bed.

▦ Patient participates in social, physical, and occupational activities to the greatest extent possible.

DOCUMENTATION

▦ Patient's bed mobility status
▦ Presence of complications
▦ Referrals for physical or occupational therapy
▦ Response to program to improve or restore bed mobility
▦ Patient's statements regarding the loss of bed mobility skills and goals for improving bed mobility
▦ Teaching provided to patient and family members
▦ Patient's and family members' demonstrated skill in carrying out bed mobility program
▦ Evaluations for expected outcomes

REFERENCES

Spagnuolo, G., Faria, C. D. C. M., da Silva, B. A., Ovando, A. C., Gomes-Osman, J., & Swarowsky, A. (2018). Are functional mobility tests responsive to group physical therapy intervention in individuals with Parkinson's disease? *NeuroRehabilitation, 42*(4), 465–472. doi:10.3233/NRE-172379

Vatwani, A. (2017). Caregiver guide and instructions for safe bed mobility. *Archives of Physical Medicine & Rehabilitation, 98*(9), 1907–1910. doi:10.1016/j.apmr.2017.03.003

Young, D. L., Seltzer, J., Glover, M., Outten, C., Lavezza, A., Mantheiy, E., ... Needham, D. M. (2018). Identifying barriers to nurse-facilitated patient mobility in the intensive care unit. *American Journal of Critical Care, 27*(3), 186–193. doi:10.4037/ajcc2018368

Impaired Physical Mobility

DEFINITION

Limitation in independent, purposeful movement of the body or of one or more extremities

RELATED FACTORS (R/T)

- Activity intolerance
- Anxiety
- Body mass index (BMI) > 75th percentile appropriate for age and gender
- Cultural belief regarding acceptable activity
- Decrease in endurance
- Decrease in muscle control
- Decrease in muscle mass
- Decrease in muscle strength
- Depression
- Disuse
- Insufficient environmental support
- Insufficient knowledge of value of physical activity
- Joint stiffness
- Malnutrition
- Pain
- Physical deconditioning
- Reluctance to initiate movement
- Sedentary lifestyle

ASSOCIATED CONDITIONS

- Alteration in bone structure integrity
- Alteration in cognitive functioning
- Alteration in metabolism
- Contractures
- Developmental delay
- Musculoskeletal impairment
- Neuromuscular impairment
- Pharmaceutical agent
- Prescribed movement restrictions
- Sensory–perceptual impairment

ASSESSMENT

- History of neuromuscular disorder or dysfunction
- Musculoskeletal status, including coordination, gait, muscle size and strength, muscle tone, range of motion (ROM), and functional mobility scale:
  0 = completely independent
  1 = requires use of equipment or device
  2 = requires help, supervision, or teaching from another person
  3 = requires help from another person and use of equipment or device
  4 = dependent; doesn't participate in activity
- Neurologic status, including level of consciousness, motor ability, and sensory ability

DEFINING CHARACTERISTICS

- Alteration in gait
- Decrease in fine motor skills
- Decrease in gross motor skills
- Decrease in range of motion
- Decrease in reaction time
- Difficulty turning
- Discomfort
- Engages in substitutions for movement
- Exertional dyspnea
- Movement-induced tremor
- Postural instability
- Slowed movement
- Spastic movement
- Uncoordinated movements

EXPECTED OUTCOMES

- Patient will maintain muscle strength and joint ROM.
- Patient will show no evidence of complications, such as contractures, venous stasis, thrombus formation, skin breakdown, and hypostatic pneumonia.
- Patient will achieve highest level of mobility (will transfer independently, will be wheelchair independent, or will ambulate with such assistive devices as walker, cane, and braces).
- Patient or family member will carry out mobility regimen.
- Patient or family member will make plans to use resources to help maintain level of functioning.

Suggested NOC Outcomes

Ambulation; Ambulation: Wheelchair; Discharge Readiness: Independent Living; Discharge Readiness: Supported Living; Mobility; Transfer Performance; Activities of Daily Living

INTERVENTIONS AND RATIONALES

S ▪ Perform ROM exercises to joints, unless contraindicated, at least once every shift. Progress from passive to active, as tolerated. *This prevents joint contractures and muscular atrophy.*

S ▪ Turn and position patient every 2 hours. Establish a turning schedule for dependent patients; post at the bedside and monitor frequency of turning. *This prevents skin breakdown by relieving pressure.*

S ▪ Place joints in functional position, use trochanter roll along the thigh, abduct the thighs, use high-top sneakers, and put a small pillow under patient's head. *These measures maintain joints in a functional position and prevent musculoskeletal deformities.*

EBP ▪ Identify the level of functioning using a functional mobility scale (see "Assessment"). Communicate patient's skill level to all staff members *to provide continuity and preserve identified level of independence.*

EBP ▪ Encourage independence in mobility by helping patient to use a trapeze and side rails, to use the unaffected leg to move the affected leg, and to perform such self-care activities as combing hair, feeding, and dressing. *This increases muscle tone and patient's self-esteem.*

EBP ▪ Place items within reach of the unaffected arm if patient has one-sided weakness or paralysis *to promote patient's independence.*

S ▪ Monitor and record daily any evidence of immobility complications (such as contractures, venous stasis, thrombus, pneumonia, and urinary tract infection). *Patients with a history of neuromuscular disorders or dysfunction may be more prone to developing complications.*

S ▪ Carry out a medical regimen to manage or prevent complications; for example, administer prophylactic heparin as ordered for venous thrombosis. *This promotes patient's health and well-being.*

S ▪ Provide progressive mobilization to the limits of patient's condition (bed mobility to chair mobility to ambulation) *to maintain muscle tone and prevent complications of immobility.* Use a transfer belt if necessary *to support patient and prevent staff injury.*

T&C ▪ Refer patient to a physical therapist for development of mobility regimen *to help rehabilitate musculoskeletal deficits.*

T&C ▪ Encourage attendance at physical therapy sessions and support activities on the unit by using the same equipment and technique. Request written mobility plans and use as reference. *All members of the health care team should reinforce learned skills in the same manner.*

EBP ▪ Instruct patient and family members in ROM exercises, transfers, skin inspection, and mobility regimen *to help prepare patient for discharge.*

EBP ▪ Demonstrate the mobility regimen and note date. Have patient and family members return mobility regimen demonstration and note date. *This ensures continuity of care and use of proper technique.*

T&C ▪ Assist in identifying resources to carry out the mobility regimen, such as the American Heart Association and the National Multiple Sclerosis Society. *These resources help provide a comprehensive approach to rehabilitation.*

Suggested NIC Interventions

Activity Therapy; Energy Management; Exercise Promotion: Strength Training; Exercise Therapy: Joint Mobility; Exercise Therapy: Muscle Control; Positioning: Wheelchair; Surveillance: Safety

EVALUATIONS FOR EXPECTED OUTCOMES

▪ Patient maintains muscle strength and joint ROM.

▪ Patient shows no evidence of contractures, venous stasis, thrombus formation, skin breakdown, hypostatic pneumonia, or other complications.

▪ Patient achieves highest mobility level possible identified by health care team (specify).

▪ Patient or family member carries out mobility regimen.

▪ Patient or family member identifies and contacts at least one resource person or group to help maintain level of functioning.

DOCUMENTATION

▪ Patient's expression of concern about loss of mobility, current status of functional abilities, and goals set for self

▪ Observations of patient's mobility status, presence of complications, and response to mobility regimen

▪ Instruction and demonstration of skills in carrying out mobility regimen

▪ Patient's response to nursing interventions

▪ Evaluations for expected outcomes

REFERENCES

Addison, O., Kundi, R., Ryan, A. S., Goldberg, A. P., Patel, R., Lal, B. K., & Prior, S. J. (2018). Clinical relevance of the modified physical performance test versus the short physical performance battery for detecting mobility impairments in older men with peripheral arterial disease. *Disability & Rehabilitation, 40*(25), 3081–3085. doi:10.1080/09638288.2017.1367966

Agahi, N., Fors, S., Fritzell, J., & Shaw, B. A. (2018). Smoking and physical inactivity as predictors of mobility impairment during late life: Exploring differential vulnerability across education level in Sweden. *Journals of Gerontology Series B: Psychological Sciences & Social Sciences, 73*(4), 675–683. doi:10.1093/geronb/gbw090

Sahrmann, S., Azevedo, D. C., & Van Dillen, L. (2017). Diagnosis and treatment of movement system impairment syndromes. *Brazilian Journal of Physical Therapy/Revista Brasileira de Fisioterapia, 21*(6), 391–399. doi:10.1016/j.bjpt.2017.08.001

Impaired Wheelchair Mobility

DEFINITION

Limitation in independent operation of wheelchair within environment

RELATED FACTORS (R/T)

- Altered mood
- Cognitive dysfunction
- Environmental constraints
- Inadequate adjustment to wheelchair size
- Inadequate knowledge of wheelchair use
- Insufficient muscle strength
- Insufficient physical endurance
- Neurobehavioral manifestations
- Obesity
- Pain
- Physical deconditioning
- Substance misuse
- Unaddressed inadequate vision

ASSOCIATED CONDITIONS

- Musculoskeletal impairment
- Neuromuscular diseases
- Vision disorders

ASSESSMENT

- Age and gender
- Vital signs
- History of neuromuscular disorder or dysfunction
- Drug history
- Musculoskeletal status, including coordination, gait, muscle size and strength, muscle tone, range of motion (ROM), and functional mobility as follows:
  - 0 = completely independent
  - 1 = requires use of equipment or device
  - 2 = requires help, supervision, or teaching from another person
  - 3 = requires help from another person and use of equipment or device
  - 4 = dependent; doesn't participate in activity

- Neurologic status, including level of consciousness, motor ability, and sensory ability
- Characteristics of patient's wheelchair (e.g., whether standard or motorized) and adequacy of wheelchair for meeting patient's needs (right size, appropriate safety features, and easy for patient to operate)
- Endurance (length of time patient can operate wheelchair before becoming fatigued)

DEFINING CHARACTERISTICS

- Difficulty bending forward to pick up object from the floor
- Difficulty folding or unfolding wheelchair
- Difficulty leaning forward to reach for something above head
- Difficulty locking brakes on manual wheelchair
- Difficulty maneuvering wheelchair sideways
- Difficulty moving wheelchair out of an elevator
- Difficulty navigating through hinged door
- Difficulty operating battery charger of power wheelchair
- Difficulty operating power wheelchair on a decline
- Difficulty operating power wheelchair on an incline
- Difficulty operating power wheelchair on curbs
- Difficulty operating power wheelchair on even surface
- Difficulty operating power wheelchair on uneven surface
- Difficulty operating wheelchair backwards
- Difficulty operating wheelchair forward
- Difficulty operating wheelchair in corners
- Difficulty operating wheelchair motors
- Difficulty operating wheelchair on a decline
- Difficulty operating wheelchair on an incline
- Difficulty operating wheelchair on curbs
- Difficulty operating wheelchair on even surface
- Difficulty operating wheelchair on stairs
- Difficulty operating wheelchair on uneven surface
- Difficulty operating wheelchair while carrying an object
- Difficulty performing pressure relief
- Difficulty performing stationary wheelie position
- Difficulty putting feet on the footplates of the wheelchair
- Difficulty rolling across side-slope while in wheelchair
- Difficulty selecting drive mode on power wheelchair
- Difficulty selecting speed on power wheelchair
- Difficulty shifting weight
- Difficulty sitting on wheelchair without losing balance
- Difficulty stopping wheelchair before bumping something
- Difficulty transferring from wheelchair
- Difficulty transferring to wheelchair
- Difficulty turning in place while on wheelie position

EXPECTED OUTCOMES

- Patient won't exhibit complications associated with impaired wheelchair mobility, such as skin breakdown, contractures, venous stasis, thrombus formation, depression, alteration in health maintenance, and falls.
- Patient will maintain or improve muscle strength and joint ROM.

- Patient will achieve highest level of independence possible with regard to wheelchair use.
- Patient will express feelings regarding alteration in ability to use wheelchair.
- Patient will maintain safety when using wheelchair.
- Patient will adapt to alteration in ability.
- Patient will participate in social and occupational activities to the greatest extent possible.
- Patient will demonstrate understanding of techniques to improve wheelchair mobility.

Suggested NOC Outcomes

Ambulation: Wheelchair; Balance; Immobility Consequences: Physiological; Immobility Consequences: Psycho-cognitive; Mobility

INTERVENTIONS AND RATIONALES

S ⬛ Perform ROM exercises for affected joints, unless contraindicated, at least once per shift. Progress from passive to active ROM as tolerated *to prevent joint contractures and muscle atrophy.*

S ⬛ Make sure patient maintains anatomically correct and functional body positioning while in the wheelchair *to promote comfort.* Explain to patient where vulnerable pressure points are and teach patient to shift and reposition own weight *to prevent skin breakdown.*

S ⬛ Assess whether patient's wheelchair is adequate to meet patient's needs *to help maintain mobility and independence.* Consider the following:
- Is the seat the right size? It should be wide and deep enough to support patient's thighs and allow patient to sit comfortably. It should be low enough so that patient's feet touch the floor but high enough to allow easy transfer from bed to chair. The chair's back should be tall enough to support patient's upper body.
- Is the chair easy for the patient to operate when weak? If the patient has little or no arm strength, the patient may need a motorized wheelchair.
- Is the chair safe? All wheelchairs have safety features, such as brakes that lock the wheels, but some safety features can be modified to meet patient's needs. For example, seat belts can be attached at the waist, hips, or chest.

S ⬛ Identify patient's level of independence using the functional mobility scale. Communicate findings to staff *to promote continuity of care and preserve the documented level of independence.*

S ⬛ Monitor and record daily evidence of complications related to impaired wheelchair mobility (contractures, venous stasis, skin breakdown, thrombus formation, depression, and alteration in health maintenance or self-care skills). *Patients with neuromuscular dysfunction are at risk for complications.*

PCC ⬛ Encourage patient to operate the wheelchair independently to the limits imposed by the patient's condition *to maintain muscle tone, prevent complications of immobility, and promote independence in self-care and health maintenance skills.*

T&C ⬛ Refer patient to a physical therapist for development of a program to enhance wheelchair mobility *to assist with rehabilitation of musculoskeletal deficits.*

T&C ⬛ Encourage attendance at physical therapy sessions and reinforce prescribed activities on the unit by using equipment, devices, and techniques used in the therapy session. Request a written copy of patient's rehabilitation program to use as a reference *to maintain continuity of care and promote patient safety.*

S ⬛ Assess patient's skin on return to bed and request a wheelchair cushion if necessary *to maintain the patient's skin integrity.*

EBP ⬛ Demonstrate techniques to promote wheelchair mobility to patient and family members, and note the date *to help prepare patient for discharge and maintain safety.* For example, teach patient and family members how to perform wheelchair push-ups. If patient can move the arms, have patient grip the arms of the chair and push down hard with hands and arms to try to raise the body off the seat. Have patient and family members perform a return demonstration *to ensure continuity of care and use of proper technique.*

T&C   ▥   Assist in identifying resources for helping patient maintain the highest level of mobility, such as a community stroke program, sports associations for people with disabilities, or the National Multiple Sclerosis Society, *to promote patient's reintegration into the community.*

Suggested NIC Interventions

Exercise Promotion: Strength Training; Exercise Therapy: Balance; Exercise Therapy: Muscle Control; Mutual Goal Setting; Positioning: Wheelchair

EVALUATIONS FOR EXPECTED OUTCOMES

▥ Patient doesn't exhibit complications associated with impaired wheelchair mobility, such as skin breakdown, contractures, venous stasis, thrombus formation, depression, alteration in health maintenance, and falls.
▥ Patient maintains or improves muscle strength and joint ROM.
▥ Patient achieves highest level of independence possible with regard to wheelchair use.
▥ Patient expresses feelings regarding alteration in ability to use wheelchair.
▥ Patient maintains safety when using wheelchair.
▥ Patient adapts to alteration in ability.
▥ Patient participates in social and occupational activities to the greatest extent possible.
▥ Patient demonstrates understanding of techniques to improve wheelchair mobility.

DOCUMENTATION

▥ Observations of changes in patient's mobility status and related complications
▥ Patient's expression of concern about loss of wheelchair mobility
▥ Patient's goals for future regarding mobility status
▥ Teaching provided to patient
▥ Patient's return demonstration of skills in carrying out wheelchair mobility program
▥ Patient's response to nursing interventions
▥ Evaluations for expected outcomes

REFERENCES

Borisoff, J. F., Ripat, J., & Chan, F. (2018). Seasonal patterns of community participation and mobility of wheelchair users over an entire year. *Archives of Physical Medicine & Rehabilitation, 99*(8), 1553–1560. doi:10.1016/j.apmr.2018.02.011

Saltan, A., Bakar, Y., & Ankarali, H. (2017). Wheeled mobility skills of wheelchair basketball players: A randomized controlled study. *Disability & Rehabilitation: Assistive Technology, 12*(4), 390–395. doi:10.1080/17483107.2016.1177857

Sol, M. E., Verschuren, O., de Groot, L., & de Groot, J. F. (2017). Development of a wheelchair mobility skills test for children and adolescents: Combining evidence with clinical expertise. *BMC Pediatrics, 17*, 1–18. doi:10.1186/s12887-017-0809-9

van der Slikke, R. M. A., de Witte, A. M. H., Berger, M. A. M., Bregman, D. J. J., & Veeger, D. J. H. E. J. (2018). Wheelchair mobility performance enhancement by changing wheelchair properties: What is the effect of grip, seat height, and mass? *International Journal of Sports Physiology & Performance, 13*(8), 1050–1058. doi:10.1123/ijspp.2017-0641

Impaired Mood Regulation

DEFINITION

A mental state characterized by shifts in mood or affect and which is comprised of a constellation of affective, cognitive, somatic, and/or physiological manifestations varying from mild to severe

RELATED FACTORS (R/T)

- Alteration in sleep pattern
- Anxiety
- Appetite change
- Hypervigilance
- Impaired social functioning
- Loneliness
- Pain
- Recurrent thoughts of death
- Recurrent thoughts of suicide
- Social isolation
- Substance misuse
- Weight change

ASSOCIATED CONDITIONS

- Chronic illness
- Functional impairment
- Psychosis

ASSESSMENT

- Vital signs
- Weight
- Presence of mental illness, medical illness, infectious disease, acquired brain injury, or developmental delay or disability
- Presence of, and, if any, the characteristics of, a relationship between mood state and therapeutic, accidental, or recreational substance use (i.e., medication, toxins, illicit/misused drugs/medication)
- Mental status examination, including appearance, affect, mood, sensorium, cognition, motor (i.e., speech, movements, gait), thought process, thought content, perceptual disturbance
- Nutritional, hydration, and elimination status
- Patterns of activity and rest
- Suicidal ideation—current, recent, past
- Thoughts or history of self-harm without suicidal intent
- Presence/absence of hope, plans for the future
- Risk of any disinhibited behavior (i.e., personal, social, sexual, financial, legal, safety)
- Developmental stage

DEFINING CHARACTERISTICS

- Changes in verbal behavior
- Disinhibition

- Dysphoria
- Excessive guilt
- Excessive self-awareness
- Excessive self-blame
- Flight of thoughts
- Hopelessness
- Impaired concentration
- Influenced self-esteem
- Irritability
- Psychomotor agitation
- Psychomotor retardation
- Sad affect
- Withdrawal

EXPECTED OUTCOMES

- The patient will not engage in self-harm and suicidal behavior.
- The patient will not engage in risky behavior.
- The patient will have a balanced pattern of activity and rest.
- The patient's food and fluid intake will meet the patient's physiologic needs.
- The patient will participate in psychoeducation.
- The patient will verbalize a realistic understanding of the meaning of own symptoms.
- The patient will identify own goals for care.
- The patient will collaborate with the nurse to create a wellness recovery plan that includes goals and positive plans for the future.
- The patient will verbalize having hope for future.
- The patient will demonstrate awareness of distorted thoughts, if present, and will identify alternative balanced thought(s).
- The patient will complete activities of daily living.

Suggested NOC Outcomes

Anxiety Level; Coping; Depression Level; Impulse; Self-control; Quality of Life; Stress Level

INTERVENTIONS AND RATIONALES

- **S** Initiate suicide and/or self-harm precautions as necessary *to ensure patient remains safe from suicide and self-harm.*
- **S** Initiate precautions to reduce risks, if any, related to disinhibition. *Patient insight into risks and potential consequences of disinhibited behavior may be limited or absent.* The disinhibited patient may require increased observation and/or frequent redirection to avoid risky behavior.
- **S** If indicated, support measures to resolve effects of substance action or substance withdrawal *to promote safe elimination of substance from the body and prevent complications of substance action or withdrawal.*
- **EBP** Ensure dietary and fluid intake to meet physiologic needs *to prevent dehydration, electrolyte imbalances, muscles loss, unhealthy weight change, elimination changes, complications of hypoglycemia. Persons with mood disturbances may not meet diet and hydration needs. Persons with mood disturbance may manifest hyperactivity or hypoactivity.*

- Encourage and support appropriate levels of rest and activity (according to patient's physiologic needs and capabilities) *to prevent complications of inactivity (e.g., skin breakdown, deep vein thrombosis, muscle atrophy, constipation) as well as to prevent complications of excessive activity (e.g., exhaustion, injury, electrolyte imbalances, exertional rhabdomyolysis).*

PCC
- Use short, simple phrases to convey instructions or questions. Permit ample time for the patient to respond, and expect the need to repeat instructions or questions at times. Tasks may need to be presented to patient for completion one step at a time and in small, simple steps. *Impaired concentration, psychomotor agitation, psychomotor retardation, or flight of ideas may inhibit processing of information and capability to remain on task.*

PCC
- Convey a nonjudgmental, supportive attitude and do not take any irritable statements/responses personally. Use effective therapeutic communication skills to avoid power struggles. *Maintenance of a therapeutic nurse–patient relationship is a key nursing responsibility.*

PCC
- Provide assistance, cues, or reminders, as needed, for the completion of activities of daily living (ADLs) *as impaired concentration, flight of ideas, psychomotor agitation, or psychomotor retardation may restrict independent skill or follow-through on ADLs.*

EBP
- Assist patient to access psychoeducation resources appropriate to patient's clinical situation *to promote understanding of etiology of patient's mood symptoms, promote engagement in care, and build self-efficacy in symptom recognition and management.*

PCC
- Engage patient to develop and enact a wellness recovery plan in own care, which includes positive goals for the future *to promote hope and engagement in self-care.*

PCC
- Assist patient in evaluating the efficacy of patient's strategies to meet goals. Emphasize gains made toward recovery goals and assist in problem-solving new solutions for strategies attempted but ineffective to meet goals *to promote self-esteem, self-efficacy, and development of problem-solving skills.*

PCC
- Assist patient with excessive guilt, excessive self-blame, or excessive self-awareness to counter distorted thinking through the best friend technique. *Excessive guilt, self-blame, or excessive self-awareness can be linked to cognitive distortions. Cognitive distortions are negative thoughts that do not truly reflect reality.*

- Ask patient to identify the specific thoughts patient has about self that link to feelings of guilt or blame, or excessive awareness of self, and then to identify what a caring and realistic best friend would tell about patient's distorted thought. *Cognitive behavioral therapy (CBT) strategies, such as the best friend technique, can help patient to become aware of the emotionally charged, distorted thoughts and to consider an alternative, more neutral, less emotionally charged thought.*

T&C
- Assist patient with referral to specialty psychotherapy resources, as indicated by patient's presentation and as determined by the clinical team. *Psychotherapies, such as CBT, interpersonal and social rhythm therapy (IPSRT), acceptance and commitment therapy (ACT), and interpersonal psychotherapy, have indications for use in persons with mood disturbances.*

Suggested NIC Interventions

Anxiety Reduction; Coping Enhancement; Emotional Support; Improved Quality of Life; Improved Well-Being; Mood Management

EVALUATIONS FOR EXPECTED OUTCOMES

- Patient remains safe from self-harm and suicidal behavior.
- Patient refrains from risky behavior.

- Patient engages in a balanced pattern of activity and rest.
- Patient's food and fluid intake meet physiologic needs.
- Patient participates in psychoeducation and verbalizes a realistic understanding of the meaning of the patient's symptoms and goals in care.
- Patient participates in creating own wellness recovery plan.
- Patient verbalizes hope and plans for future.
- Patient demonstrates awareness of distorted thinking, if present, and identifies alternative balanced thought(s).
- Patient completes ADLs.

DOCUMENTATION

- Risk assessments
- Mental status examination findings
- Observations of patient behavior and activity level
- Patient verbatim statements regarding own experience(s) of hopelessness, excessive guilt, excessive self-awareness, excessive self-blame
- Interventions implemented, including patient engagement and response
- Content of wellness recovery plan
- Relevant medical, developmental, and psychiatric history
- Referrals to other services
- Evaluations for expected outcomes

REFERENCES

El-Rasheed, A. H., ElAttar, K. S., Elrassas, H. H., Mahmoud, D. A. M., & Mohamed, S. Y. (2017). Mood regulation, alexithymia, and personality disorders in adolescent male addicts. *Addictive Disorders & Their Treatment, 16*(2), 49–58. doi:10.1097/ADT.0000000000000098

Goldschmied, J. R., Cheng, P., Hoffmann, R., Boland, E. M., Deldin, P. J., & Armitage, R. (2019). Effects of slow-wave activity on mood disturbance in major depressive disorder. *Psychological Medicine, 49*(4), 639–645. doi:10.1017/S0033291718001332

Ortiz, A., & Alda, M. (2018). The perils of being too stable: Mood regulation in bipolar disorder. *Journal of Psychiatry & Neuroscience, 43*(6), 363–365. doi:10.1503/jpn.180183

Moral Distress

DEFINITION

Response to the inability to carry out one's chosen ethical or moral decision and/or action

RELATED FACTORS (R/T)

- Conflict among decision-makers
- Conflicting information available for ethical decision-making
- Conflicting information available for moral decision-making
- Cultural incongruence
- Difficulty reaching end-of-life decision
- Difficulty reaching treatment decision
- Time constraint for decision-making

ASSOCIATED CONDITIONS

- Loss of autonomy
- Physical distance of decision-maker

ASSESSMENT

- Age
- Medical diagnosis
- Mental status
- Treatment options
- Cultural beliefs about illness and death
- Roles/relationship within the family
- Communication patterns
- Coping skills
- Values/beliefs
- Place of religion in patient's life

DEFINING CHARACTERISTIC

Anguish about acting on one's moral choice

EXPECTED OUTCOMES

- Patient and family will understand medical diagnosis, treatment regimen, and limitations related to extent of illness.
- Patient and family will identify ethical/moral dilemma.
- Patient and family will describe personal and family values and conflict with current situation.
- Patient and family will identify health care ethics resources to assist in resolution of conflict.
- Patient and family will verbalize relief from anguish, uneasiness, or distress.

Suggested NOC Outcomes

Acceptance: Health Status; Client Satisfaction; Communication; Decision-Making; Family Integrity; Family Functioning; Family Health Status; Family Integrity; Knowledge; Spiritual Health Interventions and Rationales

INTERVENTIONS AND RATIONALES

EBP ▪ Assess patient's and family's understanding of the diagnosis and prognosis, limitations, treatment options; description of their personal values; and their physical expressions of suffering. *Assessment factors assist in identifying appropriate interventions.*

PCC ▪ Establish an environment in which family members can share comfortably and openly their issues and concerns.

T&C ▪ Enlist assistance of health care ethics resources such as ethics committee or consultants. *Including experts in health care ethics will assist in identifying the patient/family values and reason for the dilemma. By identifying the source of the conflict, the process of resolution may begin, thus leading to better understanding by all parties and partial or full relief from moral suffering.*

T&C ▪ Enlist assistance of chaplain or personal clergy *to assist in the process of resolution through clarification of values related to religious views. Chaplains and personal clergy may provide a more neutral "third party" that can help defuse the situation. Personal trusted clergy might recognize or facilitate patient/family verbal and physical expressions of suffering or relief.*

EBP ▓ Educate patient and family about medical diagnosis, treatment regimen, and limitations *to help both patient and family understand the limits and read about medical treatment related to medical diagnosis.*

PCC ▓ Provide or set aside ample time for patient and family to express their feelings about the current situation. *Open, honest communication may clear misconceptions on both sides and facilitate relief from suffering in the midst of dilemma.*

PCC ▓ Acknowledge ethical/moral position of patient/family who may feel that their positions or views will go unrecognized in the midst of serious illness and high-tech treatments; they may not want to "bother" nurses and physicians with these concerns. *Acknowledging their concerns, values, and moral position allows for holistic care.*

T&C ▓ Refer, where requested, for follow-up for a family member who needs exercise, weight management, diet assistance, health screenings, and so forth. *Assisting patient in making referrals will help ensure continued efforts on the part of the patient to live a healthier lifestyle.*

Suggested NIC Interventions

Active Listening: Anger Control Assistance; Anxiety Reduction; Conflict Mediation; Consultation; Counseling; Documentation; Family Integrity Promotion; Family Support; Multidisciplinary Care Conference; Spiritual Support Family Support; Family Integrity Promotion; Family Maintenance; Truth Telling

EVALUATION OF EXPECTED OUTCOMES

▓ Family members express an understanding of the patient's diagnosis, treatment options, and prognosis.
▓ Patient and/or family describes the ethical dilemma in a way that will allow them to arrive at practical decisions about the situation.
▓ Patient and/or family can articulate how options for possible resolutions are consistent with religious beliefs and personal values.
▓ Patient and/or family consults with clergy or other trusted advisor.

DOCUMENTATION

▓ Current medical condition
▓ Changes in condition
▓ Patient's expressed wishes
▓ Discussions between nursing staff and family about the patient's condition
▓ Consultation with other professionals involved in the case

REFERENCES

Ando, M., & Kawano, M. (2018). Relationships among moral distress, sense of coherence, and job satisfaction. *Nursing Ethics, 25*(5), 571–579. doi:10.1177/0969733016660882

Foe, G., Hellmann, J., & Greenberg, R. A. (2018). Parental moral distress and moral schism in the neonatal ICU. *Journal of Bioethical Inquiry, 15*(3), 319–325. doi:10.1007/s11673-018-9858-5

Mahon, M. M., & Barker, K. L. (2018). Applying a balm: Medicating the patient to treat the (moral) distress of caregivers. *Journal of Hospice & Palliative Nursing, 20*(5), 433–441. doi:10.1097/NJH.0000000000000491

Powell, S. B., Engelke, M. K., & Swanson, M. S. (2018). Moral distress among school nurses. *Journal of School Nursing, 34*(5), 390–397. doi:10.1177/1059840517704965

Impaired Oral Mucous Membrane Integrity

DEFINITION

Injury to the lips, soft tissue, buccal cavity, and/or oropharynx

RELATED FACTORS (R/T)

- Alcohol consumption
- Cognitive dysfunction
- Decreased salivation
- Dehydration
- Depressive symptoms
- Difficulty performing oral self-care
- Inadequate access to dental care
- Inadequate knowledge of oral hygiene
- Inadequate oral hygiene habits
- Inappropriate use of chemical agent
- Malnutrition
- Mouth breathing
- Smoking
- Stressors

ASSOCIATED CONDITIONS

- Allergies
- Autosomal disorder
- Behavioral disorder
- Chemotherapy
- Decreased female hormone levels
- Decreased platelets
- Depression
- Immune system diseases
- Immunosuppression
- Infections
- Loss of oral support structure
- Mechanical factor
- Mouth abnormalities
- Nil per os (NPO) greater than 24 hours
- Oral trauma
- Radiotherapy
- Sjögren's Syndrome
- Surgical procedures
- Trauma
- Treatment regimen

ASSESSMENT

- History of oral surgery, dentures, braces, or dental problems
- History of pathologic conditions known to cause dehydration such as diabetes mellitus
- Medications, such as diuretics and antihistamines

- Vital signs
- Fluid and electrolyte status, including blood urea nitrogen level, creatinine level, intake and output, mucous membranes, serum electrolyte levels, skin turgor, and urine specific gravity
- Oral status, including inspection of oral cavity (gums and tongue), pain or discomfort, and salivation
- Nutritional status, including current weight, change from normal weight, and dietary pattern
- Psychosocial status, including change in financial status, coping skills, habits (smoking and alcohol intake), patient's perception of health problem, and recent traumatic event

DEFINING CHARACTERISTICS

- Bad taste in mouth
- Bleeding
- Cheilitis
- Coated tongue
- Decreased taste perception
- Desquamation
- Difficulty eating
- Difficulty swallowing
- Dysphonia
- Enlarged tonsils
- Geographic tongue
- Gingival hyperplasia
- Gingival pallor
- Gingival pocketing deeper than 4 mm
- Gingival recession
- Halitosis
- Hyperemia
- Macroplasia
- Mucosal denudation
- Oral discomfort
- Oral edema
- Oral fissure
- Oral lesion
- Oral mucosal pallor
- Oral nodule
- Oral pain
- Oral papule
- Oral ulcer
- Oral vesicles
- Pathogen exposure
- Presence of mass
- Purulent oral-nasal drainage
- Purulent oral-nasal exudates
- Smooth atrophic tongue
- Spongy patches in mouth
- Stomatitis
- White patches in mouth
- White plaque in mouth
- White, curd-like oral exudate
- Xerostomia

EXPECTED OUTCOMES

- Patient will have pink, moist oral mucous membranes.
- Patient will state increased comfort.
- Patient will have no complications.
- Patient will correlate precipitating factors with appropriate oral care.
- Patient will demonstrate oral hygiene practices.

Suggested NOC Outcomes

Oral Hygiene; Tissue Integrity: Skin & Mucous Membranes

INTERVENTIONS AND RATIONALES

S   Inspect patient's oral cavity every shift. Describe and document condition; report any change in status. *Regular assessments can anticipate or alleviate problems.*

EBP   Perform the prescribed treatment regimen, including administering IV or oral fluids, *to improve the condition of patient's mucous membranes.* Monitor progress, reporting favorable and adverse responses to the treatment regimen.

EBP   Establish and follow a routine oral hygiene schedule. For example, soak dentures every evening, clean with denture cream, rinse, and keep them in a properly labeled container at patient's bedside. *Routine oral hygiene can improve the condition of mucous membranes.*

EBP   Provide supportive measures, as indicated:
- Assist with oral hygiene before and after meals *to promote a feeling of comfort and well-being.*
- Use a toothbrush with suction if patient can't spit out water *to minimize risk of aspiration.*
- Provide mouthwash or gargles, as ordered, *to increase patient comfort and maintain moisture in the mouth.*
- Lubricate patient's lips frequently with water-based lubricant *to prevent cracked, irritated skin.*

EBP   Instruct patient in oral hygiene practices, if necessary. Have patient return a demonstration of the oral care routine.
- Use a soft-bristled toothbrush.
- Brush with a circular motion away from the gums.
- Include the tongue when brushing.
- Review the need for routine visits to a dentist (annually for adults). *These measures increase patient's awareness of oral hygiene practices and reduce discomfort, resulting in increased nutrition and hydration.*

EBP   Tell patient to chew gum or suck on sugarless hard candy *to stimulate salivation.*

EBP   Discuss precipitating factors, if known, and work to prevent future episodes. For example, encourage patient to avoid exercising in heat and to report effects of medication. *Patient's increased awareness of causative factors will help prevent recurrence.*

S   If oral surgery is scheduled, give the appropriate preoperative and postoperative instruction and care. Document the response. *Instruction enhances compliance with therapy.*

EBP   Encourage adherence to other aspects of health care management (controlling diabetes, changing dietary habits, and avoiding alcoholic beverages) *to control or minimize effects on mucous membranes.*

■ Encourage patient to stop smoking. *Smoking has been linked to mucous membrane breakdown and cancer.*

■ Refer patient to a dentist, dental hygienist, or other appropriate resource to correct ill-fitting dentures, modify braces, and adjust jaw wires as needed. *Regularly scheduled dental follow-up reduces the risk of trauma to oral mucous membranes.*

Suggested NIC Interventions

Fluid/Electrolyte Management; Infection Protection; Nutrition Management; Oral Health Maintenance; Oral Health Restoration

EVALUATIONS FOR EXPECTED OUTCOMES

■ Patient's total daily fluid intake equals total output.
■ Patient chews and swallows without discomfort.
■ Patient's mucous membranes remain moist, pink, and free from cuts and abrasions.
■ Patient doesn't develop complications related to extended dehydration of mucous membranes.
■ Patient discusses possible causes of alteration in oral mucous membranes, such as heat exhaustion and reactions to medication.
■ Patient discusses and demonstrates preventive measures such as regular oral hygiene.

DOCUMENTATION

■ Observations of condition, healing, and response to treatment
■ Interventions to provide supportive care and patient's response to supportive care
■ Instructions given, patient's understanding of instructions, and patient's demonstrated skill in carrying out prescribed oral care measures
■ Evaluations for expected outcomes

REFERENCES

Azuero, A., Winstead, V., Jablonski, R. A., Kolanowski, A. M., Jones, T. C., Geisinger, M. L., & Jones-Townsend, C. (2018). Randomised clinical trial: Efficacy of strategies to provide oral hygiene activities to nursing home residents with dementia who resist mouth care. *Gerodontology, 35*(4), 365–375. doi:10.1111/ger.12357
Harding, J. (2018). Oral care in cancer: Helping patients with tooth, gum and mouth problems. *British Journal of Nursing, 27*(19), 1106–1107. doi:10.12968/bjon.2018.27.19.1106
Riley, E. (2018). The importance of oral health in palliative care patients. *Journal of Community Nursing, 32*(3), 57–61.

Risk for Impaired Oral Mucous Membrane Integrity

DEFINITION

Susceptible to injury to the lips, soft tissues, buccal cavity, and/or oropharynx, which may compromise health

RISK FACTORS

■ Alcohol consumption
■ Cognitive dysfunction

- Decreased salivation
- Dehydration
- Depressive symptoms
- Difficulty performing oral self-care
- Inadequate access to dental care
- Inadequate knowledge of oral hygiene
- Inadequate oral hygiene habits
- Inappropriate use of chemical agent
- Malnutrition
- Mouth breathing
- Smoking
- Stressors

ASSOCIATED CONDITIONS

- Allergies
- Autosomal disorder
- Behavioral disorder
- Chemotherapy
- Decreased female hormone levels
- Decreased platelets
- Depression
- Immune system diseases
- Immunosuppression
- Infections
- Loss of oral support structure
- Mechanical factor
- Mouth abnormalities
- Nil per os (NPO) greater than 24 hours
- Oral trauma
- Radiotherapy
- Sjögren's Syndrome
- Surgical procedures
- Trauma
- Treatment regimen

ASSESSMENT

- Fluid intake
- Nutritional status
- Oral mucosa
- Ill-fitting dentures
- Ability to swallow
- Pain level
- Ability to provide oral hygiene

EXPECTED OUTCOMES

- Patient will have pink, moist, and intact oral mucosa.
- Patient will have no reports of oral dryness and pain.

Suggested NOC Outcomes

Hydration; Immune Status; Knowledge: Health Promotion; Nutritional Status; Self-care: Oral Hygiene

INTERVENTIONS AND RATIONALES

S ■ Assist with oral care before meals and after meals and snacks. *Good oral care can decrease risk for impaired oral mucosa.*

S ■ Avoid serving hot, cold, spicy, fried, or citrus foods. *Can damage oral mucosa.*

EBP ■ Educate about regular dental checkups. *Can ensure health of teeth and gums.*

EBP ■ Educate to breathe through nose and not mouth. *Mouth breathing can further dry the oral mucosa.*

EBP ■ Encourage 2,500 to 3,000 mL of oral intake daily unless contraindicated. *Adequate fluid intake will help prevent dehydration and dryness of mouth.*

EBP ■ Encourage patient to not smoke or use tobacco. *Smoking dries the mucosa and tobacco is an irritant to the oral mucosa.*

PCC ■ Lubricate lips. *Prevents cracking and irritation.*

S ■ Rinse mouth every 2 hours if unable to take fluid by mouth or presence of drainage or lesions. *Prevents dryness.*

S ■ Suction mouth as needed. *Can reduce risk of developing infection.*

EBP ■ Use tap water or saline to provide oral care. *Use of alcohol-based products or hydrogen peroxide will dry and damage the mouth.*

Suggested NIC Interventions

Fluid Management; Nutrition Management; Oral Health Maintenance; Oral Health Promotion

EVALUATIONS FOR EXPECTED OUTCOMES

■ Patient does not have impaired oral mucosa.
■ Patient does not report any oral dryness or pain.

DOCUMENTATION

■ Ability to provide oral hygiene
■ Evaluations for expected outcomes
■ Intake and output
■ Nutritional status
■ Oral mucosa assessment
■ Pain level

REFERENCES

Liu, W. M., Chiang, C. K., & Hwu, Y. J. (2019). Oral care for clients in long-term care. *Journal of Nursing, 66*(1), 21–26. doi:10.6224/JN.201902_66(1).04

Prendergast, V., & Hinkle, J. L. (2018). Oral care assessment tools and interventions after stroke. *Stroke, 49*(4), e153–e156. doi:10.1161/STROKEAHA.117.017045

Weintraub, J. A., Zimmerman, S., Ward, K., Wretman, C. J., Sloane, P. D., Stearns, S. C., . . . Preisser, J. S. (2018). Improving nursing home residents' oral hygiene: Results of a cluster randomized intervention trial. *Journal of the American Medical Directors Association, 19*(12), 1086–1091. doi:10.1016/j.jamda.2018.09.036

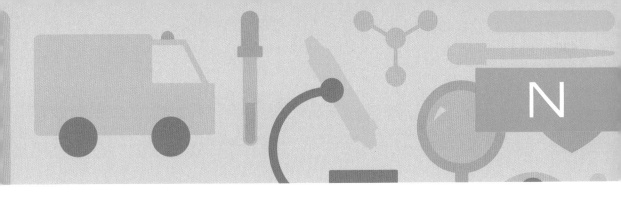

Nausea

A subjective phenomenon of an unpleasant feeling in the back of the throat and stomach, which may or may not result in vomiting

- Anxiety
- Exposure to toxin
- Fear
- Noxious environmental stimuli
- Noxious taste
- Unpleasant visual stimuli

- Biochemical dysfunction
- Esophageal disease
- Gastric distention
- Gastrointestinal irritation
- Increase in intracranial pressure (ICP)
- Intra-abdominal tumors
- Labyrinthitis
- Liver capsule stretch
- Localized tumor
- Meniere's disease
- Meningitis
- Motion sickness
- Pancreatic disease
- Pregnancy
- Psychological disorder
- Splenic capsule stretch
- Treatment regimen

- Health history, including illnesses, pregnancy, and medication use
- Nutritional status, including height, weight, fluctuations in weight, food preferences, and usual dietary patterns
- Psychosocial status, including ethnic background, family dynamics, lifestyle, perception of self, recent stressful events, and coping skills

- Aversion toward food
- Gagging sensation
- Increase in salivation
- Increase in swallowing
- Sour taste

- Patient will state reasons for nausea and vomiting.
- Patient will take steps to manage episodes of nausea and vomiting.
- Patient will ingest sufficient nutrients to maintain health.
- Patient will take steps to ensure adequate nutrition when nausea abates.
- Patient will maintain weight within specified range.

Suggested NOC Outcomes

Appetite; Comfort Level; Fluid Balance; Hydration; Nausea & Vomiting Control; Nutritional Status: Food & Fluid Intake; Suffering Severity; Symptom Control

- **PCC** Ask patient reasons for nausea or inability to eat and document explanation in patient's own words *to plan interventions.*
- Observe patient's fluid and food intake and document the findings *to assess nutrient consumption and the need for supplements.*
- **EBP** Encourage patient to eat dry, bland foods (such as dry toast or crackers) during periods of nausea *to make it possible for patient to eat.*
- **EBP** Suggest that patient avoid offensive foods and food odors, shorten food preparation time, and eat and drink slowly. *These measures may help to prevent nausea from getting worse.*
- **PCC** Administer antinausea medications as prescribed *to provide relief from nausea and allow patient to eat.*
- **EBP** Teach relaxation techniques and help patient use such techniques during mealtime *to reduce stress and divert attention from nausea, thereby helping patient eat and drink.*
- **PCC** Provide distractions when patient is feeling nauseated; for example, play favorite music, television programs, audiobooks, and so on. *Distraction helps to divert patient's attention from the unpleasant feeling of nausea.*
- **PCC** Encourage patient to make a list of best-tolerated and least-tolerated foods *to help patient choose foods wisely when nausea abates.*

Suggested NIC Interventions

Diet Staging; Fluid/Electrolyte Management; Fluid Monitoring; Medication Management; Nausea Management

- Patient states reasons for nausea and vomiting.
- Patient takes steps to manage episodes of nausea and vomiting.

▨ Patient ingests sufficient nutrients to maintain health.

▨ Patient takes steps to ensure adequate nutrition when nausea abates.

▨ Patient maintains weight within specified range.

DOCUMENTATION

▨ Patient's statements regarding nausea and its causes

▨ Episodes of nausea or vomiting

▨ Intake and output measurements

▨ Types of food and fluids ingested and patient's tolerance

▨ Nursing interventions, including teaching provided to patient

▨ Patient's response to nursing interventions

▨ Evaluations for expected outcomes

REFERENCES

Kovac, A. L. (2018). Updates in the management of postoperative nausea and vomiting. *Advances in Anesthesia, 36*(1), 81–97. doi:10.1016/j.aan.2018.07.004

Moorthy, G. S., & Letizia, M. (2018). The management of nausea at the end of life. *Journal of Hospice & Palliative Nursing, 20*(5), 442–451. doi:10.1097/NJH.0000000000000453

Sande, T. A., Laird, B. J. A., & Fallon, M. T. (2019). The management of opioid-induced nausea and vomiting in patients with cancer: A systematic review. *Journal of Palliative Medicine, 22*(1), 90–97. doi:10.1089/jpm.2018.0260

Nipple-Areolar Complex Injury

DEFINITION

Localized damage to nipple-areolar complex as a result of the breastfeeding process

RELATED FACTORS (R/T)

▨ Breast engorgement

▨ Hardened areola

▨ Improper use of milk pump

▨ Inadequate latching on

▨ Inappropriate maternal hand support of breast

▨ Inappropriate positioning of the infant during breastfeeding

▨ Inappropriate positioning of the mother during breastfeeding

▨ Ineffective infant sucking reflex

▨ Ineffective nonnutritive sucking

▨ Mastitis

▨ Maternal anxiety about breastfeeding

▨ Maternal impatience with the breastfeeding process

▨ Mother does not wait for the infant to spontaneously release the nipple

▨ Mother withdraws infant from breast without breaking the suction

▨ Nipple confusion due to use of artificial nipple

▨ Postprocedural pain

▨ Prolonged exposure to moisture

▨ Supplementary feeding

▨ Use of products that remove the natural protection of the nipple

ASSOCIATED CONDITIONS

- Ankyloglossia
- Maxillofacial abnormalities

ASSESSMENT

- Mother and infant's age
- Nipple and areolar color, texture, temperature, open or excoriated areas, and presence of swelling
- Breast engorgement
- Use of breast/milk pump
- Use of hygiene products and products for nipple care
- Positioning of infant and mother during breastfeeding
- Infant sucking reflex
- Mother's perception of breastfeeding and breastfeeding difficulties
- Cultural status, including affiliation with racial, ethnic, or religious groups

DEFINING CHARACTERISTICS

- Abraded skin
- Altered skin color
- Altered thickness of nipple-areolar complex
- Blistered skin
- Discolored skin patches
- Disrupted skin surface
- Ecchymosis
- Eroded skin
- Erythema
- Expresses pain
- Hematoma
- Macerated skin
- Scabbed skin
- Skin fissure
- Skin ulceration
- Skin vesicles
- Swelling
- Tissue exposure below the epidermis

EXPECTED OUTCOMES

- Nipple-areola will be free of pain.
- Nipple-areola will be free of infection.
- Nipple-areola will be intact and free from excoriation, abrasion, swelling, open areas.

Suggested NOC Outcomes

Breastfeeding Establishment: Infant; Breastfeeding Establishment: Maternal; Knowledge: Breastfeeding; Knowledge: Postpartum Maternal Health; Knowledge: Wound Management; Self-Management: Infection; Self-Management: Wound

S ▪ Examine the breast every shift; check nipples for inversion and for pore openings, *as anatomic conditions can lead to nipple-areolar injury, to identify problems before injury is severe.*

PCC ▪ Assess to see if the neonate is able to latch properly to the nipple to suckle. *When infant is unable to achieve a proper suckling position, wearing, bruising, blistering, or cracking of nipples may occur.*

EBP ▪ Position the mother/baby properly for baby to latch to nipple and suckle. *The couplet may need direction in assuming the best position of comfort for suckling.*

EBP ▪ Assess the neonate's mouth to determine normal anatomy of tongue and palate; assess the neonate's mouth for Candida infection. *Anatomic imperfections and thrush infection affect the neonate's ability to suckle.*

EBP ▪ Educate mother to rotate between breastfeeding and feeding expressed milk *to allow nipple-areolar wounds to heal. Depending on severity of wound, the provider may prescribe an antibiotic ointment for the affected nipple-areolar area.*

EBP ▪ For mild pain, apply warm or cool compresses. *Provides nonpharmacological pain relief.*

PCC ▪ Breastfeed using the less injured side first and limit feedings on more injured side to less than 10 minutes. *Infants generally feed more aggressively when they are hungriest.*

EBP ▪ Teach mother to detach infant by inserting the pinky finger into the corner of the infant's mouth to break the suction. *Allows easy breaking of suction.*

EBP ▪ Instruct mother to gently clean nipples. Rinse the breast after each feeding with warm water, pat with a clean towel, and air dry. *Antibacterial soaps and skincare products with alcohol or fragrances are damaging to nipple area.*

EBP ▪ Provide education about using a nipple cream, balm, gel, and/or an antibacterial ointment. *The health care provider may prescribe antibacterial ointment for an open wound.*

EBP ▪ Caution mother about use of lanolin *as lanolin can hold in excessive moisture.*

PCC ▪ If not contraindicated, administer pain medications such as ibuprofen or acetaminophen about 30 minutes before breastfeeding. *Ibuprofen and acetaminophen are considered safe to help lessen pain.*

PCC ▪ Provide encouragement and support to mother for breastfeeding. *Mother may be discouraged due to condition or pain.*

S ▪ Check with health care provider about substances and medications that can dry skin (i.e., caffeine, tobacco, nicotine, pseudoephedrine, diuretics, contraception pills). *To maintain skin integrity, avoidance of substances that are drying.*

T&C ▪ Use a multidisciplinary team approach to support the mother for nipple-areolar injury—registered nurse, lactation specialist, certified nurse midwife, pediatrician, registered dietitian, social worker. *A team approach brings expertise to address the needs of the mother and promotes health and well-being for the family unit.*

Suggested NIC Interventions

Breast Examination; Infant Care: Newborn; Skin Care: Topical Treatment; Skin Surveillance; Wound Care

▪ No patient report of nipple-areola pain.
▪ Nipple-areola does not exhibit signs and symptoms of infection.
▪ Nipple-areola area is intact and free from excoriation, abrasion, swelling, open areas.
▪ Infant is positioned to facilitate proper latch.

- Mother is positioned to facilitate proper latch.
- Mother participates in nipple-areola inspection and injury prevention techniques.

DOCUMENTATION

- Mother's expressions of breast comfort
- Assessment of factors that may create injury
- Nursing interventions and mother–infant's response to them
- Teaching and instructions given
- Referrals to support groups
- Evaluations for expected outcomes

REFERENCES

Cervellini, M. P., Coca, K. P., Gamba, M., Marcacine, K. O., & Freitas de Vilhena Abrão, A. C. (2022). Construction and validation of an instrument for classifying nipple and areola complex lesions resulting from breastfeeding. *Revista Brasileira De Enfermagem, 75*(1), 1–9. doi:10.1590/0034-7167-2021-0051

Hernández-Cordero, S., Lozada-Tequeanes, A., Fernández-Gaxiola, A. C., Shamah-Levy, T., Sachse, M., Veliz, P., & Cosío-Barroso, I. (2020). Barriers and facilitators to breastfeeding during the immediate and one month postpartum periods, among Mexican women: A mixed methods approach. *International Breastfeeding Journal, 15*, 1–12. doi:10.1186/s13006-020-00327-3

Wang, Z., Liu, Q., Min, L., & Mao, X. (2021). The effectiveness of the laid-back position on lactation-related nipple problems and comfort: A meta-analysis. *BMC Pregnancy & Childbirth, 21*(1), 1–14.

Xiao, X., Alice, Y. L., Zhu, S. N., Gong, L., Shi, H. M., & Ngai, F. W. (2020). "The sweet and the bitter": Mothers' experiences of breastfeeding in the early postpartum period: A qualitative exploratory study in China. *International Breastfeeding Journal, 15*, 1–11. doi:10.1186/s13006-020-00256-1

Risk for Nipple-Areolar Complex Injury

DEFINITION

Susceptible to localized damage to nipple-areolar complex as a result of the breastfeeding process

RISK FACTORS

- Breast engorgement
- Hardened areola
- Improper use of milk pump
- Inadequate latching on
- Inadequate nipple-areolar preparation during prenatal care
- Inappropriate maternal hand support of breast
- Inappropriate positioning of the infant during breastfeeding
- Inappropriate positioning of the mother during breastfeeding
- Ineffective infant sucking reflex
- Ineffective nonnutritive sucking
- Mastitis
- Maternal anxiety about breastfeeding
- Maternal impatience with the breastfeeding process
- Mother does not wait for the infant to spontaneously release the nipple

- Mother withdraws infant from breast without breaking the suction
- Nipple confusion due to use of artificial nipple
- Postprocedural pain
- Prolonged exposure to moisture
- Supplementary feeding
- Use of products that remove the natural protection of the nipple

ASSOCIATED CONDITIONS

- Ankyloglossia
- Maxillofacial abnormalities

ASSESSMENT

- Mother and infant's age
- Nipple and areolar color, texture, temperature, open or excoriated areas, and presence of swelling
- Breast engorgement
- Use of breast/milk pump
- Use of hygiene products and products for nipple care
- Positioning of infant and mother during breastfeeding
- Infant sucking reflex
- Mother's perception of breastfeeding and breastfeeding difficulties
- Cultural status, including affiliation with racial, ethnic, or religious groups

EXPECTED OUTCOMES

- Nipple-areola will be free of pain.
- Nipple-areola will be free of infection.
- Nipple-areola will be intact and free from excoriation, abrasion, swelling, open areas.

Suggested NOC Outcomes

Breastfeeding Establishment: Infant; Breastfeeding Establishment: Maternal; Knowledge: Breastfeeding; Knowledge: Postpartum Maternal Health; Knowledge: Wound Management; Self-Management: Infection; Self-Management: Wound

INTERVENTIONS AND RATIONALES

S ▪ Examine the breast every shift; check nipples for inversion and for pore openings, *as anatomic conditions can lead to nipple-areolar injury, to identify problems before injury is severe.*

PCC ▪ Assess to see if the neonate is able to latch properly to the nipple to suckle. *When infant is unable to achieve a proper suckling position, wearing, bruising, blistering, or cracking of nipples may occur.*

EBP ▪ Position the mother/baby properly for baby to latch to nipple and suckle. *The couplet may need direction in assuming the best position of comfort for suckling.*

EBP ▪ Assess the neonate's mouth to determine normal anatomy of tongue and palate; assess the neonate's mouth for Candida infection. *Anatomic imperfections and thrush infection affect the neonate's ability to suckle.*

EBP ▥ Educate mother about causes of nipple injuries. *Use of irritating products, cleansing nipples harshly, infant biting, bacterial infections, plugged ducts increase risk of injury.*

EBP ▥ Decrease excessive nipple moisture and allow nipples to air dry. *Air drying is less damaging to skin.*

S ▥ Instruct patient to report nipple abnormalities immediately. *Abnormalities may cause nipple injuries while breastfeeding.*

S ▥ Prevent breast engorgement. *Engorgement causes a buildup of milk and blood tissues in the breast which can lead to nipple injury.*

S ▥ Instruct mother to notify provider for fever, discharge, bleeding, inflammation, or blistering. *Signs of possible infection.*

T&C ▥ Use a multidisciplinary team approach to support the mother for nipple-areolar injury— registered nurse, lactation specialist, certified nurse midwife, pediatrician, registered dietitian, social worker. *A team approach brings expertise to address the needs of the mother and promotes health and well-being for the family unit.*

Suggested NIC Interventions

Breast Examination; Infant Care: Newborn; Skin Care: Topical Treatment; Skin Surveillance; Wound Care

EVALUATIONS FOR EXPECTED OUTCOMES

▥ No patient report of nipple-areola pain.
▥ Nipple-areola does not exhibit signs and symptoms of infection.
▥ Nipple-areola area is intact and free from excoriation, abrasion, swelling, open areas.
▥ Infant is positioned to facilitate proper latch.
▥ Mother is positioned to facilitate proper latch.
▥ Mother participates in nipple-areola inspection and injury prevention techniques.

DOCUMENTATION

▥ Mother's expressions of breast comfort
▥ Assessment of factors that may create injury
▥ Nursing interventions and mother–infant's response to them
▥ Teaching and instructions given
▥ Referrals to support groups
▥ Evaluations for expected outcomes

REFERENCES

Cervellini, M. P., Coca, K. P., Gamba, M., Marcacine, K. O., & Freitas de Vilhena Abrão, A. C. (2022). Construction and validation of an instrument for classifying nipple and areola complex lesions resulting from breastfeeding. *Revista Brasileira De Enfermagem, 75*(1), 1–9. doi:10.1590/0034-7167-2021-0051

Hernández-Cordero, S., Lozada-Tequeanes, A., Fernández-Gaxiola, A. C., Shamah-Levy, T., Sachse, M., Veliz, P., & Cosío-Barroso, I. (2020). Barriers and facilitators to breastfeeding during the immediate and one month postpartum periods, among Mexican women: A mixed methods approach. *International Breastfeeding Journal, 15*, 1–12. doi:10.1186/s13006-020-00327-3

Wang, Z., Liu, Q., Min, L., & Mao, X. (2021). The effectiveness of the laid-back position on lactation-related nipple problems and comfort: A meta-analysis. *BMC Pregnancy & Childbirth, 21*(1), 1–14.

Xiao, X., Alice, Y. L., Zhu, S. N., Gong, L., Shi, H. M., & Ngai, F. W. (2020). "The sweet and the bitter": Mothers' experiences of breastfeeding in the early postpartum period: A qualitative exploratory study in China. *International Breastfeeding Journal, 15*, 1–11. doi:10.1186/s13006-020-00256-1

Neonatal Abstinence Syndrome

DEFINITION

A constellation of withdrawal symptoms observed in newborns as a result of in-utero exposure to addicting substances, or as a consequence of postnatal pharmacological pain management

RELATED FACTORS (R/T)

To be developed

ASSESSMENT

- Gestational age
- Vital signs
- Cardiovascular status, including heart rate and rhythm
- Respiratory status, including oxygen saturation and respirations
- Gastrointestinal (GI) status, including feeding pattern, food tolerance, defecation pattern, ability to maintain adequate weight, and abdominal bloating and distention
- Neurologic status, including muscle tone, neonatal reflexes, excessive crying, lethargy, irritability, seizures, tremors, and assessments such as Brazelton Neonatal Behavioral Assessment, Dubowitz Gestational Age Assessment, and Modified Finnegan Scoring System
- Sensory status, including responsiveness to visual, tactile, and auditory stimuli and experience with pain
- Maternal history of substance misuse
- Parents' psychological status, including energy level, motivation, self-image, competence, recent life changes, experience with children, and eye contact and interaction with infant

DEFINING CHARACTERISTICS

- Diarrhea
- Disorganized infant behavior
- Disturbed sleep pattern
- Impaired comfort
- Ineffective infant feeding pattern
- Neurobehavioral stress
- Risk for aspiration
- Risk for imbalanced body temperature
- Risk for impaired attachment
- Risk for impaired skin integrity
- Risk for injury

EXPECTED OUTCOMES

- Infant will not experience complications from withdrawal of substance.
- Infant will remain free from harm.
- Infant will not experience seizure activity.
- Parents will identify means to help infant overcome behavioral disturbance.
- Parents will identify ways to improve their ability to cope with infant's responses.
- Parents will identify resources for help with infant.

Suggested NOC Outcomes

Aspiration Prevention; Comfort Status; Infant Nutritional Status; Neurological Status; Newborn Adaptation; Parent-Infant Attachment

INTERVENTIONS AND RATIONALES

S ▦ Monitor and record level of consciousness (LOC), temperature, heart rate and rhythm, and blood pressure at least every 4 hours or more often if necessary *to detect deterioration from possible hypoxia or decreased cardiac output.*

S ▦ Assess sleeping patterns *to monitor for withdrawal symptoms.*

S ▦ Use appropriate safety measures *to protect patient from injury.*

▦ Provide a gentle, soothing environment with minimal stimulation *to help calm and soothe infant.*

PCC ▦ Swaddle infant *to provide comfort.*

PCC ▦ Limit exposure to lights and noise. Cluster all care *to calm infant and promote rest.*

PCC ▦ Allow infant to engage in nonnutritive sucking, such as a pacifier *for comfort and soothing.*

EBP ▦ Monitor feeding frequency, amount, infant weight, number and weight of soiled diapers, and laboratory value *to assess nutrition status.*

EBP ▦ If inadequate weight gain, increase the frequency of feedings. A high-calorie formula may be required. *Maintaining infant weight supports neurologic function.*

EBP ▦ If diarrhea or vomiting is present, consider a lactose-free formula *to promote digestion.*

EBP ▦ Encourage breastfeeding if not contraindicated. *Breastfed babies tend to have less severe symptoms and complications.*

▦ Administer medications as prescribed *for severe withdrawal symptoms.*

PCC ▦ Convey attitude of acceptance to mother, separating individual from unacceptable behavior. *Promotes feelings of dignity and self-worth and fosters care of infant.*

PCC ▦ Assess mother's support system. *Family involvement can help patient feel more in control.*

T&C ▦ Refer the patient to a social worker for follow-up treatment after hospitalization. *Continual monitoring is usually necessary to assist family in coping with health care status.*

Suggested NIC Interventions

Aspiration Precautions; Calming Technique; Infant Care; Neurologic Monitoring; Respiratory Monitoring; Seizure Precautions; Substance Use Treatment: Drug Withdrawal

EVALUATIONS FOR EXPECTED OUTCOMES

▦ Infant does not experience complications from withdrawal of substance.
▦ Infant remains free from harm.
▦ Infant does not experience seizure activity.
▦ Parents identify means to help infant overcome behavioral disturbance.
▦ Parents identify ways to improve their ability to cope with infant's responses.
▦ Parents identify resources for help with infant.

DOCUMENTATION

▦ Infant's vital signs
▦ Assessment of body systems at risk for deterioration
▦ Observation of infant's behaviors
▦ Interventions to provide preventive or supportive care and prescribed treatment

▦ Parents' expressed feelings about caring for infant
▦ Nursing interventions and infant's response to them
▦ Evaluations for expected outcomes

REFERENCES

Corr, T. E., & Hollenbeak, C. S. (2017). The economic burden of neonatal abstinence syndrome in the United States. *Addiction, 112*(9), 1590–1599. doi:10.1111/add.13842

Dickes, L., Summey, J., Mayo, R., Hudson, J., Sherrill, W. W., & Chen, L. (2017). Potential for Medicaid savings: A state and national comparison of an innovative neonatal abstinence syndrome treatment model. *Population Health Management, 20*(6), 458–464. doi:10.1089/pop.2016.0158

MacMullen, N. J., & Samson, L. F. (2018). Neonatal abstinence syndrome: An uncontrollable epidemic. *Critical Care Nursing Clinics of North America, 30*(4), 585–596. doi:10.1016/j.cnc.2018.07.011

Wachman, E. M., Grossman, M., Schiff, D. M., Philipp, B. L., Minear, S., Hutton, E., … Whalen, B. L. (2018). Quality improvement initiative to improve inpatient outcomes for neonatal abstinence syndrome. *Journal of Perinatology, 38*(8), 1114–1122. doi:10.1038/s41372-018-0109-8

Risk for Peripheral Neurovascular Dysfunction

DEFINITION

Susceptible to disruption in the circulation, sensation, and motion of an extremity, which may compromise health

RISK FACTORS

To be developed

ASSOCIATED CONDITIONS

▦ Burn injury
▦ Fracture
▦ Immobilization
▦ Mechanical compression
▦ Orthopedic surgery
▦ Trauma
▦ Vascular obstruction

ASSESSMENT

▦ History of trauma or vascular injuries
▦ Inspection of extremities, including signs of soft tissue injury, such as abrasions, lacerations, and contusions
▦ Pain sensation, including characteristics of pain (sharp, dull, constant, or intermittent), precipitating factors, and reaction to passive stretching of affected muscles
▦ Tactile sensation in areas innervated by major nerves of upper extremities, including deltoid, radial side of forearm, palmar surface of thumb, fingers, palmar surface of little finger, and webbed space between thumb and index finger
▦ Tactile sensation in lower extremities, including medial side of foot and leg, medial side of thigh, sole of foot, and lateral aspect of leg below the knee
▦ Motor nerve function of upper extremities, including arm abduction at shoulder, arm flexion at elbow, thumb and little finger opposition, abduction and adduction of fingers, and extension of wrist and fingers

- Motor nerve function of lower extremities, including knee extension, thigh adduction, plantar flexion and dorsiflexion of ankle, and flexion and extension of toes
- Pulses in upper and lower extremities, including radial, ulnar, brachial, femoral, popliteal, posterior tibial, and dorsalis pedis; perform bilateral comparison and rank quality using following scale:
  0 = absent
  1 = very weak, barely palpable
  2 = weak, reduced
  3 = slightly weak, easily located
  4 = normal, easily located
- Vascular status, including capillary refill time, blanching, skin temperature, and skin color
- Point tenderness, especially over bony prominences
- Edema
- Increased intracompartmental pressure
- Cranial nerves (if patient has halo cast)

EXPECTED OUTCOMES

- Patient won't experience disability related to peripheral neurovascular dysfunction after injury or treatment.
- Patient will maintain circulation in extremities.
- Patient will feel and move each toe or finger after application of cast, brace, or splint.
- Patient will demonstrate correct body positioning techniques.
- Patient and family members will express understanding of risk of altered neurovascular status and need to report symptoms of impaired circulation.
- Patient will enroll in smoking-cessation program, as appropriate.
- Patient will not exhibit symptoms of neurovascular compromise.

Suggested NOC Outcomes

Circulation Status; Coordinated Movement; Neurological Status: Spinal Sensory/Motor Function; Risk Control; Risk Detection; Tissue Perfusion: Peripheral

INTERVENTIONS AND RATIONALES

- **S** Note whether patient will undergo surgery or a procedure that increases risk of peripheral neurovascular dysfunction *to anticipate complications.*
- **S** Immobilize the joints directly above and below the suspected fracture site, leaving room for pulse assessment *to facilitate monitoring of circulatory status.*
- **S** As appropriate, assess circulation before the application of the cast, brace, or splint. After application of the cast, brace, or splint, have patient move fingers and toes every 4 hours until discharge *to detect signs of impaired circulation.*
- **S** Remove the clothing around the suspected fracture site, clean the site, apply sterile dressings to open wounds, and carefully apply a cast, brace, or splint *to avoid further infection and trauma.*
- **EBP** Follow facility guidelines for the application of such devices as tourniquets, restraints, and tape *to ensure adequate circulation in affected extremity.*
- **S** If you suspect nerve compression, assess the position of the extremity that has a cast, brace, or splint. *Positioning of the extremity may affect circulation.*
- **EBP** Elevate the limb above heart level after surgery or trauma *to reduce the risk of edema.* If increased intracompartmental pressure is evident, maintain the affected limb at heart level *to reduce pressure.*

EBP ▪ If edema appears in the affected extremity, split, bivalve, slit, or cut a window in the cast and padding according to facility protocol *to avoid neurovascular impairment.*

EBP ▪ Inject prescribed neurotoxic agents (such as penicillin G, hydrocortisone, tetanus toxoid, and diazepam) away from the affected extremity and major nerves *to avoid injury.*

▪ Avoid flexing the affected extremity. *Flexion may reduce venous circulation, increasing the risk of neurovascular complications.*

EBP ▪ If patient smokes, advise enrollment in a smoking-cessation program. *Quitting smoking may enhance oxygenation, decreasing the risk of peripheral neurovascular dysfunction.*

PCC ▪ Take steps to ease patient's anxiety. *Stress may lead to vasoconstriction.*

▪ Administer and monitor the effectiveness of vasodilators, as ordered, *to control vasospasm.*

EBP ▪ If patient requires a fasciotomy to restore circulation, provide educational material that explains this emergency procedure *to reduce patient anxiety.*

EBP ▪ Instruct patient and family members in proper positioning when lying in bed and when sitting and in methods of obtaining pressure relief *to avoid pooling of blood and pressure ulcers.*

S ▪ If appropriate, discuss the cause of the injury and safety precautions *to avoid further injury.* Injuries to upper extremities usually result from industrial accidents; injuries to lower extremities, from automobile accidents.

EBP ▪ Instruct patient and family members in recognizing the symptoms of peripheral neurovascular dysfunction, including numbness, pain, and tingling. Emphasize the need to report these symptoms to a physician *to prevent onset of neurovascular damage after discharge.*

Suggested NIC Interventions

Circulatory Precautions; Exercise Promotion: Strength Training; Exercise Therapy: Joint Mobility; Peripheral Sensation Management; Positioning: Neurologic; Pressure Ulcer Prevention; Skin Surveillance; Splinting

EVALUATIONS FOR EXPECTED OUTCOMES

▪ Patient doesn't experience disability related to peripheral neurovascular dysfunction.
▪ Patient maintains circulation in extremities.
▪ Patient demonstrates ability to move each toe or finger after application of cast, brace, or splint.
▪ Patient demonstrates correct body positioning techniques.
▪ Patient and family members express understanding of risk of altered neurovascular status.
▪ Patient enrolls in smoking-cessation program, as appropriate.
▪ Patient shows no symptoms of neurovascular compromise.

DOCUMENTATION

▪ Results of neurovascular assessment (baseline and ongoing)
▪ Nature of injury or treatment
▪ History of illnesses and surgeries
▪ Symptoms of neurovascular dysfunction reported by patient and family members
▪ Patient's turning schedule
▪ Instructions provided to patient and family members at discharge
▪ Evaluations for expected outcomes

REFERENCES

Rodrigues, S., Cepeda, F. X., Toschi, D. E., Dutra, M. A. C. B., Carvalho, J. C., Costa, H. V., ... Trombetta, I. C. (2017). The role of increased glucose on neurovascular dysfunction in patients with the metabolic syndrome. *Journal of Clinical Hypertension, 19*(9), 840–847. doi:10.1111/jch.13060

Shabir, O., Berwick, J., & Francis, S. E. (2018). Neurovascular dysfunction in vascular dementia, Alzheimer's and atherosclerosis. *BMC Neuroscience, 19*(1), N.PAG. doi:10.1186/s12868-018-0465-5

Sobol, G., Gibson, P., Patel, P., Koury, K., Sirkin, M., Reilly, M., & Adams, M. (2017). Low incidence of neurovascular complications after placement of proximal tibial traction pins. *Orthopedics, 40*(6), e1004–e1008. doi:10.3928/01477447-20171012-04

Imbalanced Nutrition: Less than Body Requirements

DEFINITION

Intake of nutrients insufficient to meet metabolic needs

RELATED FACTORS (R/T)

- Altered taste perception
- Depressive symptoms
- Difficulty swallowing
- Food aversion
- Inaccurate information
- Inadequate food supply
- Inadequate interest in food
- Inadequate knowledge of nutrient requirements
- Injured buccal cavity
- Insufficient breast milk production
- Interrupted breastfeeding
- Misperception about ability to ingest food
- Satiety immediately upon ingesting food
- Sore buccal cavity
- Weakened muscles required for swallowing
- Weakened muscles required for mastication

ASSOCIATED CONDITIONS

- Body dysmorphic disorders
- Digestive system diseases
- Immunosuppression
- Kwashiorkor
- Malabsorption syndromes
- Mental disorders
- Neoplasms
- Neurocognitive disorders
- Parasitic disorders

ASSESSMENT

- Age, sex, height, and weight
- Gastrointestinal (GI) assessment, including antibiotic therapy, auscultation of bowel sounds, change in bowel habits, stool characteristics (color, amount, size, and consistency), history of GI disorder or surgery, inspection of abdomen, pain or discomfort, usual bowel elimination pattern, palpation for masses and tenderness, percussion for tympany and dullness, and nausea and vomiting

- Nutritional status, including change in type of food tolerated, financial resources, meal preparation, serum albumin level, sociocultural influences, usual dietary pattern, and weight fluctuations over past 10 years
- History of eating disorders
- Change in intrapersonal or interpersonal factors, including internal or external cues that trigger desire to eat, rate of food consumption, and stated food preference
- Cultural influences, including education level, occupation, nationality, or ethnic group; beliefs, values, and attitudes about health and illness; and health practices and customs
- Psychosocial status
- Activity level
- Coping behaviors
- Body image, including perception of observer and self-perception

DEFINING CHARACTERISTICS

- Abdominal cramping
- Abdominal pain
- Body weight below ideal weight range for age and gender
- Capillary fragility
- Constipation
- Delayed wound healing
- Diarrhea
- Excessive hair loss
- Food intake less than recommended daily allowance (RDA)
- Hyperactive bowel sounds
- Hypoglycemia
- Inadequate head circumference growth for age and gender
- Inadequate height increase for age and gender
- Lethargy
- Muscle hypotonia
- Neonatal weight gain <30 g per day
- Pale mucous membranes
- Weight loss with adequate food intake

EXPECTED OUTCOMES

- Patient will show no further evidence of weight loss.
- Patient will tolerate oral, tube, or IV feedings without adverse effects.
- Patient will take in ___ calories daily.
- Patient will gain ___ lb weekly.
- Patient will identify emotional and psychological factors that interfere with eating.
- Patient will develop plan to monitor and maintain target weight at discharge.
- Patient and family members will communicate understanding of special dietary needs.
- Patient and family members will demonstrate ability to plan diet after discharge.
- Patient will use community resources to improve nutritional status as needed.

Suggested NOC Outcomes

Nutritional Status; Nutritional Status: Food & Fluid Intake; Nutritional Status: Nutrient Intake; Symptom Severity; Weight Control

INTERVENTIONS AND RATIONALES

EBP ▦ Obtain and record patient's weight at the same time every day *to get accurate readings.*

▦ Monitor fluid intake and output *because body weight may decrease as a result of fluid loss.*

▦ Maintain parenteral fluids as ordered *to provide patient with needed fluids and electrolytes.*

EBP ▦ Provide a diet prescribed for patient's specific condition *to improve patient's nutritional status and increase weight.*

PCC ▦ Determine food preferences and provide them within the limitations of patient's prescribed diet. *This enhances compliance with diet regimen.*

PCC ▦ Provide opportunities for patient to discuss reasons for not eating *to help assess causes of eating disorder.*

EBP ▦ Offer high-protein, high-calorie supplements, such as milkshakes, custard, and ice cream. *Such foods prevent body protein breakdown and provide caloric energy.*

PCC ▦ Serve foods that require little cutting or chewing *to help prevent malingering at meals.*

PCC ▦ Provide a pleasant environment at mealtime *to enhance patient's appetite.*

▦ Keep snacks at the bedside *to give patient some control over eating time.*

▦ With some patients, begin with nutritious liquids and gradually introduce solid food. *Severely malnourished patient may not be able to chew solid foods immediately.*

PCC ▦ Avoid asking whether patient is hungry or wants to eat. Be positive in offering food. *A positive, undemanding attitude avoids confrontation with patient.*

PCC ▦ Whenever possible, sit with patient for a predetermined length of time during each meal. *This inhibits patient from dawdling during the meal and from hiding or hoarding food.*

PCC ▦ Set a target weight and have patient record daily weight *to involve patient in treatment.*

S ▦ Monitor electrolyte levels and report abnormal values. *Poor nutritional status may cause electrolyte imbalances.*

▦ If patient vomits, record amount, color, and consistency. Keep a record of all stools. *Vomitus and stool characteristics indicate status of nutrient absorption.*

T&C ▦ Refer patient to a dietitian or nutritional support team for dietary management (possible regimens include yogurt feedings and low-bulk diet). *Dietitian or nutritional support team can help patient and health care team individualize patient's diet within prescribed restrictions.*

S ▦ If bottle-feeding, record the amount ingested at each feeding. If breastfeeding, record the number of minutes the neonate nurses at each feeding as well as ingestion of any supplement *to aid in early recognition of inadequate caloric and fluid intake.*

PCC ▦ Assess the parents' knowledge of feeding techniques. As needed, teach parents how much and how often to feed neonate, how to prepare formula, how to position neonate during and after feeding, and how to burp neonate. *Early detection of knowledge deficits and appropriate instruction help eliminate misconceptions.*

PCC ▦ If patient is receiving tube feeding:
  ▦ Add food coloring if patient has an altered state of consciousness or diminished gag reflex *to help detect aspiration.*
  ▦ If possible, use a continuous infusion pump for tube feeding *to avoid diarrhea.*
  ▦ Begin the tube feeding regimen with a small amount and diluted concentration *to decrease diarrhea and improve absorption.* Increase the volume and concentration, as tolerated.
  ▦ Keep the head of the bed elevated during tube feeding *to reduce the risk of aspiration.*
  ▦ Check the feeding tube placement each shift *to verify placement in the GI tract rather than in the lungs.*

EBP ▦ If patient is receiving total parenteral nutrition:
  ▦ Ensure delivery, as prescribed. *Electrolytes, amino acids, and other nutrients must be tailored to patient's needs.*
  ▦ Monitor blood glucose levels and urine specific gravity at least once each shift.

Because glucose is the main component of total parenteral nutrition, patient may become hyperglycemic if not carefully monitored.

S ▥ Monitor bowel sounds once per shift. *Normal active bowel sounds may indicate readiness for enteral feedings; hyperactive sounds may indicate poor absorption and may be accompanied by diarrhea.*

▥ Reinforce the medical regimen by explaining to patient and family members the reasons for the present regimen. *Collaborative practice enhances patient's overall care.*

EBP ▥ Teach the principles of good nutrition for patient's specific condition. *This encourages patient and family members to participate in patient's care.*

▥ Provide or assist with oral hygiene *to help keep patient comfortable.*

EBP ▥ Provide preoperative teaching, if needed, *to reduce patient's fear and anxiety and promote understanding.*

PCC ▥ Involve family members in meal planning *to encourage them to help patient comply with the diet regimen after discharge.*

PCC ▥ Identify patients who don't have resources to eat properly or who neglect nutritional needs. *Nurses working in community settings frequently encounter patients whose nutritional needs aren't met. Nursing responsibilities include identifying these individuals and intervening on their behalf.*

T&C ▥ Depending on patient's resources, help locate soup kitchens for the homeless, senior centers that serve meals for a nominal fee, Meals on Wheels, or similar programs *to promote access to appropriate community resources.*

Suggested NIC Interventions

Energy Management; Nutritional Counseling; Nutrition Management; Nutrition Therapy; Weight Gain Assistance

EVALUATIONS FOR EXPECTED OUTCOMES

▥ Patient remains at or above specified weight.
▥ Patient doesn't develop adverse reactions from feedings, such as aspiration of food particles into lungs, diarrhea, and hyperglycemia.
▥ Patient consumes specified number of calories daily.
▥ Patient's weight increases by specified amount weekly.
▥ Patient lists emotional and psychological factors that interfere with eating.
▥ Patient states plan to monitor and maintain specific target weight after discharge.
▥ Patient and family communicate understanding of special dietary needs, either verbally or through behavior.
▥ Patient and family plan appropriate diet for patient to follow after discharge.
▥ Patient uses community resources as needed.

DOCUMENTATION

▥ Daily weight
▥ Mouth care
▥ Maintenance of nasogastric tube
▥ Intake and output
▥ Bowel sounds
▥ Blood glucose levels
▥ Urine specific gravity
▥ Patient's ability to eat

- Incidence of vomiting or diarrhea
- Presence of other complications
- Patient's statements of understanding of dietary education
- Evaluations for expected outcomes

REFERENCES

Bishop, A., Witts, S., & Martin, T. (2018). The role of nutrition in successful wound healing. *Journal of Community Nursing, 32*(4), 44–50.

de Ridder, D., Kroese, F., Evers, C., Adriaanse, M., & Gillebaart, M. (2017). Healthy diet: Health impact, prevalence, correlates, and interventions. *Psychology & Health, 32*(8), 907–941. doi:10.1080/08870446.2017.1316849

Leonard, D., Aquino, D., Hadgraft, N., Thompson, F., & Marley, J. V. (2017). Poor nutrition from first foods: A cross-sectional study of complementary feeding of infants and young children in six remote Aboriginal communities across northern Australia. *Nutrition & Dietetics, 74*(5), 436–445. doi:10.1111/1747-0080.12386

Palmeira, L., Cunha, M., & Pinto-Gouveia, J. (2018). The weight of weight self-stigma in unhealthy eating behaviours: The mediator role of weight-related experiential avoidance. *Eating & Weight Disorders, 23*(6), 785–796. doi:10.1007/s40519-018-0540-z

Readiness for Enhanced Nutrition

DEFINITION

A pattern of nutrient intake, which can be strengthened

ASSESSMENT

- Biologic factors, including age, gender, height, weight, and body mass index
- Psychological factors, including self-esteem, history of depression, and attitudes toward food and eating
- Sociocultural factors, including moral or health concerns about food and eating, financial status, and cultural background and influences of same in food choices
- Environmental factors, including ability to read and understand food labels; percentage of meals that are takeout, fast food, or eaten in restaurants; and cost of food in a particular geographical area

DEFINING CHARACTERISTIC

Expresses desire to enhance nutrition

EXPECTED OUTCOMES

- Patient will articulate present understanding of factors that enable and hinder enhanced nutritional status.
- Patient will evaluate each of the barriers to enhancing nutritional status.
- Patient will articulate the personal value of practicing positive behaviors.
- Patient will plan modifications of environment, which will reinforce change in eating habits.
- Patient will express positive feelings about self.

Suggested NOC Outcomes

Knowledge: Diet; Nutritional Status; Nutritional Status: Biochemical Measures

INTERVENTIONS AND RATIONALES

EBP **PCC** ▪ Provide patient with materials that are intellectually and culturally appropriate for enhancing nutritional knowledge. *It is important to engage patient in information-gathering before beginning to develop a plan to change behavior.*

▪ Help patient list the internal and external barriers to improving nutritional status. *Lack of understanding of patient's individual barriers, such as unclear goals, lack of skill, or lack of motivation, will prevent change from occurring.*

▪ Have patient make a list of the positive outcomes of changing the behaviors, such as wearing smaller size clothing, feeling better about being with others who are health conscious, enjoying feelings of physical and emotional well-being. *Positive reinforcers make the changes more appealing to effect.*

EBP ▪ Teach patient to read food labels, to plan meals using a standard method from the American Dietetic Association, and to shop for and stock the refrigerator and pantry with smart food choices. *New behaviors require practice in a practical sense for the kind of reinforcement that will produce the desired change.*

T&C ▪ Encourage patient to join or form some type of group *to help maintain the motivation to continue new behaviors.*

Suggested NIC Interventions

Nutrition Management; Nutritional Monitoring; Nutritional Counseling; Teaching: Prescribed Diet

EVALUATIONS FOR EXPECTED OUTCOMES

▪ Patient articulates present understanding of factors that enable and hinder enhanced nutritional status.

▪ Patient evaluates each of the barriers to enhancing nutritional status.

▪ Patient articulates the personal value of practicing positive behaviors.

▪ Patient plans modifications of environment, which will reinforce change in eating habits.

▪ Patient expresses positive feelings about self.

DOCUMENTATION

▪ Weight changes

▪ Patient's expressed attitudes toward food and eating

▪ Patient's expressed feelings about weight, body image, and emotional status

▪ Patient's participation in a group

▪ Patient's response to nursing interventions

▪ Evaluations for expected outcomes

REFERENCES

Costa de Oliveira, S., Carvalho Fernandes, A. F., Lavinas Santos, M. C., Ribeiro de Vasconcelos, E. M., & de Oliveira Lopes, M. V. (2018). Educational interventions for a healthy diet promotion during pregnancy. *Journal of Nursing UFPE/Revista de Enfermagem UFPE, 12*(4), 962–975. doi:10.5205/1981-8963-v12i4a230185p962-975-2018

Godin, L., & Sahakian, M. (2018). Cutting through conflicting prescriptions: How guidelines inform "healthy and sustainable" diets in Switzerland. *Appetite, 130*, 123–133. doi:10.1016/j.appet.2018.08.004

Hu, F. B. (2019). Nutrient supplementation no substitute for healthy diets. *Nature Reviews Cardiology, 16*(2), 77–79. doi:10.1038/s41569-018-0143-4

Vaughan, C. A., Ghosh-Dastidar, M., & Dubowitz, T. (2018). Attitudes and barriers to healthy diet and physical activity: A latent profile analysis. *Health Education & Behavior, 45*(3), 381–393. doi:10.1177/1090198117722818

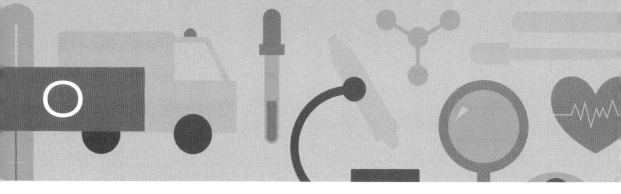

Obesity

DEFINITION

A condition in which an individual accumulates abnormal or excessive fat for age and gender that exceeds overweight

RELATED FACTORS (R/T)

- Average daily physical activity is less than recommended for gender and age
- Consumption of sugar-sweetened beverages
- Disordered eating behaviors
- Disordered eating perceptions
- Energy expenditure below energy intake based on standard assessment
- Excessive alcohol consumption
- Fear regarding lack of food supply
- Frequent snacking
- High frequency of restaurant or fried food
- Low dietary calcium intake in children
- Portion sizes larger than recommended
- Sedentary behavior occurring for ≥2 hours/day
- Shortened sleep time
- Sleep disorder
- Solid foods as major food source at <5 months of age

ASSOCIATED CONDITION

Genetic disorder

ASSESSMENT

- Health history including smoking, medications, change-of-life events, and illnesses
- Height and weight measurements
- Waist circumference measurement
- Calculate body mass index (BMI)
- Determine whether patient was overweight as a child
- Record monthly dietary history
- Record sleep schedule and habits
- Change in intrapersonal or interpersonal factors, including internal and external cues that trigger desire to eat
- Motivation to lose weight
- Rate of food consumption and stated food preference

- Psychosocial status
- Activity level
- Coping patterns
- Body image, including self-perception and perception of observer

DEFINING CHARACTERISTICS

- *Adult*: Body mass index (BMI) > 30 kg/m^2
- *Child < 2 years:* Term not used with children at this age
- *Child* 2 to 18 years: Body mass index (BMI) > 95th percentile or >30 kg/m^2 for age and gender

EXPECTED OUTCOMES

- Patient will identify internal and external cues that increase food consumption.
- Patient will plan menus appropriate to prescribed diet.
- Patient will adhere to prescribed diet.
- Patient will state plan to monitor and maintain target weight.
- Patient will identify consequences of overeating and weight gain.
- Patient will identify controllable factors that cause overeating.
- Patient will pursue weight loss that is optimal for maintenance of health.
- Patient will lose weight reasonably: 1 to 2 lb/week.
- Patient will state understanding of the need to increase activity level gradually.
- Patient will state sense of satisfaction with each new level of activity attained.

Suggested NOC Outcomes

Anxiety Level; Eating Disorder Self-Control; Exercise Participation; Nutritional Status; Weight: Body Mass

INTERVENTIONS AND RATIONALES

PCC ▪ Discuss with patient the need to lose weight. *Even a 10% decrease in body weight yields health benefits.*

PCC ▪ Help patient set realistic goals for losing weight. *This aids positive reinforcement and reduces frustration.*

PCC ▪ Support and encourage healthy patient behavior. *Creates positive relationship and reinforces healthy behaviors.*

PCC ▪ Weigh patient in a private, nonthreatening setting. *Builds trust with care team and prevents embarrassment.*

S ▪ Use medical devices and equipment specifically for obese patients. *Using equipment that is too small yields inaccurate assessment results.*

S ▪ Assess for health comorbidities, such as diabetes, skin breakdown, and hypertension. *Obesity is linked to other health concerns, which can be exacerbated by weight fluctuations.*

T&C ▪ Encourage attendance in support groups. *Support groups offer a place to share ideas and offer emotional support.*

PCC ▪ Evaluate for depression and anxiety. *Eating disorders can be linked to emotion.*

PCC ▪ Help patient identify the problem, feelings associated with eating, and circumstances in which patient turns to food. *Permanent weight loss starts with examination of factors contributing to weight gain.*

PCC ▪ Discuss patient's normal food preferences *to evaluate eating habits and include preferred foods (if nutritious) in patient's diet.*

T&C ▦ Evaluate nutritional status and refer to registered dietitian as needed. *Obese patients may be malnourished because of improper diet habits.*

EBP ▦ Discuss with patient the need for activity. *Lack of activity causes physical deconditioning and may also have a negative impact on psychological well-being.*

EBP ▦ Help patient select an exercise program (such as walking, jogging, aerobics, or swimming) appropriate to patient's age and physical condition. *Besides aiding weight loss, such activities offer an alternative to eating to alleviate stress.*

EBP ▦ Teach patient exercises for increasing strength and endurance *to improve breathing and promote general physical reconditioning.*

PCC ▦ Support and encourage activity to patient's level of tolerance *to help foster patient's independence.*

Suggested NIC Interventions

Anxiety Reduction; Behavior Modification; Exercise Promotion; Nutrition Management; Nutritional Therapy; Risk Identification; Teaching: Prescribed Diet; Weight Reduction Assistance

EVALUATIONS FOR EXPECTED OUTCOMES

▦ Patient states a desire to lose weight.
▦ Patient expresses feelings about present weight.
▦ Patient identifies cues that increase food consumption.
▦ Patient and health care professional establish weekly weight loss goal.
▦ Patient identifies a plan to increase activity level.
▦ Patient describes healthy eating pattern.
▦ Patient's blood pressure and pulse and respiratory rates remain within normal parameters.
▦ Patient expresses satisfaction with diet.
▦ Patient adheres to prescribed diet.
▦ Patient loses specified amount of weight weekly.
▦ Patient increases physical activity.

DOCUMENTATION

▦ Patient's perception of weight and body image
▦ Patient's weekly weight
▦ Patient's physical measurements, especially waist circumference
▦ Behaviors that promote or impede weight reduction
▦ Observations made while patient performs physical activities
▦ New activities patient is able to perform
▦ Evaluations for expected outcomes

REFERENCES

Brown, C. L., & Perrin, E. M. (2018). Obesity prevention and treatment in primary care. *Academic Pediatrics, 18*(7), 736–745. https://doi.org/10.1016/j.acap.2018.05.004

Hoelscher, D. M., Sharma, S. V., & Byrd-Williams, C. E. (2018). Prevention of obesity in early childhood: What are the next steps? *American Journal of Public Health, 108*(12), 1585–1587. https://doi.org/10.2105/AJPH.2018.304779

Tongvichean, T., Aungsuroch, Y., & Preechawong, S. (2019). Effect of self-management exercise program on physical fitness among people with prehypertension and obesity: A quasi experiment study. *Pacific Rim International Journal of Nursing Research, 23*(1), 6–17.

Vittrup, B., & McClure, D. (2018). Barriers to childhood obesity prevention: Parental knowledge and attitudes. *Pediatric Nursing, 44*(2), 81–94.

Risk for Occupational Injury

DEFINITION

Susceptible to sustain a work-related accident or illness, which may compromise health

RISK FACTORS

Individual

- Excessive stress
- Improper use of personal protective equipment
- Inadequate role performance
- Inadequate time management
- Ineffective coping strategies
- Insufficient knowledge
- Misinterpretation of information
- Psychological distress
- Unsafe acts or overconfidence
- Unsafe acts of unhealthy negative habits

Environmental

- Distraction from social relationships
- Exposure to biological agents
- Exposure to chemical agents
- Exposure to extremes of temperature
- Exposure to noise
- Exposure to radiation
- Exposure to teratogenic agents
- Exposure to vibration
- Inadequate physical environment
- Labor relationships
- Lack of personal protective equipment
- Night shift work rotating to day shift work
- Occupational burnout
- Physical workload
- Shift work

ASSESSMENT

- Age and gender
- Occupation and work schedule
- Physical head-to-toe examination
- Client's coping strategies
- Client's health status, including mental and physical functioning, cognitive abilities, sensory perception, response to stimuli, and motor skills
- Health history, including accidents, falls, and exposure to environmental hazards
- Environmental factors, including work environment, electrical wiring, lighting, utilities, fire precautions, presence of toxic or noxious substances, and special safety needs
- Knowledge level, including understanding of occupational safety precautions

EXPECTED OUTCOMES

- Client will remain free from physical injury.
- Client will follow safety precautions in and out of the work area.
- Client will develop strategy to maintain safety.

Suggested NOC Outcomes

Adherence Behavior; Compliance Behavior; Knowledge: Personal Safety; Personal Safety Behavior; Risk Control; Risk Detection

INTERVENTIONS AND RATIONALES

S ■ Assist client in identifying situations and hazards that can cause accidents *to increase client's awareness of potential dangers.*

PCC ■ Assess and document any motor, mental, or sensory deficits *to identify specific safety needs.*

QI ■ Monitor facility employee injuries, illnesses, and work-related hospitalizations to develop plan to improve work safety environment.

S ■ Encourage client to wear all the required personal protective equipment (PPE) consistently *for protection from hazards related to specific work area.*

EBP ■ Instruct client to use the correct lifting procedures *for back protection and to prevent hernias.*

S ■ Encourage client to keep all work areas clean and free from trash and debris. *Clutter, trash, and debris are potential fall and fire hazards.*

S ■ Encourage client to follow all safety procedures; do not skip safety procedures because they are inconvenient. *Safety procedures are in place to prevent injury.*

EBP ■ Provide client teaching as needed. Possible topics may include personal health, exposure risk, and PPE use. *Education can help client take steps to prevent injury.*

S ■ Encourage client to report potential safety hazards from environment *to decrease possibility of injury.*

S ■ Encourage client to immediately report malfunctioning equipment to appropriate personnel for replacement or repair *to help prevent accidents.*

■ Encourage participation in risk management groups. *Early detection of safety risks prevents injury.*

T&C ■ Refer client to appropriate resources such as the National Institute for Occupational Safety and Health (NIOSH) and Occupational Safety and Health Administration (OSHA) for more information about identifying and removing safety hazards. *This enables client to maintain the environment to achieve optimal safety level.*

Suggested NIC Interventions

Body Mechanics Promotion; Environmental Management: Safety; Environmental Management: Worker Safety; Risk Identification

EVALUATIONS FOR EXPECTED OUTCOMES

- Client remains free from physical injury.
- Client identifies and eliminates safety hazards in work area.
- Client demonstrates prevention and safety precautions.
- Client describes learned safety measures.

DOCUMENTATION

- Client's statements about situations that cause accidents and injuries
- Client's lack of awareness of, or disregard for, safety hazards
- Assessment of work environment
- Observation of physical findings
- Client's knowledge of safety practices
- Client's cognitive deficits that inhibit learning or attention to safety hazards
- Interventions to help client recognize and eliminate safety hazards
- Client's response to nursing interventions
- Evaluations for expected outcomes

REFERENCES

Dzhambov, A., & Dimitrova, D. (2017). Occupational noise exposure and the risk for work-related injury: A systematic review and meta-analysis. *Annals of Work Exposures & Health, 61*(9), 1037–1053. doi:10.1093/annweh/wxx078

Leibler, J. H., & Perry, M. J. (2017). Self-reported occupational injuries among industrial beef slaughterhouse workers in the Midwestern United States. *Journal of Occupational & Environmental Hygiene, 14*(1), 23–30. doi:10.1080/15459624.2016.1211283

Salminen, S., Perttula, P., Hirvonen, M., Perkiö-Mäkelä, M., & Vartia, M. (2017). Link between haste and occupational injury. *Work, 56*(1), 119–124. doi:10.3233/WOR-162471

Ugolini, A., Parodi, G. B., Casali, C., Silvestrini, B. A., & Giacinti, F. (2018). Work-related traumatic dental injuries: Prevalence, characteristics and risk factors. *Dental Traumatology, 34*(1), 36–40. doi:10.1111/edt.12376

Risk for Other-Directed Violence

DEFINITION

Susceptible to behaviors in which an individual demonstrates that he or she can be physically, emotionally, and/or sexually harmful to others

RISK FACTORS

- Access to weapon
- Impulsiveness
- Negative body language
- Pattern of indirect violence
- Pattern of other-directed violence
- Pattern of threatening violence
- Pattern of violent antisocial behavior
- Suicidal behavior

ASSOCIATED CONDITIONS

- Alteration in cognitive functioning
- Neurologic impairment
- Pathologic intoxication
- Perinatal complications
- Prenatal complications
- Psychotic disorder

ASSESSMENT

- Age
- Gender
- Recent stressors and coping strategies
- Patient history, including health history, substance abuse history (type and effects on mental status), and previous episodes of violence (circumstances, behavior, arrests)
- Reactions of family members to episodes of violence
- Mental status examination (with emphasis on insight and judgment)
- Physical findings, including neurologic examination
- Laboratory studies, including electroencephalography, toxicology screening, and blood chemistry

EXPECTED OUTCOMES

- Patient will maintain control over anger.
- Patient will successfully re-channel hostility into socially acceptable behaviors.
- Patient will discuss angry feelings and will verbalize ways to tolerate frustration appropriately.
- Patient will express need for long-term treatment by appropriate professional.

Suggested NOC Outcomes

Abuse Cessation; Abusive Behavior Self-Restraint; Aggression Self-Control; Impulse Self-Control

INTERVENTIONS AND RATIONALES

PCC ■ Maintain a low level of stimuli in patient's environment *to avoid increasing agitation and provoking violent behavior.*

S ■ Remove all objects from the environment that patient could use to injure others *to provide for patient's safety and protect potential victims of violence.*

PCC ■ Instruct staff members to maintain and convey a calm attitude toward patient. *Anxiety is contagious and can be transferred to patient. A calm attitude reinforces a feeling of safety.*

PCC ■ Explain in a firm, calm voice that you'll help patient remain in control. *Communicating willingness to help patient maintain self-control encourages patient to take control of own behavior.*

PCC ■ Set limits on patient's behavior *to reinforce the expectation that patient will act in a responsible, controlled manner.*

PCC ■ Express understanding of patient's feelings and encourage open discussion *to provide support, reassurance, and positive reinforcement for desirable behaviors.*

EBP ■ Administer prescribed medications to help patient control aggressive behavior and remain calm. Monitor for effectiveness. *When used appropriately, medications commonly remove the need for physical restraint.*

EBP ■ Explain the medication program to patient *to promote compliance* and make sure patient takes medications as prescribed *to help keep patient calm.*

S ■ According to facility policy, restrain or seclude patient as necessary *to prevent serious injury to self or others.* Use seclusion or restraint only after less restrictive measures have failed. Both measures require a physician's order as well as accurate documentation.

PCC ■ Establish a daily routine of strenuous exercise and encourage patient to adhere to it. *Exercise provides an alternative way to handle frustration.*

▓ Encourage patient to gradually begin discussing hostile feelings *to help develop more appropriate ways of dealing with hostility.*

 ▓ Refer patient for appropriate long-term treatment, for example, to a drug or alcohol rehabilitation center, psychiatrist, or psychologist. *Patient may require help from specialized professionals or agencies.*

Suggested NIC Interventions

> *Anger Control Assistance; Behavior Management; Environmental Management: Violence Prevention; Impulse Control Training*

EVALUATIONS FOR EXPECTED OUTCOMES

▓ Patient behaves in nonaggressive manner.
▓ Patient re-channels hostility by participating in strenuous physical exercise on daily basis.
▓ Patient states what precipitates anger and describes consequences of failing to control it.
▓ Patient expresses need for ongoing treatment.

DOCUMENTATION

▓ Patient behaviors that indicate escalating agitation
▓ Other observations about patient's verbal and nonverbal behavior
▓ Factors that precipitate acts of violence
▓ Nursing interventions performed to reduce or prevent violent behavior
▓ Nursing interventions performed to ensure safety of other patients and staff members
▓ Patient's response to nursing interventions
▓ Referrals to specialized professionals and agencies
▓ Evaluations for expected outcomes

REFERENCES

Harford, T. C., Yi, H.-Y., Chen, C. M., & Grant, B. F. (2018). Substance use disorders and self- and other-directed violence among adults: Results from the national survey on drug use and health. *Journal of Affective Disorders, 225*, 365–373. doi:10.1016/j.jad.2017.08.021

Katz, J. (2018). Bystander training as leadership training: Notes on the origins, philosophy, and pedagogy of the mentors in violence prevention model. *Violence Against Women, 24*(15), 1755–1776. doi:10.1177/1077801217753322

Morphet, J., Griffiths, D., Beattie, J., Velasquez Reyes, D., & Innes, K. (2018). Prevention and management of occupational violence and aggression in healthcare: A scoping review. *Collegian, 25*(6), 621–632. doi:10.1016/j.colegn.2018.04.003

Morrall, P., Worton, K., & Antony, D. (2018). Why is murder fascinating and why does it matter to mental health professionals? *Mental Health Practice, 21*(7), 34–39. doi:10.7748/mhp.2018.e1249

Overweight

DEFINITION

A condition in which an individual accumulates abnormal or excessive fat for age and gender

RELATED FACTORS (R/T)

▓ Average daily physical activity is less than recommended for gender and age
▓ Consumption of sugar-sweetened beverages

- Disordered eating behaviors
- Disordered eating perceptions
- Energy expenditure below energy intake based on standard assessment
- Excessive alcohol consumption
- Fear regarding lack of food supply
- Frequent snacking
- High frequency of restaurant or fried food
- Insufficient knowledge of modifiable factors
- Low dietary calcium intake in children
- Portion size larger than recommended
- Sedentary behavior occurring for >2 hours/day
- Shortened sleep time
- Sleep disorder
- Solid foods as a major source at <5 months of age

ASSOCIATED CONDITION

Genetic disorder

ASSESSMENT

- Health history, including family history of overweight
- Body measurements, including height, weight, and body mass index (BMI) or percentile on growth chart
- Dietary habits including food preferences and normal dietary intake
- Activity level
- Sedentary level
- Psychosocial status, including behavior, mood, stressors, coping mechanisms, and support systems (family, friends)

DEFINING CHARACTERISTICS

- *Adult*: Body mass index (BMI) > 25 kg/m^2
- *Child < 2 years:* Weight-for-length > 95th percentile
- *Child 2 to 18 years:* Body mass index (BMI) > 85th percentile or 25 kg/m^2 but <95th percentile or 30 kg/m^2 for age and gender

EXPECTED OUTCOMES

- Patient will identify internal and external factors contributing to weight gain.
- Patient will state need to lose weight.
- Patient will lose weight.
- Patient will express feelings regarding dietary regimen and current weight.
- Patient will identify internal and external cues that lead to increased food consumption.
- Patient will plan meals appropriate for prescribed diet.
- Patient will adhere to prescribed diet.
- Patient will participate in regular physical activity.
- Patient will achieve weight goal.
- Patient will state understanding of dietary and physical activity recommendations.
- Patient will participate in meal and activity planning and weight monitoring.

Suggested NOC Outcomes

Anxiety Level; Eating Disorder Self-Control; Exercise Participation; Nutritional Status; Weight: Body Mass

INTERVENTIONS AND RATIONALES

PCC ▪ With input from patient, set a realistic weight goal. *Involvement in the decision-making process improves compliance with plan of care.*

PCC ▪ Instruct patient to keep a food diary *to have an accurate record of intake.*

T&C ▪ Have a dietitian calculate caloric intake patient will require to reach a healthy weight *to allow planning of appropriate diet.*

PCC ▪ Determine patient's food preferences *to evaluate eating habits and to include preferred foods, if nutritional, in patient's diet.*

▪ Weigh patient weekly or as prescribed *to monitor the effectiveness of the diet.*

EBP ▪ Encourage a diet of foods low in calories and fat, high in complex carbohydrates and fiber, and rich in lean proteins and fruits and vegetables. *This encourages patient to eat food that provides energy without causing weight gain.*

PCC ▪ Encourage patient to express feelings about dietary changes to assess perception of the problem. Help patient identify emotions associated with food and situations that trigger eating episodes. *Permanent weight maintenance requires an understanding of the risk factors that contribute to weight gain.*

PCC ▪ Give patient emotional support and positive feedback for adhering to the prescribed diet. *This will foster compliance and help ensure adherence to the diet.*

EBP ▪ Discuss the importance of incorporating physical activity into lifestyle. Help patient select activities appropriate for age and physical condition. *Physical activity aids in weight loss and offers an alternative to eating to alleviate stress.*

T&C ▪ Refer patient as appropriate to resources for health coaching, behavior modification, or cognitive therapy *to prevent relapse into high-risk eating behaviors.*

Suggested NIC Interventions

Anxiety Reduction; Behavior Modification; Exercise Promotion; Nutrition Management; Nutritional Therapy; Risk Identification; Teaching: Prescribed Diet; Weight Reduction Assistance

EVALUATIONS FOR EXPECTED OUTCOMES

▪ Patient identifies internal and external factors contributing to weight gain.
▪ Patient states need to lose weight.
▪ Patient loses weight.
▪ Patient monitors weight and sustains target weight.
▪ Patient expresses feelings regarding dietary regimen and current weight.
▪ Patient identifies internal and external cues that lead to increased food consumption.
▪ Patient plans meals appropriate for prescribed diet.
▪ Patient adheres to prescribed diet.
▪ Patient participates in regular physical activity.
▪ Patient achieves weight goal.
▪ Patient states understanding of dietary and physical activity recommendations.
▪ Patient will participate in meal and activity planning and weight monitoring.

DOCUMENTATION

- Patient's expression of feelings about weight, eating, and dietary regimen
- Patient's weight and height
- Patient's body measurements plotted on growth chart
- Ability of patient to maintain target weight
- Foods consumed by patient
- Physical activity performed by patient
- Behaviors that promote or impede weight maintenance
- Family participation in care
- Evaluations for expected outcomes

REFERENCES

Gogia, R., & Begum, R. (2018). To study the effectiveness of occupational therapy in children with overweight/obesity and its impact upon quality of life. *Indian Journal of Physiotherapy & Occupational Therapy, 12*(4), 166–170. doi:10.5958/0973-5674.2018.00100.4

Lane-Tillerson, C. (2018). Evaluating the efficacy of a behavior modification program in overweight African American adolescents. Revisiting the literature. *ABNF Journal, 29*(4), 112–116.

Solgaard Nielsen, S., & Reffstrup Christensen, J. (2018). Occupational therapy for adults with overweight and obesity: Mapping interventions involving occupational therapists. *Occupational Therapy International*, 1–17. doi:10.1155/2018/7412686

Risk for Overweight

DEFINITION

Susceptible to excessive fat accumulation for age and gender, which may compromise health

RISK FACTORS

- Average daily physical activity is less than recommended for gender and age
- Consumption of sugar-sweetened beverages
- Disordered eating behaviors
- Disordered eating perceptions
- Energy expenditure below energy intake based on standard assessment
- Excessive alcohol consumption
- Fear regarding lack of food supply
- Frequent snacking
- High frequency of restaurant or fried food
- Insufficient knowledge of modifiable factors
- Low dietary calcium intake in children
- Portion size larger than recommended
- Sedentary behavior occurring for >2 hours/day
- Shortened sleep time
- Sleep disorder
- Solid foods as a major source at <5 months of age

ASSOCIATED CONDITION

Genetic disorder

- Health history, including family history of overweight
- Body measurements, including height, weight, and body mass index (BMI) or percentile on growth chart
- Dietary habits, including food preferences and normal dietary intake
- Activity level
- Sedentary level
- Psychosocial status, including behavior, mood, stressors, coping mechanisms, and support systems (family, friends)

- Patient will identify internal and external factors contributing to potential weight gain.
- Patient will plan to monitor weight and sustain target weight.
- Patient will express feelings regarding dietary regimen and current weight.
- Patient will identify internal and external cues that lead to increased food consumption.
- Patient will plan meals appropriate for prescribed diet.
- Patient will adhere to prescribed diet.
- Patient will participate in regular physical activity.
- Patient will maintain weight goal.
- Patient will state understanding of dietary and physical activity recommendations.
- Patient participates in meal and activity planning and weight monitoring.

Suggested NOC Outcomes

Anxiety Level; Eating Disorder Self-Control; Exercise Participation; Nutritional Status; Weight: Body Mass

PCC ▪ With input from patient, set a realistic weight goal. *Involvement in the decision-making process improves compliance with plan of care.*

PCC ▪ Instruct patient to keep a food diary *to have an accurate record of intake.*

T&C ▪ Have a dietitian calculate caloric intake that patient will require to reach a healthy weight *to allow planning of appropriate diet.*

PCC ▪ Determine patient's food preferences *to evaluate eating habits and to include preferred foods, if nutritional, in patient's diet.*

▪ Weigh patient weekly or as prescribed *to monitor the effectiveness of the diet.*

EBP ▪ Encourage a diet of foods low in calories and fat, high in complex carbohydrates and fiber, and rich in lean proteins and fruits and vegetables. *This encourages patient to eat food that provides energy without causing weight gain.*

PCC ▪ Encourage patient to express feelings about dietary changes to assess perception of the problem. Help patient identify emotions associated with food and situations that trigger eating episodes. *Permanent weight maintenance requires an understanding of the risk factors that contribute to weight gain.*

PCC ▪ Give patient emotional support and positive feedback for adhering to the prescribed diet. *This will foster compliance and help ensure adherence to the diet.*

EBP ▪ Discuss the importance of incorporating physical activity into lifestyle. Help patient select activities appropriate for age and physical condition. *Physical activity aids in weight loss and offers an alternative to eating to alleviate stress.*

T&C ▓ Refer patient, as appropriate, to resources for health coaching, behavior modification, or cognitive therapy *to prevent relapse into high-risk eating behaviors.*

Suggested NIC Interventions

Anxiety Reduction; Behavior Modification; Exercise Promotion; Nutrition Management; Nutritional Therapy; Risk Identification; Teaching: Prescribed Diet; Weight Reduction Assistance

EVALUATIONS FOR EXPECTED OUTCOMES

▓ Patient identifies internal and external factors contributing to potential weight gain.
▓ Patient monitors weight and sustains target weight.
▓ Patient expresses feelings regarding dietary regimen and current weight.
▓ Patient identifies internal and external cues that lead to increased food consumption.
▓ Patient plans meals appropriate for prescribed diet.
▓ Patient adheres to prescribed diet.
▓ Patient participates in regular physical activity.
▓ Patient maintains weight goal.
▓ Patient states understanding of dietary and physical activity recommendations.
▓ Patient participates in meal and activity planning and weight monitoring.

DOCUMENTATION

▓ Patient's expression of feelings about weight, eating, and dietary regimen
▓ Patient's weight and height
▓ Patient's body measurements plotted on growth chart
▓ Ability of patient to maintain target weight
▓ Foods consumed by patient
▓ Physical activity performed by patient
▓ Behaviors that promote or impede weight maintenance
▓ Family participation in care
▓ Evaluations for expected outcomes

REFERENCES

Bagherniya, M., Taghipour, A., Sharma, M., Sahebkar, A., Contento, I. R., Keshavarz, S. A., … Safarian, M. (2018). Obesity intervention programs among adolescents using social cognitive theory: A systematic literature review. *Health Education Research, 33*(1), 26–39. doi:10.1093/her/cyx079

Helseth, S., Riiser, K., Holmberg Fagerlund, B., Misvær, N., & Glavin, K. (2017). Implementing guidelines for preventing, identifying and treating adolescent overweight and obesity-School nurses' perceptions of the challenges involved. *Journal of Clinical Nursing, 26*(23–24), 4716–4725. doi:10.1111/jocn.13823

Warehime, S., Dinkel, D., Snyder, K., & Lee, J.-M. (2018). Postpartum physical activity and sleep levels in overweight, obese and normal-weight mothers. *British Journal of Midwifery, 26*(6), 400–408. doi:10.12968/bjom.2018.26.6.400

Zhou, T., Sun, D., Heianza, Y., Li, X., Champagne, C. M., LeBoff, M. S., … Qi, L. (2018). Genetically determined vitamin D levels and change in bone density during a weight-loss diet intervention: The preventing overweight using novel dietary strategies (POUNDS lost) trial. *American Journal of Clinical Nutrition, 108*(5), 1129–1134. doi:10.1093/ajcn/nqy197

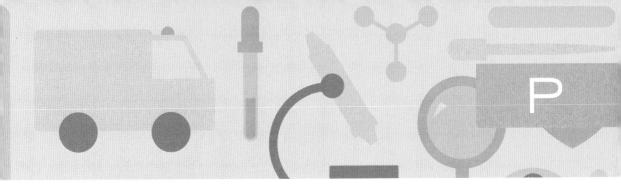

Acute Pain

Unpleasant sensory and emotional experience associated with actual or potential tissue damage, or described in terms of such damage (International Association for the Study of Pain); sudden or slow onset of any intensity from mild to severe with an anticipated or predictable end, and with a duration of less than 3 months

- Biological injury agent
- Chemical injury agent
- Physical injury agent

- Age
- Gender
- Descriptive characteristics of pain, including location, quality, intensity on a scale of 1 to 10, temporal factors, and sources of relief
- History of exposure to physical, biologic, or chemical agents as a cause of pain
- Physiologic variables, such as age and pain tolerance
- Psychological variables, such as body image, personality, previous experience with pain, anxiety, and secondary gain
- Sociocultural variables, including cognitive style, culture or ethnicity, attitude and values, sex, and birth order
- Environmental variables, such as setting and time

- Appetite change
- Change in physiologic parameter
- Diaphoresis
- Distraction behavior
- Evidence of pain using standardized pain behavior checklist for those unable to communicate verbally
- Expressive behavior
- Facial expression of pain
- Guarding behavior
- Hopelessness
- Narrowed focus

- Positioning to ease pain
- Protective behavior
- Proxy report of pain behavior/activity changes
- Pupil dilation
- Self-focused
- Self-report of intensity using standardized pain scale
- Self-report of pain characteristics using standardized pain instrument

EXPECTED OUTCOMES

- Patient will rate pain on a scale of 1 to 10 on a standardized scale.
- Patient will express relief from pain within a reasonable time after intervention.
- Patient will identify specific characteristics of pain.
- Patient will help develop a plan for pain control.
- Patient will identify measures effective in relieving pain.
- Patient will articulate factors that intensify pain and will modify behavior accordingly.
- Patient will state and carry out appropriate interventions for pain relief.
- Patient will decrease amount and frequency of pain medication needed.
- Patient will state satisfaction with pain management regimen.
- Patient will use available resources to understand pain phenomenon and will cooperate with treatment plan.

Suggested NOC Outcomes

Anxiety Level; Comfort Level; Pain Control; Pain: Disruptive Effects; Pain Level; Sleep

INTERVENTIONS AND RATIONALES

S Assess patient's signs and symptoms of pain behavioral cues and administer pain medication as prescribed. Monitor and record the medication's effectiveness and adverse effects. *Assessment allows for care plan modification, as needed.*

PCC Use a pain scale when assessing pain. *Although pain is subjective, when using the scale you can compare patient's perception of pain from one assessment to another.*

EBP Using a pain flowchart, record the time of medication administration and results of pain assessment every hour until the next dose to monitor the therapy's effectiveness.

PCC Return to patient in 30 minutes to check intervention effectiveness. *This establishes trusting–caring relationship that encourages accurate communication.*

PCC Demonstrate acceptance when patient reveals pain. *This helps establish a trusting relationship with patient and encourages open expression of feelings. A patient may deny pain to appear "good."*

PCC Perform comfort measures to promote relaxation, such as massage, bathing, repositioning, and relaxation techniques. *These measures reduce muscle tension or spasm, redistribute pressure on body parts, and help patient focus on nonpain-related subjects.*

PCC Plan activities with patient to provide distraction, such as reading, crafts, television, and visits, *to help patient focus on nonpain-related matters.*

EBP Provide patient with information to help increase pain tolerance; for example, reasons for pain and length of time it will last. *This educates patient and encourages compliance in trying alternative pain relief measures.*

PCC Manipulate the environment to promote periods of uninterrupted rest. This promotes health, well-being, and increased energy level important to pain relief.

EBP ▦ Apply heat or cold, as ordered (specify), *to minimize or relieve pain.*

PCC ▦ Help patient into a comfortable position and use pillows to splint or support painful areas as appropriate *to reduce muscle tension or spasm and to redistribute pressure on body parts.*

PCC ▦ Collaborate with patient in administering prescribed analgesics when alternative methods of pain control are inadequate. *Gaining patient's trust and involvement helps ensure compliance and may reduce medication intake.*

PCC ▦ Encourage patient to report which pain relief measures prove most effective *to give patient a sense of control and promote effective modification of therapy.*

PCC ▦ Try to anticipate the onset of pain. Provide prescribed medication before painful procedures such as dressing changes or activities such as deep breathing. *Careful pain management can improve relief and may enable the patient to cope better with procedures.*

T&C ▦ Consider the services of a psychiatric mental health professional to help patient and staff members establish a realistic plan to resolve the problem. *Patients who remain helpless, unmotivated, uncooperative, and manipulative are self-destructive. Underlying causes should be explored.*

EBP ▦ Discuss with patient possible association between exacerbation of pain and patient's identified stressors. *This helps patient explore exacerbating emotional or environmental factors that may affect pain.*

PCC ▦ Ask patient to help establish goals and develop plan for pain control. *This gives patient a sense of control.*

PCC ▦ Provide patient with positive feedback about progress toward reaching goals *to improve motivation and encourage compliance.*

PCC ▦ Spend at least 15 minutes/shift allowing patient to express feelings, *which will help give patient a sense of control.*

EBP ▦ When possible, allow patient to use alternative pain treatments from patient's culture (such as acupuncture) as a substitute for or complement to Western treatments *to promote nonpharmacologic pain management.*

Suggested NIC Interventions

Analgesic Administration; Anxiety Reduction; Coping Enhancement; Emotional Support; Hope Instillation; Medication Management; Pain Management; Positioning; Sleep Enhancement

EVALUATIONS FOR EXPECTED OUTCOMES

▦ Patient identifies most effective pain relief measures.

▦ Patient's pain rating is documented (using a scale of 1 to 10) before administering medication and 30 to 45 minutes afterward.

▦ Patient articulates factors that intensify pain and modifies behavior accordingly.

▦ Patient carries out alternative pain control measures such as heat or cold applications.

▦ Patient reports more than 4 hours' sleep nightly (reports of less than 4 hours require further assessment).

▦ Patient decreases amount and frequency of pain medication within 72 hours.

▦ Patient discusses characteristics of pain, including location, duration, and frequency.

▦ Patient reports achieving pain relief with analgesia or other measures.

▦ Patient participates in development of health care plan and discusses modifications.

▦ Patient acknowledges that pain may be related to emotional factors and lists stressors that may exacerbate pain.

▦ Patient states satisfaction with pain management regimen.

DOCUMENTATION

- Patient's description of physical pain, pain relief, and feelings about pain
- Observations of patient's physical, psychological, and sociocultural responses to pain
- Comfort measures and medications provided to reduce pain and effectiveness of interventions
- Information provided to patient about pain and pain relief
- Other interventions performed to assist patient with pain control
- Evaluations for expected outcomes

REFERENCES

Drake, G., & de C. Williams, A. C. (2017). Nursing education interventions for managing acute pain in hospital settings: A systematic review of clinical outcomes and teaching methods. *Pain Management Nursing, 18*(1), 3–15. doi:10.1016/j.pmn.2016.11.001

Fitzgerald, S. (2017). Assessment and management of acute pain in older people: Barriers and facilitators to nursing practice. *Australian Journal of Advanced Nursing, 35*(1), 48–57.

Shuman, C. J., Xie, X.-J., Herr, K. A., & Titler, M. G. (2018). Sustainability of evidence-based acute pain management practices for hospitalized older adults. *Western Journal of Nursing Research, 40*(12), 1749–1764. doi:10.1177/0193945917738781

Urman, R. D., Böing, E. A., Khangulov, V., Fain, R., Nathanson, B. H., Wan, G. J., … Cirillo, J. (2019). Analysis of predictors of opioid-free analgesia for management of acute post-surgical pain in the United States. *Current Medical Research & Opinion, 35*(2), 283–289. doi:10.1080/03007995.2018.1481376

Chronic Pain

DEFINITION

Unpleasant sensory and emotional experience associated with actual or potential tissue damage, or described in terms of such damage (International Association for the Study of Pain); sudden or slow onset of any intensity from mild to severe, constant, or recurring without an anticipated or predictable end, and a duration of greater than 3 months

RELATED FACTORS (R/T)

- Alteration in sleep pattern
- Emotional distress
- Fatigue
- Increase in body mass index
- Ineffective sexuality pattern
- Injury agent
- Malnutrition
- Nerve compression
- Prolonged computer use
- Repeated handling of heavy loads
- Social isolation
- Whole-body vibration

ASSOCIATED CONDITIONS

- Chronic musculoskeletal condition
- Confusion
- Crush injury
- Damage to the nervous system
- Fracture

- Genetic disorder
- Imbalance of neurotransmitters, neuromodulators, and receptors
- Immune disorder
- Impaired metabolic functioning
- Ischemic condition
- Muscle injury
- Post-trauma-related condition
- Prolonged increase in cortisol level
- Spinal cord injury
- Tumor infiltration

ASSESSMENT

- Descriptive characteristics of pain, including location, quality, intensity on a scale of 1 to 10, temporal factors, duration, precipitating factors (food, alcohol, activity, and stress), and comfort factors
- Physiologic variables, such as general health state, length of pain, organ system involvement, pain tolerance, disability (work, family, or social), and pain interventions (such as injection, traction, ice, physical therapy, and transcutaneous electrical nerve stimulation)
- Psychological variables, such as age, self-esteem, self-worth, role (worker, husband, breadwinner), coping behavior (appropriate or inappropriate), secondary gains (disability insurance, workmen's compensation, litigation), suffering (emotional component), manipulative behavior, dependence on others or on system, and previous hospital experience
- Sociocultural variables, including educational level, motivation, culture or ethnicity, sex, values and beliefs, pain behaviors, financial distress, and religion
- Environmental variables, such as setting and time
- Pharmacologic variables, including type of drugs, amount used in 1 day, use of illicit drugs, and use of alcohol

DEFINING CHARACTERISTICS

- Alteration in ability to continue previous activities
- Alteration in sleep pattern
- Anorexia
- Evidence of pain using standardized pain behavior checklist for those unable to communicate verbally
- Facial expression of pain
- Proxy report of pain behavior/activity changes
- Self-focused
- Self-report of intensity using standardized pain scale
- Self-report of pain characteristics using standardized pain instrument

EXPECTED OUTCOMES

- Patient will rate pain on a scale of 1 to 10 on a standardized scale.
- Patient will identify characteristics of pain and pain behaviors.
- Patient will develop pain management program that includes activity and rest schedule, exercise program, and medication regimen that isn't pain contingent.
- Patient will state relationship of increasing pain to stress, activity, and fatigue.

Suggested NOC Outcomes

Comfort Level; Depression Level; Depression Self-Control; Pain Control; Pain Level; Quality of Life; Sleep; Symptom Control

INTERVENTIONS AND RATIONALES

S ▪ Assess patient's physical symptoms of pain, physical complaints, and daily activities. Administer pain medication, as prescribed. Monitor and record the effectiveness and adverse effects of medication. (Keep in mind that pain behavior and pain talk may be inconsistent.) *Correlating patient's pain behavior with activities, time of day, and visits may be useful in modifying tasks.*

EBP ▪ Provide instruction about amount of pain medication needed to control symptoms and allow patient to remain active. *Teaching patient about medications may help to increase the accuracy of dosage necessary to provide pain relief.*

PCC ▪ Develop a behavior-oriented care plan; for instance, set up a plan to follow the activity schedule. *Behavioral–cognitive measures can help patient modify learned pain behaviors.*

EBP ▪ Teach patient how to use relaxation techniques, guided imagery, massage, or music therapy to relieve pain. *These methods work as an adjunct to medications, increase self-help, and foster independence.*

EBP ▪ Teach patient and family members such techniques as massage, application of ice, and exercise *to relieve pain and foster independence.*

PCC ▪ Work closely with staff and patient's family *to achieve pain management goals and maximize patient's cooperation.*

EBP ▪ Use behavior modification; for example, spend time with patient only if the discussion includes no pain talk. Use contingency rewards for decreasing pain talk and pain behavior. *Reducing pain talk helps patient refocus on other, more important matters.*

PCC ▪ Encourage self-care activities. Develop a schedule. *This helps patient gain a sense of control and reduces dependence on caregivers and society.*

PCC ▪ Establish a specific time to talk with patient about pain and its psychological and emotional effects *to establish a trusting, supportive relationship that encompasses patient's physiologic, emotional, social, sexual, and financial concerns.*

Suggested NIC Interventions

Analgesic Administration; Behavior Modification; Biofeedback; Emotional Support; Mood Management; Pain Management; Patient Contracting; Simple Massage

EVALUATIONS FOR EXPECTED OUTCOMES

▪ Patient maintains activity diary and pain-level chart that rates severity of pain on a scale of 1 to 10.
▪ Patient maintains pain management program that includes activity and rest schedule, exercise program, and medication regimen.
▪ Patient states that stress, activity, and fatigue may increase pain.

DOCUMENTATION

▪ Patient's description of physical pain, pain relief, and feelings about pain
▪ Pain talk and pain behavior and affect

- Relationship of reports of pain to activities
- Treatments and pain talk
- Time out of bed
- Comfort measures initiated by nurse, patient, or family members
- Response to interventions
- Response to pharmacologic agents
- Interaction with staff
- Evaluations for expected outcomes

REFERENCES

Ahuja, D., Bharati, S. J., Mishra, S., & Bhatnagar, S. (2017). Chronic cancer pain: Diagnostic dilemma and management challenges. *Indian Journal of Palliative Care, 23*(4), 480–483. doi:10.4103/IJPC .IJPC_74_17

Geurts, J. W., Willems, P. C., Lockwood, C., Kleef, M., Kleijnen, J., & Dirksen, C. (2017). Patient expectations for management of chronic non-cancer pain: A systematic review. *Health Expectations, 20*(6), 1201–1217. doi.org/10.1111/hex.12527

Gilmartin-Thomas, J. F., Bell, J. S., Liew, D., Arnold, C. A., Buchbinder, R., Chapman, C., ... McNeil, J. (2019). Chronic pain medication management of older populations: Key points from a national conference and innovative opportunities for pharmacy practice. *Research in Social & Administrative Pharmacy, 15*(2), 207–213. doi:10.1016/j.sapharm.2018.03.060

Oosterhaven, J., Wittink, H., Mollema, J., Kruitwagen, C., & Deville, W. (2019). Predictors of dropout in interdisciplinary chronic pain management programmes: A systematic review. *Journal of Rehabilitation Medicine (Stiftelsen Rehabiliteringsinformation), 51*(1), 2–10. doi:10.2340/16501977-2502

Chronic Pain Syndrome

DEFINITION

Recurrent or persistent pain that has lasted at least 3 months, and that significantly affects daily functioning or well-being

RELATED FACTORS (R/T)

- Body mass index above normal range for age and gender
- Fear of pain
- Fear-avoidance beliefs
- Inadequate knowledge of pain management behaviors
- Negative affect
- Sleep disturbances

ASSESSMENT

- Characteristics of pain: location, quality, intensity on a scale of 1 to 10, duration, precipitating factors (food, alcohol, activity, and stress), and comfort factors
- Physiologic variables: general health state, length of pain, organ system involvement, pain tolerance, disability (work, family, or social), and pain interventions (such as injection, traction, ice, physical therapy, and transcutaneous electrical nerve stimulation)
- Psychological variables: age, self-esteem, self-worth, depression, poor sleep quality, fatigue, decreased libido, role (worker, husband, breadwinner), coping behavior (appropriate or inappropriate), suffering (emotional component), manipulative behavior, dependence on others or on system, and previous hospital experience

■ Sociocultural variables: educational level, motivation, culture or ethnicity, sex, values and beliefs, pain behaviors, financial distress, and religion

■ Use of medications including type of drug, amount used in 1 day, and/or use of illicit drugs

■ Use of alcohol

■ Environment

DEFINING CHARACTERISTICS

■ Anxiety (00146)

■ Constipation (00011)

■ Disturbed sleep pattern (00198)

■ Fatigue (00093)

■ Fear (00148)

■ Impaired mood regulation (00241)

■ Impaired physical mobility (00085)

■ Insomnia (00095)

■ Social isolation (00053)

■ Stress overload (00177)

EXPECTED OUTCOMES

■ Patient will develop pain management program that includes activity and rest schedule, exercise program, and medication regimen that isn't pain contingent.

■ Patient will state relationship of increasing pain to stress, activity, and fatigue.

■ Patient will state desire to participate in self-care behavior or activities.

Suggested NOC Outcomes

Agitation Level; Anxiety Level; Appetite; Client Satisfaction: Pain Control; Comfort Status; Depression Level; Fatigue Level; Personal Well-Being; Quality of Life

INTERVENTIONS AND RATIONALES

PCC ■ Assess patient's physical symptoms of pain, physical complaints, and daily activities. *Knowing patterns is essential in developing a pain management plan.*

EBP ■ Administer pain medication, as prescribed. Monitor and record the effectiveness and adverse effects of medication. (Keep in mind that pain behavior and pain talk may be inconsistent.) *Medicating pain before it is out of control fosters better pain management.*

EBP ■ Provide instruction about amount of pain medication needed to control symptoms and allow the patient to remain active. *Teaching patient about medications may help increase the accuracy of dosage necessary to provide pain relief.*

PCC ■ Develop a behavior-oriented care plan; for instance, set up a plan to follow the activity schedule. *Behavioral–cognitive measures can help patient modify learned pain behaviors.*

EBP ■ Teach patient how to use relaxation techniques, guided imagery, massage, or music therapy to relieve pain. *These methods work as an adjunct to medications, increase self-help, and foster independence.*

■ Teach patient and family members techniques such as massage, application of ice, and exercise *to relieve pain and foster independence.*

T&C ■ Work closely with patient, patient's family, and staff *to achieve pain management goals and maximize patient's cooperation.*

PCC ■ Encourage self-care activities. Develop a schedule. *This helps patient gain a sense of control and reduces dependence on caregivers and society.*

Suggested NIC Interventions

Analgesic Administration; Coping Enhancement; Guided Imagery; Mood Management; Positioning; Relaxation Therapy

EVALUATIONS FOR EXPECTED OUTCOMES

- Patient maintains activity diary and pain-level chart that rates severity of pain on a scale of 1 to 10.
- Patient maintains pain management program that includes activity and rest schedule, exercise program, and medication regimen.
- Patient states that stress, activity, and fatigue may increase pain.
- Patient participates in self-care activities.

DOCUMENTATION

- Patient's description of physical pain, pain rating, pain relief, and feelings about pain
- Comfort measures initiated by nurse, patient, or family members
- Response to interventions
- Response to pharmacologic agents
- Interaction with others
- Evaluations for expected outcomes

REFERENCES

Doiron, R. C., & Nickel, J. C. (2018). Management of chronic prostatitis/chronic pelvic pain syndrome. *Canadian Urological Association Journal, 12*(6 Suppl. 3), S161–S163. doi:10.5489/cuai.5325

Majeed, M. H., Ali, A. A., & Sudak, D. M. (2019). Psychotherapeutic interventions for chronic pain: Evidence, rationale, and advantages. *International Journal of Psychiatry in Medicine, 54*(2), 140–149. doi:10.1177/0091217418791447

McClintock, A. S., McCarrick, S. M., Garland, E. L., Zeidan, F., & Zgierska, A. E. (2019). Brief mindfulness-based interventions for acute and chronic pain: A systematic review. *Journal of Alternative & Complementary Medicine, 25*(3), 265–278. doi:10.1089/acm.2018.0351

Williams, A., Dongen, J. M., Kamper, S. J., O'Brien, K. M., Wolfenden, L., Yoong, S. L., ... van Dongen, J. M. (2019). Economic evaluation of a healthy lifestyle intervention for chronic low back pain: A randomized controlled trial. *European Journal of Pain, 23*(3), 621–634. doi:10.1002/ejp.1334

Labor Pain

DEFINITION

Sensory and emotional experience that varies from pleasant to unpleasant, associated with labor and childbirth

RELATED FACTORS (R/T)

Behavioral Factors

- Insufficient fluid intake
- Supine position

Cognitive Factors

- Fear of childbirth
- Inadequate knowledge about childbirth

- Inadequate preparation to deal with labor pain
- Low self-efficacy
- Perception of labor pain as nonproductive
- Perception of labor pain as negative
- Perception of labor pain as threatening
- Perception of labor pain as unnatural
- Perception of pain as meaningful

Social Factors

- Interference in decision-making
- Unsupportive companionship

Unmodified Environmental Factors

- Noisy delivery room
- Overcrowded delivery room
- Turbulent environment

ASSOCIATED CONDITIONS

- Cervical dilation
- Depression
- Fetal expulsion
- High maternal trait anxiety
- Prescribed mobility restriction
- Prolonged duration of labor

ASSESSMENT

- Characteristics of pain, including intensity on 0 to 10 scale, location, quality, duration, and alleviating factors
- Behavioral response to pain
- Assessment of vital signs
- Understanding and expectations of labor and delivery

DEFINING CHARACTERISTICS

- Altered blood pressure
- Altered heart rate
- Altered muscle tension
- Altered neuroendocrine functioning
- Altered respiratory rate
- Altered urinary functioning
- Anxiety
- Appetite change
- Diaphoresis
- Distraction behavior
- Expressive behavior
- Facial expression of pain
- Narrow focus
- Nausea
- Perineal pressure

- Positioning to ease pain
- Protective behavior
- Pupil dilation
- Reports altered sleep–wake cycle
- Self-focused
- Uterine contraction
- Vomiting

EXPECTED OUTCOMES

- Patient will identify characteristics of pain and will describe intensifying factors.
- Patient will modify behavior to decrease pain.
- Patient will express decrease in intensity of discomfort.
- Patient will experience satisfaction with pain control during labor and delivery.

Suggested NOC Outcomes

Anxiety Level; Client Satisfaction: Pain Control; Comfort Status; Comfort Status: Physical; Nausea & Vomiting Severity; Vital Signs

INTERVENTIONS AND RATIONALES

S ▪ Orient patient on admission to the labor and delivery suite. Show patient her room and explain the operations of her bed and call bell. Explain admission protocol and the labor process. *These measures will allay the patient's initial anxiety.*

PCC ▪ Assess patient's knowledge of the labor and delivery process and her current anxiety level *to plan supportive strategies.*

EBP ▪ Explain available analgesics and anesthesia to patient and support person. *Awareness of available medications will reduce anxiety.*

EBP ▪ Explain available nonpharmacologic pain reductions strategies available to patient and support person. *Awareness of available methods will reduce anxiety.*

PCC ▪ Encourage the support person to stay with patient in labor *as a woman in labor will respond more readily to supportive measures offered by a familiar caring person.*

EBP ▪ Assist patient and support person in techniques to decrease the discomfort of labor:
  - Conscious relaxation. *During labor, relaxation enables the patient to use coping techniques.*
  - Concentration on an internal or external focal point. *A focal point allows controlled thoughts while breathing.*
  - Slow, deep chest breathing. *Deep chest breathing creates a sense of relaxation during contractions.*
  - Shallow chest breathing: slow panting-like breaths. *Slow breathing avoids hyperventilation. Shallow chest breathing lifts the diaphragm from the uterus during contractions, decreasing the intensity of the contractions.*
  - Effleurage. *This technique stimulates large-diameter sensory nerve fibers and interferes with the transmission of pain impulses to the brain.*

PCC ▪ In the first stage of labor, provide patient with diversional activities *to decrease anxiety.*

PCC ▪ As labor progresses, modify the environment to reduce distractions (close the door, turn off television, and close curtains). *These measures help patient concentrate during the active phase of labor.*

EBP ▪ If needed, apply sacral pressure to the patient, *to decrease back pain.*

PCC ▪ Assist patient with position changes and use pillows to make her more comfortable. Assure all body parts are supported and joints are slightly flexed. *Frequent position changes promote comfort, prevent stiffness, and prevent pressure ulcers.*

S ▪ Assess for bladder distention and encourage patient to void every 2 hours. *A distended bladder increases discomfort during contractions.*

PCC ▪ Provide frequent mouth care. According to facility protocol, provide ice chips, water-based jelly, or a wet 4″ × 4″ gauze swab for dry lips *to relieve dry mouth and lips caused by breathing techniques and nothing-by-mouth status.*

PCC ▪ Apply a cool damp cloth to patient's forehead *to relieve diaphoresis.*

PCC ▪ Change patient's gown and linens as needed *to ease discomfort caused by diaphoresis or vaginal discharge.*

PCC ▪ Encourage patient to rest and relax between contractions to decrease fatigue. *Fatigue worsens pain perception and decreases patient's ability to cope with contractions.*

EBP ▪ Discuss with patient and support person which pain medications are available if alternative pain control methods prove inadequate. *Patient may need prescribed analgesics to cope with the labor process.*

Suggested NIC Interventions

Calming Technique; Energy Management; Environmental Management: Comfort; Guided Imagery; Massage; Medication Administration; Medication Management; Music Therapy; Pain Management; Positioning; Relaxation Therapy; Simple Massage; Support System Enhancement

EVALUATIONS FOR EXPECTED OUTCOMES

▪ Patient identifies characteristics of pain and describes intensifying factors.
▪ Patient modifies behavior to decrease pain, including using breathing techniques, asking for analgesia when needed, and assuming a more comfortable position.
▪ Patient reports decrease in intensity of discomfort.
▪ Patient expresses satisfaction with her pain control during childbirth.

DOCUMENTATION

▪ Patient's childbirth preparation and plans for pain control while giving birth
▪ Patient's description of pain
▪ Observation of patient's response to labor
▪ Nursing interventions to decrease discomfort
▪ Patient's response to nursing interventions
▪ Evaluations for expected outcomes

REFERENCES

Arnold, M. J., & Dhaliwal, S. (2019). Complementary and integrative treatments for pain management in labor. *American Family Physician, 99*(3), 154–156.

Lennon, R. (2018). Pain management in labour and childbirth: Going back to basics. *British Journal of Midwifery, 26*(10), 637–641. doi:10.12968/bjom.2018.26.10.637

Sanders, R. A., & Lamb, K. (2017). Non-pharmacological pain management strategies for labour: Maintaining a physiological outlook. *British Journal of Midwifery, 25*(2), 78–85. doi:10.12968/bjom.2017.25.2.78

Impaired Parenting

DEFINITION

Limitation of primary caregiver to nurture, protect, and promote optimal growth and development of the child, through a consistent, empathic exercise of authority and appropriate behavior in response to the child's needs

RELATED FACTORS (R/T)

- Altered parental role
- Decreased emotion recognition abilities
- Depressive symptoms
- Difficulty managing complex treatment regimen
- Dysfunctional family processes
- Emotional vacillation
- High use of Internet-connected devices
- Inadequate knowledge about child development
- Inadequate knowledge about child health maintenance
- Inadequate parental role model
- Inadequate problem-solving skills
- Inadequate social support
- Inadequate transportation
- Inattentive to child's needs
- Increased anxiety symptoms
- Low self-efficacy
- Marital conflict
- Nonrestorative sleep–wake cycle
- Perceived economic strain
- Social isolation
- Substance misuse
- Unaddressed intimate partner violence

ASSOCIATED CONDITIONS

Parent

- Depression
- Mental disorders

Infant or Child

- Behavioral disorder
- Complex treatment regimen
- Emotional disorder
- Neurodevelopmental disabilities

ASSESSMENT

- Parental status, including age, degree of apprehension, developmental state, family roles, and relationship with spouse or significant other
- Gender and health status of other children
- Parents' knowledge of child care and normal growth and development
- Previous bonding history

- Interaction of parent and infant or child, including care practices, eye contact, smiling, touching, verbalization, visual and voice responses, and response to appearance, disabilities, and gender of child
- Psychosocial status, including financial stressors and previous experience, work demands, and support of family, friends, and significant other

DEFINING CHARACTERISTICS

Parental Externalizing Symptoms

- Hostile parenting behaviors
- Impulsive behaviors
- Intrusive behaviors
- Negative communication

Parental Internalizing Symptoms

- Decreased engagement in parent–child relations
- Decreased positive temperament
- Decreased subjective attention quality
- Extreme mood swings
- Failure to provide safe home environment
- Inadequate response to infant behavioral cues
- Inappropriate child-care arrangements
- Rejects child
- Social alienation

Infant or Child

- Anxiety
- Conduct problems
- Delayed cognitive development
- Depressive symptoms
- Difficulty establishing healthy intimate interpersonal relations
- Difficulty functioning socially
- Difficulty regulating emotion
- Extreme mood alterations
- Low academic performance
- Obesity
- Role reversal
- Somatic complaints
- Substance misuse

EXPECTED OUTCOMES

- Parents will establish eye, physical, and verbal contact with infant or child.
- Parents will communicate feelings and anxieties about child's condition and parenting skills.
- Parents will express willingness to care for child and will demonstrate competent parenting skills.
- Parents will voice satisfaction with infant or child.
- Parents will demonstrate correct feeding, bathing, and dressing techniques.
- Parent will express willingness to work to maintain relationship with other parent.
- Parents will state plans for well-child care.
- Parents will express knowledge of developmental norms.

- Parents will provide play activities for child.
- Parents will identify ways to express anger and frustration that don't harm child.

Suggested NOC Outcomes

Caregiver Performance: Direct Care; Child Development: Middle Childhood; Family Coping; Family Functioning; Parenting: Early/Middle Childhood Physical Safety; Parent–Infant Attachment; Parenting Performance

INTERVENTIONS AND RATIONALES

PCC ▪ Involve parents in the care of infant or child immediately *to promote attachment to child.*
PCC ▪ Provide opportunities for caretaking by allowing parents to share a room with their infant or child or by extending visitation periods. *Participation in care increases parent's feeling of self-esteem and self-worth.*
EBP ▪ Educate parents about
  - normal growth and development
  - breastfeeding or bottle-feeding techniques
  - infant care, such as bathing and dressing
  - routine well-child care
  - signs and symptoms of illness
  - child's need for tactile and sensory stimulation. *Knowledge of normal growth and development may decrease unrealistic expectations and increase chances of successful parenting.*
  ▪ When caring for child in parents' presence, act as a role model for effective parenting skills. *Lack of knowledge of routine child care practices and growth and developmental norms significantly contributes to child abuse. Demonstration is a more effective means of teaching parenting skills than lecturing.*
PCC ▪ Encourage questions about care taking and provide appropriate information *to allay anxiety and monitor knowledge retention.*
PCC ▪ Assess parents' level of understanding of child's condition and their expectations *to clear up misunderstandings, allow for prompt intervention, and promote realistic planning.*
PCC ▪ Encourage parents to express their anxieties related to child's condition and their parenting skills *to identify and clarify misconceptions.*
PCC ▪ Praise parents when they display appropriate parenting skills *to provide positive reinforcement.*
T&C ▪ Refer parents to a family support group and other community resources such as Parents Anonymous. *Battering parents typically lack a support system and have a sense of being alone. A support group may help ease isolation.*
T&C ▪ Refer parents to social services as needed *to help ensure comprehensive care.*
PCC ▪ Encourage verbalization of infant's or child's impact on family life. *Ventilation of feelings helps parents deal more effectively with the stress of child care.*
S ▪ Be alert for signs and symptoms of child abuse, including neglect, uncleanliness, and frequent accidents or withdrawn, fearful behavior on the part of the child. Report actual or suspected child abuse to appropriate authorities. *Reporting child abuse is your professional duty. The United States legally requires nurses to report abuse.*

Suggested NIC Interventions

Attachment Promotion; Coping Enhancement; Family Integrity Promotion; Family Process Maintenance; Family Support; Mutual Goal Setting; Parent Education: Childrearing Family; Role Enhancement

- Parents make appropriate physical, verbal, and eye contact when interacting with infant or child.
- Parents make statements indicating satisfaction with infant or child.
- Parents demonstrate correct feeding, bathing, and dressing techniques.
- Parent expresses willingness to maintain relationship with other parent.
- Parents bring infant for routine well-child care.
- Parents verbalize knowledge of developmental norms.
- Parents provide play activities for child.
- Parents identify ways to express anger and frustration that don't harm child.

DOCUMENTATION

- Parents' expressions of feelings about child
- Parents' expressions of concern about their performance as parents
- Observation of parental visits, bonding, care taking, and knowledge level
- Instructions given to parents and parents' understanding of their responsibilities
- Infant's weight
- Evaluations for expected outcomes

REFERENCES

Bond, D. K., & Borelli, J. L. (2017). Maternal attachment insecurity and poorer proficiency savoring memories with their children: The mediating role of rumination. *Journal of Social & Personal Relationships, 34*(7), 1007–1030. doi:10.1177/0265407516664995

Cassé, J. F. H., Finkenauer, C., Oosterman, M., van der Geest, V. R., & Schuengel, C. (2018). Family conflict and resilience in parenting self-efficacy among high-risk mothers. *Journal of Interpersonal Violence, 33*(6), 1008–1029. doi:10.1177/0886260515614280

Håkansson, U., Söderström, K., Watten, R., Skårderud, F., & Øie, M. G. (2018). Parental reflective functioning and executive functioning in mothers with substance use disorder. *Attachment & Human Development, 20*(2), 181–207. doi:10.1080/14616734.2017.1398764

Ng-Knight, T., Shelton, K. H., Frederickson, N., McManus, I. C., & Rice, F. (2018). Maternal depressive symptoms and adolescent academic attainment: Testing pathways via parenting and self-control. *Journal of Adolescence, 62*, 61–69. doi:10.1016/j.adolescence.2017.11.003

Risk for Impaired Parenting

DEFINITION

Primary caregiver susceptible to a limitation to nurture, protect, and promote optimal growth and development of the child, through a consistent, empathic exercise of authority and appropriate behavior in response to the child's needs

RISK FACTORS

- Altered parental role
- Decreased emotion recognition abilities
- Depressive symptoms
- Difficulty managing complex treatment regimen
- Dysfunctional family processes
- Emotional vacillation
- High use of Internet-connected devices

- Inadequate knowledge about child development
- Inadequate knowledge about child health maintenance
- Inadequate parental role model
- Inadequate problem-solving skills
- Inadequate social support
- Inadequate transportation
- Inattentive to child's needs
- Increased anxiety symptoms
- Low self-efficacy
- Marital conflict
- Nonrestorative sleep–wake cycle
- Perceived economic strain
- Social isolation
- Substance misuse
- Unaddressed intimate partner violence

ASSOCIATED CONDITIONS

Parent

- Depression
- Mental disorders

Infant or Child

- Behavioral disorder
- Complex treatment regimen
- Emotional disorder
- Neurodevelopmental disabilities

ASSESSMENT

- Ages of caregiver and child
- Caregiver's psychosocial status, including developmental state, educational level, family roles, presence or absence of spouse or significant other, financial stressors, previous parenting experience, work demands, and support of family, friends, or significant other
- Interaction between caregiver and infant or child, including care practices, eye contact, response to appearance and gender of infant, smiling, touching, verbalization, and visual and voice responses

EXPECTED OUTCOMES

- Caregiver will establish eye, physical, and verbal contact with infant or child.
- Caregiver will demonstrate correct feeding, bathing, and dressing techniques.
- Caregiver will state plans to bring infant or child to clinic for routine physical and psychological examinations.
- Caregiver will express understanding of developmental norms.
- Caregiver will provide age-appropriate play activities.

Suggested NOC Outcomes

Caregiver Performance: Direct Care; Family Coping; Family Functioning; Parenting Performance

- Assess the amount of developmental stimulation provided by caregiver. For example, use the Home Observation for Measurement of the Environment (HOME) Inventory on a home visit *to assess whether the home environment is developmentally stimulating.*
- Instruct caregiver in the basics of infant and child care. *Research shows that the primary source of information about parenting is caregiver's own parents. If a caregiver lacks an effective role model, you may need to supply basic information about parenting.*
- When caring for child in the caregiver's presence, act as a role model for effective parenting skills. Demonstrate comfort measures, such as rocking infant, and show caregiver how to hold infant in an *en face* position *to familiarize caregiver with routine childcare practices.*
- **EBP** Teach caregiver about normal growth and development and identify ages at which child should master developmental tasks such as rolling over, crawling, and walking. *This will help caregiver monitor child's growth and development and practice appropriate safety precautions, such as blocking stairways, securing crib side rails, and preventing other accidents.* Also discuss problematic behaviors associated with specific ages, such as colic, temper tantrums, and sleeping difficulties, *to further enhance caregiver's understanding of developmental norms.*
- **EBP** Discuss child's need for tactile and sensory stimulation. Demonstrate play activities that promote developmental skills, such as shaking a rattle in front of an infant to build eye-and-hand coordination or placing a mobile above an infant to encourage visual tracking and trunk and head control. *Sensory experiences promote cognitive development.*
- **PCC** Familiarize caregiver with techniques for detecting symptoms of illness in infant or child, including *knowledge of how to monitor the child's health status will assist in the diagnosis and early treatment of problems.*
  - taking temperatures and reading thermometers
  - assessing child's respiratory status
  - observing for behavioral cues of illness, such as increased crying, rubbing ears, or drawing legs to abdomen.
- **PCC** Encourage caregiver to ask questions about infant and child care. Identify the questions parents commonly ask about infant care, such as cord care, feeding techniques, and bathing. Reassure caregiver that other parents also need to ask basic questions. *A caregiver who lacks effective parenting role models may not know what questions to ask or may hesitate to ask questions because of embarrassment.*
- **PCC** Praise caregiver for display of appropriate parenting skills *to provide positive reinforcement.*
- **S** Emphasize the importance of making regular visits to a health care professional, even when child appears healthy. *Routine visits allow early detection of developmental delays and provision of preventive care, such as immunizations.*
- **T&C** As necessary, refer caregiver and family to a physician, nurse practitioner, or social services for follow-up *to ensure continuity of care.*

Suggested NIC Interventions

Counseling; Family Integrity Promotion: Childbearing Family; Family Process Maintenance; Family Support; Parenting Promotion

- Caregiver makes appropriate eye, physical, and verbal contact with infant or child.
- Caregiver demonstrates correct feeding, bathing, and dressing techniques.

- Caregiver brings infant or child to clinic for routine examinations.
- Caregiver expresses understanding of developmental norms and accurately assesses child's developmental status and needs.
- Caregiver provides age-appropriate play activities.

DOCUMENTATION

- Evidence of neglect of infant or child
- Observations of caregiver's skills and knowledge level
- Presence or absence of caregiver–child bonding behaviors
- Questions asked by caregiver about care of infant or child
- Instructions given to caregiver and caregiver's response
- Evaluations for expected outcomes

REFERENCES

Behbahani, M., Zargar, F., Assarian, F., & Akbari, H. (2018). Effects of mindful parenting training on clinical symptoms in children with attention deficit hyperactivity disorder and parenting stress: Randomized controlled trial. *Iranian Journal of Medical Sciences, 43*(6), 596–604.

Guttmannova, K., Hill, K. G., Bailey, J. A., Hartigan, L. A., Small, C. M., & Hawkins, J. D. (2017). Parental alcohol use, parenting, and child on-time development. *Infant & Child Development, 26*(5). doi:10.1002/icd.2013

Han, J. W., & Lee, H. (2018). Effects of parenting stress and controlling parenting attitudes on problem behaviors of preschool children: Latent growth model analysis. *Journal of Korean Academy of Nursing, 48*(1), 109–121. doi:10.4040/jkan.2018.48.1.109

Thompson, W. C. A., Scott, K. L., Dyson, A., & Lishak, V. (2018). Are we in this together? Post-separation co-parenting of fathers with and without a history of domestic violence. *Child Abuse Review, 27*(2), 137–149. doi:10.1002/car.2510

Readiness for Enhanced Parenting

DEFINITION

A pattern of primary caregiver to nurture, protect, and promote optimal growth and development of the child, through a consistent, empathic exercise of authority and appropriate behavior in response to the child's needs, which can be strengthened

ASSESSMENT

- Parental status that includes parents' age and maturity, parental role models during childhood, role satisfaction, adjustment to parental role, ability to relate appropriately to various age levels of children, willingness to adjust to various age needs, social support available, education needs of parent, present parenting skills, coping mechanisms, knowledge of child care and growth and development, discipline methods utilized, bonding and attachment issues
- Family status, including relationship of parents to each other, relationship of parents to children and to other dependent person(s), sibling relationships, spirituality, community involvement, age-appropriate safety issues, nutritional status, health care practices
- Psychosocial status including financial, single-parent or dual-parent family, educational level, employment, environment, stressors, affection and concern, consistency and reliability of parenting techniques

- Expresses desire to enhance acceptance of child
- Expresses desire to enhance attention quality
- Expresses desire to enhance child health maintenance
- Expresses desire to enhance child-care arrangements
- Expresses desire to enhance engagement with child
- Expresses desire to enhance home environmental safety
- Expresses desire to enhance mood stability
- Expresses desire to enhance parent–child relations
- Expresses desire to enhance patience
- Expresses desire to enhance positive communication
- Expresses desire to enhance positive parenting behaviors
- Expresses desire to enhance positive temperament
- Expresses desire to enhance response to infant behavioral cues

- Parents will express satisfaction in role of parent.
- Parents will express confidence in ability to parent.
- Home will exhibit signs of safe and functional environment.
- Child care or dependent persons care routines will be adequate.
- Children and dependent persons will appear nutritionally healthy.
- Family will appear to be physically healthy.
- Family will express belief in a higher spiritual power.
- Family will express enjoying spending time together.
- Parents will demonstrate consistency and effectiveness related to discipline.
- Family will express confidence in social and community resources available related to family needs.

Suggested NOC Outcomes

Parent–Infant Attachment; Parenting: Psychosocial Safety

PCC ■ Discuss with parents their perceptions and philosophy related to the role of parents in a family. *Verbalizing perceptions and beliefs provides an opportunity to clarify parents' thinking.*

PCC ■ Offer parents an opportunity to express their doubts or convictions about the adequacy of their parenting skills. *An open and receptive attitude provides an atmosphere for increased trust and enhanced learning.*

PCC ■ Support family efforts as they adapt to the ever-changing issues of family needs. *Recognition of and appreciation for one's efforts enhances motivation to continue to improve skills.*

S ■ Observe the home environment and discuss the issues of safety and cleanliness if needed. *Family members need to have privacy and a sense of personal space as well as an environment that's free from environmental hazards, both chemical and physical.*

PCC ■ Request that parents describe a typical day with normal routines related to family dynamics and functioning. *This provides a concrete example for reflection of family functioning.*

PCC ▦ Discuss the food likes and dislikes of the family. *Parents need to be aware of nutritional preferences in order to increase family compliance for change.*

EBP ▦ Review the elements of a well-balanced diet for the various age groups represented in the family. *Different ages and developmental levels have different nutritional needs.*

PCC ▦ Discuss health care beliefs and practices with regard to the health maintenance of all family members. *Knowledge of sound health care practices enhances the well-being of family members.*

▦ Explore family's value system as well as their spiritual beliefs and practices. *Spirituality and values provide a basis for ethical and moral reasoning and an enhanced meaning to life.*

PCC ▦ Encourage family to "play" together. *Laughter and joy increase enjoyment and bonding as well as growth in the family unit.*

PCC ▦ Praise the family for traditions and activities that they do together. *Sharing meaningful activities increases loyalty, security, and a sense of belonging for family members.*

EBP ▦ Engage parents in a discussion of discipline practices and offer suggestions to enhance their present skills. *Discipline needs to be consistent, loving, and have reasonable guidelines. Children want and need limits so as to feel secure and safe.*

T&C ▦ Explore parents' perception of social support and community resources available to the family. *Social support and community resources provide guidance and positive reinforcement for parenting techniques and are a source of assistance and strength when families are experiencing stress.*

Suggested NIC Interventions

Developmental Enhancement: Child; Family Integrity Promotion: Childbearing Family; Family Involvement Promotion

EVALUATIONS FOR EXPECTED OUTCOMES

▦ Parents state enjoyment and satisfaction in the role of parent.
▦ Parents relate a positive sense of self and confidence in their ability to parent.
▦ Home environment is clean and free from chemical and physical hazards.
▦ Family functions in a structured and goal-oriented direction.
▦ Family members express participating in regular health and dental checkups.
▦ Family members express belief in a higher power and participation in their spiritual community.
▦ Family members look forward to family traditions, especially those related to holidays and vacations, and to spending time together as a family at school and community activities.
▦ Children are provided with consistent structure and guidelines; they express awareness of family rules and belief that those rules are fair.
▦ Family utilizes various social support venues as well as community resources to meet the needs of the family and individual family members.

DOCUMENTATION

▦ Parents' feelings and concerns about parenting
▦ Discipline methods described by parents
▦ Interventions to assist family with identifying nutritional needs of various age groups
▦ Health care teaching for family with different age groups
▦ Parents' perception of social and community support and resources
▦ Evaluations for expected outcomes

REFERENCES

Bhusiri, P., Phuphaibul, R., Suwonnaroop, N., & Viwatwongkasem, C. (2018). Effects of parenting skills training program for aggressive behavior reduction among school-aged children: A quasi-experimental study. *Pacific Rim International Journal of Nursing Research, 22*(4), 332–346.

Julian, M. M., Muzik, M., Kees, M., Valenstein, M., Dexter, C., & Rosenblum, K. L. (2018). Intervention effects on reflectivity explain change in positive parenting in military families with young children. *Journal of Family Psychology, 32*(6), 804–815. doi:10.1037/fam0000431

Norona, A. N., & Baker, B. L. (2017). The effects of early positive parenting and developmental delay status on child emotion dysregulation. *Journal of Intellectual Disability Research, 61*(2), 130–143. doi:10.1111/jir.12287

Risk for Perioperative Hypothermia

DEFINITION

Susceptible to an inadvertent drop in core body temperature below 36° C/96.8° F occurring 1 hour before to 24 hours after surgery, which may compromise health

RISK FACTORS

- Anxiety
- Body mass index below normal range for age and gender
- Environmental temperature <21 °C/69.8 °F
- Inadequate availability of appropriate warming equipment
- Wound area uncovered

ASSOCIATED CONDITIONS

- Acute hepatic failure
- Anemia
- Burns
- Cardiovascular complications
- Chronic renal impairment
- Combined regional and general anesthesia
- Neurologic disorder
- Pharmaceutical preparations
- Trauma

ASSESSMENT

- Body weight
- Environment temperature
- Patient temperature
- Patient's thermal comfort level
- Skin assessment

EXPECTED OUTCOMES

- Patient will maintain normothermia before surgery.
- Patient will maintain normothermia during surgery.
- Patient will maintain normothermia after surgery.

Suggested NOC Outcomes

Neurological Status: Autonomic; Thermoregulation; Vital Signs; Risk Control: Hypothermia

INTERVENTIONS AND RATIONALES

EBP ▪ Implement passive warming measures such as cotton blankets, surgical drapes, plastic sheeting, and reflective blankets during the intraoperative period. *Decreases risk of subsequent hypothermia.*

EBP ▪ Increase ambient temperature to between 20° C and 25° C. *Ambient temperature can reduce risk of heat loss through convection.*

S ▪ Measure patient's temperature 1 to 2 hours before start of anesthesia and either continuously or every 15 minutes during surgery and every hour postsurgery. *Monitor for higher risk for hypothermia.*

EBP ▪ Prewarm IV infusions. *May reduce the risk of subsequent hypothermia.*

EBP ▪ Prewarm patient 20 to 30 minutes before surgery. *Counteracts decline in temperature.*

Suggested NIC Interventions

Comfort Level; Fluid Management; Hypothermia Treatment; Temperature Regulation; Vital Signs Monitoring

EVALUATIONS FOR EXPECTED OUTCOMES

▪ Patient expresses thermal comfort level.
▪ Patient maintains normothermic body temperature.

DOCUMENTATION

▪ Environmental temperature
▪ Use of passive warming measures
▪ Vital signs

REFERENCES

Duff, J., Walker, K., Edward, K., Ralph, N., Giandinoto, J., Alexander, K., ... Stephenson, J. (2018). Effect of a thermal care bundle on the prevention, detection and treatment of perioperative inadvertent hypothermia. *Journal of Clinical Nursing, 27*(5–6), 1239–1249. doi:10.1111/jocn.14171

Rosenkilde, C., Vamosi, M., Lauridsen, J. T., & Hasfeldt, D. (2017). Efficacy of prewarming with a self-warming blanket for the prevention of unintended perioperative hypothermia in patients undergoing hip or knee arthroplasty. *Journal of PeriAnesthesia Nursing, 32*(5), 419–428. doi:10.1016/j.jopan.2016.02.007

Steelman, V. M., Chae, S., Duff, J., Anderson, M. J., & Zaidi, A. (2018). Warming of irrigation fluids for prevention of perioperative hypothermia during arthroscopy: A systematic review and meta-analysis. *Arthroscopy: The Journal of Arthroscopy & Related Surgery, 34*(3), 930–942.e2. doi.org/10.1016/j.arthro.2017.09.024

Risk for Perioperative-Positioning Injury

DEFINITION

Susceptible to inadvertent anatomical and physical changes as a result of posture or positioning equipment used during an invasive/surgical procedure, which may compromise health

RISK FACTOR

- Decreased muscle strength
- Dehydration
- Factors identified by standardized, validated screening tool
- Inadequate access to appropriate equipment
- Inadequate access to appropriate support surfaces
- Inadequate availability of equipment for individuals with obesity
- Malnutrition
- Obesity
- Prolonged nonanatomic positioning of limbs
- Rigid support surface

ASSOCIATED CONDITIONS

- Diabetes mellitus
- Edema
- Emaciation
- General anesthesia
- Immobilization
- Neuropathy
- Sensoriperceptual disturbance from anesthesia
- Vascular diseases

ASSESSMENT

- Reason for surgery
- Type of surgery and its expected length
- Health status, including age, weight, vital signs, nutritional status, integumentary status, musculoskeletal status, hydration status, temperature, peripheral vascular status, neurologic status, and smoking history
- Laboratory studies, including hematocrit and hemoglobin levels, complete blood count, electrolyte levels, urinalysis, blood coagulation studies, and liver function tests
- Mobility status, including range of motion (ROM), presence of prosthesis, and limb abnormality, impairment, or injury
- Current medical treatments, including radiation therapy, chemotherapy, and steroid therapy

EXPECTED OUTCOMES

- Patient will maintain effective breathing patterns.
- Patient will maintain adequate cardiac output.
- Patient's surgical positioning will facilitate gas exchange.
- Patient won't show evidence of neurologic, musculoskeletal, or vascular compromise.
- Patient will maintain tissue integrity.

Suggested NOC Outcomes

Blood Coagulation; Circulation Status; Cognitive Orientation; Neurological Status; Respiratory Status: Ventilation; Thermoregulation; Tissue Integrity: Skin & Mucous Membranes; Tissue Perfusion: Peripheral

S ▪ Document and report the results of the preoperative nursing assessment. Identify factors predisposing patient to tissue injury. *This information guides interventions.*

▪ Use appropriate mode of patient transportation (stretcher, patient bed, wheelchair, or crib) *to ensure patient safety.*

S ▪ Make sure an adequate number of staff members assist with transferring patient—at least two for moving patient onto an operating room bed, and at least four for moving anesthetized patient off operating room bed. *Adequate staffing enhances safety.*

S ▪ Check the operating room bed before surgery for proper functioning. *Intraoperative bed malfunction can result in increased anesthesia time and a more difficult surgical approach.*

S ▪ Ensure proper positioning.

Supine Position

S ▪ Check patient's neck and spine for proper alignment *to avoid trauma.*

▪ Check that patient's legs are straight and ankles uncrossed. *Crossed ankles cause pressure on tissue, vessels, and nerves.*

S ▪ Place a safety strap 5 cm above patient's knees, tight enough to restrain without compromising superficial venous return. *Applied too tightly, the safety strap may cause venous thrombosis or compression of tibial, peroneal, or sciatic nerves.*

EBP ▪ Secure patient's arms at sides with a draw sheet with palms down, making sure no part of the arm or hand extends over the mattress. Alternatively, secure patient's arms on padded arm boards at less than a 90-degree angle from the body, with palms supinated. *Hyperextension can cause injury to the brachial plexus. Supination of palms minimizes pressure.*

EBP ▪ Apply eye pads if patient's eyelids won't remain closed or if surgery is being performed on the head, neck, or chest. If allowed to remain open, the eye may dry out and become infected. *Corneal abrasions may result from drapes and other foreign material rubbing against the eye.*

EBP ▪ If surgery is expected to last more than 2 hours or if patient is predisposed to a pressure injury, place padding under patient's occiput, scapulae, olecranon, sacrum, coccyx, and calcaneus *to protect potential pressure points.* Apply a padded footboard *to support patient's feet, avoid plantar flexion, and prevent stretching of the tibial nerve and subsequent foot drop.*

EBP ▪ Unless contraindicated, place a foam doughnut or small pillow under patient's head *to prevent stretching of the neck muscles.*

Prone Position

S ▪ Make sure at least four staff members assist when turning patient *to ensure safety.*

S ▪ Check the lower eye and ear for excessive pressure. Apply eye pads. *Head support helps maintain cervical and thoracic spine alignment. Checking the dependent ear and eye lowers the risk of pressure injury. Pads protect the eyes.*

EBP ▪ Place patient's arms on arm boards extended in front beside patient's head with the elbows slightly flexed and palms pronated *to prevent strain on the shoulder, elbows, and wrist joints.*

S ▪ Check for proper alignment of the neck and spine *to avoid trauma.*

S ▪ Check a female patient's breasts and male patient's genitalia for excessive pressure from chest rolls or a laminectomy brace *to avoid soft tissue and nerve injury.*

EBP ▪ Check the bilateral pulses of upper and lower extremities. *The top and bottom edges of chest rolls or a laminectomy brace may compress radial and femoral arteries.*

EBP ▪ Place padding under patient's knees *to avoid injury to soft tissue and knee joint.*

EBP ▪ Place a pillow under patient's ankles *to avoid putting pressure on toes and feet, stretching the tibial nerve, or causing plantar flexion.*

Lateral Position

S ▪ Make sure at least four staff members assist when turning patient *to ensure safety.*

S ▪ Check patient's neck and spine for proper alignment *to avoid trauma.*

S ▪ Check patient's dependent eye and ear for excessive pressure. Apply eye pads. *Head supports help maintain cervical and thoracic spine alignment. Checking the dependent ear and eye lowers the risk of pressure injury. Pads protect patient's eyes.*

EBP ▪ Place a small roll under patient's dependent lower axilla *to relieve pressure on chest and axilla, allow for adequate chest expansion, and prevent compression of the brachial plexus by the humeral head.*

EBP ▪ Place patient's lower arm on arm board at less than 90-degree angle from the body, with palm supinated. Place patient's upper arm on an elevated padded support at less than a 90-degree angle from the body with palm pronated, and apply restraints *to avoid injury to brachial plexus.*

EBP ▪ Place the bottom leg flexed at the hip and knee and the top leg straight. *Flexing the bottom leg provides greater stability for the torso, decreases pressure on the lateral aspect of the lower leg, and prevents the bony areas of the knees and ankles from pressing against each other.*

EBP ▪ Place pillows between patient's knees and ankles *to support the top leg, prevent strain on the top hip, and pad pressure points on the medial aspects of both legs.*

EBP ▪ Place padding under the lateral aspects of patient's bottom knee and ankle *to reduce the risk of tissue injury to the area over the lateral malleolus of the ankle and peroneal nerve damage (foot drop).*

EBP ▪ Place a safety strap across patient's upper thighs or wide tape over the hips. Attach a strap or tape to the bed *to ensure safety.*

Lithotomy Position

EBP ▪ Secure patient's arms on arm boards or at the sides. If the arms are placed at patient's sides, position the fingers away from the break in the table *to prevent the fingers from becoming compressed in the bed mechanism.*

S ▪ Check patient's neck and spine for proper alignment *to avoid trauma.*

EBP ▪ Position the stirrups at equal height and attach them to the bed securely to prevent accidental movement. *Uneven leg flexion and hip abduction can cause strain on the lumbar and sacral areas.*

EBP ▪ Place the loop straps of the post stirrup behind patient's ankle and under the foot. Pad the post portion of the stirrup if it could come in contact with the leg. *Loop straps support and secure the legs.*

EBP ▪ Pad popliteal knee support stirrups *to prevent possible thrombosis of superficial vessels and pressure injury to femoral and obturator nerves.*

EBP ▪ With the help of a coworker, raise and lower patient's legs simultaneously and slowly to prevent ankle and knee injury and hip dislocation. *Lowering legs too quickly may cause sudden hypotension.*

S ▪ Assess patient position following each positional change *to ensure proper body alignment and adequate padding and support.*

S ▪ Apply restraints after positioning patient *to prevent falls and injury.*

Suggested NIC Interventions

Aspiration Precautions; Bleeding Reduction: Wound; Circulatory Care: Arterial Insufficiency; Circulatory Care: Venous Insufficiency; Embolus Care: Pulmonary; Fluid Management; Hemodynamic Regulation; Infection Control: Intraoperative; Positioning: Intraoperative; Skin Surveillance; Surgical Precautions; Temperature Regulation: Intraoperative

▦ Patient maintains effective breathing patterns. Patient's position doesn't restrict ventilation. Patient has adequate chest expansion.

▦ Patient maintains adequate cardiac output. Patient doesn't experience any significant episodes of hypertension or hypotension.

▦ Patient's positioning allows for adequate gas exchange, as evidenced by patient's ventilation–perfusion ratio and oxygen saturation.

▦ Patient shows no evidence of neurologic, musculoskeletal, or vascular compromise. Patient's mobility status and ROM remain at preoperative levels. Patient doesn't experience pain, numbness, tingling, or weakness in positioned body parts.

▦ Patient's tissue integrity remains intact; skin doesn't become reddened, discolored, ulcerated, edematous, or excoriated.

▦ Results of preoperative nursing assessment
▦ Operative procedure, type of anesthesia, and surgical positioning
▦ Surgical times, including time patient entered operating room, time incision was made, time incision was closed, and time patient left operating room
▦ Method of patient transport and transfer
▦ Estimated intraoperative blood loss
▦ Types and placement of padding, restraints, and positional devices
▦ Intraoperative repositioning of patient
▦ Intraoperative insertion of permanent or temporary implants
▦ Peripheral pulses
▦ Evaluations for expected outcomes

REFERENCES

Burlingame, B. L. (2017). Guideline implementation: Positioning the patient. *AORN Journal, 106*(3), 227–237. doi:10.1016/j.aorn.2017.07.010

Spader, C. (2018). Changing times and perioperative pressure injury prevention: Longer surgeries and new patient populations require a keener focus on prevention. *American Nurse Today*, 24–25.

Spruce, L. (2017). Back to basics: Preventing perioperative pressure injuries. *AORN Journal, 105*(1), 92–99. doi:10.1016/j.aorn.2016.10.018

Woodfin, K. O., Johnson, C., Parker, R., Mikach, C., Johnson, M., & McMullan, S. P. (2018). Use of a novel memory aid to educate perioperative team members on proper patient positioning technique. *AORN Journal, 107*(3), 325–332. doi:10.1002/aorn.12075

Disturbed Personal Identity

Inability to maintain an integrated and complete perception of self

▦ Alteration in social role
▦ Cult indoctrination
▦ Cultural incongruence
▦ Discrimination
▦ Dysfunctional family processes
▦ Low self-esteem
▦ Mania states

- Perceived prejudice
- Stages of growth

ASSOCIATED CONDITIONS

- Dissociative identity disorder
- Organic brain disorder
- Pharmaceutical agent
- Psychiatric disorder

ASSESSMENT

- Choices of vocation, sexual orientation, religious orientation, and friendships
- Ability to defend choices regarding long-range goals, to recognize alternatives, and to appreciate consequences
- Comfort level with decisions made about long-range goals
- Degree of anxiety or depression about long-range goals
- Loss of interest or social isolation from usual activities or friends
- Level of irritability about long-range goals
- Sleep difficulties
- Changes in eating habits
- Rape trauma
- Family status, including method of dealing with general conflicts, level of patient's communication with parents, handling of negotiations regarding restriction of freedom, degree of patient's separation from family, tolerance of patient's expressed opinions, reaction of parents to patient's long-range goals, and age-appropriateness of dating, curfew regulation, and money responsibilities
- Family and cultural standards related to separation issues

DEFINING CHARACTERISTICS

- Alteration in body image
- Confusion about cultural values
- Confusion about goals
- Confusion about ideological values
- Delusional description of self
- Feeling of emptiness
- Feeling of strangeness
- Fluctuating feelings about self
- Gender confusion
- Inability to distinguish between internal and external stimuli
- Inconsistent behavior
- Ineffective coping strategies
- Ineffective relationships
- Ineffective role performance

EXPECTED OUTCOMES

- Patient will establish trusting relationship with caregiver.
- Patient's issues will be discussed.
- Family's issues will be discussed.
- Patient will establish a firm, positive sense of self and personal identity.

- Patient will choose long-range goals using problem-solving techniques and will be comfortable with choices.
- Family will accept patient's choices of long-range goals.

Suggested NOC Outcomes

Distorted Thought Self-Control; Identity; Personal Well-Being; Self-Esteem

INTERVENTIONS AND RATIONALES

PCC - Assess patient alone without family *to gather baseline data and begin a therapeutic relationship.*

PCC - Explain your role as a patient advocate; negotiate rules of interaction, including confidentiality and depth and breadth of discussion *to establish your role as a resource for patient rather than as family's agent.*

PCC - Explore personal identity issues distressing to patient *to isolate issues into smaller, more solvable units.*

PCC - Help patient identify own values, beliefs, hopes, dreams, skills, and interests. *Patient's deficits may lie in a lack of self-exploration, problem-solving methods used, or separation issues with parents.*

PCC - Instruct patient to write about feelings in a journal and to list coping strategies. *Journaling can help patient maintain self-control and may increase insight.*

PCC - Integrate personal identity issues into decisions and choices *to help patient develop skill in problem-solving methods.*

PCC - Help patient identify the likely consequences of each choice. *Discussion and explanation aid problem-solving skills.*

EBP - Promote choices with the most likelihood of success. *Specific instructions can help patient gain problem-solving ability and maturity.*

PCC - Encourage family conferences to explore potential reactions to patient's choices, and promote support for patient's independent decision-making. *Meetings can help patient and family members identify problems and find better ways to interact. Meetings also allow patient and family members to ventilate true feelings in a safe environment.*

T&C - Encourage peer support groups *to explore and share personal identity experiences. Adolescents and young adults commonly accept support from peers more readily than from older adults.*

T&C - Promote outpatient counseling and family meetings as appropriate to reinforce progress. *Establishing outpatient support systems can reduce regression.*

PCC - Listen to patient's personal values and beliefs, but remain nonjudgmental, even if patient's values and beliefs differ from those of your own. *Remaining nonjudgmental but attentive shows your support.*

T&C - Refer patients to mental health services for medication and symptom management. *Disturbed personal identity may require ongoing mental health care.*

Suggested NIC Interventions

Delusion Management; Environmental Management: Violence Prevention; Hallucination Management; Reality Orientation

EVALUATIONS FOR EXPECTED OUTCOMES

- Patient openly discusses concerns with caregiver.
- Patient describes personal identity struggles.

- Family members discuss their reactions to patient's personal identity choices.
- Patient describes values, beliefs, skills, and interests in a positive way.
- Patient identifies choices and possible alternatives, postulates consequences, and makes decisions about long-range goals.
- Family members accept patient's choices of long-range goals.

DOCUMENTATION

- Assessment of patient's initial issues and problem-solving ability, including family's reactions, as well as assessment of level of separation achieved by patient
- Patient's level of emotional distress and changes in sleep and eating, initially and as hospitalization continues
- Patient's progress in problem solving and making choices
- Patient–family interactions and content of family meetings
- Patient's interaction in peer-group meetings
- Outpatient resources identified and suggested to patient and family members
- Evaluations for expected outcomes

REFERENCES

Albert Sznitman, G., Van Petegem, S., & Zimmermann, G. (2019). Exposing the role of coparenting and parenting for adolescent personal identity processes. *Journal of Social & Personal Relationships*, 36(4), 1233–1255. doi:10.1177/0265407518757707
Lannegrand-Willems, L., Chevrier, B., Perchec, C., & Carrizales, A. (2018). How is civic engagement related to personal identity and social identity in late adolescents and emerging adults? A person-oriented approach. *Journal of Youth & Adolescence*, 47(4), 731–748. doi:10.1007/s10964-018-0821-x
Meca, A., Sabet, R. F., Farrelly, C. M., Benitez, C. G., Schwartz, S. J., Gonzales-Backen, M., ... Lorenzo-Blanco, E. I. (2017). Personal and cultural identity development in recently immigrated Hispanic adolescents: Links with psychosocial functioning. *Cultural Diversity & Ethnic Minority Psychology*, 23(3), 348–361. doi:10.1037/cdp0000129
Notini, L., Gillam, L., & Pang, K. C. (2018). Facial feminization surgery: Private, personal identity, compensatory justice, and resource allocation. *American Journal of Bioethics*, 18(12), 12–15. doi:10.1 080/15265161.2018.1531168

Risk for Disturbed Personal Identity

DEFINITION

Susceptible to the inability to maintain an integrated and complete perception of self, which may compromise health

RISK FACTORS

- Alteration in social role
- Cult indoctrination
- Cultural incongruence
- Discrimination
- Dysfunctional family processes
- Low self-esteem
- Manic states
- Perceived prejudice
- Stages of growth

ASSOCIATED CONDITIONS

- Dissociative identity disorder
- Organic brain disorder
- Pharmaceutical agent
- Psychiatric disorder

ASSESSMENT

- Choices of vocation, sexual orientation, religious orientation, and friendships
- Ability to defend choices regarding long-range goals, to recognize alternatives, and to appreciate consequences
- Comfort level with decisions made about long-range goals
- Degree of anxiety or depression about long-range goals
- Loss of interest in or social isolation from usual activities or friends
- Level of irritability about long-range goals
- Sleep difficulties
- Changes in eating habits
- Family status, including method of dealing with general conflicts, level of patient's communication with family members/others, handling of negotiations regarding restriction of freedom, degree of patient's separation from family, tolerance of patient's expressed opinions, reaction to patient's long-range goals, and age-appropriateness of dating, curfew regulation, and money responsibilities
- Family and cultural standards

EXPECTED OUTCOMES

- Patient will actively participate in milieu therapies.
- Patient will maintain safety and report any thoughts of suicide to staff.
- Patient will perform relaxation techniques during periods of stress.
- Patient will verbalize understanding of the need for long-term therapy.

Suggested NOC Outcomes

Anxiety Control; Coping; Depression Level; Distorted Thought Control; Impulse Control; Self-Esteem; Substance Addiction Consequences

INTERVENTIONS AND RATIONALES

- **S** Assess patient for thoughts of suicide *as patient may require immediate safety precautions and psychological support.*
- **S** Assess for history of previous or current medical conditions, substance abuse, and any pharmacologic side effects. *Brain trauma, organic brain disorders, substance abuse, or medication side effects can present with similar symptoms.*
- **PCC** Work with patient to identify triggers that provoke anxiety. *Patient may not remember or be aware of the events that trigger patient's symptoms and will need assistance in identifying them.*
- **PCC** Provide patient with emotional support and reassurance of safety during episodes of dissociation *as the symptoms patient is experiencing can be disturbing and anxiety provoking in and of themselves.*
- **EBP** Reorient patient as necessary *in order to reduce anxiety related to confusion.*

EBP ▪ Educate patient on positive coping mechanisms such as cognitive therapies and relaxation techniques, and assist patient in applying these techniques. *Assisting patient with relaxation therapies during times of anxiety decreases anxiety and helps assure patient of the efficacy of these coping mechanisms.*

PCC ▪ Dedicate quality time to patient in a therapeutic and consistent manner *in order to help patient feel safe, allow time for open expression of feelings, and develop a trusting relationship.*

T&C ▪ Refer patient for long-term therapy and educate patient regarding the length of treatment. *Patient may not be aware that long-term treatment may be necessary.*

T&C ▪ Refer patient to support groups in the community *as this will help the patient to realize that he or she is not alone and because these groups provide further anxiety prevention strategies and support.*

Suggested NIC Interventions

Anxiety Reduction; Coping Enhancement; Decision-Making Support; Risk Identification; Self-Esteem Enhancement; Substance Use Prevention; Suicide Prevention; Relaxation Therapy

EVALUATIONS FOR EXPECTED OUTCOMES

▪ Patient participates in milieu therapy.
▪ Patient expresses no thoughts of suicide.
▪ Patient uses appropriate stress management techniques.
▪ Patient verbalizes need for long-term therapy.

DOCUMENTATION

▪ Results of assessment for suicidal ideation
▪ Assessment of health history and use/reaction to medications
▪ Patient's responses to therapeutic actions
▪ Patient–family interactions and content of family meetings
▪ Cognitive therapies and relaxation techniques used
▪ Outpatient resources identified and suggested to patient
▪ Evaluations for expected outcomes

REFERENCES

Albert Sznitman, G., Van Petegem, S., & Zimmermann, G. (2019). Exposing the role of coparenting and parenting for adolescent personal identity processes. *Journal of Social & Personal Relationships, 36*(4), 1233–1255. doi:10.1177/0265407518757707

Craig, S. L., Iacono, G., Paceley, M. S., Dentato, M. P., & Boyle, K. E. H. (2017). Intersecting sexual, gender, and professional identities among social work students: The importance of identity integration. *Journal of Social Work Education, 53*(3), 466–479. doi:10.1080/10437797.2016.1272516

Meca, A., Sabet, R. F., Farrelly, C. M., Benitez, C. G., Schwartz, S. J., Gonzales-Backen, M., ... Lorenzo-Blanco, E. I. (2017). Personal and cultural identity development in recently immigrated Hispanic adolescents: Links with psychosocial functioning. *Cultural Diversity & Ethnic Minority Psychology, 23*(3), 348–361. doi:10.1037/cdp0000129

Risk for Poisoning

DEFINITION

Susceptible to accidental exposure to, or ingestion of, drugs or dangerous products in sufficient doses, which may compromise health

RISK FACTORS

External

- Access to dangerous product
- Access to illicit drugs potentially contaminated by poisonous additives
- Access to pharmaceutical agent
- Occupational setting without adequate safeguards

Internal

- Emotional disturbance
- Inadequate precautions against poisoning
- Insufficient knowledge of pharmacological agents
- Insufficient knowledge of poisoning prevention
- Insufficient vision

ASSOCIATED CONDITION

Alteration in cognitive function

ASSESSMENT

- Age
- Gender
- Drug history, including use of prescription and over-the-counter medications
- Use of alcoholic beverages
- Health history, including accidents, allergies, exposure to pollutants, falls, hyperthermia, hypothermia, poisoning, sensory or perceptual changes (auditory, gustatory, kinesthetic, olfactory, tactile, and visual), and trauma
- Circumstances surrounding present situation that might lead to injury
- Neurologic status, including level of consciousness (LOC), mental status, and orientation
- Psychosocial history, including age, habits (drug or alcohol use), occupation, and personality
- Laboratory studies, including clotting factors, hemoglobin levels and hematocrit, platelet count, white blood cell count, and toxicology screening

EXPECTED OUTCOMES

- Patient won't ingest or be exposed to dangerous substances.
- Patient will communicate an understanding of need for self-protection.
- Patient and family members will state method for safekeeping of potentially dangerous products.

Suggested NOC Outcomes

Personal Safety Behavior; Safe Home Environment; Risk Control: Drug Use; Risk Detection

INTERVENTIONS AND RATIONALES

S Observe, record, and report falls, seizures, and unsafe practices to ensure implementation of appropriate interventions. *Overdose of certain medications (such as phenothiazines) can cause such neurologic problems as seizures.*

EBP Instruct patient or family member in the drug regimen, including the reasons for taking drugs, safety precautions, and how to monitor the effectiveness of drugs, *to increase compliance.*

S ▪ Regularly review and document patient's medication regimen *to monitor medication use, assess whether certain medications should be discontinued, and monitor for drug interactions.*

EBP ▪ Instruct patient or family member to store drugs in a secure area away from the bedside *to prevent accidental ingestion. Many older patients keep medications at their bedside to decrease the need to arise during the night.*

S ▪ If color-coding medications, use only bright, contrasting colors. *Older patients can't distinguish pastel colors well.*

▪ Help patient or family member identify behaviors that contribute to the risk of toxicity, such as obtaining prescriptions from various health care providers or using different pharmacies, *to raise awareness of potential hazards.*

PCC ▪ Encourage patient or family member to retain a primary physician who coordinates care. *Older patients with multiple health problems may receive care from various providers who are unaware of each other's treatment plans and medication regimens.*

EBP ▪ Provide instructions for the use of medications, including quantity, frequency, and number of doses, *to enhance understanding of the medication regimen and increase compliance.* Make sure the instructions are clearly written in black or blue ink. *Older patients can read black or blue ink more easily.*

S ▪ Make sure all medication labels are inscribed in large print and include dosage instructions *to avoid medication errors.*

PCC ▪ Help patient maintain an accurate and effective system for following the medication regimen, such as a check-off calendar system or separate pill boxes labeled for each day of the week, *to reduce errors.* Encourage the patient to work with a pharmacist when developing this system.

S ▪ Monitor and record patient's respiratory status *because certain poisons can cause respiratory depression.*

S ▪ Monitor and record neurologic status *because excessive toxic exposure can cause coma.* Patient may have pinpoint or dilated pupils, depending on the type of drug or poison ingested and the length of time patient has been hypoxic.

S ▪ Monitor vital signs, intake and output, and LOC. Record and report any changes. Severe hypotension may develop following overdose. *It may be related to central nervous system defect, direct myocardial depression, or vasodilation. Marked hyperthermia can occur with salicylate overdose, which affects the metabolic rate. Dehydration may develop in some patients from an increased respiratory rate, sweating, vomiting, and urine losses.*

S ▪ Remove dangerous or potentially dangerous products from the environment *to avoid injury.*

S ▪ Observe, record, and report falls, seizures, and unsafe practices to ensure implementation of appropriate interventions. *Overdose of certain medications can cause such neurologic problems as seizures.*

S ▪ Check the settings on oxygen flow meters every hour on patients known to retain carbon dioxide (e.g., some patients with chronic obstructive pulmonary disease). *This avoids carbon dioxide narcosis from excessive oxygen therapy in poorly ventilated patients; if unchecked, patient may stop breathing.*

EBP ▪ Monitor patient's urine and serum toxicity levels, when indicated, *to reduce the risk of toxicity. Age-related changes in body function may lead to decreased renal, liver, and GI clearance of drugs, increasing the patient's risk of toxicity. Also, various drugs commonly used by the older patient increase the risk of toxicity from drug interactions.*

EBP ▪ Teach patient about the harmful and potentially lethal effects of abusing drugs, alcohol, or other dangerous substances *to enhance knowledge and foster better informed decisions.* Provide appropriate written materials. *Written materials reinforce teaching and allow review after discharge.*

EBP ▪ Teach parents and caregivers to be alert for stomach aches, irritability, and headaches. *These may be early signs of poisoning.*

EBP ▦ Provide patient and family members with information about such specific products as medications, oxygen, and total parenteral nutrition. Tailor instructions to a specific product and patient's ability to learn self-care. *This enables patient and family members to identify and alter environmental or lifestyle factors to achieve optimum health level.*

T&C ▦ Identify available community resources to help prevent or treat substance abuse. *Support services and groups can provide the patient with safe settings in which to explore problems and feelings and develop adaptive methods of coping.*

Suggested NIC Interventions

Environmental Management: Safety; Environmental Risk Protection; Health Education; Home Maintenance Assistance; Surveillance: Safety; Vital Signs Monitoring; Medication Management; Risk Identification

EVALUATIONS FOR EXPECTED OUTCOMES

▦ Patient doesn't report or exhibit signs or symptoms resulting from exposure to or ingestion of dangerous substances.
▦ Patient doesn't experience episodes of toxicity.
▦ Patient requests information on protection from dangerous products.
▦ Patient and family members describe method for safekeeping of potentially dangerous products.

DOCUMENTATION

▦ Patient's statements that indicate potential for injury
▦ Physical findings
▦ Record of falls, seizures, and unsafe practices
▦ Observations or knowledge of unsafe practices
▦ Interventions to treat toxicity or other injury
▦ Factors that increase patient's risk of drug toxicity
▦ Knowledge deficits and learning objectives
▦ Teaching topics, materials, and methods
▦ Interventions performed to prevent injury
▦ Patient's response to nursing interventions
▦ Referrals to community resources or professionals for ongoing counseling
▦ Evaluations for expected outcomes

REFERENCES

Nistor, N., Frasinariu, O. E., Rugină, A., Ciomaga, I. M., Jităreanu, C., & Ştreangă, V. (2018). Epidemiological study on accidental poisonings in children from northeast Romania. *Medicine, 97*(29), 1–4. doi:10.1097/MD.0000000000011469

Prashar, A., & Ramesh, M. (2018). Assessment of pattern and outcomes of pesticides poisoning in a tertiary care hospital. *Tropical Medicine & International Health, 23*(12), 1401–1407. doi:10.1111/tmi.13156

Sinha, A., Raheja, H., & Kupfer, Y. (2018). Myocardial infarction after accidental minoxidil poisoning. *American Journal of Therapeutics, 25*(2), e279–e281. doi:10.1097/MJT.0000000000000536

Post-Trauma Syndrome

DEFINITION

Sustained maladaptive response to a traumatic, overwhelming event

- Diminished ego strength
- Environment not conducive to needs
- Exaggerated sense of responsibility
- Insufficient social support
- Perceives event as traumatic
- Self-injurious behavior
- Survivor role

- Age
- Gender
- Education level
- History and circumstances of accident or trauma
- Patient's perception of event
- Physical injuries sustained, including cardiopulmonary, musculoskeletal, genitourinary, and integumentary
- Neurologic status
- Emotional reactions, including grief reaction, self-concept, and sleep pattern
- Cognitive reactions, including concentration, memory, and orientation
- Behavioral reactions, including available support systems, clergy, coping patterns, family members, problem-solving ability, and social interactions
- Available support systems

- Aggression
- Alienation
- Alteration in concentration
- Alteration in mood
- Anger
- Anxiety
- Avoidance behavior
- Compulsive behavior
- Denial
- Depression
- Dissociative amnesia
- Enuresis
- Exaggerated startle response
- Fear
- Flashbacks
- Gastrointestinal irritation
- Grieving
- Guilt
- Headache
- Heart palpitations
- History of detachment
- Hopelessness
- Horror
- Hypervigilance

- Intrusive dreams
- Intrusive thoughts
- Irritability
- Neurosensory irritability
- Nightmares
- Panic attacks
- Rage
- Reports of feeling numb
- Repression
- Shame
- Substance misuse

EXPECTED OUTCOMES

- Patient will recover or be rehabilitated from physical injuries to the extent possible.
- Patient will state feelings and fears related to traumatic accident or event.
- Patient will express feelings of anger, blame, fear, and guilt.
- Patient will express feelings of safety.
- Patient will use available support systems.
- Patient will use effective coping mechanisms to reduce fear.
- Patient will mobilize support systems and professional resources, as needed.
- Patient will maintain or reestablish adaptive social interactions with family members.

Suggested NOC Outcomes

Anxiety Self-Control; Body Image; Coping; Depression Level; Fear Self-Control; Hope; Impulse Self-Control; Quality of Life; Self-Esteem; Stress Level

INTERVENTIONS AND RATIONALES

EBP - Follow the medical regimen to manage physical injuries. *Attention to physical needs supports healing of the body.*

S - Monitor mental status, reorienting patient to surroundings and interpreting reality as often as necessary, *to alleviate psychic numbing, a characteristic symptom of assault.*

PCC - Instruct patient in at least one fear-reducing behavior, such as seeking support from others when frightened, *to help the patient gain a sense of mastery over the current situation.*

PCC - Provide emotional support:

  PCC - Visit patient frequently *to reduce patient's fear of being alone.*

  PCC - Be available to listen *to respond empathetically to patient's feelings.*

  PCC - Accept and encourage the statement of patient's feelings *to reassure patient that feelings are appropriate and valid.*

  S - Assure patient of personal safety, and take the measures needed to ensure it. *Frequent nightmares or flashbacks may cause patient to question the safety of his or her environment.*

  PCC - Avoid care-related activities or environmental stimuli that may intensify symptoms associated with trauma (loud noises, bright lights, abrupt entrances into patient's room, or painful procedures or treatment). *Environmental stimuli can easily intensify flashbacks to a traumatic event.*

  S - Reorient patient to surroundings and reality as frequently as necessary. *Post-trauma psychic numbing impairs orientation, memory, and reality perception.*

  PCC - Instruct patient in at least one fear-reducing behavior such as seeking support from others when frightened. *As patient learns to reduce fears, coping skills will increase.*

- Support patient's family members:
  - **PCC** ▪ Provide time for them to express feelings.
  - ▪ Help family understand patient's reactions. *This reduces their anxiety and gives them a chance to help patient.*
- **T&C** ▪ Offer referrals to other support persons or groups, including clergy, mental health professionals, and trauma support groups. *Referrals help patient to regain a sense of universality, reduce isolation, share fears, and deal constructively with feelings.*
- **PCC** ▪ Recognize that patient's culture may affect patient's response to trauma; remain supportive and nonjudgmental *to show your support for and acceptance of patient's response to trauma.*
- **PCC** ▪ Help patient identify support persons who can be trusted, such as a therapist, clergy person, or school nurse, *to help prevent further episodes of violence.*
- **T&C** ▪ Make appropriate referrals to mental health professionals and social service agencies *to ensure the patient's safety in the community.*

Suggested NIC Interventions

Active Listening; Anxiety Reduction; Coping Enhancement; Counseling; Forgiveness Facilitation; Mood Management; Security Enhancement; Socialization Enhancement; Support Group; Support System Enhancement

EVALUATIONS FOR EXPECTED OUTCOMES

- Patient resumes usual activities of daily living to extent possible.
- Patient expresses feelings associated with traumatic event.
- Patient expresses feelings of anger, blame, fear, and guilt.
- Patient expresses feeling of safety.
- Patient interacts with supportive people to alleviate distress.
- Patient demonstrates use of at least one fear-reducing behavior (specify).
- Patient interacts with family members in beneficial manner.

DOCUMENTATION

- Patient's perception of traumatic event
- Observations of patient's behavior
- Observations of patient's social interaction with others
- Interventions
- Patient's responses to nursing interventions
- Referrals to other support persons or groups
- Evaluations for expected outcomes

REFERENCES

Bonnan-White, J., Hetzel-Riggin, M. D., Diamond-Welch, B. K., & Tollini, C. (2018). "You blame me, therefore I blame me": The importance of first disclosure partner responses on trauma-related cognitions and distress. *Journal of Interpersonal Violence, 33*(8), 1260–1286. doi:10.1177/0886260515615141

Cascio, K. A. (2019). Providing trauma-informed care to women exiting prostitution: assessing programmatic responses to severe trauma. *Journal of Trauma & Dissociation, 20*(1), 100–113. doi:10.1080/15299732.2018.1502713

Frost, R., Hyland, P., McCarthy, A., Halpin, R., Shevlin, M., & Murphy, J. (2019). The complexity of trauma exposure and response: Profiling PTSD and CPTSD among a refugee sample. *Psychological Trauma: Theory, Research, Practice & Policy, 11*(2), 165–175. doi:10.1037/tra0000408

Risk for Post-Trauma Syndrome

DEFINITION

Susceptible to sustained maladaptive response to a traumatic, overwhelming event, which may compromise health

RISK FACTORS

- Diminished ego strength
- Environment not conducive to needs
- Exaggerated sense of responsibility
- Insufficient social support
- Perceives event as traumatic
- Self-injurious behavior
- Survivor role

ASSESSMENT

- Age and gender
- History of traumatic event, including circumstances, losses incurred (financial, property, physical integrity, close relationships), effect of trauma on social interactions, and grief reaction
- Health history, including previous traumatic events, patient's characteristic perception of such events and coping responses, and alcohol or substance abuse
- Mental status, including cognitive and emotional function, problems with concentration, memory, orientation, mood, and behavior
- Changes in appetite, self-image, sleep pattern, or sexual drive
- Available sources of support, including friends, family, caregivers, and community resources

EXPECTED OUTCOMES

- Patient won't develop chronic post-trauma response, substance abuse, or other mental health disorders.
- Patient will express understanding of post-trauma response.
- Patient's response to trauma won't be characterized by avoidance, numbness, or intrusiveness.
- Patient will express feelings of safety.
- Patient will employ effective coping skills.
- Patient will reach out to appropriate sources of support to reduce fear.

Suggested NOC Outcomes

Coping; Depression Level; Depression Self-Control; Risk Detection; Social Support; Spiritual Health; Stress Level

INTERVENTIONS AND RATIONALES

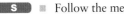

- Follow the medical regimen *to treat medical problems associated with the traumatic event.*
- Assess patient's baseline mental status and monitor changes in cognitive and psychosocial function *to detect the need for intervention as soon as possible.*

PCC ▪ Listen actively to patient's statements about the traumatic event *to encourage a trusting relationship and open discussion.*

PCC ▪ Communicate your acceptance of patient's fears and feelings related to the traumatic event *to reassure patient that feelings are appropriate and valid.*

PCC ▪ Reassure patient of safety of the environment. *Patient may be reluctant to express lingering fears and require reassurance.*

PCC ▪ Avoid nursing care or environmental stimuli that may worsen or initiate symptoms (such as loud noises, bright lights, and painful procedures) *to avoid triggering flashbacks to the traumatic event.* Also, warn patient to avoid disruptive stimuli.

PCC ▪ Caution patient before you make physical contact and avoid approaching patient from behind *to avoid actions that may be misinterpreted and that may trigger reexperience of the traumatic event.*

PCC ▪ Explore with patient strategies to reduce the traumatic response, such as having a support person call patient on a regular basis and using stress-reducing techniques when experiencing increased fear and anxiety, *to strengthen coping skills and foster a sense of control.*

EBP ▪ Teach patient that a post-trauma response may occur immediately or days, weeks, or years after a trauma *to alert patient to the risk of post-trauma response.*

PCC ▪ Help patient increase awareness of people, places, and events that trigger or reduce a post-trauma response *to encourage patient to take an active role in treatment.*

PCC ▪ Provide opportunities for patient to discuss the trauma periodically, based on patient's needs and willingness to talk *to prevent the development of post-trauma response.*

PCC ▪ Encourage family members and friends to express their perceptions and feelings about the traumatic event and reactions they see in patient *to aid assessment.*

EBP ▪ Provide teaching to family members, friends, and caregivers about the signs and symptoms of post-trauma response and interventions they can use *to promote involvement with rather than withdrawal from patient.*

T&C ▪ Explore uses of appropriate community resources and make referrals according to patient's and family members' needs *to ensure continuity of care and decrease patient's isolation.*

Suggested NIC Interventions

Coping Enhancement; Hope Instillation; Mood Management; Self-Awareness Enhancement

EVALUATIONS FOR EXPECTED OUTCOMES

▪ Patient doesn't develop chronic post-trauma response, substance abuse, or other mental health disorders.

▪ Patient expresses understanding of post-trauma response.

▪ Patient's response to trauma isn't characterized by avoidance, numbness, or intrusiveness.

▪ Patient expresses feelings of safety.

▪ Patient employs effective coping skills and reaches out to appropriate sources of support to reduce fear.

DOCUMENTATION

▪ Patient's perception of the traumatic event

▪ Observation of patient's behavior, coping skills, and use of support systems

▪ Patient's response to nursing care activities

▪ Patient's communication patterns with friends, family, and others and their responses

▪ Teaching provided to patient and family

- Referrals for ongoing support
- Evaluations for expected outcomes

REFERENCES

Peng, H. T., Tenn, C., Vartanian, O., Rhind, S. G., Jarmasz, J., Tien, H., & Beckett, A.; LT-SIM study group. (2018). Biological response to stress during battlefield trauma training: Live tissue versus high-fidelity patient simulator. *Military Medicine, 183*(9/10), e349–e356. doi:10.1093/milmed/usx236

Scoglio, A. A. J., Rudat, D. A., Garvert, D., Jarmolowski, M., Jackson, C., & Herman, J. L. (2018). Self-compassion and responses to trauma: The role of emotion regulation. *Journal of Interpersonal Violence, 33*(13), 2016–2036. doi:10.1177/0886260515622296

Streb, M., Conway, M. A., & Michael, T. (2017). Conditioned responses to trauma reminders: How durable are they over time and does memory integration reduce them? *Journal of Behavior Therapy & Experimental Psychiatry, 57*, 88–95. doi:10.1016/j.jbtep.2017.04.005

Readiness for Enhanced Power

DEFINITION

A pattern of participating knowingly in change for well-being, which can be strengthened

ASSESSMENT

- Patient's perception of present state of power
- Patient's perception of ability to enhance power
- Support systems, including family members, friends, clergy
- Patient's ability to identify choices
- Patient's readiness for change to occur
- Reliance on health care system to resolve complaints or assume power

DEFINING CHARACTERISTICS

- Expresses desire to enhance awareness of possible changes
- Expresses desire to enhance identification of choices that can be made for change
- Expresses desire to enhance independence with actions for change
- Expresses desire to enhance involvement in change
- Expresses desire to enhance knowledge for participation in change
- Expresses desire to enhance participation in choices for daily living
- Expresses desire to enhance participation in choices for health
- Expresses desire to enhance power

EXPECTED OUTCOMES

- Patient will express perceived control in influencing health outcomes.
- Patient will participate in choices that enhance care and well-being.
- Patient will develop a plan for adjusting to significant life changes.

Suggested NOC Outcomes

Family Resiliency; Health Beliefs: Perceived Control; Personal Autonomy; Psychosocial Adjustment: Life Change

PCC ▦ Assess patient's understanding of need for changes to improve well-being; *knowledge increases power in independent decisions for change.*

PCC ▦ Assess patient's participation in choices to be made *to enhance care and well-being.*

PCC ▦ Assist patient in acquiring knowledge necessary for positive decision-making. *Making positive decisions that produce benefits will reinforce health-seeking behaviors.*

PCC ▦ Help patient to involve family, community, clergy, and friends with changes to the care plan *to increase patient's perceived control to affect maximal self-care outcomes.*

PCC ▦ Work with patient to help develop a plan that takes into account the resources identified as being helpful to patient in attaining an optimal level of self-care. *This will help patient maintain control of own decision-making about health while using the input of others whom patient trusts.*

Suggested NOC Outcomes

Assertiveness Training; Coping Enhancement; Self-Modification Assistance; Self-Responsibility Facilitation

▦ Patient expresses understanding of the need for changes to improve well-being.

▦ Patient participates in choices that enhance own care and well-being.

▦ Patient develops a plan for adjusting to significant life changes.

▦ Patient's understanding of needed changes for own care and well-being

▦ Patient's choices that enhance own care and well-being

▦ Patient's knowledge to make ongoing changes to own care and well-being

▦ Evaluations for expected outcomes

REFERENCES

Akpotor, M. E., & Johnson, E. A. (2018). Client empowerment: A concept analysis. *International Journal of Caring Sciences, 11*(2), 743–750.

Daruwalla, Z., Thakkar, V., Aggarwal, M., Kiasatdolatabadi, A., Guergachi, A., & Keshavjee, K. (2019). Patient empowerment: The role of technology. *Studies in Health Technology & Informatics, 257,* 70–74. doi:10.3233/978-1-61499-951-5-70

Ghomi, R., Vasli, P., Hosseini, M., & Ahmadi, F. (2019). Effect of an empowerment program on the caring behaviors of mothers with preterm infants: the health belief model approach. *International Journal of Health Promotion & Education, 57*(2), 55–66. doi:10.1080/14635240.2018.1549959

Larsen, T., & Sagvaag, H. (2018). Empowerment and pathologization: A case study in Norwegian mental health and substance abuse services. *Health Expectations, 21*(6), 1231–1240. doi:10.1111/hex.12828

Powerlessness

A state of actual or perceived loss of control or influence over factors or events that affect one's well-being, personal life, or the society (adapted from American Psychology Association)

▦ Anxiety

▦ Caregiver role strain

- Dysfunctional institutional environment
- Impaired physical mobility
- Inadequate interest in improving one's situation
- Inadequate interpersonal relations
- Inadequate knowledge to manage a situation
- Inadequate motivation to improve one's situation
- Inadequate participation in treatment regimen
- Inadequate social support
- Ineffective coping strategies
- Low self-esteem
- Pain
- Perceived complexity of treatment regimen
- Perceived social stigma
- Social marginalization

ASSOCIATED CONDITIONS

- Cerebrovascular disorders
- Cognition disorders
- Critical illness
- Progressive illness
- Unpredictability of illness trajectory

ASSESSMENT

- Age
- Gender
- Level of education
- Occupation
- Ethnic group
- Nature of the medical diagnosis
- Mobility
- Behavioral responses (verbal and nonverbal), including calmness or agitation, anger, independence or dependence, interest or apathy, and satisfaction or dissatisfaction
- Usual coping strategies
- Past experiences with hospitalization
- Knowledge, including current understanding of physical condition and physical, mental, and emotional readiness to learn
- Family status, including marital status; developmental stage; socioeconomic status; support systems; history of physical, sexual, or emotional support; and family health history
- Environment, including equipment and supplies, health care professionals and personnel, lighting, location of patient's personal belongings, noise, privacy, and space
- Number and types of stressors
- Social factors
- Spiritual beliefs and value system

DEFINING CHARACTERISTICS

- Delayed recovery
- Depressive symptoms
- Expresses doubt about role performance
- Expresses frustration about inability to perform previous activities
- Expresses lack of purpose in life

- Expresses shame
- Fatigue
- Loss of independence
- Reports inadequate sense of control
- Social alienation

EXPECTED OUTCOMES

- Patient will identify feelings of powerlessness associated with the present situation.
- Patient will acknowledge fears, feelings, and concerns about current situation.
- Patient will describe modifications or adjustments to the environment that allow feelings of control.
- Patient will participate in self-care activities (specify).
- Patient will make decisions related to care.
- Patient will identify life situations over which the patient has no control.
- Patient will develop a plan to take control of life.
- Patient will state feelings of regained control.

Suggested NOC Outcomes

Anxiety Level; Decision-Making; Depression Self-Control; Family Participation in Professional Care; Fear Level; Health Beliefs; Self-Esteem; Social Involvement; Social Support

INTERVENTIONS AND RATIONALES

PCC ▪ Encourage patient to express feelings and concerns. Set aside time for discussions with patient about daily events. *This helps patient bring vaguely understood emotions into focus.*

PCC ▪ Accept patient's feelings of powerlessness as normal. *This indicates respect for patient and enhances feelings of self-worth.*

EBP ▪ Identify and develop patient's coping mechanisms, strengths, and resources for support. *By making use of coping skills, patient can reduce anxiety and fears and successfully undergo grieving necessary to come to terms with chronic illness.*

PCC ▪ Discuss situations that provoke feelings of anger, anxiety, and powerlessness *to identify areas patient can control and to prevent anger from being inappropriately directed at self or others.*

PCC ▪ Encourage participation in self-care. Provide positive reinforcement for patient's activities. Encourage patient to take an active role as a member of the health care team. *This enhances patient's sense of control and reduces passive and dependent behavior.*

PCC ▪ Provide as many opportunities as possible for patient to make decisions about self-care (for instance, positioning, choosing an injection site, and visiting) *to communicate respect for patient and enhance feelings of independence.*

▪ Help patient learn about the health condition, treatment, and prognosis *to help patient feel in control.*

PCC ▪ Acknowledge the importance of patient's space:
  - Verbally delineate patient's space.
  - Orient patient to personal space.
  - If patient is immobilized, ask for instructions regarding placement of personal belongings.
  - If possible, allow patient to walk around the space and arrange personal belongings. *These measures enhance patient's potential for regaining sense of power.*

`PCC` ▪ Reduce irritating noises if possible and explain the reasons for alarms and other disturbances. *Excessive sensory stimuli can cause disorientation, hallucinations, and delusional thinking.*

`PCC` ▪ Modify the environment when possible to meet patient's self-care needs *to promote patient's sense of control over environment.*

`PCC` ▪ Decrease unpredictable events by discussing rules, policies, procedures, and schedules with patient. *Fear of the unknown interferes with patient's ability to cope.*

`PCC` ▪ Encourage family members to support patient without taking control *to increase patient's feelings of self-worth.*

`EBP` ▪ Reinforce patient's rights as stated in Patient's Bill of Rights *to protect patient's right to make decisions about health care treatment.*

`PCC` ▪ Identify and arrange to accommodate patient's spiritual needs. *Spirituality enables patient to gain courage and resist despair.*

`EBP` ▪ Explain treatments and procedures, and encourage patient to participate in planning personal care. Provide choices for when and how activities will occur (such as bathing, eating, and getting out of bed). *This increases patient's feeling of powerfulness and reduces passivity and dependence on caregiver.*

`PCC` ▪ Provide as many situations as possible in which patient can take control (such as positioning, choosing an injection site, and visiting) *to help reduce potential for maladaptive coping behaviors.*

`PCC` ▪ Encourage participation in self-care. Provide positive reinforcement for patient's activities *to encourage increasing participation in self-care in the future.*

`PCC` ▪ Respect and show your acceptance of patient's cultural beliefs about health. The belief that each patient has the personal authority and responsibility *to try to reach optimal well-being is a Western value not shared by all cultures.*

`T&C` ▪ Contact social services *to ensure the patient receives legal and financial support as needed.*

Suggested NIC Interventions

Anxiety Reduction; Cognitive Restructuring; Decision-Making Support; Family Presence Facilitation; Mutual Goal Setting; Presence; Self-Esteem Enhancement; Values Clarification

EVALUATIONS FOR EXPECTED OUTCOMES

▪ Patient verbalizes positive and negative feelings about current situation.
▪ Patient expresses feelings of lack of control.
▪ Patient discusses feelings of powerlessness.
▪ Patient demonstrates increased control by participating in decisions related to health care.
▪ Patient's environment is adjusted to enhance feelings of control.
▪ Patient performs self-care measures to the extent possible.
▪ Patient expresses feelings of regained control.

DOCUMENTATION

▪ Patient's expressions of anger, frustration, and sense of lack of control over environment
▪ Patient's interest in surroundings, participation in self-care, verbalization of understanding, and demonstration of skill in relation to medical diagnosis
▪ Patient's responses to opportunities to participate in own care
▪ Interventions to promote patient's control over environment
▪ Patient's response to nursing interventions
▪ Evaluations for expected outcomes

REFERENCES

Agner, J., & Braun, K. L. (2018). Patient empowerment: A critique of individualism and systematic review of patient perspectives. *Patient Education & Counseling, 101*(12), 2054–2064. doi:10.1016/j .pec.2018.07.026

Huang, Y., Yang, Y., Ni, P., Xiao, X., Ye, J., Kui, G., & Xie, T. (2018). Translation and validation of the Chinese powerlessness assessment tool. *Wound Repair & Regeneration, 26*(2), 200–205. doi:10.1111/ wrr.12626

Wermström, J., Ryrlén, E., & Axelsson, Å. B. (2017). From powerlessness to striving for control— experiences of invasive treatment while awake. *Journal of Clinical Nursing, 26*(7–8), 1066–1073. doi:10.1111/jocn.13440

Risk for Powerlessness

DEFINITION

Susceptible to a state of actual or perceived loss of control or influence over factors or events that affect one's well-being, personal life, or the society, which may compromise health (adapted from American Psychology Association)

RISK FACTORS

- Anxiety
- Caregiver role strain
- Dysfunctional institutional environment
- Impaired physical mobility
- Inadequate interest in improving one's situation
- Inadequate interpersonal relations
- Inadequate knowledge to manage a situation
- Inadequate motivation to improve one's situation
- Inadequate participation in treatment regimen
- Inadequate social support
- Ineffective coping strategies
- Low self-esteem
- Pain
- Perceived complexity of treatment regimen
- Perceived social stigma
- Social marginalization

ASSOCIATED CONDITIONS

- Cerebrovascular disorders
- Cognition disorders
- Critical illness
- Progressive illness
- Unpredictability of illness trajectory

ASSESSMENT

- Age, gender
- Nature of the medical diagnosis
- Mobility
- Behavioral responses

- Past experiences and hospitalization
- Knowledge, including understanding of present situation
- Coping skill
- Support system

EXPECTED OUTCOMES

- The patient will make decisions regarding course of action.
- The patient will decrease level of anxiety by changing response to stressors.
- The patient will participate in self-care activities.
- The patient will describe modifications or adjustments to the environment that allow feelings of control.
- The patient will discuss factors in the illness-related regimen over which control can be maintained.
- The patient will demonstrate ability to plan for controllable factors.
- The patient will express feeling of maintaining control.
- The patient will accept and adapt to lifestyle.

Suggested NOC Outcomes

Anxiety Level; Body Image; Coping; Endurance; Information Processing; Personal Autonomy; Risk Control; Social Support

INTERVENTIONS AND RATIONALES

PCC Assess for high-risk behaviors; health-promoting activities; coping skills; activities of daily living, including rest and sleep; sensory perception; decision-making skills; and sexuality patterns. *Assessment information helps identify appropriate interventions.*

PCC Modify environment when possible *to meet patient's self-care needs to promote sense of control over the environment.*

S Orient patient to space by walking with patient around space and assisting with placement of personal belongings.

EBP Teach patient about risk factors and other aspects of the patient's medical condition *to help patient feel in control of personal care.*

PCC Be present when patient is facing situations in which the patient feels powerlessness *to help patient cope.*

PCC Encourage patient to express concerns. Set aside time for discussions with patient about daily events. *This helps patient to focus on vaguely understood emotions.*

Discuss situations that provoke feelings of anxiety, anger, and powerlessness *to identify areas of patient concern and to prevent anger from being inappropriately directed at self.*

PCC Encourage participation in self-care. Provide patient with as many decisions as possible with regard to self-care (such as positioning, choosing an injection site, and receiving visitors) *to communicate respect for patient and enhance feelings of independence.*

PCC Provide positive environment for patient's activities. Encourage patient to take an active role as a member of patient's health care team. *This enhances patient's sense of control and reduces passive and dependent behavior.*

PCC Encourage family members to support patient without taking control *to increase patient's feelings of self-worth.*

PCC Arrange to accommodate patient's spiritual needs. *Spiritual assistance may help patient gain courage and resist despair.*

▥ Refer to mental health professional *for additional assistance with coping*. Refer patient to community resources *that may offer assistance to the patient when needed*.
 ▥ Offer written information that can be referred to when needed.

Suggested NIC Interventions

Decision-Making Support; Risk Control; Presence; Self-Assistance

EVALUATION OF EXPECTED OUTCOMES

▥ Patient will be able to express feelings that may lead to powerlessness.
▥ Patient will identify changes in the environment that allow feelings of control.
▥ Patient participates regularly in self-care activities.

DOCUMENTATION

▥ Patient's behavioral responses to current situation (e.g., anger, frustration, crying)
▥ Degree of independence with which patient attends to self-care activities
▥ Interventions to provide patient with control over the environment
▥ Patient's response to nursing intervention

REFERENCES

Alves Silva, R., Lima Martins, Á. K., Barreto de Castro, N., Viana, A. V., Butcher, H. K., & Martins da Silva, V. (2017). Analysis of the concept of powerlessness in individuals with stroke. *Investigacion & Educacion En Enfermeria, 35*(3), 306–319. doi:10.17533/udea.iee.v35n3a07

Cardoso Silva, Y., Silva, K. L., & Menezes Brito, M. J. (2018). Power relationships in home care: Tensions and contradictions between professionals, users and caregivers. *Journal of Nursing UFPE/Revista de Enfermagem UFPE, 12*(4), 897–907. doi:10.5205/1981-8963-v12i4a110272p896-907-2018

Goodridge, D., Isinger, T., & Rotter, T. (2018). Patient family advisors' perspectives on engagement in health-care quality improvement initiatives: Power and partnership. *Health Expectations, 21*(1), 379–386. doi:10.1111/hex.12633

Lynch, F. R. (2018). Prospects for senior power. *Generations, 42*(4), 65–72.

Adult Pressure Injury

DEFINITION

Localized damage to the skin and/or underlying tissue of an adult, as a result of pressure, or pressure in combination with shear (European Pressure Ulcer Advisory Panel, 2019)

RELATED FACTORS (R/T)

External Factors

▥ Altered microclimate between skin and supporting surface
▥ Excessive moisture
▥ Inadequate access to appropriate equipment
▥ Inadequate access to appropriate health services
▥ Inadequate availability of equipment for individuals with obesity
▥ Inadequate caregiver knowledge of pressure injury prevention strategies
▥ Increased magnitude of mechanical load
▥ Pressure over bony prominence
▥ Shearing forces

- Surface friction
- Sustained mechanical load
- Use of linen with insufficient moisture wicking property

Internal Factors

- Decreased physical activity
- Decreased physical mobility
- Dehydration
- Dry skin
- Hyperthermia
- Inadequate adherence to incontinence treatment regimen
- Inadequate adherence to pressure injury prevention plan
- Inadequate knowledge of pressure injury prevention strategies
- Protein-energy malnutrition
- Smoking
- Substance misuse

Other Factors

- Factors identified by standardized, validated screening tool

ASSOCIATED CONDITIONS

- Anemia
- Cardiovascular diseases
- Central nervous system diseases
- Chronic neurologic conditions
- Critical illness
- Decreased serum albumin level
- Decreased tissue oxygenation
- Decreased tissue perfusion
- Diabetes mellitus
- Edema
- Elevated C-reactive protein
- Hemodynamic instability
- Hip fracture
- Immobilization
- Impaired circulation
- Intellectual disability
- Medical devices
- Peripheral neuropathy
- Pharmaceutical preparations
- Physical trauma
- Prolonged duration of surgical procedure
- Sensation disorders
- Spinal cord injuries

ASSESSMENT

- Age
- Integumentary status, including color, elasticity, hygiene, lesions, moisture, sensation, temperature, texture, turgor, and quantity and distribution of hair

- Musculoskeletal status, including muscle strength and mass, joint mobility, paralysis, and range of motion
- Bowel and bladder continence
- Nutritional status, including appetite, dietary intake, hydration, current weight, and change from normal weight
- Hemoglobin and serum albumin levels and hematocrit
- Injuries
- Chronic diseases
- Circulation, especially to bony areas
- Medications
- Body type and weight
- Use of medical devices (e.g., leg braces, oxygen tubing, cervical collar)
- History of previous skin breakdown
- Risk assessment tool (Braden)

DEFINING CHARACTERISTICS

- Blood-filled blister
- Erythema
- Full-thickness tissue loss
- Full-thickness tissue loss with exposed bone
- Full-thickness tissue loss with exposed muscle
- Full-thickness tissue loss with exposed tendon
- Localized heat in relation to surrounding tissue
- Pain at pressure points
- Partial thickness loss of dermis
- Purple localized area of discolored intact skin
- Ulcer is covered by eschar
- Ulcer is covered by slough

EXPECTED OUTCOMES

- Patient will have intact skin.
- Patient's bony prominences will have limited contact with bedding and mattress.
- Patient will have adequate nutrition.
- Patient will maintain adequate circulation to skin.
- Patient will explain skin care regimen.
- Patient and family members will demonstrate skin care regimen.

Suggested NOC Outcomes

Circulation Status; Fluid Balance; Neurological Status: Peripheral; Nutritional Status; Physical Aging; Risk Control: Infectious Process; Tissue Integrity: Skin and Mucous Membranes; Tissue Perfusion: Peripheral; Wound Healing: Primary Intention; Wound Healing; Secondary Intention

INTERVENTIONS AND RATIONALES

- **S** Inspect patient's skin every shift; document skin condition and report status changes. *Early detection of changes prevents or minimizes skin breakdown.*
- **S** At regular intervals, monitor skin over bony prominences for redness and blanching. *Regular monitoring of the patient's skin helps to identify problems early.*

EBP ▦ Use pressure redirecting devices, as needed, such as a foam mattress, alternating pressure mattress, gel headrests, sheepskin, pillows, and padding. *Devices redirect pressure and assist in avoiding discomfort and skin breakdown.*

S ▦ Keep patient's skin clean and dry; lubricate, as needed. Do not use irritating soap, and rinse skin well. *These measures alleviate skin dryness, promote comfort, and reduce the risk of irritation and skin breakdown.*

S ▦ Protect bony prominences with foam padding. *Prominences have little subcutaneous fat and are prone to breakdown; using foam padding may help promote skin integrity.*

S ▦ Lift patient's body, whenever required, using a lifting sheet, if needed. Avoid shearing force. *Shearing force results when tissues slide against each other; a lifting sheet reduces sliding.*

EBP ▦ Keep linen dry, clean, and free from wrinkles or crumbs. Change wet bed linens and incontinence pads immediately. *Dry, smooth linens help prevent excoriation and skin breakdown.*

EBP ▦ Monitor nutritional intake; maintain adequate hydration. *Anemia (less than 10 mg hemoglobin) and low serum albumin concentrations (less than 2 mg) are associated with the development of pressure injury. Hydration helps maintain skin integrity.*

EBP ▦ Use a risk assessment tool such as the Braden scale to continually assess risk as patient's condition changes. *Systematic monitoring helps to identify problems early.*

S ▦ Change patient's position at least every 2 hours; follow turning schedule posted at bedside. Monitor frequency of turning. *These measures reduce pressure on tissues, promote circulation, and help prevent skin breakdown.*

EBP ▦ Indicate the risk factor potential on patient's chart and care plan, and reevaluate weekly, using an accepted form such as the Braden Scale. *The risk factor score helps evaluate treatment progress.*

EBP ▦ Explain the importance of practicing preventive skin care measures *to encourage compliance with skin care regimen.*

PCC ▦ Supervise patient and patient's family in preventive skin care measures. Give constructive feedback. *Practice helps improve skill in managing the skin care regimen.*

Suggested NIC Interventions

Bathing; Circulatory Precautions; Electrolyte Management; Positioning; Pressure Ulcer Prevention; Skin Care: Topical Treatments; Skin Surveillance; Wound Care

EVALUATIONS FOR EXPECTED OUTCOMES

▦ Patient's skin remains intact.
▦ Patient maintains adequate hydration.
▦ Patient maintains adequate circulation to skin.
▦ Patient lists preventive skin care measures.
▦ Patient and family members demonstrate skin care measures.
▦ Patient and family members understand need to avoid prolonged pressure, obtain adequate nutrition, prevent incontinence, and consistently perform skin care measures.

DOCUMENTATION

▦ Nutritional screening
▦ Pressure injury treatment plan
▦ Braden or other skin assessment index
▦ Application of barrier creams and peri care

- Use of pressure redistribution devices
- Repositioning and frequency
- Education for the patient and family regarding pressure injury prevention and treatment
- Evaluations for expected outcomes

REFERENCES

Rivera, J., Donohoe, E., Deady-Rooney, M., Douglas, M., & Samaniego, N. (2020). Implementing a pressure injury prevention bundle to decrease hospital-acquired pressure injuries in an adult critical care unit: An evidence-based, pilot initiative. *Wound Management & Prevention, 66*(10), 20. doi:10.25270/wmp.2020.10.2028

Stone, A. (2020). Preventing pressure injuries in nursing home residents using a low-profile alternating pressure overlay: A point-of-care trial. *Advances in Skin & Wound Care, 33*(10), 533. doi:10.1097/01.ASW.0000695756.80461.64

Tschannen, D., & Anderson, C. (2020). The pressure injury predictive model: A framework for hospital-acquired pressure injuries. *Journal of Clinical Nursing, 29*(7–8), 1398–1421. doi:10.1111/jocn.15171

Wang, I., Walker, R., & Gillespie, B. M. (2019). Pressure injury prevention for surgery: Results from a prospective, observational study in a tertiary hospital. Implementing pressure injury prevention in a perioperative setting. *AORN Journal, 109*(3), 392–397. doi:10.1002/aorn.12629

Risk for Adult Pressure Injury

DEFINITION

Adult susceptible to localized damage to the skin and/or underlying tissue, as a result of pressure, or pressure in combination with shear, which may compromise health (European Pressure Ulcer Advisory Panel, 2019)

RISK FACTORS

External Factors

- Altered microclimate between skin and supporting surface
- Excessive moisture
- Inadequate access to appropriate equipment
- Inadequate access to appropriate health services
- Inadequate availability of equipment for individuals with obesity
- Inadequate caregiver knowledge of pressure injury prevention strategies
- Increased magnitude of mechanical load
- Pressure over bony prominence
- Shearing forces
- Surface friction
- Sustained mechanical load
- Use of linen with insufficient moisture wicking property

Internal Factors

- Decreased physical activity
- Decreased physical mobility
- Dehydration
- Dry skin
- Hyperthermia
- Inadequate adherence to incontinence treatment regimen
- Inadequate adherence to pressure injury prevention plan

- Inadequate knowledge of pressure injury prevention strategies
- Protein-energy malnutrition
- Smoking
- Substance misuse

Other Factors

- Factors identified by standardized, validated screening tool

ASSOCIATED CONDITIONS

- Anemia
- Cardiovascular diseases
- Central nervous system diseases
- Chronic neurologic conditions
- Critical illness
- Decreased serum albumin level
- Decreased tissue oxygenation
- Decreased tissue perfusion
- Diabetes mellitus
- Edema
- Elevated C-reactive protein
- Hemodynamic instability
- Hip fracture
- Immobilization
- Impaired circulation
- Intellectual disability
- Medical devices
- Peripheral neuropathy
- Pharmaceutical preparations
- Physical trauma
- Prolonged duration of surgical procedure
- Sensation disorders
- Spinal cord injuries

ASSESSMENT

- Age
- Integumentary status, including color, elasticity, hygiene, lesions, moisture, sensation, temperature, texture, turgor, and quantity and distribution of hair
- Musculoskeletal status, including muscle strength and mass, joint mobility, paralysis, and range of motion
- Bowel and bladder continence
- Nutritional status, including appetite, dietary intake, hydration, current weight, and change from normal weight
- Hemoglobin and serum albumin levels and hematocrit
- Injuries
- Chronic diseases
- Circulation, especially to bony areas
- Medications
- Body type and weight
- Use of medical devices (e.g., leg braces, oxygen tubing, cervical collar)

- History of previous skin breakdown
- Risk assessment tool (Braden)

EXPECTED OUTCOMES

- Patient will not experience a pressure ulcer.
- Patient's bony prominences will have limited contact with bedding and mattress.
- Patient will have adequate nutrition.
- Patient will maintain adequate circulation to skin.
- Patient will explain skin care regimen.
- Patient and family members will demonstrate skin care regimen.

Suggested NOC Outcomes

> Circulation Status; Fluid Balance; Neurological Status: Peripheral; Nutritional Status; Physical Aging; Tissue Perfusion: Peripheral

INTERVENTIONS AND RATIONALES

S • Inspect patient's skin every shift; document skin condition and report status changes. *Early detection of changes prevents or minimizes skin breakdown.*

S • At regular intervals, monitor skin over bony prominences for redness and blanching. *Regular monitoring of patient's skin helps to identify problems early.*

EBP • Use pressure redirecting devices, as needed, such as a foam mattress, alternating pressure mattress, gel headrests, sheepskin, pillows, and padding. *Devices redirect pressure and assist in avoiding discomfort and skin breakdown.*

S • Keep patient's skin clean and dry; lubricate, as needed. Don't use irritating soap, and rinse skin well. *These measures alleviate skin dryness, promote comfort, and reduce the risk of irritation and skin breakdown.*

S • Protect bony prominences with foam padding. *Prominences have little subcutaneous fat and are prone to breakdown; using foam padding may help promote skin integrity.*

S • Lift patient's body, whenever required, using a lifting sheet, if needed. Avoid shearing force. *Shearing force results when tissues slide against each other; a lifting sheet reduces sliding.*

EBP • Keep linen dry, clean, and free from wrinkles or crumbs. Change wet bed linens and incontinence pads immediately. *Dry, smooth linens help prevent excoriation and skin breakdown.*

EBP • Monitor nutritional intake; maintain adequate hydration. *Anemia (<10 mg hemoglobin) and low serum albumin concentrations (<2 mg) are associated with the development of pressure ulcers. Hydration helps maintain skin integrity.*

EBP • Use a risk assessment tool such as the Braden Scale to continually assess risk as patient's condition changes. *Systematic monitoring helps to identify problems early.*

S • Change patient's position at least every 2 hours; follow turning schedule posted at bedside. Monitor frequency of turning. *These measures reduce pressure on tissues, promote circulation, and help prevent skin breakdown.*

EBP • Indicate the risk factor potential on patient's chart and care plan, and reevaluate weekly, using an accepted form such as the Braden Scale. *The risk factor score helps evaluate treatment progress.*

EBP • Explain the importance of practicing preventive skin care measures *to encourage compliance with skin care regimen.*

PCC • Supervise patient and patient's family in preventive skin care measures. Give constructive feedback. *Practice helps improve skill in managing the skin care regimen.*

Suggested NIC Interventions

Bathing; Circulatory Precautions; Electrolyte Monitoring; Positioning; Pressure Management; Skin Care: Topical Treatments

EVALUATIONS FOR EXPECTED OUTCOMES

- Patient's skin remains intact.
- Patient's weight remains within established limits.
- Patient maintains adequate hydration.
- Patient maintains adequate circulation to skin.
- Patient lists preventive skin care measures.
- Patient and family members demonstrate skin care measures.
- Patient and family members understand need to avoid prolonged pressure, obtain adequate nutrition, prevent incontinence, and consistently perform skin care measures.

DOCUMENTATION

- Nutritional screening
- Pressure ulcer prevention plan
- Braden or other skin assessment index
- Application of barrier creams and peri care
- Use of pressure redistribution devices
- Repositioning and frequency
- Education for the patient and family regarding pressure ulcer prevention and treatment

REFERENCES

Ahtiala, M., Soppi, E., & Tallgren, M. (2018). Specific risk factors for pressure ulcer development in adult critical care patients—A retrospective cohort study. *EWMA Journal, 19*(1), 35–42.

Aloweni, F., Ang, S. Y., Fook, C. S., Agus, N., Yong, P., Goh, M. M., ... Soh, R. C. (2019). A prediction tool for hospital-acquired pressure ulcers among surgical patients: Surgical pressure ulcer risk score. *International Wound Journal, 16*(1), 164–175. doi:10.1111/iwj.13007

Deng, X., Yu, T., & Hu, A. (2017). Predicting the risk for hospital-acquired pressure ulcers in critical care patients. *Critical Care Nurse, 37*(4), e1–e11. doi:10.4037/ccn2017548

National Pressure Ulcer Advisory Panel. (2007). Updated pressure ulcer stages. Retrieved from http://www.npuap.org/resources/educational-and-clinical-resources/pressure-ulcer-categorystaging-illustrations.

Patton, D., Moore, Z., O'Connor, T., Shanley, E., De Oliveira, A. L., Vitoriano, A., ... Nugent, L. E. (2018). Using technology to advance pressure ulcer risk assessment and self-care: Challenges and potential benefits. *EWMA Journal, 19*(2), 23–27.

Child Pressure Injury

DEFINITION

Localized damage to the skin and/or underlying tissue of a child or adolescent, as a result of pressure, or pressure in combination with shear (European Pressure Ulcer Advisory Panel, 2019)

RELATED FACTORS (R/T)

External Factors

- Altered microclimate between skin and supporting surface
- Difficulty for caregiver to lift patient completely off bed

- Excessive moisture
- Inadequate access to appropriate equipment
- Inadequate access to appropriate health services
- Inadequate access to appropriate supplies
- Inadequate access to equipment for children with obesity
- Inadequate caregiver knowledge of appropriate methods for removing adhesive materials
- Inadequate caregiver knowledge of appropriate methods for stabilizing devices
- Inadequate caregiver knowledge of modifiable factors
- Inadequate caregiver knowledge of pressure injury prevention strategies
- Increased magnitude of mechanical load
- Pressure over bony prominence
- Shearing forces
- Surface friction
- Sustained mechanical load
- Use of linen with insufficient moisture wicking property

Internal Factors

- Decreased physical activity
- Decreased physical mobility
- Dehydration
- Difficulty assisting caregiver with moving self
- Difficulty maintaining position in bed
- Difficulty maintaining position in chair
- Dry skin
- Hyperthermia
- Inadequate adherence to incontinence treatment regimen
- Inadequate adherence to pressure injury prevention plan
- Inadequate knowledge of appropriate methods for removing adhesive materials
- Inadequate knowledge of appropriate methods for stabilizing devices
- Protein-energy malnutrition
- Water–electrolyte imbalance

Other Factors

- Factors identified by standardized, validated screening tool

ASSOCIATED CONDITIONS

- Alkaline skin pH
- Altered cutaneous structure
- Anemia
- Cardiovascular diseases
- Decreased level of consciousness
- Decreased serum albumin level
- Decreased tissue oxygenation
- Decreased tissue perfusion
- Diabetes mellitus
- Edema
- Elevated C-reactive protein
- Frequent invasive procedures
- Hemodynamic instability

- Immobilization
- Impaired circulation
- Intellectual disability
- Medical devices
- Pharmaceutical preparations
- Physical trauma
- Prolonged duration of surgical procedure
- Sensation disorders
- Spinal cord injuries

ASSESSMENT

- Age
- Integumentary status, including color, elasticity, hygiene, lesions, moisture, sensation, temperature, texture, turgor, and quantity and distribution of hair
- Musculoskeletal status, including muscle strength and mass, joint mobility, paralysis, and range of motion
- Bowel and bladder continence
- Nutritional status, including appetite, dietary intake, hydration, current weight, and change from normal weight
- Hemoglobin and serum albumin levels and hematocrit
- Injuries
- Chronic diseases
- Circulation, especially to bony areas
- Medications
- Body type and weight
- Use of medical devices (e.g., leg braces, oxygen tubing, cervical collar)
- History of previous skin breakdown
- Risk assessment tool (Braden)

DEFINING CHARACTERISTICS

- Blood-filled blister
- Erythema
- Full-thickness tissue loss
- Full-thickness tissue loss with exposed bone
- Full-thickness tissue loss with exposed muscle
- Full-thickness tissue loss with exposed tendon
- Localized heat in relation to surrounding tissue
- Pain at pressure points
- Partial thickness loss of dermis
- Purple localized area of discolored intact skin
- Ulcer is covered by eschar
- Ulcer is covered by slough

EXPECTED OUTCOMES

- Child will have intact skin.
- Child's bony prominences will have limited contact with bedding and mattress.
- Child will have adequate nutrition.
- Child will maintain adequate circulation to skin.
- Family members will demonstrate skin care regimen.

Suggested NOC Outcomes

Circulation Status; Fluid Balance; Neurological Status: Peripheral; Nutritional Status; Physical Aging; Risk Control: Infectious Process; Tissue Integrity: Skin and Mucous Membranes; Tissue Perfusion: Peripheral; Wound Healing: Primary Intention; Wound Healing; Secondary Intention

INTERVENTIONS AND RATIONALES

S ▪ Inspect child's skin every shift; document skin condition and report status changes. *Early detection of changes prevents or minimizes skin breakdown.*

S ▪ At regular intervals, monitor skin over bony prominences for redness and blanching. *Regular monitoring of the child's skin helps to identify problems early.*

EBP ▪ Use pressure redirecting devices, as needed, such as a foam mattress, alternating pressure mattress, gel headrests, sheepskin, pillows, and padding. *Devices redirect pressure and assist in avoiding discomfort and skin breakdown.*

S ▪ Keep child's skin clean and dry; lubricate, as needed. Do not use irritating soap, and rinse skin well. *These measures alleviate skin dryness, promote comfort, and reduce the risk of irritation and skin breakdown.*

S ▪ Protect bony prominences with foam padding. *Prominences have little subcutaneous fat and are prone to breakdown; using foam padding may help promote skin integrity.*

S ▪ Lift child's body, whenever required, using a lifting sheet, if needed. Avoid shearing force. *Shearing force results when tissues slide against each other; a lifting sheet reduces sliding.*

EBP ▪ Keep linen dry, clean, and free from wrinkles or crumbs. Change wet bed linens and incontinence pads immediately. *Dry, smooth linens help prevent excoriation and skin breakdown.*

EBP ▪ Monitor nutritional intake; maintain adequate hydration. *Anemia (less than 10 mg hemoglobin) and low serum albumin concentrations (less than 2 mg) are associated with the development of pressure injury. Hydration helps maintain skin integrity.*

EBP ▪ Use a risk assessment tool such as the Braden scale to continually assess risk as child's condition changes. *Systematic monitoring helps to identify problems early.*

S ▪ Change child's position at least every 2 hours; follow turning schedule posted at bedside. Monitor frequency of turning. *These measures reduce pressure on tissues, promote circulation, and help prevent skin breakdown.*

EBP ▪ Indicate the risk factor potential on child's chart and care plan, and reevaluate weekly, using an accepted form such as the Braden Scale. *The risk factor score helps evaluate treatment progress.*

S ▪ Avoid tight fitting clothes. *Tight clothes may rub on child's skin creating a friction injury.*

S ▪ Remove braids, beads, head bands, barrettes or extensions *to prevent pressure sores when child is in bed.*

EBP ▪ Encourage weight shifting at least every 15 to 30 minutes when your child is sitting in a chair *to avoid extended time on pressure areas.*

EBP ▪ Do not use donut type devices. *May increase pressure in some areas.*

▪ Limit time on toilet seat to less than 15 minutes. *Extended time on seat causes pressure on thighs.*

S ▪ Instruct parents to call provider when skin redness or color change lasts more than 30 minutes after changing positions or there are new signs of skin irritation. *To identify possible problem areas.*

EBP ▪ Explain the importance of practicing preventive skin care measures *to encourage compliance with skin care regimen.*

PCC ▪ Supervise child and child's family in preventive skin care measures. Give constructive feedback. *Practice helps improve skill in managing the skin care regimen.*

Suggested NIC Interventions

Bathing; Circulatory Precautions; Electrolyte Management; Positioning; Pressure Ulcer Prevention; Skin Care: Topical Treatments; Skin Surveillance; Wound Care

EVALUATIONS FOR EXPECTED OUTCOMES

- Child's skin remains intact.
- Child maintains adequate hydration.
- Child maintains adequate circulation to skin.
- Patients/family members list preventive skin care measures.
- Family members demonstrate skin care measures.
- Family members understand need to avoid prolonged pressure, obtain adequate nutrition, prevent incontinence, and consistently perform skin care measures.

DOCUMENTATION

- Nutritional screening
- Pressure injury treatment plan
- Braden or other skin assessment index
- Application of barrier creams and peri care
- Use of pressure redistribution devices
- Repositioning and frequency
- Education regarding pressure injury prevention and treatment
- Evaluations for expected outcomes

REFERENCES

Delmore, B., Deppisch, M., Sylvia, C., Luna-Anderson, C., & Nie, A. M. (2019). Pressure injuries in the pediatric population: A national pressure ulcer advisory panel white paper. *Advances in Skin & Wound Care, 32*(9), 394. doi:10.1097/01.ASW.0000577124.58253.66

Jackson, J. E., Kirkland-Kyhn, H., Kenny, L., Beres, A. L., & Mateev, S. (2021). Reducing hospital-acquired pressure injuries among pediatric patients receiving ECMO: A retrospective study examining quality improvement outcomes. *Wound Management & Prevention, 67*(9), 14. doi:10.25270/wmp.2021.9.1424

Sullivan, C. B., Puricelli, M. D., & Smith, R. J. (2021). What is the best approach to prevent advanced-stage pressure injuries after pediatric tracheotomy? *The Laryngoscope, 131*(6), 1196–1197. doi:10.1002/lary.28878

Xiao, C., Pan, L., Lin, Y., Ye, L., Liang, H., Tao, J., & Luo, Y. (2021). A model for predicting 7-day pressure injury outcomes in paediatric patients: A machine learning approach. *Journal of Advanced Nursing, 77*(3), 1304–1314. doi:10.1111/jan.14680

Risk for Child Pressure Injury

DEFINITION

Child or adolescent susceptible to localized damage to the skin and/or underlying tissue, as a result of pressure, or pressure in combination with shear, which may compromise health (European Pressure Ulcer Advisory Panel, 2019)

RISK FACTORS

External Factors

- Altered microclimate between skin and supporting surface
- Difficulty for caregiver to lift patient completely off bed

- Excessive moisture
- Inadequate access to appropriate equipment
- Inadequate access to appropriate health services
- Inadequate access to appropriate supplies
- Inadequate access to equipment for children with obesity
- Inadequate caregiver knowledge of appropriate methods for removing adhesive materials
- Inadequate caregiver knowledge of appropriate methods for stabilizing devices
- Inadequate caregiver knowledge of modifiable factors
- Inadequate caregiver knowledge of pressure injury prevention strategies
- Increased magnitude of mechanical load
- Pressure over bony prominence
- Shearing forces
- Surface friction
- Sustained mechanical load
- Use of linen with insufficient moisture wicking property

Internal Factors

- Decreased physical activity
- Decreased physical mobility
- Dehydration
- Difficulty assisting caregiver with moving self
- Difficulty maintaining position in bed
- Difficulty maintaining position in chair
- Dry skin
- Hyperthermia
- Inadequate adherence to incontinence treatment regimen
- Inadequate adherence to pressure injury prevention plan
- Inadequate knowledge of appropriate methods for removing adhesive materials
- Inadequate knowledge of appropriate methods for stabilizing devices
- Protein-energy malnutrition
- Water–electrolyte imbalance

Other Factors

- Factors identified by standardized, validated screening tool

ASSOCIATED CONDITIONS

- Alkaline skin pH
- Altered cutaneous structure
- Anemia
- Cardiovascular diseases
- Decreased level of consciousness
- Decreased serum albumin level
- Decreased tissue oxygenation
- Decreased tissue perfusion
- Diabetes mellitus
- Edema
- Elevated C-reactive protein
- Frequent invasive procedures

- Hemodynamic instability
- Immobilization
- Impaired circulation
- Intellectual disability
- Medical devices
- Pharmaceutical preparations
- Physical trauma
- Prolonged duration of surgical procedure
- Sensation disorders
- Spinal cord injuries

ASSESSMENT

- Age
- Integumentary status, including color, elasticity, hygiene, lesions, moisture, sensation, temperature, texture, turgor, and quantity and distribution of hair
- Musculoskeletal status, including muscle strength and mass, joint mobility, paralysis, and range of motion
- Bowel and bladder continence
- Nutritional status, including appetite, dietary intake, hydration, current weight, and change from normal weight
- Hemoglobin and serum albumin levels and hematocrit
- Injuries
- Chronic diseases
- Circulation, especially to bony areas
- Medications
- Body type and weight
- Use of medical devices (e.g., leg braces, oxygen tubing, cervical collar)
- History of previous skin breakdown
- Risk assessment tool (Braden)

EXPECTED OUTCOMES

- Child will have intact skin.
- Child's bony prominences will have limited contact with bedding and mattress.
- Child will have adequate nutrition.
- Child will maintain adequate circulation to skin.
- Family members will verbalize pressure injury risk factors.
- Family members will demonstrate skin care regimen.

Suggested NOC Outcomes

Circulation Status; Fluid Balance; Immobility Consequences: Physiological; Neurological Status: Peripheral; Nutritional Status; Physical Aging; Risk Control: Pressure Injury; Tissue Integrity: Skin and Mucous Membranes; Tissue Perfusion: Peripheral

INTERVENTIONS AND RATIONALES

- **S** Inspect child's skin every shift; document skin condition and report status changes. *Early detection of changes prevents or minimizes skin breakdown.*
- **S** At regular intervals, monitor skin over bony prominences for redness and blanching. *Regular monitoring of the child's skin helps to identify problems early.*

EBP ▪ Use pressure redirecting devices, as needed, such as a foam mattress, alternating pressure mattress, gel headrests, sheepskin, pillows, and padding. *Devices redirect pressure and assist in avoiding discomfort and skin breakdown.*

S ▪ Keep child's skin clean and dry; lubricate, as needed. Don't use irritating soap, and rinse skin well. *These measures alleviate skin dryness, promote comfort, and reduce the risk of irritation and skin breakdown.*

S ▪ Protect bony prominences with foam padding. *Prominences have little subcutaneous fat and are prone to breakdown; using foam padding may help promote skin integrity.*

S ▪ Lift child's body, whenever required, using a lifting sheet, if needed. Avoid shearing force. *Shearing force results when tissues slide against each other; a lifting sheet reduces sliding.*

EBP ▪ Keep linen dry, clean, and free from wrinkles or crumbs. Change wet bed linens and incontinence pads immediately. *Dry, smooth linens help prevent excoriation and skin breakdown.*

EBP ▪ Monitor nutritional intake; maintain adequate hydration. *Anemia (less than 10 mg hemoglobin) and low serum albumin concentrations (less than 2 mg) are associated with the development of pressure injury. Hydration helps maintain skin integrity.*

EBP ▪ Use a risk assessment tool such as the Braden scale to continually assess risk as child's condition changes. *Systematic monitoring helps to identify problems early.*

S ▪ Change child's position at least every 2 hours; follow turning schedule posted at bedside. Monitor frequency of turning. *These measures reduce pressure on tissues, promote circulation, and help prevent skin breakdown.*

EBP ▪ Indicate the risk factor potential on child's chart and care plan, and reevaluate weekly, using an accepted form such as the Braden Scale. *The risk factor score helps evaluate treatment progress.*

S ▪ Avoid tight fitting clothes. *Tight clothes may rub on child's skin creating a friction injury.*

S ▪ Remove braids, beads, head bands, barrettes or extensions *to prevent pressure sores when child is in bed.*

EBP ▪ Encourage weight shifting at least every 15 to 30 minutes when your child is sitting in a chair *to avoid extended time on pressure areas.*

EBP ▪ Do not use donut type devices. *May increase pressure in some areas.*

▪ Limit time on toilet seat to less than 15 minutes. *Extended time on seat causes pressure on thighs.*

S ▪ Instruct parents to call provider when skin redness or color change lasts more than 30 minutes after changing positions or there are new signs of skin irritation. *To identify possible problem areas.*

EBP ▪ Explain the importance of practicing preventive skin care measures *to encourage compliance with skin care regimen.*

PCC ▪ Supervise child and child's family in preventive skin care measures. Give constructive feedback. *Practice helps improve skill in managing the skin care regimen.*

Suggested NIC Interventions

Bathing; Circulatory Precautions; Electrolyte Monitoring; Positioning; Pressure Management; Pressure Ulcer Care; Pressure Ulcer Prevention; Risk Identification; Skin Care: Topical Treatments; Skin Surveillance

EVALUATIONS FOR EXPECTED OUTCOMES

▪ Child's skin remains intact.

▪ Child maintains adequate hydration.

- Child maintains adequate circulation to skin.
- Patients/family members list preventive skin care measures.
- Family members demonstrate skin care measures.
- Family members understand need to avoid prolonged pressure, obtain adequate nutrition, prevent incontinence, and consistently perform skin care measures.

DOCUMENTATION

- Nutritional screening
- Pressure injury treatment plan
- Braden or other skin assessment index
- Application of barrier creams and peri care
- Use of pressure redistribution devices
- Repositioning and frequency
- Education regarding pressure injury prevention and treatment
- Evaluations for expected outcomes

REFERENCES

Delmore, B., Deppisch, M., Sylvia, C., Luna-Anderson, C., & Nie, A. M. (2019). Pressure injuries in the pediatric population: A national pressure ulcer advisory panel white paper. *Advances in Skin & Wound Care, 32*(9), 394. doi:10.1097/01.ASW.0000577124.58253.66

Jackson, J. E., Kirkland-Kyhn, H., Kenny, L., Beres, A. L., & Mateev, S. (2021). Reducing hospital-acquired pressure injuries among pediatric patients receiving ECMO: A retrospective study examining quality improvement outcomes. *Wound Management & Prevention, 67*(9), 14. doi:10.25270/wmp.2021.9.1424

Sullivan, C. B., Puricelli, M. D., & Smith, R. J. (2021). What is the best approach to prevent advanced-stage pressure injuries after pediatric tracheotomy? *The Laryngoscope, 131*(6), 1196–1197. doi:10.1002/lary.28878

Xiao, C., Pan, L., Lin, Y., Ye, L., Liang, H., Tao, J., & Luo, Y. (2021). A model for predicting 7-day pressure injury outcomes in paediatric patients: A machine learning approach. *Journal of Advanced Nursing, 77*(3), 1304–1314. doi:10.1111/jan.14680

Neonatal Pressure Injury

DEFINITION

Localized damage to the skin and/or underlying tissue of a neonate, as a result of pressure, or pressure in combination with shear (European Pressure Ulcer Advisory Panel, 2019)

RELATED FACTORS (R/T)

External Factors

- Altered microclimate between skin and supporting surface
- Excessive moisture
- Inadequate access to appropriate equipment
- Inadequate access to appropriate health services
- Inadequate access to appropriate supplies
- Inadequate caregiver knowledge of appropriate methods for removing adhesive materials
- Inadequate caregiver knowledge of appropriate methods for stabilizing devices
- Inadequate caregiver knowledge of modifiable factors
- Inadequate caregiver knowledge of pressure injury prevention strategies
- Increased magnitude of mechanical load
- Pressure over bony prominence
- Shearing forces

- Surface friction
- Sustained mechanical load
- Use of linen with insufficient moisture wicking property

Internal Factors

- Decreased physical mobility
- Dehydration
- Dry skin
- Hyperthermia
- Water–electrolyte imbalance

Other Factors

- Factors identified by standardized, validated screening tool

ASSOCIATED CONDITIONS

- Anemia
- Decreased serum albumin level
- Decreased tissue oxygenation
- Decreased tissue perfusion
- Edema
- Immature skin integrity
- Immature skin texture
- Immature stratum corneum
- Immobilization
- Medical devices
- Nutritional deficiencies related to prematurity
- Pharmaceutical preparations
- Prolonged duration of surgical procedure
- Significant comorbidity

ASSESSMENT

- Age
- Integumentary status, including color, elasticity, hygiene, lesions, moisture, sensation, temperature, texture, turgor, and quantity and distribution of hair
- Musculoskeletal status, including muscle strength and mass, joint mobility, paralysis, and range of motion
- Nutritional status, including appetite, dietary intake, hydration, current weight, and change from normal weight
- Hemoglobin and serum albumin levels and hematocrit
- Injuries
- Circulation, especially to bony areas
- Medications
- Use of medical devices (e.g., oxygen tubing)
- Risk assessment tool (The Neonatal Skin Condition Score [NSCS])

DEFINING CHARACTERISTICS

- Blood-filled blister
- Erythema

- Full-thickness tissue loss
- Full-thickness tissue loss with exposed bone
- Full-thickness tissue loss with exposed muscle
- Full-thickness tissue loss with exposed tendon
- Localized heat in relation to surrounding tissue
- Maroon localized area of discolored intact skin
- Partial thickness loss of dermis
- Purple localized area of discolored intact skin
- Skin ulceration
- Ulcer is covered by eschar
- Ulcer is covered by slough

EXPECTED OUTCOMES

- Neonate will have intact skin.
- Neonate's bony prominences will have limited contact with bedding and mattress.
- Neonate will have adequate nutrition.
- Neonate will maintain adequate circulation to skin.
- Family members will demonstrate skin care regimen.

Suggested NOC Outcomes

Circulation Status; Fluid Balance; Neurological Status: Peripheral; Nutritional Status; Physical Aging; Risk Control: Infectious Process; Tissue Integrity: Skin and Mucous Membranes; Tissue Perfusion: Peripheral; Wound Healing: Primary Intention; Wound Healing; Secondary Intention

INTERVENTIONS AND RATIONALES

EBP ▪ Determine the cause of the skin breakdown and remove, if able, the cause. *Eliminating the pressure source is the first step in treatment.*

EBP ▪ Cleanse area the skin breakdown with sterile water or normal saline every 4 to 6 hours and allow to air dry. *Keeping the affected area clean prevents risk of infection. Air drying prevents further breakdown.*

EBP ▪ Apply topical agents as prescribed by the provider. *Most topical agents are prescribed in consideration of gestational age, skin condition, and toxic potential.*

EBP ▪ Apply dressings as prescribed by wound care/wound ostomy provider. *Dressings should only be applied when prescribed, adhesives and some types of materials can cause further breakdown.*

EBP ▪ Assess nutritional status and ensure adequate nutrient intake of additional calories, protein, vitamin C, vitamin A, zinc, magnesium, copper, and iron. *Skin healing requires additional nutrients.*

T&C ▪ Request consult with dietitian *to provide assessment and nutrition care needs.*

PCC EBP ▪ Educate family on the causes and risk factors for pressure ulcer development and prevention. *Family can assist in monitoring for injuries and planning care.*

Suggested NIC Interventions

Bathing; Circulatory Precautions; Electrolyte Management; Positioning; Pressure Ulcer Prevention; Skin Care: Topical Treatments; Skin Surveillance; Wound Care

EVALUATIONS FOR EXPECTED OUTCOMES

- Neonate's skin remains intact.
- Neonate maintains adequate hydration.
- Neonate maintains adequate circulation to skin.
- Patients/family members list preventive skin care measures.
- Family members demonstrate skin care measures.
- Family members understand the need to avoid prolonged pressure, obtain adequate nutrition, prevent incontinence, and consistently perform skin care measures.

DOCUMENTATION

- Nutritional screening
- Pressure injury treatment plan
- Braden or other skin assessment index
- Application of barrier creams and peri care
- Use of pressure redistribution devices
- Repositioning and frequency
- Education regarding pressure injury prevention and treatment
- Evaluations for expected outcomes

REFERENCES

Lawrence, C., Mohr, L. D., Geistkemper, A., Murphy, S., & Fleming, K. (2021). Sustained reduction of nasal pressure injuries in the neonatal intensive care unit with the use of bubble continuous positive airway pressure: A quality improvement project. *Journal of Wound, Ostomy & Continence Nursing, 48*(2), 101–107.

Marufu, T. C., Setchell, B., Cutler, E., Dring, E., Wesley, T., Banks, A., … Manning, J. C. (2021). Pressure injury and risk in the inpatient paediatric and neonatal populations: A single centre point-prevalence study. *Journal of Tissue Viability, 30*(2), 231–236.

Nie, A. M. (2020). Creating a pediatric and neonatal pressure injury prevention program when evidence was sparse or absent: A view from here. *Journal of Wound, Ostomy & Continence Nursing, 47*(4), 353–355.

Razmus, I. S., & Keep, S. M. (2021). Neonatal intensive care nursing pressure injury prevention practices: A descriptive survey. *Journal of Wound, Ostomy & Continence Nursing, 48*(5), 394–402.

Risk for Neonatal Pressure Injury

DEFINITION

Neonate susceptible to localized damage to the skin and/or underlying tissue, as a result of pressure, or pressure in combination with shear, which may compromise health (European Pressure Ulcer Advisory Panel, 2019)

RISK FACTORS

External Factors

- Altered microclimate between skin and supporting surface
- Excessive moisture
- Inadequate access to appropriate equipment
- Inadequate access to appropriate health services
- Inadequate access to appropriate supplies
- Inadequate caregiver knowledge of appropriate methods for removing adhesive materials
- Inadequate caregiver knowledge of appropriate methods for stabilizing devices
- Inadequate caregiver knowledge of modifiable factors

- Inadequate caregiver knowledge of pressure injury prevention strategies
- Increased magnitude of mechanical load
- Pressure over bony prominence
- Shearing forces
- Surface friction
- Sustained mechanical load
- Use of linen with insufficient moisture wicking property

Internal Factors

- Decreased physical mobility
- Dehydration
- Dry skin
- Hyperthermia
- Water–electrolyte imbalance

Other Factors

- Factors identified by standardized, validated screening tool

ASSOCIATED CONDITIONS

- Anemia
- Decreased serum albumin level
- Decreased tissue oxygenation
- Decreased tissue perfusion
- Edema
- Immature skin integrity
- Immature skin texture
- Immature stratum corneum
- Immobilization
- Medical devices
- Nutritional deficiencies related to prematurity
- Pharmaceutical preparations
- Prolonged duration of surgical procedure
- Significant comorbidity

ASSESSMENT

- Age
- Integumentary status, including color, elasticity, hygiene, lesions, moisture, sensation, temperature, texture, turgor, and quantity and distribution of hair
- Musculoskeletal status, including muscle strength and mass, joint mobility, paralysis, and range of motion
- Nutritional status, including appetite, dietary intake, hydration, current weight, and change from normal weight
- Hemoglobin and serum albumin levels and hematocrit
- Injuries
- Circulation, especially to bony areas
- Medications
- Use of medical devices (e.g., oxygen tubing)
- Risk assessment tool (The Neonatal Skin Condition Score [NSCS])

- Neonate will have intact skin.
- Neonate's bony prominences will have limited contact with bedding and mattress.
- Neonate will have adequate nutrition.
- Neonate will maintain adequate circulation to skin.
- Family members will demonstrate skin care regimen.

Suggested NOC Outcomes

Circulation Status; Fluid Balance; Immobility Consequences: Physiological; Neurological Status: Peripheral; Nutritional Status; Physical Aging; Risk Control: Pressure Injury; Tissue Integrity: Skin and Mucous Membranes; Tissue Perfusion: Peripheral

- **EBP** Keep bedding and clothing dry and wrinkle free. *Moisture and wrinkle increase the risk of skin breakdown.*
- **PCC** Change diaper immediately upon soiling, use barrier cream *to protect skin from injury and treat any excoriation.*
- **PCC** Assess skin in diaper area for rash. *Identify and treat yeast infections as needed.*
- **EBP** Place critically ill or infant younger than 32 weeks on synthetic sheepskin that is covered with a blanket. *Redistributes pressure and reduces sheering forces.*
- **EBP** Place gel pillows under back infants head as needed. *Reduces pressure on back of head.*
- **EBP** Reposition infant every two to four hours and as needed to redistribute pressure.
- **EBP** Lift infant carefully and avoid sliding infant across bedding *to prevent friction or sheer injury.*
- **EBP** Assess and examine skin under medical devices at least every 12 hours *to observe for blanching or redness.*
- **EBP** Change pulse oximeter sites a minimum of every 12 hours or more frequently as needed and rotate transcutaneous monitor sites regularly *to prevent restriction of circulation.*
- **EBP** Monitor fit and/or use of protective barrier of nasal cannula/nasal device pressure *can be damaging to the nares and erode the nasal septum.*
- **S** Prevent infant from lying on lines or on other hard objects while in bed *to prevent uneven surfaces.*
- **EBP** Assess nutritional status and ensure adequate nutrient intake of additional calories, protein, vitamin C, vitamin A, zinc, magnesium, copper, and iron. *Skin healing requires additional nutrients.*
- **T&C** Request consultation with dietitian *to provide assessment and nutrition care needs.*
- **PCC EBP** Educate family on the causes and risk factors for pressure ulcer development and prevention. *Family can assist in monitoring for injuries and planning care.*

Suggested NIC Interventions

Bathing; Circulatory Precautions; Electrolyte Monitoring; Positioning; Pressure Management; Pressure Ulcer Care; Pressure Ulcer Prevention; Risk Identification; Skin Care: Topical Treatments; Skin Surveillance

- Neonate's skin remains intact.
- Neonate maintains adequate hydration.
- Neonate maintains adequate circulation to skin.

- Patients/family members list preventive skin care measures.
- Family members demonstrate skin care measures.
- Family members understand need to avoid prolonged pressure, obtain adequate nutrition, prevent incontinence, and consistently perform skin care measures.

DOCUMENTATION

- Nutritional screening
- Pressure injury treatment plan
- Braden or other skin assessment index
- Application of barrier creams and peri care
- Use of pressure redistribution devices
- Repositioning and frequency
- Education regarding pressure injury prevention and treatment
- Evaluations for expected outcomes

REFERENCES

Lawrence, C., Mohr, L. D., Geistkemper, A., Murphy, S., & Fleming, K. (2021). Sustained reduction of nasal pressure injuries in the neonatal intensive care unit with the use of bubble continuous positive airway pressure: A quality improvement project. *Journal of Wound, Ostomy & Continence Nursing, 48*(2), 101–107.

Marufu, T. C., Setchell, B., Cutler, E., Dring, E., Wesley, T., Banks, A., ... & Manning, J. C. (2021). Pressure injury and risk in the inpatient paediatric and neonatal populations: A single centre point-prevalence study. *Journal of Tissue Viability, 30*(2), 231–236.

Nie, A. M. (2020). Creating a pediatric and neonatal pressure injury prevention program when evidence was sparse or absent: A view from here. *Journal of Wound, Ostomy & Continence Nursing, 47*(4), 353–355.

Razmus, I. S., & Keep, S. M. (2021). Neonatal intensive care nursing pressure injury prevention practices: A descriptive survey. *Journal of Wound, Ostomy & Continence Nursing, 48*(5), 394–402.

Ineffective Protection

DEFINITION

Decrease in the ability to guard self from internal or external threats such as illness or injury

RELATED FACTORS (R/T)

- Depressive symptoms
- Difficulty managing complex treatment regimen
- Hopelessness
- Inadequate vaccination
- Ineffective health self-management
- Low self-efficacy
- Malnutrition
- Physical deconditioning
- Substance misuse

ASSOCIATED CONDITIONS

- Blood coagulation disorders
- Immune system diseases
- Neoplasms

- Pharmaceutical preparations
- Treatment regimen

ASSESSMENT

- Vital signs
- Health maintenance, including high-risk behaviors and health-promoting activities
- Patient's knowledge of present condition, including diagnosis, treatment, prevention of complications, and management of adverse effects
- Coping skills, including physical, psychosocial, and spiritual strengths
- Mobility status
- Comfort level, including symptom management
- Activities of daily living, including rest, sleep, and exercise
- Cardiovascular status, including heart rate, rhythm, heart sounds, blood pressure, peripheral pulses, and electrocardiogram results
- Neurologic status, including sensory perception, decision-making abilities, and thought processes
- Respiratory status, including gas exchange and breathing patterns
- Nutritional status, including food preferences, modifications in diet, and weight changes
- Bowel and bladder elimination patterns
- Protective mechanisms, including immune, hematopoietic, integumentary, and sensorimotor systems
- Laboratory studies, including white blood cell count and differential, erythrocyte sedimentation rate, immunoelectrophoresis, enzyme-linked immunosorbent assay, and cultures of blood, body fluid, sputum, urine, and wound exudate
- Sexuality patterns

DEFINING CHARACTERISTICS

- Altered sweating
- Anorexia
- Chilling
- Coughing
- Disorientation
- Dyspnea
- Expresses itching
- Fatigue
- Impaired physical mobility
- Impaired tissue healing
- Insomnia
- Leukopenia
- Low serum hemoglobin level
- Maladaptive stress response
- Neurosensory impairment
- Pressure injury
- Psychomotor agitation
- Thrombocytopenia
- Weakness

EXPECTED OUTCOMES

- Patient won't experience chills, fever, or other signs and symptoms of illness.
- Patient will demonstrate use of protective measures, including conservation of energy, maintenance of balanced diet, and attainment of adequate rest.

- Patient will demonstrate effective coping skills.
- Patient will demonstrate personal cleanliness and will maintain clean environment.
- Patient will maintain safe environment.
- Patient will demonstrate increased strength and resistance.
- Patient's immune system response will improve.

Suggested NOC Outcomes

Abuse Protection; Immune Status; Immunization Behavior; Knowledge: Infection Control; Knowledge: Personal Safety

INTERVENTIONS AND RATIONALES

- **PCC** Spend as much time as possible with patient *to provide comfort and support.*
- **PCC** Promote personal and environmental cleanliness *to decrease threat from microorganisms.*
- **S** Monitor vital signs. *This allows for early detection of complications.*
- **S** Institute safety precautions *to reduce risk of falls, cuts, or other injuries and subsequent infection, bleeding, and impaired healing.*
- **EBP** Teach protective measures, including the need to conserve energy, obtain adequate rest, and eat a balanced diet. Adequate sleep and nutrition enhance immune function. *Energy conservation can help decrease the weakness caused by anemia.*
- **PCC** Provide relief for symptoms (fever, chills, myalgia, weakness). *Discomfort interferes with rest, disturbs nutritional intake, and places added stress on patient.*
- **EBP** Teach patient coping strategies, including stress management and relaxation techniques. *Relaxation and decreased stress can increase immune function, thereby improving strength and resistance.*

Suggested NIC Interventions

Coping Enhancement; Environmental Management: Safety; Infection Control; Infection Protection; Nutritional Counseling; Positioning; Risk Identification

EVALUATIONS FOR EXPECTED OUTCOMES

- Patient doesn't develop petechiae, epistaxis, melena, hematuria, fever, cough, redness, drainage, pallor, headache, weakness, or dizziness. Vital signs remain within normal limits.
- Patient demonstrates a normal pattern of rest, activity, and sleep.
- Patient consumes an adequate diet.
- Patient reports being able to cope effectively.
- Patient demonstrates personal cleanliness and maintains clean environment.
- Patient uses safety precautions to avoid falls and other injuries.
- Patient demonstrates increased strength and resistance.
- Patient's immune system response improves.

DOCUMENTATION

- Patient's understanding of abnormal blood profiles
- Patient's description of measures to prevent or manage complications
- Observations of patient's behavior, including health-promoting and high-risk activities

- Signs and symptoms of decreased immune resistance in body systems assessed (cardiopulmonary, neurologic, gastrointestinal, genitourinary, and integumentary)
- Observations of infection or bleeding
- Interventions to assist with coping strategies and health maintenance and promotion
- Patient's response to interventions
- Evaluations for expected outcomes

REFERENCES

Anakaraonye, A. R., Mann, E. S., Annang Ingram, L., & Henderson, A. K. (2019). Black US college women's strategies of sexual self-protection. *Culture, Health & Sexuality, 21*(2), 160–174. doi:10.1080/13691058.2018.1459844

Juanjuan, L., Yanjin, H., & Ling, Z. (2017). Application of protection motivation intervention in risk factors self-management of elderly with cardiovascular disease. *Chinese Nursing Research, 31*(34), 4388–4391. doi:10.3969/j.issn.1009-6493.2017.34.020

Konkle-Parker, D., Fouquier, K., Portz, K., Wheeless, L., Arnold, T., Harris, C., & Turan, J. (2018). Women's decision-making about self-protection during sexual activity in the deep south of the USA: A grounded theory study. *Culture, Health & Sexuality, 20*(1), 84–98. doi:10.1080/13691058.2017.1331468

Tangcharoensathien, V., Chandrasiri, O., Waleewong, O., & Rajatanavin, N. (2019). Overcoming internal challenges and external threats to noncommunicable disease control. *Bulletin of the World Health Organization, 97*(2), 74–74A. doi:10.2471/BLT.18.228809

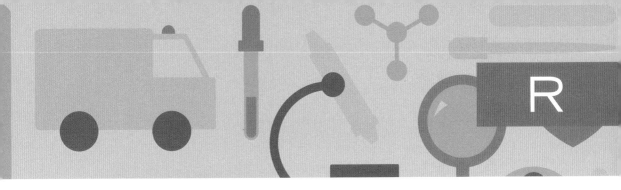

Rape-Trauma Syndrome

DEFINITION

Sustained maladaptive response to a forced, violent, sexual penetration against the victim's will and consent

RELATED FACTORS (R/T)

To be developed

ASSESSMENT

- History and circumstances of traumatic event
- Physical injuries sustained, including genitourinary, integumentary, musculoskeletal, and neurologic
- Emotional reactions, including grief reaction, changes in self-concept, and spiritual distress
- Support systems available to patient, including clergy, family members, and friends
- Problem-solving techniques usually employed by patient

DEFINING CHARACTERISTICS

- Aggression
- Agitation
- Alteration in sleep pattern
- Anger
- Anxiety
- Change in relationship(s)
- Confusion
- Denial
- Dependency
- Depression
- Disorganization
- Dissociative identity disorder
- Embarrassment
- Fear
- Guilt
- Helplessness
- History of suicide attempt
- Humiliation

- Hyperalertness
- Impaired decision-making
- Low self-esteem
- Mood swings
- Muscle spasm
- Muscle tension
- Nightmares
- Paranoia
- Perceived vulnerability
- Phobias
- Physical trauma
- Powerlessness
- Self-blame
- Sexual dysfunction
- Shame
- Shock
- Substance abuse
- Thoughts of revenge

EXPECTED OUTCOMES

- Patient will recover from physical injuries to fullest extent possible.
- Patient will express feelings and fears.
- Patient will use support systems.

Suggested NOC Outcomes

Abuse Protection; Abuse Recovery: Emotional; Coping

INTERVENTIONS AND RATIONALES

PCC   Explain assessment procedures to patient *to reduce the level of fear associated with data gathering after a rape.*

EBP   Follow the medical regimen to manage physical injuries caused by the traumatic event. *This is the first step in meeting patient's hierarchy of needs and depends on the extent of patient's other injuries and the intensity of the psychological response.*

EBP   Follow the facility's protocol regarding legal responsibilities. Be aware of the potential legal issues of rape and of the role nurses may play as witnesses in legal proceedings. *These steps will help protect patient's legal rights.*

PCC   Provide emotional support:
- Be available to listen. *Active listening allows an empathetic response to patient's feelings while being aware of one's own thoughts and behaviors.*
- Accept patient's feelings *to let him or her know any feelings are valid and acceptable.*
- Approach patient in a warm, caring manner *to cultivate trust and cooperation.*
- Provide privacy during the physical examination and interviewing process. *To protect patient's rights, no information should be released without prior consent.*
- Assure patient of his or her safety and take all necessary measures to ensure it. *This reduces patient's fears of repeated assault.*

PCC   Support patient's family members in their reactions to the traumatic event:
- Provide time for them to express their feelings and concerns.
- Help them understand patient's reactions.

Giving them time to talk and providing accurate information helps them support their loved one.

T&C ▪ Offer referral to other support persons or groups, such as clergy, a crisis center, mental health professionals, rape counselors, and Women Organized Against Rape. *This will help patient express feelings and develop coping skills.*

Suggested NIC Interventions

Abuse Protection Support; Anxiety Reduction; Crisis Intervention; Rape-Trauma Treatment; Self-Esteem Enhancement

EVALUATIONS FOR EXPECTED OUTCOMES

▪ Patient recovers from physical injuries.
▪ Patient expresses feelings common to rape victims, such as anger, blame, humiliation, and fear of disease or pregnancy.
▪ Patient contacts local mental health, rape counseling, or crisis center.

DOCUMENTATION

▪ Patient's expressions of feelings about herself and traumatic event
▪ Physical findings and treatment
▪ Observations of family's interaction with patient
▪ Referrals to support persons
▪ Patient's response to nursing interventions
▪ Evaluations for expected outcomes

REFERENCES

Brown, A. L. (2019). The effects of exposure to negative social reactions and participant gender on attitudes and behavior toward a rape victim. *Violence Against Women, 25*(2), 208–222. doi:10.1177/1077801218761603

Keefe, J. R., Wiltsey Stirman, S., Cohen, Z. D., DeRubeis, R. J., Smith, B. N., & Resick, P. A. (2018). In rape trauma PTSD, patient characteristics indicate which trauma-focused treatment they are most likely to complete. *Depression & Anxiety (1091–4269), 35*(4), 330–338. doi:10.1002/da.22731

Kilimnik, C. D., & Terry, P. H. (2018). Understanding sexual consent and nonconsensual sexual experiences in undergraduate women: The role of identification and rape myth acceptance. *Canadian Journal of Human Sexuality, 27*(3), 195–206. doi:10.3138/cjhs.2017-0028

Mukamana, D., Brysiewicz, P., Collins, A., & Rosa, W. (2018). Genocide rape trauma management: An integrated framework for supporting survivors. *Advances in Nursing Science, 41*(1), 41–56. doi:10.1097/ANS.0000000000000177

Ineffective Relationship

DEFINITION

A pattern of mutual partnership that is insufficient to provide for each other's needs

RELATED FACTORS (R/T)

▪ Ineffective communication skills
▪ Stressors
▪ Substance misuse
▪ Unrealistic expectations

Alteration in cognitive functioning in one partner

- Coping status, including method of dealing with general conflicts, level of patient's communication with family and others; handling of negotiations regarding restriction of freedom, degree of patient's separation from family, tolerance of patient's expressed opinions, reaction to patient's long-range goals; and age-appropriateness of dating, curfew regulation, and money responsibilities
- Family and cultural standards
- Family status, including family composition; responsibilities assumed in caring for family members (including patient); and ability of family to meet their physical, social, emotional, and economic needs
- Individual's past response to crises, including stress management and communication patterns to express anger, affection, and confrontation
- Sociological factors, including job satisfaction, presence of support systems, or hobbies

- Delay in meeting of developmental goals appropriate for family life cycle stage
- Dissatisfaction with complementary relationship between partners
- Dissatisfaction with emotional need fulfillment between partners
- Dissatisfaction with idea sharing between partners
- Dissatisfaction with information sharing between partners
- Dissatisfaction with physical need fulfillment between partners
- Inadequate understanding of partner's compromised functioning
- Insufficient balance in autonomy between partners
- Insufficient balance in collaboration between partners
- Insufficient mutual respect between partners
- Insufficient mutual support in daily activities between partners
- Partner not identified as support person
- Unsatisfying communication with partner

- Patient will actively participate in activities that build cohesion with partner/family.
- Patient will express understanding of role as an individual, partner, and/or member of the family.
- Patient will identify negative behaviors that contribute to the dysfunction of the patient's relationship(s) and a desire to change them.
- Patient will verbalize positive aspects of own relationship(s).

Suggested NOC Outcomes

Abusive Behavior Self-Control; Coping; Family Functioning; Role Performance; Psychosocial Adjustment: Social Support; Substance Addiction Consequences

- `PCC` Assess patient and involve family and other health care providers as appropriate *as they can provide additional information and/or perspectives of which patient may not be aware.*

PCC ■ Assess patient and family for signs of addiction or abuse *as both can contribute negatively to the physiologic and psychological status of the patient and partner/family and the status of their relationship.*

PCC ■ Assist patient with cognitive therapies that develop positive coping skills to help build self-esteem *as this fosters self-confidence and a positive attitude toward personal relationships.*

EBP ■ Educate patient and partner/family regarding importance of everyone following through with the treatment plan *as joint participation is necessary to facilitate a successful outcome.*

PCC ■ Provide a safe environment and assist patient and partner/family in communicating openly regarding positive aspects of their relationship *in order to help facilitate positive interaction.*

PCC ■ Work with patient and partner/family to set up a treatment plan. *Encouraging patient to work with partner/family helps to create cohesiveness and mutual support in implementing the treatment plan.*

T&C ■ Work with outside agencies/programs if abuse or addiction is a factor *in order to ensure patient and partner/family safety.*

Suggested NIC Interventions

Anxiety Reduction; Abuse Protection Support; Coping Enhancement; Complex Relationship Building; Family Support; Role Enhancement; Sexual Counseling; Substance Use Treatment; Support Group

EVALUATIONS FOR EXPECTED OUTCOMES

■ Patient participates in activities.
■ Patient identifies negative behaviors and states plans for their resolution.
■ Patient verbalizes positive aspects of relationships.

DOCUMENTATION

■ Assessment of patient's relationships and evidence of addiction or drug abuse
■ Patient's progress in problem solving and making choices
■ Patient–family interactions and content of family meetings
■ Patient's response to interventions
■ Outpatient resources identified and suggested to patient and family members
■ Evaluations for expected outcomes

REFERENCES

Coyne, S. M., Nelson, D. A., Carroll, J. S., Smith, N. J., Chongming, Y., Holmgren, H. G., ... Yang, C. (2017). Relational aggression and marital quality: A five-year longitudinal study. *Journal of Family Psychology, 31*(3), 282–293. doi:10.1037/fam0000274

Ha, T., Otten, R., McGill, S., & Dishion, T. J. (2019). The family and peer origins of coercion within adult romantic relationships: A longitudinal multimethod study across relationships contexts. *Developmental Psychology, 55*(1), 207–215. doi:10.1037/dev0000630

McKiernan, A., Ryan, P., McMahon, E., Bradley, S., & Butler, E. (2018). Understanding young people's relationship breakups using the dual processing model of coping and bereavement. *Journal of Loss & Trauma, 23*(3), 192–210. doi:10.1080/15325024.2018.1426979

Miano, A., Weber, T., Roepke, S., & Dziobek, I. (2018). Childhood maltreatment and context dependent empathic accuracy in adult romantic relationships. *Psychological Trauma: Theory, Research, Practice & Policy, 10*(3), 309–318. doi:10.1037/tra0000296

Risk for Ineffective Relationship

DEFINITION

Susceptible to developing a pattern that is insufficient for providing a mutual partnership to provide for each other's needs

RISK FACTORS

- Ineffective communication skills
- Stressor
- Substance abuse
- Unrealistic expectations

ASSOCIATED CONDITION

- Alteration in cognitive functioning in one partner

ASSESSMENT

- Coping status, including method of dealing with general conflicts, level of patient's communication with family and others; handling of negotiations regarding restriction of freedom, degree of patient's separation from family; tolerance of patient's expressed opinions, reaction to patient's long-range goals; and age-appropriateness of dating, curfew regulation, and money responsibilities
- Family and cultural standards
- Family status, including family composition; responsibilities assumed in caring for family members (including patient); and ability of family to meet their physical, social, emotional, and economic needs
- Individual's past response to crises, including stress management and communication patterns to express anger, affection, and confrontation
- Sociological factors, including job satisfaction, presence of support systems, or hobbies

EXPECTED OUTCOMES

- Patient will actively participate in activities that help build cohesion with partner/family.
- Patient will express understanding of own role as an individual, a partner, and/or member of the family.
- Patient will identify healthy coping mechanisms that will support the patient as an individual, a partner, and/or family member.
- Patient will verbalize desire to work with partner/family in developing healthy communication skills.

Suggested NOC Outcomes

Family Functioning; Family Integrity; Role Performance; Psychosocial Adjustment; Life Change; Social Interaction Skills; Social Support

INTERVENTIONS AND RATIONALES

PCC ▪ Assess patient and partner/family, *since the partner/family can provide additional information/perspectives of which patient may not be aware.*

PCC ■ Assess support system and availability. *The partner may travel frequently, and immediate family may not live in proximity to patient, which can cause emotional strain.*

PCC ■ Assist patient and partner/family to identify positive activities that they can participate in together *to help build cohesion.*

■ Assist patient with cognitive therapies and stress reduction techniques. *Positive coping skills can help foster self-confidence and a positive attitude and positive behaviors toward personal relationships.*

■ Educate patient and partner/family regarding the need for family treatment, *as the partner/family is also affected by the status of the relationship, and only together can they begin to repair the relationship.*

PCC ■ Provide a safe environment and assist patient and partner/family in communicating openly *in order to help facilitate a positive interaction.*

PCC ■ Work with patient and partner/family to ensure that the treatment plan is sensitive to their cultural practices and developmental needs *in order to help build unity and confidence in their ability to follow-through with the treatment plan.*

Suggested NIC Interventions

Anxiety Reduction; Abuse Protection Support; Complex Relationship Building; Family Support; Role Enhancement; Sexual Counseling; Substance Use Treatment; Support Group

EVALUATIONS FOR EXPECTED OUTCOMES

■ Patient participates in activities.
■ Patient verbalizes accurate knowledge of role in family.
■ Patient states effective coping strategies.
■ Patient and family demonstrate improved communication.

DOCUMENTATION

■ Assessment of family dynamics
■ Cognitive therapies and stress reduction techniques used
■ Referrals to family treatment modalities
■ Changes in relationship
■ External agencies contacted by patient
■ Evaluations for expected outcomes

REFERENCES

Joel, S., Impett, E. A., Spielmann, S. S., & MacDonald, G. (2018). How interdependent are stay/leave decisions? On staying in the relationship for the sake of the romantic partner. *Journal of Personality and Social Psychology, 115*(5), 805–824. doi:10.1037/pspi0000139

Moroz, S., Chen, S., Daljeet, K. N., & Campbell, L. (2018). The dark triad and break-up distress. *Personality and Individual Differences, 132,* 52–59. doi:10.1016/j.paid.2018.05.022

Zhang, S., Baams, L., van de Bongardt, D., & Dubas, J. S. (2018). Intra- and inter-individual differences in adolescent depressive mood: The role of relationships with parents and friends. *Journal of Abnormal Child Psychology, 46*(4), 811–824. doi:10.1007/s10802-017-0321-6

Readiness for Enhanced Relationship

DEFINITION

A pattern of mutual partnership to provide for each other's needs, which can be strengthened

ASSESSMENT

- Sexual status, including usual patterns of sexuality
- Patient's health status, support systems, expressed concerns regarding relationship
- Communication patterns

DEFINING CHARACTERISTICS

- Expresses desire to enhance autonomy between partners
- Expresses desire to enhance collaboration between partners
- Expresses desire to enhance communication between partners
- Expresses desire to enhance emotional need fulfillment for each partner
- Expresses desire to enhance mutual respect between each partner
- Expresses desire to enhance satisfaction with complementary relationship between partners
- Expresses desire to enhance satisfaction with emotional need fulfillment for each partner
- Expresses desire to enhance satisfaction with idea sharing between partners
- Expresses desire to enhance satisfaction with information sharing between partners
- Expresses desire to enhance satisfaction with physical need fulfillment for each partner
- Expresses desire to enhance understanding of partner's functional deficit (e.g., physical, psychological, social)

EXPECTED OUTCOMES

- Patient will communicate effectively with partner and family members.
- Patient will articulate ways to mutually meet physical and emotional needs of partner and self.
- Patient will participate in appropriate counseling (premarital, preconceptual, sexual) as needed.
- Patient will verbalize that relationships are characterized by well-balanced autonomy and self-efficacy.

Suggested NOC Outcomes

Family Functioning; Role Performance; Sexual Functioning; Social Interaction Skills

INTERVENTIONS AND RATIONALES

- **PCC** Assess communication techniques and effectiveness of couple and family *to be able to counsel and/or refer appropriately as needed.*
- **T&C** Suggest that patient and partner/family members attend counseling sessions as appropriate for their life cycle stage. *Patients may need permission from a health care professional in order to feel comfortable seeking relationship assistance.*
- Teach patient and family members normal family life cycle stages *so that they can better understand what is normal and are able to anticipate challenges.*
- **PCC** Encourage patient and family members to share information and ideas *in order to enhance communication.*
- **T&C** Refer as needed to colleagues in other disciplines such as social workers or counselors *to facilitate enhanced communication.*

Suggested NIC Interventions

Family Integrity Promotion; Family Support; Preconceptual Counseling; Sexual Counseling; Socialization Enhancement; Support System Enhancement

EVALUATIONS FOR EXPECTED OUTCOMES

- Patient communicates effectively with partner and family.
- Patient states ways to meet physical and emotional needs of partner and self.
- Patient actively participates in recommended counseling.

DOCUMENTATION

- Patient's statement of improved communication with partner/family members
- Patient's participation in recommended counseling
- Referrals to other disciplines
- Evaluations for expected outcomes

REFERENCES

Chilwarwar, V., & Sriram, S. (2018). Exploring gender differences in choice of marriage partner among individuals with visual impairment. *Sexuality and Disability*. doi:10.1007/s11195-018-9536-x

Diamond, R. M., Brimhall, A. S., & Elliott, M. (2018). Attachment and relationship satisfaction among first married, remarried, and post-divorce relationships. *Journal of Family Therapy, 40*, S111–S127. doi:10.1111/1467-6427.12161

Lawrence, E. M., Rogers, R. G., Zajacova, A., & Wadsworth, T. (2018). Marital happiness, marital status, health, and longevity. *Journal of Happiness Studies: An Interdisciplinary Forum on Subjective Well-being*. doi:10.1007/s10902-018-0009-9

Impaired Religiosity

DEFINITION

Impaired ability to exercise reliance on beliefs and/or participate in rituals of a particular faith tradition

RELATED FACTORS (R/T)

- Anxiety
- Cultural barrier to practicing religion
- Depression
- Environmental barrier to practicing religion
- Fear of death
- Ineffective caregiving
- Ineffective coping strategies
- Insecurity
- Insufficient social support
- Insufficient sociocultural interaction
- Insufficient transportation
- Pain
- Spiritual distress

ASSOCIATED CONDITION

Illness

ASSESSMENT

- Age, gender, sex
- Religious affiliation, beliefs/values
- Usual religious practices, support system

DEFINING CHARACTERISTICS

- Desire to reconnect with previous belief pattern
- Desire to reconnect with previous customs
- Difficulty adhering to prescribed religious beliefs
- Difficulty adhering to prescribed religious rituals
- Distress about separation from faith community
- Questioning of religious belief patterns
- Questioning of religious customs

EXPECTED OUTCOMES

- Patient will describe conflicts with his or her religious beliefs and the effects of his or her illness on these beliefs.
- Patient will accept counsel of a person trained in spirituality.
- Patient will engage in religious practices to the extent that it is therapeutic.
- Patient will express satisfaction with ability to practice patient's religion.

Suggested NOC Outcomes

Hope; Motivation; Quality of Life; Spiritual Health

INTERVENTIONS AND RATIONALES

PCC ▪ Assess spiritual or religious beliefs; religious affiliation; importance of religion in daily life; religious involvement of family; religious dietary restrictions; importance of religion in helping with usual coping. *Assessment information helps identify appropriate interventions.*

PCC ▪ Approach patient in a nonjudgmental way when he or she is discussing religious beliefs or spiritual needs. *The nurse's beliefs may differ radically, but it is a professional responsibility to assist patient in an ethically sensitive way.*

PCC ▪ Help patient list the religious practices most important to him or her *to determine what is possible to provide in the hospital.*

PCC ▪ Acquire simple-to-obtain items, such as books, pictures, CD, cross, *to provide comfort to the patient.*

PCC ▪ Confirm that patient's spiritual needs are being satisfied *so that modifications can be made in the plan.*

PCC ▪ Involve family members in helping meet patient's spiritual needs if patient agrees. *If family members have strong spiritual beliefs, they can be a help to one another in times of pain and difficulty.*

PCC ▪ Encourage patient and family to express feelings associated with diagnosis, treatment, and recovery. *Expression of feelings helps patient and family cope with treatment.*

PCC ▪ Schedule time to spend with the family. *They need time with health care providers to ask questions.*

T&C ▪ Suggest a referral to a clergy person or faith community nurse *so that the person can discuss deeper spiritual issues.*

Suggested NIC Interventions

Religious Ritual Enhancement; Coping Enhancement; Hope Instillation; Active Listening; Spiritual Growth; Spiritual Support

EVALUATIONS FOR EXPECTED OUTCOMES

▨ Patient expresses understanding about how illness impacts patient's religious beliefs.
▨ Patient works with staff to modify plan as needed.
▨ Patient requests whatever resources patient thinks will help meet present needs.
▨ Family and clergy visit to provide support.

DOCUMENTATION

▨ Assessment of patient's perspectives on religiosity
▨ Practices that are meaningful to the patient
▨ Visits from clergy
▨ Modifications to the plan

REFERENCES

Ames, D., Erickson, Z., Youssef, N. A., Arnold, I., Adamson, C. S., Sones, A. C., ... Koenig, H. G. (2019). Moral injury, religiosity, and suicide risk in U.S. veterans and active duty military with PTSD symptoms. *Military Medicine, 184*(3/4), e271–e278. doi:10.1093/milmed/usy148

Bolton, C., Lane, C., Keezer, R., & Smith, J. (2018). The transformation of religiosity in individuals with cognitive impairment. *Journal of Religion, Spirituality & Aging.* doi:10.1080/15528030.2018 .1534706

Lin, C., Saffari, M., Koenig, H. G., & Pakpour, A. H. (2018). Effects of religiosity and religious coping on medication adherence and quality of life among people with epilepsy. *Epilepsy & Behavior, 78,* 45–51. doi:10.1016/j.yebeh.2017.10.008

McClintock, C. H., Anderson, M., Svob, C., Wickramaratne, P., Neugebauer, R., Miller, L., & Weissman, M. M. (2018). Multidimensional understanding of religiosity/spirituality: Relationship to major depression and familial risk. *Psychological Medicine.* doi:10.1017/S0033291718003276

Readiness for Enhanced Religiosity

DEFINITION

A pattern of reliance on religious beliefs and/or participation in rituals of a particular faith tradition, which can be strengthened

ASSESSMENT

▨ Age, gender, marital status
▨ Health history
▨ Support systems (family, clergy)
▨ Communication skills
▨ Cultural factors
▨ Religious affiliation
▨ Spiritual beliefs and practices that are important to patient
▨ Perceptions of faith, life, death, and suffering

DEFINING CHARACTERISTICS

▨ Expresses desire to enhance belief patterns used in the past
▨ Expresses desire to enhance connection with a religious leader
▨ Expresses desire to enhance forgiveness
▨ Expresses desire to enhance participation in religious experiences
▨ Expresses desire to enhance participation in religious practices

- Expresses desire to enhance religious customs used in the past
- Expresses desire to enhance religious options
- Expresses desire to enhance use of religious material

EXPECTED OUTCOMES

- Patient will articulate all that infuses strength and hope.
- Patient will discuss aspects of religion that are important to the patient.
- Patient will list how staff can facilitate patient's participation in religious practices.
- Patient will request or agree to talk to a spiritual professional.
- Patient will express a feeling of peace with provided religious opportunities.

Suggested NOC Outcomes

Health Beliefs; Health-Promoting Behavior; Hope; Motivation; Quality of Life; Spiritual Health

INTERVENTIONS AND RATIONALES

- **PCC** Perform a thorough spiritual assessment *to develop a holistic home care plan.*
- **PCC** Help patient list the religious practices most important to patient *to determine what's possible to provide in the home.*
- **PCC** Acquire simple-to-obtain items, such as a Bible, *to comfort patient while planning more complex support.*
- **EBP** Encourage guided imagery, prayer, and meditations *as methods of enhancing spiritual experiences.*
- **T&C** Suggest a referral *to clergy so patient may discuss deeper spiritual issues.*
- **T&C** Consider having a congregational nurse or faith community nurse visit weekly *to provide ongoing spiritual care.*
- **PCC** Confirm that patient's spiritual needs are being satisfied *if modifications are made to the plan.*

Suggested NIC Interventions

Presence; Religious Ritual Enhancement; Spiritual Growth Facilitation; Spiritual Support; Values Clarification

EVALUATIONS FOR EXPECTED OUTCOMES

- Patient describes sources of strength and hope.
- Patient discusses aspects of religion that are of deep personal importance.
- Patient receives the assistance needed to participate in religious practices.
- Patient talks to a spiritual professional.
- Patient expresses peace with the ongoing attention to personal spiritual needs.

DOCUMENTATION

- Assessment of spiritual needs
- Religious practices to enjoy at home
- Efforts to obtain resources to satisfy patient's needs
- Visits by spiritual professional
- Patient's responses to interventions
- Evaluations for expected outcomes

REFERENCES

Peres, M. F. P., Kamei, H. H., Tobo, P. R., & Lucchetti, G. (2018). Mechanisms behind religiosity and spirituality's effect on mental health, quality of life and well-being. *Journal of Religion & Health, 57*(5), 1842–1855. doi:10.1007/s10943-017-0400-6

Purnell, M. C., Johnson, M. S., Jones, R., Calloway, E. B., Hammond, D. A., Hall, L. A., & Spadaro, D. C. (2019). Spirituality and religiosity of pharmacy students. *American Journal of Pharmaceutical Education, 83*(1), 28–33.

Schuurmans-Stekhoven, J. B. (2019). Auspicious or suspicious—Does religiosity really promote elder well-being? Examining the belief-as-benefit effect among older Japanese. *Archives of Gerontology & Geriatrics, 81*, 129–135. doi:10.1016/j.archger.2018.12.005

Risk for Impaired Religiosity

DEFINITION

Susceptible to an impaired ability to exercise reliance on religious beliefs and/or participate in rituals of a particular faith tradition, which may compromise health

RISK FACTORS

- Insufficient transportation
- Pain
- Anxiety
- Depression
- Fear of death
- Ineffective caregiving
- Ineffective coping strategies
- Insecurity
- Insufficient social support
- Cultural barrier to practicing religion
- Environmental barrier to practicing religion
- Insufficient sociocultural interaction
- Spiritual distress

ASSOCIATED CONDITION

Illness

ASSESSMENT

- Age, gender
- Religious affiliation, beliefs, practices; importance of religion in daily life
- Environmental assessment of present living circumstances
- Support systems (family, clergy)

EXPECTED OUTCOMES

- Patient will articulate those religious practices that are of deep personal importance.
- Patient will decide what changes to patient's practices are realistic and acceptable.
- Patient will cope with the limitations imposed by current circumstances.
- Patient will make use of the available spiritual resources.
- Patient will express satisfaction with ability to practice patient's religion.

Suggested NOC Outcomes

Health Beliefs; Health-Promoting Behavior; Hope; Motivation; Quality of Life; Spiritual Health

INTERVENTIONS AND RATIONALES

PCC ■ Perform a thorough spiritual assessment *to develop a holistic care plan.*

PCC ■ Help patient list the religious practices that carry the most personal meaning and importance *to determine what's possible to provide for the patient.*

PCC ■ If patient desires, acquire simple-to-obtain items, such as a Bible, *to comfort patient while planning more complex support.*

PCC ■ Help patient explore modifications to patient's activities without compromising spiritual comfort. *Decision-making promotes feelings of independence and control.*

PCC ■ Explain available resources *to prepare for developing a realistic plan.*

PCC ■ Have patient list options for participation in religious activities *to promote optimism or acceptance in present situation.*

PCC ■ Check daily, then weekly, *to assess patient's level of satisfaction with the plan.*

T&C ■ Work with family, friends, or clergy *to provide appropriate spiritual support.*

Suggested NIC Interventions

Active Listening; Emotional Support; Hope Instillation; Presence; Religious Addiction Prevention; Religious Ritual Enhancement; Spiritual Growth Facilitation; Spiritual Support; Values Clarification

EVALUATIONS FOR EXPECTED OUTCOMES

■ Patient expresses satisfaction with the religious activities that are provided.

■ Patient participates in practicing those religious activities that are available.

■ Patient asks to modify plan as needed.

■ Family and clergy visit and support.

■ Patient expresses feelings of health and wholeness.

DOCUMENTATION

■ Thorough spiritual assessment

■ Religious practices that are meaningful to patient

■ Religious practices that can be provided in the present situation

■ Patient's satisfaction with options

■ Patient's participation in religious and other kinds of activities

■ Evaluations for expected outcomes

REFERENCES

Ames, D., Erickson, Z., Youssef, N. A., Arnold, I., Adamson, C. S., Sones, A. C., ... Koenig, H. G. (2019). Moral injury, religiosity, and suicide risk in U.S. veterans and active duty military with PTSD symptoms. *Military Medicine, 184*(3/4), e271–e278. doi:10.1093/milmed/usy148

Martin, N., Baralt, L., & Garrido-Ortega, C. (2018). What's religion got to do with it? Exploring college students' sexual and reproductive health knowledge and awareness of sexual and reproductive health services in relation to their gender and religiosity. *Journal of Religion & Health, 57*(5), 1856–1875. doi:10.1007/s10943-017-0432-y

Stevens, J. M., Arzoumanian, M. A., Greenbaum, B., Schwab, B. M., & Dalenberg, C. J. (2019). Relationship of abuse by religious authorities to depression, religiosity, and child physical abuse history in a college sample. *Psychological Trauma: Theory, Research, Practice & Policy, 11*(3), 292–299. doi:10.1037/tra0000421

Relocation Stress Syndrome

DEFINITION

Physiologic and/or psychosocial disturbance following transfer from one environment to another

RELATED FACTORS (R/T)

- Ineffective coping strategies
- Insufficient predeparture counseling
- Insufficient support system
- Language barrier
- Move from one environment to another
- Powerlessness
- Significant environmental change
- Social isolation
- Unpredictability of experience

ASSOCIATED CONDITIONS

- Compromised health status
- Deficient mental competence
- Impaired psychosocial functioning

ASSESSMENT

- Reason for transfer or relocation
- Nature of relocation
- Physical and mental status of patient, including health condition, cognitive functioning, and functional abilities
- Financial resources
- Support systems, including family, friends, and health care workers
- Resources available to help prepare for relocation
- Conditions in original environment versus conditions in new environment
- Coping and problem-solving abilities, including educational level, past experiences with relocation, and participation in recreational activities or hobbies

DEFINING CHARACTERISTICS

- Alienation
- Aloneness
- Alteration in sleep pattern
- Anger
- Anxiety
- Concern about relocation
- Dependency
- Depression
- Fear
- Frustration
- Increase in illness
- Increase in physical symptoms
- Increase in verbalization of needs

- Insecurity
- Loneliness
- Loss of identity
- Loss of self-worth
- Low self-esteem
- Pessimism
- Preoccupation
- Unwillingness to move
- Withdrawal

EXPECTED OUTCOMES

- Patient will request information about new environment.
- Patient will communicate understanding of relocation.
- Patient and family members will take steps to prepare for relocation.
- Patient will use available resources.
- Patient will express satisfaction with adjustment to new environment.

Suggested NOC Outcomes

Anxiety Self-Control; Coping; Depression Level; Depression Self-Control; Loneliness Severity; Psychosocial Adjustment: Life Change; Quality of Life; Stress Level

INTERVENTIONS AND RATIONALES

PCC ▪ Assign a primary nurse to patient *to provide a consistent, caring, and accepting environment that enhances patient's adjustment and well-being.*

PCC ▪ Help patient and family members prepare for relocation. Conduct group discussions, provide pictures of the new setting, and communicate any additional information that will ease transition *to help patient cope with a new environment.*

PCC ▪ If possible, allow patient and family members to visit the new location and provide introductions to the new staff. *The more familiar the environment, the less stress patient will experience during relocation.*

PCC ▪ Assess patient's needs for additional health care services before relocation *to ensure that patient receives appropriate care in the new environment.*

T&C ▪ Communicate all aspects of patient's discharge plan to appropriate staff members at the new location *to ensure continuity of care.*

EBP ▪ Educate family members about relocation stress syndrome and its potential effects *to encourage family members to provide needed emotional support throughout the transition period.*

PCC ▪ Encourage patient to express emotions associated with relocation *to provide opportunity to correct misconceptions, answer questions, and reduce anxiety.*

PCC ▪ Reassure patient that family members and friends know the patient's new location and will continue to visit *to reduce feelings of abandonment and anxiety.*

Suggested NIC Interventions

Active Listening; Coping Enhancement; Counseling; Hope Instillation; Mood Management; Presence; Sleep Enhancement; Self-Responsibility Facilitation; Spiritual Support

EVALUATIONS FOR EXPECTED OUTCOMES

- Patient requests information about new environment.
- Patient expresses understanding of relocation process.
- Patient and family members complete preparations for relocation.
- Patient makes use of available resources to smooth transition to new environment.
- Patient expresses feelings associated with adjustment to new environment.

DOCUMENTATION

- Evidence of patient's emotional distress over relocation
- Patient's needs in preparing for relocation
- Available resources and support systems
- Intervention to prepare patient and family members for relocation and patient's and family members' responses
- Discharge plan instructions communicated to new staff
- Evaluations for expected outcomes

REFERENCES

Lee, S., Oh, H., Suh, Y., & Seo, W. (2017). A tailored relocation stress intervention programme for family caregivers of patients transferred from a surgical intensive care unit to a general ward. *Journal of Clinical Nursing, 26*(5–6), 784–794. doi:10.1111/jocn.13568

Lin, L.-J., & Yen, H.-Y. (2018). The benefits of continuous leisure participation in relocation adjustment among residents of long-term care facilities. *Journal of Nursing Research (Lippincott Williams & Wilkins), 26*(6), 427–437. doi:10.1097/jnr.0000000000000263

Salcioglu, E., Ozden, S., & Ari, F. (2018). The role of relocation patterns and psychosocial stressors in posttraumatic stress disorder and depression among earthquake survivors. *Journal of Nervous and Mental Disease, 206*(1), 19–26.

Risk for Relocation Stress Syndrome

DEFINITION

Susceptible to physiological and/or psychosocial disturbance following transfer from one environment to another that may compromise health

RISK FACTORS

- Ineffective coping strategies
- Insufficient predeparture counseling
- Insufficient support system
- Language barrier
- Move from one environment to another
- Powerlessness
- Significant environmental change
- Social isolation
- Unpredictability of experience

ASSOCIATED CONDITIONS

- Compromised health status
- Deficient mental competence
- Impaired psychosocial functioning

ASSESSMENT

- Consideration of transfer or relocation
- Nature of possible relocation
- Physical and mental status of patient, including health condition, cognitive functioning, and functional abilities
- Financial resources
- Support systems, including family, friends, and health care workers
- Resources available to help prepare for relocation
- Conditions in original environment versus conditions in new environment
- Coping and problem-solving abilities, including educational level, past experiences with relocation, and participation in recreational activities or hobbies

EXPECTED OUTCOMES

- Patient will request information about new environment.
- Patient will participate in decision-making regarding relocation.
- Patient will communicate understanding of need for relocation.
- Patient will take steps to prepare for relocation along with family members or partner.
- Patient will express satisfaction with adjustment to new environment.

Suggested NOC Outcomes

Loneliness Severity; Psychosocial Adjustment: Life Change; Quality of Life; Stress Level

INTERVENTIONS AND RATIONALES

- Assess patient's needs for additional health care services before relocation *to ensure that patient receives appropriate care in the new environment.*
- **PCC** If possible, include patient in the decision-making process regarding potential location, dates, and circumstances of relocation *to promote a feeling of participation in choices, which will allow a feeling of control.*
- **PCC** If possible, allow patient and family members to visit the new location and provide introductions to the new staff. *The more familiar the environment, the less stress patient will experience during relocation.*
- **EBP** Educate family members about relocation stress syndrome and its potential effects *to encourage family members to provide needed emotional support throughout the transition period.*
- **PCC** Help patient and family members prepare for relocation. Conduct group discussions, provide pictures of setting, and communicate any information that will ease transition *to help patient with the new environment.*
- **PCC** Encourage patient to express emotions associated with relocation *to provide an opportunity to correct misconceptions, answer questions, and reduce anxiety.*
- **T&C** Communicate all aspects of patient's discharge plan to appropriate staff members at the new location *to ensure continuity of care.*
- **PCC** Reassure patient that family members and friends know the new location and will continue to visit *to reduce feelings of abandonment and anxiety.*

Suggested NIC Interventions

Active Listening; Coping Enhancement; Self-Responsibility Facilitation; Spiritual Support

EVALUATIONS FOR EXPECTED OUTCOMES

▥ Patient requests information about new environment.
▥ Patient expresses understanding of relocation process.
▥ Patient and family members complete preparations for relocation.
▥ Patient makes use of available resources to smooth transition to new environment.
▥ Patient expresses feelings associated with adjustment to new environment.

DOCUMENTATION

▥ Evidence of patient's emotional distress over relocation
▥ Patient's needs in preparing for relocation
▥ Available resources and support systems
▥ Intervention to prepare patient and family members for relocation and patient's and family members' responses
▥ Discharge plan instructions communicated to new staff
▥ Evaluations for expected outcomes

REFERENCES

Haapakangas, A., Hongisto, V., Varjo, J., & Lahtinen, M. (2018). Benefits of quiet workspaces in open-plan offices—Evidence from two office relocations. *Journal of Environmental Psychology, 56,* 63–75. doi:10.1016/j.jenvp.2018.03.003

Salcioglu, E., Ozden, S., & Ari, F. (2018). The role of relocation patterns and psychosocial stressors in posttraumatic stress disorder and depression among earthquake survivors. *Journal of Nervous & Mental Disease, 206*(1), 19–26. doi:10.1097/NMD.0000000000000627

Smetcoren, A. S., De Donder, L., Dury, S., De Witte, N., Kardol, T., & Verte, D. (2017). Refining the push and pull framework: identifying inequalities in residential relocation among older adults. *Ageing & Society, 37*(1), 90–112. doi:10.1017/S0144686X15001026

Impaired Resilience

DEFINITION

Decreased ability to recover from perceived adverse or changing situations, through a dynamic process of adaptation

RELATED FACTORS (R/T)

▥ Community violence
▥ Disruption in family rituals
▥ Disruption in family roles
▥ Disturbance in family dynamics
▥ Dysfunctional family processes
▥ Inadequate resources
▥ Inconsistent parenting
▥ Ineffective family adaptation
▥ Insufficient impulse control
▥ Insufficient resources
▥ Insufficient social support
▥ Multiple coexisting adverse situations
▥ Perceived vulnerability
▥ Substance misuse

ASSOCIATED CONDITION

Psychological disorder

ASSESSMENT

- Patient's perception of problem, coping mechanisms, problem-solving ability, decision-making competencies, relationships, family system
- Health history, history of chronic illness
- Activity status, nutritional status, sleep patterns
- Cultural status, including affiliation with racial, ethnic, or religious groups

DEFINING CHARACTERISTICS

- Decreased interest in academic activities
- Decreased interest in vocational activities
- Depression
- Guilt
- Impaired health status
- Ineffective coping strategies
- Ineffective integration
- Ineffective sense of control
- Low self-esteem
- Renewed elevation of distress
- Shame
- Social isolation

EXPECTED OUTCOMES

- Patient will adapt to new or changing situation.
- Patient will have interest in academic activities.
- Patient will identify personal strengths.
- Patient will integrate into new environment.
- Patient will engage in activities that promote health.
- Patient will identify strategies that have been successful in previous times of stress.

Suggested NOC Outcomes

Role Performance; Effective/Enhanced Resilience; Knowledge: Health Behavior

INTERVENTIONS AND RATIONALES

PCC ▪ Explore with patient what maladaptive behaviors patient is exhibiting due to impaired individual resilience. *Patient must take ownership of behaviors before change can take place.*
- Assist patient in making a list of strengths and resources with contact information and the parameters for contacting those resources. *Planning for needs decreases anxiety and increases self-care.*

EBP ▪ Instruct patient to engage in positive health behaviors. *Adequate sleep, nutritional intake, and activity improve decision-making.*

PCC ▪ Encourage patient to wait to make life-changing decisions until the current crisis is over. *Decision-making is impaired during times of crisis.*

T&C ▓ Refer patients to mental health resources in the event of maladaptive coping or safety risk. *Individuals with impaired individual resilience face an increased risk of physical and mental illness.*

Suggested NIC Interventions

Anxiety Reduction; Coping Enhancement; Decision-Making Support; Spiritual Support

EVALUATIONS FOR EXPECTED OUTCOMES

▓ Patient expresses adjustment to new or changing situation.
▓ Patient engages in academic activities.
▓ Patient identifies at least three personal strengths that lead to increased resilience.
▓ Patient shares strategies that were successful during other stressful periods.
▓ Patient states activities that will promote health.

DOCUMENTATION

▓ Patient's expressions of feelings regarding current crisis
▓ Patient's planned health promotion behaviors
▓ Patient's understanding of available resources if needed
▓ Evaluations for expected outcomes

REFERENCES

Ayed, N., Toner, S., & Priebe, S. (2018). Conceptualizing resilience in adult mental health literature: A systematic review and narrative synthesis. *Psychology and Psychotherapy: Theory, Research and Practice.* doi:10.1111/papt.12185

Greup, S. R., Kaal, S. E. J., Jansen, R., Manten-Horst, E., Thong, M. S. Y., van, d. G., ... Husson, O. (2018). Post-traumatic growth and resilience in adolescent and young adult cancer patients: An overview. *Journal of Adolescent and Young Adult Oncology, 7*(1), 1–14. doi:10.1089/jayao.2017.0040

Rook, C., Smith, L., Johnstone, J., Rossato, C., López Sánchez, G. F., Suárez, A. D., & Roberts, J. (2018). Reconceptualising workplace resilience—A cross-disciplinary perspective. *Anales De Psicología, 34*(2), 332–339. doi:10.6018/analesps.34.2.299371

Risk for Impaired Resilience

DEFINITION

Susceptible to decreased ability to recover from perceived adverse or changing situations, through a dynamic process of adaptation, which may compromise health

RISK FACTORS

▓ Community violence
▓ Disruption in family rituals
▓ Disruption in family roles
▓ Disturbance in family dynamics
▓ Dysfunctional family processes
▓ Inadequate resources
▓ Inconsistent parenting

- Ineffective family adaptation
- Insufficient impulse control
- Insufficient resources
- Insufficient social support
- Multiple coexisting adverse situations
- Perceived vulnerability
- Substance misuse

ASSOCIATED CONDITION

Psychological disorder

ASSESSMENT

- Patient perception of problem, coping mechanisms, problem-solving ability, decision-making competencies, relationships, family system
- Health history, history of chronic illness
- Activity status, nutritional status, sleep patterns
- Cultural status, including affiliation with racial, ethnic, or religious groups

EXPECTED OUTCOMES

- Patient will identify available support systems to maintain resilience.
- Patient will identify healthy coping strategies.
- Patient will verbalize belief in self to withstand current situation.
- Patient will engage in activities that promote health.
- Patient will identify strategies that have been helpful in previous times of stress.

Suggested NOC Outcomes

Role Performance; Effective/Enhanced Resilience

INTERVENTIONS AND RATIONALES

PCC ▪ Evaluate previous mechanisms of effective coping in difficult situations. *Assimilating current situation to previous successes enhances resilience.*

PCC ▪ Assist patient in making a list of strengths and resources. Be knowledgeable of cultural aspects of resilience. *Cultural relevance is critical to all aspects of patient care.*

PCC ▪ Instruct patient to engage in positive self-talk: "I can handle this" or "I will accomplish one thing today and celebrate it." *A positive outlook increases endorphins and enhances self-efficacy.*

EBP ▪ Encourage patient to maintain activities of health promotion, including adequate sleep, nutritious eating, and activity. *Maintaining adequate self-care enhances resilience.*

T&C ▪ Refer patients to mental health resources in the event of maladaptive coping or safety risk. *Risk of compromised resilience may lead to actual compromised resilience.*

Suggested NIC Interventions

Anxiety Reduction; Coping Enhancement; Decision-Making Support; Spiritual Support

EVALUATIONS FOR EXPECTED OUTCOMES

- Patient acknowledges previous strategies of effective coping in difficult situations.
- Patient makes list of strengths and resources, including cultural considerations.
- Patient engages in positive self-talk.
- Patient engages in positive health promotion activities.

DOCUMENTATION

- Patient's acknowledgment of effective strategies
- Patient's list of strengths and resources
- Patient's identified health promotion activities
- Evaluations for expected outcomes

REFERENCES

Ergün, G., Gümüş, F., & Dikeç, G. (2018). Examining the relationship between traumatic growth and psychological resilience in young adult children of parents with and without a mental disorder. *Journal of Clinical Nursing, 27*(19–20), 3729–3738. doi:10.1111/jocn.14533

Eshel, Y., Kimhi, S., Lahad, M., Leykin, D., & Goroshit, M. (2018). Risk factors as major determinants of resilience: A replication study. *Community Mental Health Journal, 54*(8), 1228–1238. doi:10.1007/s10597-018-0263-7

Park, S., & Schepp, K. G. (2018). A theoretical model of resilience capacity: Drawn from the words of adult children of alcoholics. *Nursing Forum, 53*(3), 314–323. doi:10.1111/nuf.12255

Readiness for Enhanced Resilience

DEFINITION

A pattern of ability to recover from perceived adverse or changing situations, through a dynamic process of adaptation, which can be strengthened

ASSESSMENT

Patient's perception of situation, coping mechanisms, problem-solving ability, decision-making competencies, relationships, family system

DEFINING CHARACTERISTICS

- Expresses desire to enhance available resources
- Expresses desire to enhance communication skills
- Expresses desire to enhance environmental safety
- Expresses desire to enhance goal setting
- Expresses desire to enhance involvement in activities
- Expresses desire to enhance own responsibility for action
- Expresses desire to enhance positive outlook
- Expresses desire to enhance progress toward goal
- Expresses desire to enhance relationship with others
- Expresses desire to enhance resilience
- Expresses desire to enhance self-esteem
- Expresses desire to enhance sense of control
- Expresses desire to enhance support system

- Expresses desire to enhance use of conflict management strategies
- Expresses desire to enhance use of coping skills
- Expresses desire to enhance use of resource

EXPECTED OUTCOMES

- Patient will identify available support systems to maintain resilience.
- Patient will identify healthy coping strategies.
- Patient will verbalize belief in self to withstand current situation.
- Patient will engage in activities that promote health.
- Patient will identify strategies that have been helpful in previous times of stress.
- Patient will identify impact of resilience on personal growth.

Suggested NOC Outcomes

Enhanced Self-Esteem; Enhanced Personal Potential; Knowledge: Health Behavior

INTERVENTIONS AND RATIONALES

- **PCC** ▪ Explore with patient the process and growth in mastering a situation or crisis that enhanced patient's resilience. *Mastery of responses in crisis situations can generalize to future situations.*
- **PCC** ▪ Listen therapeutically to patient's self-exploration and mastery. *Active listening is the key to the therapeutic alliance and accurate assessment.*
- **PCC** ▪ Instruct patient to journal experiences for future reflection. *Journaling is a therapeutic tool for self-exploration and expansion.*
- **PCC** ▪ Guide patient in reviewing life goals that might now be attainable. *Personal potential is maximized in an environment of resilience.*
- **PCC** ▪ Encourage patient to assist others or get involved to enrich the lives of others. *Humans benefit from shared positive experiences.*

Suggested NIC Interventions

Coping Enhancement; Enhanced Human Potential

EVALUATIONS FOR EXPECTED OUTCOMES

- Patient acknowledges previous strategies of effective coping in difficult situations.
- Patient makes list of strengths and resources, including cultural considerations.
- Patient engages in positive self-talk.
- Patient engages in positive health promotion activities.
- Patient identifies the impact of resilience toward growth.

DOCUMENTATION

- Patient's acknowledgment of readiness for increased resilience
- Patient's statements regarding the impact of resilience on personal growth
- Patient's feelings of resilience
- Evaluations for expected outcomes

REFERENCES

Cleary, M., Kornhaber, R., Thapa, D. K., West, S., & Visentin, D. (2018). The effectiveness of interventions to improve resilience among health professionals: A systematic review. *Nurse Education Today, 71*, 247–263. doi:10.1016/j.nedt.2018.10.002

Foster, K., Cuzzillo, C., & Furness, T. (2018). Strengthening mental health nurses' resilience through a workplace resilience programme: A qualitative inquiry. *Journal of Psychiatric and Mental Health Nursing.* doi:10.1111/jpm.12467

Kinman, G., & Grant, L. (2017). Building resilience in early-career social workers: Evaluating a multi-modal intervention. *British Journal of Social Work, 47*(7), 1979–1998. doi:10.1093/bjsw/bcw164

Parental Role Conflict

DEFINITION

Parental experience of role confusion and conflict in response to crisis

RELATED FACTORS (R/T)

- Interruptions in family life due to home care regimen
- Intimidated by invasion modalities
- Intimidated by restrictive modalities
- Parent–child separation

ASSESSMENT

- Parental age
- Child age
- Parental status, including age and maturity; apprehension, fear, and guilt; coping mechanisms employed; developmental state of family and other children; knowledge of normal growth and development of children; past response to crises; understanding of child's present condition; spiritual practices of parents and family; stability of parental relationship; and support systems available to parent
- Available support systems, including other family members, friends, visiting nurses, and community resources
- Parent–child relationship before development of special needs and any changes that have occurred
- Parent–child interaction, including eye contact, response to appearance (such as bandages, deformities, and hospital equipment), smiling, touching, and verbalization
- Child's health status, including severity of illness and health care needs
- Child's level of development

DEFINING CHARACTERISTICS

- Anxiety
- Concern about change in parental role
- Concern about family
- Disruption in caregiver routine
- Fear
- Frustration
- Guilt
- Perceived inadequacy to provide for child's needs

▨ Perceived loss of control over decisions relating to child
▨ Reluctance to participate in usual caregiving activities

EXPECTED OUTCOMES

▨ Parents will communicate feelings about present situation.
▨ Parents will participate in their child's daily care.
▨ Parents will seek out and accept external support, education, and assistance in caring for child at home.
▨ Parents will begin to provide physical, emotional, and developmental care to child at home.
▨ Parents will seek assistance in meeting their own emotional and developmental needs.
▨ Parents will express feelings of greater control and ability to contribute more to child's well-being.
▨ Parents will express knowledge of child's developmental needs.
▨ Parents will hold, touch, and convey warmth and affection to child.
▨ Parents will use available support systems or agencies to assist in coping.

Suggested NOC Outcomes

Caregiver Adaptation to Patient Institutionalization; Caregiver Home Care Readiness; Coping; Family Coping; Family Normalization

INTERVENTIONS AND RATIONALES

PCC ▨ Orient parents or primary caregivers to the hospital environment, visiting procedures, medical equipment, and staff. *Familiarity decreases anxiety.*

PCC ▨ Provide family-centered care by obtaining parents' input for child's care. *Parents can meet many of child's needs better than staff.*

▨ Involve parents in child's care conferences and in the physical care of child. *Participation may decrease parents' feelings of helplessness.*

▨ Promote the emotional well-being of parents by providing respite care, encouraging parents to spend time away from child to enhance their marital relationship, and providing information about additional sources of support. *Encouraging parents to pay attention to their own emotional needs will enhance their ability to care for their child.*

▨ Listen to parents, child, and siblings openly and without passing judgment *to gain their trust.*

PCC ▨ Help parents develop realistic expectations of their child and formulate achievable short-term goals based on child's needs and abilities *to reduce frustration and feelings of helplessness.*

PCC ▨ Ensure attention to all of child's normal health needs, including dental care, immunizations, safety, and educational and nutritional needs. *A chronically ill child needs total health care, not just illness-related interventions.*

EBP ▨ Advocate normal growth and development for child with special needs. Encourage visits by friends and discourage overprotective behavior *to help child obtain social acceptance. Increased social interaction will encourage parents, siblings, and others to view child as a unique individual instead of a burden. This, in turn, will help promote child's self-esteem.*

EBP ▨ Teach parents normal childhood physical and psychological development *to prepare parents to deal with changes.*

PCC ▨ Encourage parental involvement in appropriate support groups or agencies when necessary or ordered. *Such groups can provide emotional support and help reduce feelings of being overwhelmed.*

- Ask parents if they have questions about child's status and provide information, as requested, *to reduce feelings of helplessness.*
- Provide for the needs of parents, as appropriate. Offer facilities for showering, sleeping, and eating. Be available to care for child if parents need an opportunity to rest. *Helping parents meet their needs will empower them to meet child care demands.*
- Act as a liaison between family and the multidisciplinary health care team, equipment vendors, community agencies, and third-party payers. *An organized approach with one central coordinator decreases stress for family and enhances continuity of care.*

Suggested NOC Outcomes

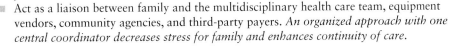

Caregiver Support; Coping Enhancement; Family Involvement Promotion; Family Presence Facilitation; Family Process Maintenance; Role Enhancement

EVALUATIONS FOR EXPECTED OUTCOMES

- Parents communicate feelings about present situation.
- Parents participate in their child's daily care.
- Parents express feelings of control in present situation.
- Parents communicate knowledge of child's developmental needs.
- Parents seek out and use community resources to assist in meeting child's physical, psychological, and educational needs.
- Parents seek help to meet their own emotional and developmental needs.
- Parents express feelings of greater control and capability in meeting child's needs.
- Parents hold, touch, and express warmth and affection to child.
- Parents contact support systems or community agencies to assist in coping.

DOCUMENTATION

- Observations of parents' ability to cope and their level of involvement in child's hospital care and daily needs
- Interventions performed to help parents lower stress and cope with situation
- Referrals to outside agencies or support groups
- Family members' expressions of feelings about their role in caring for child at home
- Observations of parent–child interaction
- Nursing interventions to resolve parental role conflict
- Parents', child's, and siblings' responses to interventions
- Child's medical and emotional state
- Evaluations for expected outcomes

REFERENCES

Agarwal, I. B., & Agarwal, P. C. (2018). Role of parents in the development of social competency among adolescents. *Journal of Human Behavior in the Social Environment.* doi:10.1080/10911359.2018.1465004

Camisasca, E., Miragoli, S., Di Blasio, P., & Grych, J. (2017). Children's coping strategies to inter-parental conflict: The moderating role of attachment. *Journal of Child & Family Studies,* 26(4), 1099–1111. doi:10.1007/s10826-016-0645-9

Giroux, C. M., Wilson, L. A., & Corkett, J. K. (2019). Parents as partners: investigating the role(s) of mothers in coordinating health and education activities for children with chronic care needs. *Journal of Interprofessional Care,* 33(2), 243–251. doi:10.1080/13561820.2018.1531833

Kuntsche, S., & Kuntsche, E. (2019). Being old fashioned in a modern world: Gender role attitudes moderate the relation between role conflicts and alcohol use of parents. *Drug & Alcohol Dependence,* 195, 90–93. doi:10.1016/j.drugalcdep.2018.11.025

Ineffective Role Performance

DEFINITION

A pattern of behavior and self-expression that does not match the environmental context, norms, and expectations

RELATED FACTORS (R/T)

- Alteration in body image
- Conflict
- Depression
- Domestic violence
- Fatigue
- Inadequate role model
- Inappropriate linkage with the health care system
- Insufficient resources
- Insufficient rewards
- Insufficient role preparation
- Insufficient role socialization
- Insufficient support system
- Low self-esteem
- Pain
- Stressors
- Substance misuse
- Unrealistic role expectations

ASSOCIATED CONDITIONS

- Neurological defect
- Personality disorder
- Physical illness
- Psychosis

ASSESSMENT

- Age
- Gender
- Patient's perception of social, vocational, and family roles
- Health history, including medical diagnosis, course and severity of illness, and reason for hospitalization
- Neurologic status, including level of consciousness, memory, mental status, orientation, and cognitive and perceptual functioning
- Physical disabilities or limitations
- Coping behaviors
- Patient's perception of illness and its effect on social, cultural, and vocational roles
- Psychosocial status, including current stressors, support systems, hobbies, interests, work history, educational background, and changes in role function
- Family status, including roles of family members, effect of illness on patient's family, and family's understanding of patient's illness

DEFINING CHARACTERISTICS

- Alteration in role perception
- Anxiety
- Change in capacity to resume role
- Change in others' perception of role
- Change in self-perception of role
- Change in usual pattern of responsibility
- Depression
- Discrimination
- Domestic violence
- Harassment
- Inappropriate development expectations
- Ineffective adaptation to change
- Ineffective coping strategies
- Ineffective role performance
- Insufficient confidence
- Insufficient external support for role enactment
- Insufficient knowledge of role requirements
- Insufficient motivation
- Insufficient opportunity for role enactment
- Insufficient self-management
- Insufficient skills
- Pessimism
- Powerlessness
- Role ambivalence
- Role conflict
- Role confusion
- Role denial
- Role dissatisfaction
- Role strain
- System conflict
- Uncertainty

EXPECTED OUTCOMES

- Patient will express feelings about diminished ability to perform usual roles.
- Patient and family members will recognize and state feelings about limitations imposed by illness.
- Patient will discuss plans to reevaluate social, family, and vocational roles and adapt them to present physical and mental status.
- Patient will make decisions about course of treatment and management of illness.
- Patient will continue to function in usual roles as much as possible.
- Patient will express feelings of making productive contribution to self-care, to others, or to environment.

Suggested NOC Outcomes

Caregiver Lifestyle Disruption; Coping; Depression Level; Psychomotor Energy; Psychosocial Adjustment: Life Change; Role Performance

INTERVENTIONS AND RATIONALES

PCC ◼ If possible, assign the same nurse to patient each shift *to establish rapport and foster development of a therapeutic relationship.*

PCC ◼ Discuss with patient factors that make it difficult to fulfill patient's usual vocational or social role. How does patient feel about no longer being in the usual role? *Discussion helps patient gain insight and rationally define problems and potential solutions.*

PCC ◼ Spend ample time with patient each shift *to foster a sense of safety and decrease loneliness.*

◼ Provide opportunities for patient to express thoughts and feelings *to help patient identify how altered role performance has affected patient's life.*

PCC ◼ Encourage patient to explore strengths. *Having patient talk about existing strengths will help in identifying new strengths patient needs to develop to succeed in a new role.*

PCC ◼ Convey a belief in patient's ability to develop the necessary coping skills. *By projecting a positive attitude, you can help patient gain confidence.*

◼ Be aware of patient's emotional vulnerability and allow open expression of all emotions. *An accepting attitude will help patient deal with the effects of chronic illness and loss of functioning.*

PCC ◼ Provide opportunities for patient to make decisions and encourage patient to maintain personal responsibilities. *Showing respect for patient's decision-making ability enhances feelings of independence.*

PCC ◼ Encourage patient to participate in self-care activities, keeping in mind patient's physical and emotional limitations. *Involvement in self-care promotes optimal functioning.*

EBP ◼ Assess patient's knowledge of illness and educate patient about condition, treatment, and prognosis. *Education helps patient cope with effects of illness more effectively.*

PCC ◼ Encourage patient to recognize personal strengths and to use them. *This will help maintain optimal functioning and foster a healthier self-image.*

PCC ◼ Encourage patient to continue to fulfill life roles within the constraints posed by illness. *This will help patient maintain a sense of purpose and preserve connections with other people.*

◼ Encourage patient to participate in his or her care as an active member of the health care team. *This will help establish mutually accepted goals between patient and caregivers. Patient who participates in care is more likely to take an active role in other aspects of life.*

PCC ◼ Help family members identify their feelings about patient's decreased role functioning. Encourage participation in a support group. *Relatives of patient may need social support, information, and an outlet for ventilating feelings.*

PCC ◼ Offer patient and family members a realistic assessment of patient's illness, and communicate hope for the immediate future. *Education helps promote patient safety and security and helps family members plan for future health care requirements.*

EBP ◼ Educate patient and family members about managing illness, controlling environmental factors that affect patient's health, and redefining roles *to promote optimal functioning. Through education, family members may become resources in patient's care.*

T&C ◼ Investigate support groups and other community resources *to help the patient find new outlets for forming social relationships.*

Suggested NIC Interventions

Anticipatory Guidance; Caregiver Support; Coping Enhancement; Family Process Maintenance; Role Enhancement; Hope Instillation

EVALUATIONS FOR EXPECTED OUTCOMES

- Patient shares feelings about illness and altered role performance in a constructive manner.
- Patient describes plans to adapt to role changes related to aging and chronic illness.
- Patient and family members understand role changes that are occurring because of chronic illness and express their feelings about these limitations.
- Patient demonstrates increased functioning by making decisions about health care and participating in planning and implementing aspects of personal care.
- Patient demonstrates ability to perceive options and uses options to function in usual roles as much as possible.
- Patient expresses feelings of having made productive contribution to self-care, to others, or to the environment.

DOCUMENTATION

- Observations of patient's physical, emotional, and mental status
- Patient's thoughts and feelings about illness and diminished role capacity
- Nursing interventions performed to help patient understand change in role functioning
- Patient's response to nursing interventions
- Health teaching, counseling, and precautions taken to maintain or enhance patient's level of functioning
- Referrals to sources of support for patient and family members
- Evaluations for expected outcomes

REFERENCES

Agree, E. M. (2017). Social changes in women's roles, families, and generational ties. *Generations, 41*(2), 63–70.

DePasquale, N., Polenick, C. A., Hinde, J., Bray, J. W., Zarit, S. H., Moen, P., ... Almeida, D. M. (2018). Health behavior among men with multiple family roles: The moderating effects of perceived partner relationship quality. *American Journal of Men's Health, 12*(6), 2006–2017. doi:10.1177/1557988316660088

Duxbury, L., Stevenson, M., & Higgins, C. (2018). Too much to do, too little time: Role overload and stress in a multi-role environment. *International Journal of Stress Management, 25*(3), 250–266. doi:10.1037/str0000062

Prendeville, P., & Kinsella, W. (2019). The role of grandparents in supporting families of children with autism spectrum disorders: A family systems approach. *Journal of Autism & Developmental Disorders, 49*(2), 738–749. doi:10.1007/s10803-018-3753-0

Caregiver Role Strain

DEFINITION

Difficulty in fulfilling care responsibilities, expectations, and/or behaviors for family or significant others

RELATED FACTORS (R/T)

Care Receiver

- Condition inhibits conversation
- Dependency
- Discharged home with significant needs

- Increase in care needs
- Problematic behavior
- Substance misuse
- Unpredictability of illness trajectory
- Unstable health condition

Caregiver

- Physical conditions
- Substance misuse
- Unrealistic self-expectations
- Competing role commitments
- Ineffective coping strategies
- Inexperience with caregiving
- Insufficient emotional resilience
- Insufficient energy
- Insufficient fulfillment of others' expectations
- Insufficient fulfillment of self-expectations
- Insufficient knowledge about community resources
- Insufficient privacy
- Insufficient recreation
- Isolation
- Not developmentally ready for caregiver role
- Stressors

Caregiver–Care Receiver Relationship

- Abusive relationship
- Codependency
- Pattern of ineffective relationships
- Presence of abuse
- Unrealistic care receiver expectations
- Violent relationship

Caregiving Activities

- Around-the-clock care responsibilities
- Change in nature of care activities
- Complexity of care activities
- Excessive caregiving activities
- Extended duration of caregiving required
- Inadequate physical environment for providing care
- Insufficient assistance
- Insufficient equipment for providing care
- Insufficient respite for caregiver
- Insufficient time
- Unpredictability of care situation

Family Processes

- Family isolation
- Ineffective family adaptation

- Pattern of family dysfunction
- Pattern of family dysfunction prior to the caregiving situation
- Pattern of ineffective family coping

Socioeconomic

- Alienation
- Difficulty accessing assistance
- Difficulty accessing community resources
- Difficulty accessing support
- Insufficient community resources
- Insufficient social support
- Insufficient transportation
- Social isolation

ASSOCIATED CONDITIONS

Care Receiver

- Alteration in cognitive functioning
- Chronic illness
- Congenital disorder
- Illness severity
- Psychiatric disorder
- Psychological disorder

Caregiver

- Alteration in cognitive functioning
- Health impairment
- Psychological disorder

ASSESSMENT

- Caregiver's age, sex, level of education, occupation, and marital status
- Caregiver's physical and mental status, including chronic health problems, self-care abilities, mobility limitations, and level of cognitive function
- Care recipient's physical and mental status, including illness, self-care limitations, mobility limitations, and level of cognitive function
- Patient's physical and mental status, including history of psychiatric illness, self-care limitations, and level of cognitive function
- Support systems, including financial resources, family members and friends, community services, health-related services such as geriatric day care, and home health aides
- Home environment, including layout, structural barriers, need for equipment or assistive devices, and availability of transportation
- Cultural, ethnic, and religious background
- Perceived and actual obligations of caregiver
- Caregiver's personal strengths, including coping and problem-solving abilities and participation in diversional activities or hobbies
- Family roles, coping patterns, family alliances, goals, and values

DEFINING CHARACTERISTICS

Caregiving Activities

- Apprehensiveness about future ability to provide care
- Apprehensiveness about future health of care receiver
- Apprehensiveness about potential institutionalization of care receiver
- Apprehensiveness about well-being of care receiver if unable to provide care
- Difficulty completing required tasks
- Difficulty performing required tasks
- Dysfunctional change to caregiving activities
- Preoccupation with care routine

Caregiver Health Status: Physiologic

- Fatigue
- Gastrointestinal distress
- Headache
- Hypertension
- Rash
- Weight change

Caregiver Health Status: Emotional

- Alteration in sleep pattern
- Anger
- Depression
- Emotional vacillation
- Frustration
- Impatience
- Ineffective coping strategies
- Insufficient time to meet personal needs
- Nervousness
- Somatization
- Stressors

Caregiver Health Status: Socioeconomic

- Change in leisure activities
- Low work productivity
- Refusal of career advancement
- Social isolation

Caregiver–Care Receiver Relationship

- Difficulty watching care receiver with illness
- Grieving changes in relationship with care receiver
- Uncertainty about changes in relationship with care receiver

Family Processes

- Concern about family member(s)
- Family conflict

- Caregiver will fulfill role responsibilities/activities/behaviors to best of ability.
- Caregiver will describe current stressors.
- Caregiver will discuss how patient's illness has altered established roles and responsibilities within family.
- Caregiver will identify which stressors can and can't be controlled.
- Caregiver will refrain from using destructive coping mechanisms, such as substance abuse and physical or mental abuse of care recipient.
- Caregiver will identify formal and informal sources of support.
- Caregiver will show evidence of using support systems.
- Caregiver will report increased ability to cope with stress.

Suggested NOC Outcomes

Caregiver Emotional Health; Caregiver Lifestyle Disruption; Caregiver Physical Health; Caregiver Stressors; Caregiver Well-Being; Caregiving Endurance Potential; Family Support During Treatment; Role Performance

PCC
- Help caregiver to identify current stressors in order *to evaluate the causes of role strain.*
- Assist caregiver to clarify needs, set individual goals, and develop plans to meet them. *This will instill in each person a sense of empowerment and control over life.*

PCC
- Using a nonjudgmental approach, help caregiver evaluate which stressors are controllable and which aren't *to begin to develop strategies to reduce stress.*

PCC
- Encourage caregiver to discuss coping skills used to overcome similar stressful situations in the past *to build confidence for managing the current situation.*

T&C
- Encourage caregiver to participate in a support group. Provide information on organizations such as Alzheimer's Association, Children of Aging Parents, Al-Anon, the referral service of the community AIDS task force, etc., *to foster mutual support and provide an opportunity for caregiver to discuss personal feelings with empathetic listeners.*

- Encourage discussion among family members about role changes and added responsibilities that have occurred as a result of the patient's health status *to establish open and honest communication among family members.*

- Encourage discussion of family's past experience with crises, comparing them with the present situation *to help family see they have survived difficulties together and encourage them to seek viable solutions.*

PCC
- Encourage family members to retain involvement with social and religious networks *to avoid feelings of isolation and abandonment.*

T&C
- Help caregiver identify informal sources of support, such as family members, friends, church groups, and community volunteers, *to provide resources for obtaining an occasional or regularly scheduled respite.*

T&C
- Help caregiver identify available formal support services, such as home health agencies, municipal or county social services, hospital social workers, physicians, clinics, and day care centers, *to enhance coping by providing a reliable structure for support.*

- If caregiver seems overly anxious or distraught, gently point out facts about care recipient's mental and physical condition. *Many times, especially when care recipient is a family member, caregiver's perspective is clouded by a long history of emotional involvement. Your input may help caregiver view the situation more objectively.*

T&C ▦ If you believe that excessive emotional involvement is hindering caregiver's ability to function, consider recommending Codependents Anonymous, a support group for people whose preoccupation with a relationship leads to chronic suffering and diminished effectiveness, *to provide support.*

▦ Refer family to appropriate professional services *to ensure their needs are being met. Caregiver support groups may provide the family with helpful strategies that have worked for others facing the same problems.*

Suggested NIC Interventions

Active Listening; Caregiver Support; Coping Enhancement; Counseling; Normalization Promotion; Role Enhancement; Support Group; Home Maintenance Assistance

EVALUATIONS FOR EXPECTED OUTCOMES

▦ Caregiver identifies and develops a realistic appraisal of each stressful situation.
▦ Caregiver adjusts to changes in roles and responsibilities.
▦ Caregiver doesn't exhibit signs of stress.
▦ Caregiver uses community resources, as needed.
▦ Caregiver describes emotional response to each stressful situation.
▦ Caregiver identifies sources of support.
▦ Caregiver uses available support systems.
▦ Caregiver uses appropriate coping skills for each stressful situation.
▦ Caregiver attends support groups or seeks other forms of professional assistance.

DOCUMENTATION

▦ Stressors (perceived and actual) identified by caregiver
▦ Role adjustment and flexibility of family members
▦ Coping patterns
▦ Observations of caregiver's response to stressful situations
▦ Referrals provided
▦ Caregiver's use of informal and formal support systems
▦ Coping strategies identified by caregiver and nurse
▦ Evidence of improvement in caregiver's ability to cope
▦ Response to nursing interventions
▦ Evaluations for expected outcomes

REFERENCES

Besser, L. M., & Galvin, J. E. (2018). Perceived burden among caregivers of patients with frontotemporal degeneration in the United States. *International Psychogeriatrics.* doi:10.1017/S104161021800159X

Kajiwara, K., Noto, H., & Yamanaka, M. (2018). Changes in caregiving appraisal among family caregivers of persons with dementia: A longitudinal study over 12 months. *Psychogeriatrics, 18*(6), 460–467. doi:10.1111/psyg.12360

Leonidou, C., & Giannousi, Z. (2018). Experiences of caregivers of patients with metastatic cancer: What can we learn from them to better support them? *European Journal of Oncology Nursing, 32,* 25–32. doi:10.1016/j.ejon.2017.11.002

Liu, H., Yang, C., Wang, Y., Hsu, W., Huang, T., Lin, Y., ... Shyu, Y. L. (2017). Balancing competing needs mediates the association of caregiving demand with caregiver role strain and depressive symptoms of dementia caregivers: A cross-sectional study. *Journal of Advanced Nursing, 73*(12), 2962–2972. doi:10.1111/jan.13379

Risk for Caregiver Role Strain

DEFINITION

Susceptible to difficulty in fulfilling care responsibilities, expectations, and/or behaviors for family or significant others, which may compromise health

RISK FACTORS

Care Receiver

- Dependency
- Discharged home with significant needs
- Increase in care needs
- Problematic behavior
- Substance misuse
- Unpredictability of illness trajectory
- Unstable health condition

Caregiver

- Substance misuse
- Unrealistic self-expectations
- Competing role commitments
- Ineffective coping strategies
- Inexperience with caregiving
- Insufficient emotional resilience
- Insufficient energy
- Insufficient fulfillment of others' expectations
- Insufficient fulfillment of self-expectations
- Insufficient knowledge about community resources
- Insufficient privacy
- Insufficient recreation
- Isolation
- Not developmentally ready for caregiver role
- Physical conditions
- Stressors

Caregiver–Care Receiver Relationship

- Abusive relationship
- Codependency
- Pattern of ineffective relationships
- Presence of abuse
- Unrealistic care receiver expectations
- Violent relationship

Caregiving Activities

- Around-the-clock care responsibilities
- Change in nature of care activities
- Complexity of care activities
- Excessive caregiving activities

- Extended duration of caregiving required
- Inadequate physical environment for providing care
- Insufficient assistance
- Insufficient equipment for providing care
- Insufficient respite for caregiver
- Insufficient time
- Unpredictability of care situation

Family Processes

- Family isolation
- Ineffective family adaptation
- Pattern of family dysfunction
- Pattern of family dysfunction prior to the caregiving situation
- Pattern of ineffective family coping

Socioeconomic

- Alienation
- Difficulty accessing assistance
- Difficulty accessing community resources
- Difficulty accessing support
- Insufficient community resource
- Insufficient social support
- Insufficient transportation
- Social isolation

ASSOCIATED CONDITIONS

Care Receiver

- Alteration in cognitive functioning
- Chronic illness
- Congenital disorder
- Illness severity
- Psychological disorder
- Psychiatric disorder

Caregiver

- Alteration in cognitive functioning
- Health impairment
- Psychological disorder

ASSESSMENT

- Caregiver's age, gender, and general health
- Caregiver's physical and mental status, including chronic health problems, self-care abilities, mobility limitations, and level of cognitive function
- Care recipient's physical and mental status, including illness, self-care limitations, mobility limitations, and level of cognitive function
- Family status, including role performance and perception of role within family

- Support systems, including financial resources, family members and friends, community services, and health-related services, such as geriatric day care and home health aides
- Home environment, including layout, structural barriers, need for equipment or assistive devices, and availability of transportation
- Cultural, ethnic, and religious background
- Perceived and actual obligations of caregiver
- Caregiver's personal strengths, including usual coping and problem-solving abilities and participation in diversional activities or hobbies

EXPECTED OUTCOMES

- Caregiver will report reduced stress related to caregiver duties.
- Caregiver will identify current stressors.
- Caregiver will realistically describe current obligations and challenges that lie ahead.
- Caregiver will distinguish obligations that must be fulfilled from those that can be controlled or limited.
- Caregiver will identify appropriate coping strategies and will state plans to incorporate strategies into daily routine.
- Caregiver will state intention to contact formal and informal sources of support.
- Caregiver will contact sources of support to help provide care.
- Caregiver will allot time each day for respite, recreation, and personal developmental activities.
- Caregiver will report satisfaction with ability to cope with stress caused by caregiving responsibilities.

Suggested NOC Outcomes

Caregiver Emotional Health; Caregiver Home Care Readiness; Caregiver Lifestyle Disruption; Caregiver–Patient Relationship; Caregiver Physical Health; Caregiver Stressors; Caregiving Endurance Potential; Rest

INTERVENTIONS AND RATIONALES

PCC ▪ Help caregiver identify current stressors. Ask whether stress is likely to increase or decrease in the future *to evaluate the risk of caregiver role strain.*

PCC ▪ Encourage caregiver to discuss coping skills used to overcome similar stressful situations in the past *to bolster caregiver's confidence in ability to manage current situation and explore ways to apply coping strategies before caregiver becomes overwhelmed.*

T&C ▪ Help caregiver identify informal sources of support, such as family members, friends, church groups, and community volunteers, *to plan for an occasional or regularly scheduled respite.*

T&C ▪ Help caregiver identify available formal support services, such as home health agencies, municipal or county social services, hospital social workers, physicians, clinics, and day care centers, *to help lessen risk of strain on caregiver.*

PCC ▪ Encourage caregiver to discuss hobbies or diversional activities. *Incorporating enjoyable activities into the daily or weekly schedule will discipline caregiver to take needed breaks from caregiving responsibilities and thereby diminish stress.*

T&C ▪ Encourage caregiver to participate in a support group. Provide information on organizations such as Alzheimer's Association, Children of Aging Parents, Al-Anon, or the referral service of the community task force for AIDS, etc., *to foster mutual support and provide an outlet for expressing feelings before frustration becomes overwhelming.*

T&C ▦ If caregiver seems overly anxious or distraught, gently point out facts about care recipient's mental and physical condition. *Many times, especially when care recipient is a family member, caregiver's perspective is clouded by a long history of emotional involvement. Your input may help caregiver view the situation more objectively.* If you believe that excessive emotional involvement is hindering caregiver's ability to function, consider recommending Codependents Anonymous, a support group for people whose preoccupation with a relationship leads to chronic suffering and diminished effectiveness, *to provide support.*

Suggested NIC Interventions

Caregiver Support; Coping Enhancement; Exercise Promotion; Home Maintenance Assistance; Referral; Respite Care; Role Enhancement; Support Group

EVALUATIONS FOR EXPECTED OUTCOMES

▦ Caregiver identifies and develops a realistic appraisal of each stressful situation.
▦ Caregiver describes coping strategies used in stressful situations.
▦ Caregiver develops realistic assessment of situation.
▦ Caregiver distinguishes obligations that must be fulfilled from those the caregiver can control or limit.
▦ Caregiver identifies and uses adaptive coping strategies.
▦ Caregiver uses available support systems.
▦ Caregiver incorporates recreational activities into daily routine.
▦ Caregiver reports satisfaction in coping with stress.

DOCUMENTATION

▦ Current stressors identified by caregiver
▦ Risk factors (developmental, physiologic, psychological, and situational) for caregiver role strain identified by nurse
▦ Caregiver's statements indicating intention to take action to minimize stress, such as seeking help from support services, participating in a caregiver support group, and scheduling time for recreational activities
▦ Coping strategies identified by caregiver and nurse
▦ Observations of caregiver's response to stressful situations
▦ Referrals provided
▦ Evaluations for expected outcomes

REFERENCES

Ariza-Vega, P., Ortiz-Piña, M., Kristensen, M. T., Castellote-Caballero, Y., & Jiménez-Moleón, J. J. (2019). High perceived caregiver burden for relatives of patients following hip fracture surgery. *Disability & Rehabilitation, 41*(3), 311–318. doi:10.1080/09638288.2017.1390612

Liu, H., Yang, C., Wang, Y., Hsu, W., Huang, T., Lin, Y., … Shyu, Y. L. (2017). Balancing competing needs mediates the association of caregiving demand with caregiver role strain and depressive symptoms of dementia caregivers: A cross-sectional study. *Journal of Advanced Nursing, 73*(12), 2962–2972. doi:10.1111/jan.13379

Paúl, C., Teixeira, L., Duarte, N., Pires, C. L., & Ribeiro, O. (2019). Effects of a community intervention program for dementia on mental health: The importance of secondary caregivers in promoting positive aspects and reducing strain. *Community Mental Health Journal, 55*(2), 296–303. doi:10.1007/s10597-018-0345-6

Wang, T., & Anderson, J. A. (2018). Predicting caregiver strain to improve supports for the caregivers of children with emotional and behavioral disorders. *Journal of Family Issues, 39*(4), 896–916. doi:10.1177/0192513X16683986

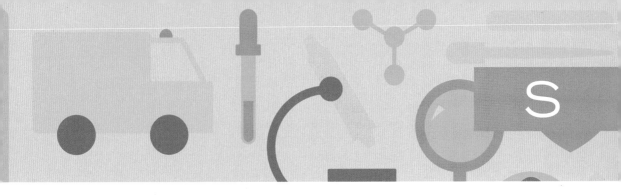

Bathing Self-Care Deficit

Inability to independently or complete cleansing activities

- Anxiety
- Decrease in motivation
- Environmental barrier
- Pain
- Weakness

- Alteration in cognitive functioning
- Impaired ability to perceive body part
- Impaired ability to perceive spatial relationships
- Musculoskeletal impairment
- Neuromuscular impairment
- Perceptual disorders

- Age
- History of injury or disease associated with musculoskeletal impairment, neurologic, sensory, or psychological impairment
- Self-care abilities, including knowledge and use of adaptive equipment, preparation of equipment and supplies, and technical or mechanical skills
- Musculoskeletal status, including coordination; functional ability; gait; mechanical restriction (such as cast, splint, and traction); muscle tone, size, and strength; range of motion; and tremors
- Neurologic status, including cognition, communication ability, insight or judgment, level of consciousness, memory, sensory and motor ability, and orientation
- Psychosocial status, including coping mechanisms, family members, lifestyle, patient's perceptions of health problem and self, and personality

- Impaired ability to access bathroom
- Impaired ability to access water

- Impaired ability to dry body
- Impaired ability to gather bathing supplies
- Impaired ability to regulate bath water
- Impaired ability to wash body

EXPECTED OUTCOMES

- Patient will demonstrate ability to perform bathing.
- Patient will have bathing self-care needs met.
- Patient will have few, if any, complications.
- Patient and family members will carry out self-care program daily.
- Patient will communicate feelings about limitations.
- Patient and family members will demonstrate correct use of assistive devices.
- Patient and family members will carry out bathing and hygiene program daily.

Suggested NOC Outcomes

Adaptation to Physical Disability; Energy Conservation; Pain Level; Self-Care: Activities of Daily Living (ADLs); Self-Care: Bathing; Self-Care: Hygiene; Self-Care: Oral Hygiene

INTERVENTIONS AND RATIONALES

- Assess patient's functional, cognitive, and perceptual level at established intervals. Document and report any changes. *Ongoing assessment allows you to identify changing needs and adjust interventions accordingly.*
- **PCC** Observe patient's functional, perceptual, and cognitive level every shift; document and report any changes. *Careful observation helps you adjust nursing actions to meet patient's needs.*
- **EBP** Perform the prescribed treatment for underlying condition. Monitor patient's progress, reporting favorable and adverse responses to treatment. *Applying therapy consistently aids patient's independence.*
- **PCC** Encourage patient to voice feelings and concerns about self-care deficits *to help patient achieve the highest functional level possible.*
- **PCC** Monitor the completion of bathing and hygiene daily, offering direction and instruction as needed. Praise patient's accomplishments. *Reinforcement and rewards may encourage renewed effort.*
- **PCC** Allow ample time to perform self-care. Encourage child to complete each task. Provide constructive feedback. *Rushing creates unnecessary stress and promotes failure. Completing a task without assistance promotes self-confidence. Positive feedback encourages progress.*
- **PCC** Provide privacy for self-care activities. *Providing privacy fosters patient dignity.*
- **S** Provide safety equipment such as nonslip mats, grab bars, and shower seats *to promote safety.*
- **S** Provide assistive devices, such as a long-handled toothbrush, for bathing and hygiene; instruct patient on use. *Appropriate assistive devices encourage independence.*
- **PCC** Assist with or perform bathing and hygiene daily. Assist only when patient has difficulty *to promote feeling of independence.*
- **EBP** Instruct patient and family members in bathing and hygiene techniques (you can give family members written instructions). Have patient and family members demonstrate bathing and hygiene under supervision. *Return demonstration identifies problem areas and increases patient's and family members' self-confidence.*
- **T&C** As needed, refer patient to a psychiatric liaison nurse, support group, or home health care agency. *These extra resources will reinforce activities planned to meet patient's needs.*

Suggested NIC Interventions

Bathing; Behavior Modification; Discharge Planning; Ear Care; Foot Care; Hair Care; Nail Care; Self-Care Assistance; Teaching: Individual

EVALUATIONS FOR EXPECTED OUTCOMES

- Patient meets bathing self-care needs.
- Patient accepts help from staff if needed.
- Patient participates in activities that minimize risk of such complications as infection and skin integrity alteration.
- Patient expresses feelings about self-care deficit. If unable to meet own needs, patient seeks assistance from a family member or the staff within 24 hours.
- Patient or family members demonstrate appropriate use of assistive devices.
- Patient follows daily bathing and hygiene program. Family members assist, as needed.

DOCUMENTATION

- Patient's expression of feelings and concerns about self-care limitations and their impact on body image and lifestyle
- Patient's willingness to participate in bathing and hygiene routine
- Observations of patient's impaired ability to perform self-care
- Patient's response to treatment of underlying condition
- Interventions to provide supportive care
- Patient's response to nursing interventions
- Instructions to patient and family members and their understanding of instructions and demonstrated skill in carrying out self-care functions
- Evaluations for expected outcomes

REFERENCES

Greiman, L., Fleming, S. P., Ward, B., Myers, A., & Ravesloot, C. (2018). Life starts at home: Bathing, exertion and participation for people with mobility impairment. *Archives of Physical Medicine & Rehabilitation, 99*(7), 1289–1294.

Ramos de Aguiar Prado, A., Ramos, R. L., Pimenta Lopes Ribeiro, O. M., Almeida de Figueiredo, N. M., Martins, M. M., & Alves Machado, W. C. (2017). Bath for dependent patients: Theorizing aspects of nursing care in rehabilitation. *Revista Brasileira de Enfermagem, 70*(6), 1337–1342.

Vining, R. D., Gosselin, D. M., Thurmond, J., Case, K., & Bruch, F. R. (2017). Interdisciplinary rehabilitation for a patient with incomplete cervical spinal cord injury and multimorbidity: A case report. *Medicine, 96*(34), 1–6.

Zwakhalen, S. M. G., Hamers, J. P. H., Metzelthin, S. F., Ettema, R., Heinen, M., de Man, V. G. J. M., … Schuurmans, M. J. (2018). Basic nursing care: The most provided, the least evidence based—A discussion paper. *Journal of Clinical Nursing, 27*(11–12), 2496–2505.

Dressing Self-Care Deficit

DEFINITION

Inability to independently put on or remove clothing

RELATED FACTORS (R/T)

- Anxiety
- Decrease in motivation

- Discomfort
- Environmental barrier
- Fatigue
- Pain
- Weakness

ASSOCIATED CONDITIONS

- Alteration in cognitive functioning
- Musculoskeletal impairment
- Neuromuscular impairment
- Perceptual disorders

ASSESSMENT

- History of neurologic, sensory, psychological, or musculoskeletal impairment
- Age
- Self-care abilities, including knowledge and use of adaptive equipment, preparation of equipment and supplies, and technical or mechanical skills
- Musculoskeletal status, including coordination; functional ability; gait; mechanical restriction (such as cast, splint, and traction); muscle tone, size, and strength; range of motion; and tremors
- Neurologic status, including cognition, communication ability, insight or judgment, level of consciousness, memory, motor and sensory ability, and orientation
- Psychosocial status, including coping mechanisms, family members, lifestyle, patient's perceptions of health problem and self, and personality

DEFINING CHARACTERISTICS

- Impaired ability to choose clothing
- Impaired ability to fasten clothing
- Impaired ability to gather clothing
- Impaired ability to maintain appearance
- Impaired ability to pick up clothing
- Impaired ability to put clothing on lower body
- Impaired ability to put clothing on upper body
- Impaired ability to put on various items of clothing
- Impaired ability to remove clothing item
- Impaired ability to use assistive device
- Impaired ability to use zipper

EXPECTED OUTCOMES

- Patient will have dressing self-care needs met.
- Patient will have few, if any, complications.
- Patient will communicate feelings about limitations.
- Patient and family members will demonstrate correct use of assistive devices.
- Patient and family members will carry out dressing program daily.
- Patient and family members will identify resources to help cope with problems and discharge.

Suggested NOC Outcomes

Self-Care: Dressing; Self-Care: Grooming; Self-Care: Activities of Daily Living (ADLs)

INTERVENTIONS AND RATIONALES

`PCC` ■ Assess patient's functional, cognitive, and perceptual level at periodic intervals. Document and report any changes. *Ongoing assessment allows you to identify changing needs and adjust interventions accordingly.*

`PCC` ■ Observe patient's functional, perceptual, and cognitive level every shift; document and report any changes. *Careful observation helps you adjust nursing actions to meet patient's needs.*

`EBP` ■ Perform the prescribed treatment for the underlying musculoskeletal condition. Monitor patient's progress, reporting favorable and adverse responses to treatment. *Applying therapy consistently aids patient's independence.*

`PCC` ■ Encourage patient to voice feelings and concerns about self-care deficits *to help patient achieve the highest functional level.*

`PCC` ■ Provide privacy *to enhance patient's dignity.*

`PCC` ■ Provide enough time for patient to perform dressing and grooming. *Rushing creates unnecessary stress and promotes failure.*

`PCC` ■ Monitor patient's abilities to dress and groom daily. *This identifies problem areas before they become sources of frustration.*

`PCC` ■ Encourage family members to provide clothing patient can easily manage. Patient may benefit from clothing slightly larger than regular size and Velcro straps. *Such clothing makes independent dressing easier.*

`S` ■ Provide necessary assistive devices, such as a long-handled shoehorn and zipper pull as needed. Instruct patient on use. *Appropriate assistive devices encourage independence.*

`PCC` ■ Assist with or perform dressing and grooming: fasten clothes, comb hair, and clean nails. Provide help only when patient has difficulty *to promote feeling of independence.*

`EBP` ■ Instruct patient and family members in dressing and grooming techniques (you can give family members written instructions). Have patient and family members demonstrate dressing and grooming techniques under supervision. *Return demonstration reveals problem areas and increases self-confidence.*

`T&C` ■ As needed, refer patient to a psychiatric liaison nurse, support group, or home health care agency. *Extra resources reinforce activities planned to meet patient's needs.*

Suggested NIC Interventions

Body Image Enhancement; Energy Management; Self-Care Teaching: Individual; Hair Care; Self-Care Assistance: Dressing/Grooming; Skin Surveillance

EVALUATIONS FOR EXPECTED OUTCOMES

■ Patient meets dressing self-care needs.
■ Patient accepts help from staff if needed.
■ Patient participates in activities designed to minimize risk of complications.
■ Patient expresses feelings about self-care limitations.
■ Patient and family members demonstrate appropriate use of assistive devices.
■ Patient follows daily dressing and grooming program. Family members assist, as needed.

DOCUMENTATION

■ Patient's expression of feelings and concerns about self-care limitations and their impact on body image and lifestyle
■ Patient's willingness to participate in dressing and grooming

- Observations of patient's impaired ability to perform dressing and grooming
- Interventions to provide supportive care
- Patient's response to nursing interventions
- Instructions given to patient and family members, their understanding of instructions, and their demonstrated skill in carrying out self-care functions
- Evaluations for expected outcomes

REFERENCES

Buse, C., & Twigg, J. (2018). Dressing disrupted: Negotiating care through the materiality of dress in the context of dementia. *Sociology of Health & Illness, 40*(2), 340–352.

Kosar, C. M., Thomas, K. S., Gozalo, P. L., & Mor, V. (2018). Higher level of obesity is associated with intensive personal care assistance in the nursing home. *Journal of the American Medical Directors Association, 19*(11), 1015–1019.

Raffaele, B., Biagioli, V., Cirillo, L., De Marinis, M. G., & Matarese, M. (2018). Cross-validation of the Self-care Ability Scale for Elderly (SASE) in a sample of Italian older adults. *Scandinavian Journal of Caring Sciences, 32*(4), 1398–1408. doi:10.1111/scs.12585

Feeding Self-Care Deficit

DEFINITION

Inability to eat independently

RELATED FACTORS (R/T)

- Anxiety
- Decrease in motivation
- Discomfort
- Environmental barrier
- Fatigue
- Pain
- Weakness

ASSOCIATED CONDITIONS

- Alteration in cognitive functioning
- Musculoskeletal impairment
- Neuromuscular impairment
- Perceptual disorders

ASSESSMENT

- Age
- History of neurologic, sensory, psychological or musculoskeletal impairment
- Self-care abilities, including knowledge and use of adaptive equipment, preparation of equipment and supplies, and technical and mechanical skills
- Musculoskeletal status, including coordination; functional ability; gait; mechanical restriction (such as cast, splint, and traction); muscle tone, size, and strength; range of motion; and tremors
- Psychosocial status, including coping mechanisms, family members, lifestyle, motivation, patient's perception of health problem and self, and personality

DEFINING CHARACTERISTICS

- Impaired ability to bring food to mouth
- Impaired ability to chew food
- Impaired ability to get food onto utensil
- Impaired ability to handle utensils
- Impaired ability to manipulate food in mouth
- Impaired ability to open containers
- Impaired ability to pick up cup
- Impaired ability to prepare food
- Impaired ability to self-feed a complete meal
- Impaired ability to self-feed in an acceptable manner
- Impaired ability to swallow food
- Impaired ability to swallow sufficient amount of food
- Impaired ability to use assistive device

EXPECTED OUTCOMES

- Patient will have feeding self-care needs met.
- Patient will have few, if any, complications.
- Patient will express feelings about feeding limitations.
- Patient and family members will demonstrate correct use of assistive devices.
- Patient and family members will carry out feeding program daily.
- Patient and family members will identify resources to help cope with problems and discharge.

Suggested NOC Outcomes

Nutritional Status; Self-Care: Activities of Daily Living (ADLs); Self-Care: Eating; Swallowing Status

INTERVENTIONS AND RATIONALES

PCC ▪ Assess patient's functional, cognitive, and perceptual level at periodic intervals. Document and report any changes. *Ongoing assessment allows you to identify changing needs and adjust interventions accordingly.*

PCC ▪ Observe patient's functional, perceptual, and cognitive level every shift; document and report changes. *Careful observation helps you adjust nursing actions to meet patient's needs.*

EBP ▪ Perform the prescribed treatment for the underlying condition. Monitor patient's progress and report responses. *Applying therapy consistently aids patient's independence.*

S ▪ Weigh patient weekly and record weight. Report a change of more than 1 lb/week *to ensure adequate nutrition and fluid balance.*

S ▪ Monitor and record breath sounds every 4 hours *to check for aspiration of food.* Report crackles, wheezes, or rhonchi.

PCC ▪ Encourage patient to express feelings and concerns about feeding deficits *to help patient achieve the highest functional level.* Provide emotional support to help patient come to terms with self-care deficit and achieve the highest functional level.

PCC ▪ Initiate an ordered feeding program:
  - Determine the types of food best handled by patient *to encourage patient's feelings of independence.*

▧ Place patient in high Fowler position to feed *to aid swallowing and digestion.* Support weakened extremities and wash patient's face and hands before meals.

▧ Provide assistive devices; instruct patient on their use *to allow more independence.*

▧ Supervise or assist at each meal—for example, cut food into small pieces. *This aids chewing, swallowing, and digestion and reduces the risk of choking or aspiration.*

▧ Feed patient slowly. *Rushing causes stress, reducing digestive activity and causing intestinal spasms.*

▧ Keep suction equipment at the bedside *to remove aspirated foods, if necessary.*

▧ Instruct patient and family members in feeding techniques and equipment. *This aids understanding and encourages compliance.*

▧ Record the percentage of food consumed *to ensure adequate nutrition.*

PCC ▧ Encourage patient to carry out the aspects of feeding according to patient's abilities. *This gives patient a sense of achievement and control.*

T&C ▧ Refer patient to a psychiatric liaison nurse, support group, or such community agencies as Visiting Nurse Association and Meals on Wheels. *Additional resources reinforce activities planned to meet patient's needs.*

Suggested NIC Interventions

Fluid Management; Nutrition Management; Nutritional Monitoring; Self-Care Assistance: Feeding; Swallowing Therapy; Aspiration Precautions; Family Involvement Promotion

EVALUATIONS FOR EXPECTED OUTCOMES

▧ Patient meets feeding self-care needs.

▧ Patient accepts help from staff if needed.

▧ Patient participates in activities designed to minimize risk of complications.

▧ Patient and family members demonstrate proper use of assistive devices.

▧ Patient follows daily self-care feeding program. Family members provide assistance, as needed.

▧ Patient and family members identify and contact available support resources, as needed.

DOCUMENTATION

▧ Patient's expression of feelings and concerns about inability to feed self

▧ Observations of patient's impaired ability to perform self-care

▧ Patient's response to treatment

▧ Patient's weight

▧ Patient's intake

▧ Interventions to provide supportive care

▧ Instructions given to patient and family members, their understanding of instructions, and their demonstrated skill in carrying out self-care functions

▧ Patient's response to interventions

▧ Evaluations for expected outcomes

REFERENCES

Batchelor, M. M. K., McConnell, E. S., Amella, E. J., Anderson, R. A., Bales, C. W., Silva, S., … Colon, E. C. S. (2017). Experimental comparison of efficacy for three handfeeding techniques in dementia. *Journal of the American Geriatrics Society, 65*(4), e89–e94. doi:10.1111/jgs.14728

Roberts, H., Pilgrim, A., Jameson, K., Cooper, C., Sayer, A., & Robinson, S. (2017). The impact of trained volunteer mealtime assistants on the dietary intake of older female in-patients: The

Southampton Mealtime Assistance Study. *Journal of Nutrition, Health & Aging, 21*(3), 320–328. doi:10.1007/s12603-016-0791-1

Sakamoto, M., Watanabe, Y., Edahiro, A., Motokawa, K., Shirobe, M., Hirano, H., ... Yoshihara, A. (2019). Self-feeding ability as a predictor of mortality Japanese nursing home residents: A two-year longitudinal study. *Journal of Nutrition, Health & Aging, 23*(2), 157–164. doi:10.1007/s12603-018-1125-2

Toileting Self-Care Deficit

DEFINITION

Inability to independently perform tasks associated with bowel and bladder elimination

RELATED FACTORS (R/T)

- Anxiety
- Decrease in motivation
- Discomfort
- Environmental barrier
- Fatigue
- Pain
- Weakness

ASSOCIATED CONDITIONS

- Alteration in cognitive functioning
- Musculoskeletal impairment
- Neuromuscular impairment
- Perceptual disorders

ASSESSMENT

- Age
- History of neurologic, sensory, psychological, or musculoskeletal impairment
- Self-care abilities, including knowledge and use of adaptive equipment, preparation of equipment and supplies, and technical or mechanical skills
- Musculoskeletal status, including coordination; functional ability; gait; mechanical restriction (such as cast, splint, and traction); muscle tone, size, and strength; range of motion; and tremors
- Neurologic status, including cognition, communication ability, insight or judgment, level of consciousness, memory, motor and sensory ability, and orientation
- Psychosocial status, including coping mechanisms, family members, lifestyle, patient's perceptions of health problem and self, and personality

DEFINING CHARACTERISTICS

- Impaired ability to complete toilet hygiene
- Impaired ability to flush toilet
- Impaired ability to manipulate clothing for toileting
- Impaired ability to reach toilet
- Impaired ability to rise from toilet
- Impaired ability to sit on toilet

EXPECTED OUTCOMES

- Patient will have toileting self-care needs met.
- Patient will have few, if any, complications.
- Patient will communicate feelings about limitations.
- Patient and family members will demonstrate correct use of assistive devices.
- Patient and family members will carry out toileting program daily.
- Patient and family members will identify resources to help cope with problems and discharge from facility.

Suggested NOC Outcomes

Self-Care: Activities of Daily Living (ADLs); Self-Care: Hygiene; Self-Care: Toileting

INTERVENTIONS AND RATIONALES

PCC ■ Observe patient's functional, perceptual, and cognitive level every shift; document and report any changes. *Careful observation helps you adjust nursing actions to meet patient's needs.*

EBP ■ Perform the prescribed treatment for the underlying condition. Monitor patient's progress, reporting favorable and adverse responses to treatment. *Applying therapy consistently aids patient's independence.*

PCC ■ Encourage patient to voice feelings and concerns about self-care deficits *to help patient achieve the highest functional level possible.*

S ■ Monitor intake and output and skin condition; record episodes of incontinence. *Accurate intake and output records can identify potential imbalances.*

S ■ Use assistive devices, as needed, such as an external catheter at night, a bedpan or urinal every 2 hours during the day, and adaptive equipment for bowel care. Instruct on use. As control improves, reduce the use of assistive devices. *Assisting at an appropriate level helps maintain patient's self-esteem.*

PCC ■ Assist with toileting only if needed. Allow patient to perform independently as much as possible *to promote independence.*

EBP ■ Instruct patient and family members in toileting routine (you can give family members written instructions). Have patient and family members demonstrate toileting routine under supervision. *Return demonstration identifies problem areas and increases patient's self-confidence.*

PCC ■ Provide positive, constructive feedback when assisting with toileting. *Reinforcement and rewards may enhance self-esteem.*

PCC ■ Assist with toileting, giving simple instructions one at a time, *to aid comprehension.*

PCC ■ Complete urinary and bowel care if patient can't do so. Follow urinary and bowel elimination plans. *Monitoring success or failure of toileting plans helps identify and resolve problem areas.*

T&C ■ As needed, refer patient to a psychiatric liaison nurse, support group, or home health care agency. *Extra resources reinforce activities planned to meet patient's needs.*

Suggested NIC Interventions

Bowel Training; Self-Care Assistance: Toileting; Urinary Elimination Management; Bowel Incontinence Care

- Patient meets toileting self-care needs.
- Patient accepts help from staff if needed.
- Patient and family members express feelings about self-care deficit. If unable to meet own needs, patient seeks assistance from family member or staff within 24 hours.
- Patient and family members demonstrate appropriate use of assistive devices.
- Patient follows toileting program daily. Family members assist, as needed.
- Patient and family members identify and contact available support resources, as needed.

- Patient's expression of feelings and concerns about self-care limitations and their impact on body image and lifestyle
- Patient's willingness to participate in self-care
- Observations of patient's ability to perform toileting routine and patient's response to treatment
- Patient's intake and output
- Interventions to provide supportive care
- Instructions given to patient and family members, their understanding of instructions, and their demonstrated skill in carrying out self-care functions
- Patient's response to nursing interventions
- Evaluations for expected outcomes

REFERENCES

Imanishi, M., Tomohisa, H., & Higaki, K. (2017). Impact of continuous in-home rehabilitation on quality of life and activities of daily living in elderly clients over 1 year. *Geriatrics & Gerontology International, 17*(11), 1866–1872. doi:10.1111/ggi.12978

King, E. C., Holliday, P. J., & Andrews, G. J. (2018). Care challenges in the bathroom: The views of professional care providers working in clients' homes. *Journal of Applied Gerontology, 37*(4), 493–515. doi:10.1177/0733464816649278

Rojas, J., Joseph, J., Liu, B., Srikumaran, U., & McFarland, E. G. (2018). Can patients manage toileting after reverse total shoulder arthroplasty? A systematic review. *International Orthopaedics, 42*(10), 2423–2428. doi:10.1007/s00264-018-3900-4

Readiness for Enhanced Self-Care

A pattern of performing activities for oneself to meet health-related goals, which can be strengthened

- Patient's perception of adequacy of self-care
- Patient's attitude toward use of health care services
- Self-care abilities, including knowledge and use of adaptive equipment, preparation of equipment and supplies, and technical and mechanical skills
- Neurologic status, including cognition, communication ability, insight or judgment, level of consciousness, memory, sensory and motor ability, and orientation
- Psychosocial status, including coping mechanisms, family members, lifestyle, patient's perceptions of self, and personality

DEFINING CHARACTERISTICS

- Expresses desire to enhance independence with health
- Expresses desire to enhance independence with life
- Expresses desire to enhance independence with personal development
- Expresses desire to enhance independence with well-being
- Expresses desire to enhance knowledge of self-care strategies
- Expresses desire to enhance self-care

EXPECTED OUTCOMES

- Patient will demonstrate positive decision-making toward maximizing potential for self-care.
- Patient will express satisfaction with independence in assuming responsibility for planning self-care.
- Patient and family members will involve staff, family, and community in developing strategies for self-care.
- Patient will monitor self-care measures taken for effectiveness and make alterations as needed.

Suggested NOC Outcomes

Self-Care: Activities of Daily Living (ADLs); Adherence Behavior; Client Satisfaction: Functional Assistance; Health Beliefs: Perceived Ability to Perform

INTERVENTIONS AND RATIONALES

- **PCC** Assess patient's satisfaction with level of self-care *to support general well-being.*
- **PCC** Assess current ability to provide self-care *to establish a baseline.*
- **PCC** Assess effectiveness of self-care measures *to identify the need for adjustments.*
- **PCC** Assist patient in developing plan *to promote autonomous decision-making to increase patient's responsibility for facilitating care.*
- **EBP** Provide information that supports implementation of a program to sustain health-seeking behavior *to promote patient autonomy in self-care.*
- **PCC** Encourage health team, family, and community efforts to participate in patient's self-care initiatives *to promote satisfactory mutual goal setting and group efforts.*
- **T&C** Encourage patient and his or her family to participate in support networks that promote patient independence where possible *to promote patient and family resilience.*
- **T&C** Develop a referral list for community resources to promote patient's enhanced self-care.

Suggested NIC Interventions

Mutual Goal Setting; Resiliency Promotion; Self-Responsibility Facilitation

EVALUATIONS FOR EXPECTED OUTCOMES

- Patient meets self-care needs.
- Patient expresses awareness of need to maintain independence in health management.
- Patient makes positive decisions to maximize self-care abilities.
- Patient expresses satisfaction with independence in self-care.
- Patient develops and maintains a plan for enhanced self-care.
- Patient involves staff, family, and community in developing strategies for self-care.
- Patient monitors self-care and changes needed.

DOCUMENTATION

- Patient's expression of self-care needs
- Observations of patient's impaired ability to perform self-care activities
- Interventions to provide supportive care
- Patient's response to nursing interventions
- Evaluations for expected outcomes

REFERENCES

Jeong, H. W., & So, H. S. (2018). Structural equation modeling of self-care behaviors in kidney transplant patients based on self-determination theory. *Journal of Korean Academy of Nursing, 48*(6), 731–742. doi:10.4040/jkan.2018.48.6.731

Nadrian, H., Shojafard, J., Mahmoodi, H., Rouhi, Z., & Rezaeipandari, H. (2018). Cognitive determinants of self-care behaviors among patients with heart failure: A path analysis. *Health Promotion Perspectives, 8*(4), 275–282. doi:10.15171/hpp.2018.39

Shad, F. S., Rahnama, M., Abdollahimohammad, A., Ahmadi, S., & Sima, D. (2018). An investigation into the impact of Orem's self-care program on life satisfaction in hemodialysis patients: A clinical trial study. *Medical-Surgical Nursing Journal, 7*(4), 1–6. doi:10.5812/msnj.88795

Readiness for Enhanced Self-Concept

DEFINITION

A pattern of perceptions or ideas about the self, which can be strengthened

ASSESSMENT

- Age
- Gender
- Developmental stage
- Health problems
- Past experience with health care system
- Mental status
- Belief system (norms, values, religion)
- Social interaction patterns
- Family system
- Perception of self (past and present), including body image, coping mechanisms, problem-solving ability, and self-worth

DEFINING CHARACTERISTICS

- Acceptance of limitations
- Acceptance of strengths
- Actions congruent with verbal expressions
- Expresses confidence in abilities
- Expresses desire to enhance role performance
- Expresses desire to enhance self-concept
- Expresses satisfaction with body image
- Expresses satisfaction with personal identity
- Expresses satisfaction with sense of worth
- Expresses satisfaction with thoughts about self

▤ Patient will articulate long- and short-term goals.
▤ Patient will express motivation necessary to achieve goals.
▤ Patient will develop realistic plan to achieve stated goals.
▤ Patient will practice self-management strategies needed to be successful.
▤ Patient will evaluate progress and modify behavior as needed.

Suggested NOC Outcomes

Body Image; Neglect Recovery; Personal Autonomy; Self-Esteem

EBP ▤ Provide patient with materials and resources on health-related issues that affect the individual's attitude. *Knowledge will enhance or inhibit patient's motivation or resolve.*

EBP ▤ Answer questions related to written material *so patient is adequately prepared to establish realistic goals.*

PCC ▤ Assist patient in writing long- and short-term goals. *These goals can serve as tools for self-evaluation as new behaviors are being practiced.*

PCC ▤ Have patient list one or two realistic, practical behaviors that will facilitate achieving goals. *The more positive the behaviors are, the greater the chance patient has of being successful.*

PCC ▤ Assist patient to determine positive rewards for successful behavioral changes. *Reinforcement is needed for new behavior to continue.*

Suggested NIC Interventions

Hope Instillation; Self-Awareness Enhancement; Self-Responsibility Facilitation

▤ Patient has realistic goals and workable plan for change.
▤ Patient responds positively to changes in self-concept.
▤ Patient demonstrates interest in evaluating progress.
▤ Patient shows a willingness to modify plan to continue reaching goals.

▤ Patient's expressions of self-concept
▤ Patient's adherence to plan
▤ Modifications to plan
▤ Patient's response to nursing interventions
▤ Evaluations for expected outcomes

REFERENCES

Maïano, C., Coutu, S., Morin, A. J. S., Tracey, D., Lepage, G., & Moullec, G. (2019). Self-concept research with school-aged youth with intellectual disabilities: A systematic review. *Journal of Applied Research in Intellectual Disabilities, 32*(2), 238–255. doi:10.1111/jar.12543

Xu, Q., Li, S., & Yang, L. (2019). Perceived social support and mental health for college students in mainland China: The mediating effects of self-concept. *Psychology, Health & Medicine, 24*(5), 595–604. doi:10.1080/13548506.2018.1549744

Wong, A. E., & Vallacher, R. R. (2018). Reciprocal feedback between self-concept and goal pursuit in daily life. *Journal of Personality, 86*(3), 543–554. doi:10.1111/jopy.12334

Risk for Self-Directed Violence

DEFINITION

Susceptible to behaviors in which an individual demonstrates that he or she can be physically, emotionally, and/or sexually harmful to self

RISK FACTORS

- Behavioral cues of suicidal intent
- Conflict about sexual orientation
- Conflict in interpersonal relationship(s)
- Employment concern
- Engaged in autoerotic sexual acts
- Insufficient personal resources
- Social isolation
- Suicidal ideation
- Suicidal plan
- Verbal cues of suicidal intent

ASSOCIATED CONDITIONS

- Mental health issue
- Physical health issue
- Psychological disorder

ASSESSMENT

- Age
- Gender
- Developmental stage
- Race
- Religion
- Marital status (widowed, divorced, married, or single)
- Life situation, including isolation (living alone or in urban area) and recent retirement, unemployment, or move to new area
- Recent stressors, including divorce, death of spouse, and relocation
- Availability of weapons or toxic substances
- Mood and affect, including persistent depression; feelings of worthlessness, hopelessness, helplessness, isolation, inadequacy, and humiliation; deterioration in school work; and flat, distant, remote affect
- Behavioral changes, including loss of interest in personal appearance, overeating or eating too little, verbal or written cues or preoccupation with death, threats of suicide, acting out (such as sexual promiscuity, delinquency, or running away), low energy level, sleep disturbances, frequent naps, irritability, somatic and physical complaints, antisocial or self-destructive behavior, tendency to be accident-prone, and acts of self-mutilation
- Psychological status, including loss of interest in hobbies and preferred activities, refusal to attend school (cutting class and truancy), social withdrawal and isolation, academic problems, and feelings of rejection by peers and social group

EXPECTED OUTCOMES

- Patient won't harm self.
- Patient will discuss sadness, despair, and other feelings.
- Patient will acknowledge suicidal thoughts.

- Patient will receive referral to mental health professional.
- Patient will report decreased desire to kill self.
- Patient will discuss appropriate coping skills to avoid future suicidal episodes.
- Patient will discuss feelings that precipitated suicide attempt.
- Patient will attend therapy sessions with mental health professional.
- Patient will describe available resources for crisis prevention and management.
- Patient will report improved feelings of self-worth.

Suggested NOC Outcomes

Depression Self-Control; Impulse Self-Control; Mood Equilibrium; Quality of Life; Self-Mutilation Restraint; Suicide Self-Restraint; Will to Live

INTERVENTIONS AND RATIONALES

S ▪ Take all suicide threats seriously. *Early intervention reduces the likelihood of a suicide attempt.*

PCC ▪ Ask patient directly, "Have you thought about killing yourself?" If patient says yes, ask, "What do you plan to do?" *Suicide risk increases if patient has a definite plan.*

S ▪ Assess for signs of suicidal thinking that warrant further investigation, such as sudden hoarding of medications, giving away possessions, sudden interest in guns, and despondent remarks, *to determine if patient is at risk for suicide.*

S ▪ Remove any objects that the adolescent could use for self-inflicted injury, such as razors, belts, glass objects, and pills, *to ensure safety.*

S ▪ Arrange supervision (preferably one-on-one) for patient according to facility policy. This ensures compliance with legal requirements *to protect patient while demonstrating staff concern.*

PCC ▪ Make a contract with patient against self-harm for a specific period. Continue negotiating until there's no evidence of suicidal ideation. *A contract puts the subject of suicide in the open, places some responsibility for safety on the patient, and demonstrates your regard for the patient as worthwhile.*

S ▪ Supervise administration of all prescribed medications and be aware of their actions and possible adverse effects. *Medications may be a treatment alternative. By watching as they're administered, you prevent patient from hoarding doses (sometimes called "cheeking"), thus ensuring patient's safety.*

PCC ▪ Set aside time for listening to patient *to communicate that you care.*

PCC ▪ Assess patient for signs and symptoms of depression, such as a persistent depressed mood, diminished interest in daily activities, sleep disturbances, inappropriate guilt, loss of energy, poor concentration, changes in appetite, psychomotor retardation or agitation, and a passive wish for death. *Elderly patients are at increased risk for depression. Depression increases in frequency and intensity with advancing age. Factors that contribute to an increase in depression include changes in neurotransmitter levels, multiple losses, diminished health, and decreased resources. Depression may also occur in the early stages of dementia.*

PCC ▪ Discuss the problems that led patient to this episode of depression. *Talking about specific events may help patient achieve catharsis and develop appropriate coping skills.* Events that may contribute to depression in older patients include recent major loss, experience of rejection by or isolation from family or friends, recent disability, loss of partner, loss of sexual function, and loss of social, family, or occupational role.

PCC ▪ Recognize patient's feelings of inadequacy and take steps to bolster self-esteem. Encourage patient to participate in a life review, revisit places where significant past events took place, put together a scrapbook, research family genealogy, or attend family, class, or church reunions. *These activities help patient experience emotions, which ultimately promotes improved self-esteem.*

PCC ▪ Avoid comparing patient with others *to reduce stereotyping and foster individuality.*

PCC ▪ Support patient but don't give false reassurances that everything will work out. Let patient know that, although no easy answer exists, help is available and you'll help find alternative solutions *to ease despair.*

PCC ▪ Convey a caring, nonjudgmental attitude when talking with patient. *This demonstrates your unconditional positive regard and helps establish a trusting relationship.*

PCC ▪ Listen carefully as patient talks. Don't challenge patient's statements or reinforce denial of the current situation. *This communicates caring, support, and understanding without reinforcing denial, which usually masks underlying suicidal feelings.*

PCC ▪ Encourage patient to set a goal of cooperating with psychiatric intervention. *Ambivalence about psychiatric care or refusal to attend sessions indicates that patient is still in denial.*

T&C ▪ Help patient identify community resources *to obtain continued therapy and support after hospitalization.*

T&C ▪ Provide patient and patient's family members with telephone numbers for crisis prevention centers, suicide hotlines, counselors, and other community support services. *Having many alternatives for support helps reduce the patient's anxiety.*

Suggested NIC Interventions

Behavior Management: Self-Harm; Counseling; Crisis Intervention; Family Involvement Promotion; Mutual Goal Setting; Suicide Prevention; Support Group

EVALUATIONS FOR EXPECTED OUTCOMES

▪ Patient doesn't harm self.
▪ Patient expresses feelings and thoughts in way that promotes healing process.
▪ Patient discusses events that led up to current crisis.
▪ Patient acknowledges suicidal thoughts.
▪ Patient receives referral to mental health professional.
▪ Patient states experiencing fewer suicidal thoughts.
▪ Patient expresses understanding the importance of increased social support and improved coping skills in avoiding future suicidal episodes.
▪ Patient discusses feelings and reasons for attempting suicide.
▪ Patient attends counseling sessions with mental health professional.
▪ Patient describes crisis prevention resources, such as hotline telephone number, local crisis center, or name of therapist.
▪ Patient expresses improved sense of self-worth.

DOCUMENTATION

▪ Patient's description of feelings before and after suicide attempt
▪ Observations of patient's behavior, mood, and affect
▪ Nursing interventions to reduce or prevent self-destructive behavior
▪ Patient's response to interventions
▪ Evaluations for expected outcomes

REFERENCES

Gupta, D., & Kumar, S. (2018). Suicide: Managing self-directed violence? *Indian Journal of Community Health*, 30(4), 411–414.

Hoffberg, A. S., Spitzer, E., Mackelprang, J. L., Farro, S. A., & Brenner, L. A. (2018). Suicidal self-directed violence among homeless US veterans: A systematic review. *Suicide & Life-Threatening Behavior*, 48(4), 481–498. doi:10.1111/sltb.12369

Holliday, R., Wortzel, H., & Matarazzo, B. (2018). Words matter: The language of suicidal self-directed violence. *Psychiatric Times*, 35(12), 8–9.

Chronic Low Self-Esteem

DEFINITION

Long-standing negative perception of self-worth, self-acceptance, self-respect, competence, and attitude toward self

RELATED FACTORS (R/T)

- Decreased mindful acceptance
- Difficulty managing finances
- Disturbed body image
- Fatigue
- Fear of rejection
- Impaired religiosity
- Inadequate affection received
- Inadequate attachment behavior
- Inadequate family cohesiveness
- Inadequate group membership
- Inadequate respect from others
- Inadequate sense of belonging
- Inadequate social support
- Ineffective communication skills
- Insufficient approval from others
- Low self-efficacy
- Maladaptive grieving
- Negative resignation
- Repeated negative reinforcement
- Spiritual incongruence
- Stigmatization
- Stressors
- Values incongruent with cultural norms

ASSOCIATED CONDITION

- Depression
- Functional impairment
- Mental disorders
- Physical illness

ASSESSMENT

- Reason for hospitalization or outpatient treatment
- Age
- Gender
- Developmental stage
- Family system, including marital status, role in family, and sibling position
- Perception of health problem
- Past experience with health care system
- Mental status, including abstract thinking, affect, communication, general appearance, judgment or insight, memory, mood, orientation, perception, and thinking process
- Belief system, including norms, religion, and values
- Social interaction pattern
- Social and occupational history

- Perception of self (past and present), including body image, coping mechanisms, problem-solving ability, and self-worth
- Past experience with crisis
- Past history of treatment for psychosocial disturbance, including hospitalization, medication, psychotherapy, and suicidal ideation, plans, and attempts
- Neurovegetative signs, including ability to experience pleasure, appetite, energy level, and sleep

DEFINING CHARACTERISTICS

- Dependent on others' opinions
- Depressive symptoms
- Excessive guilt
- Excessive seeking of reassurance
- Expresses loneliness
- Hopelessness
- Insomnia
- Loneliness
- Nonassertive behavior
- Overly conforming behaviors
- Reduced eye contact
- Rejects positive feedback
- Reports repeated failures
- Rumination
- Self-negating verbalizations
- Shame
- Suicidal ideation
- Underestimates ability to deal with situation

EXPECTED OUTCOMES

- Patient will voice positive feelings about self.
- Patient will gradually join in self-care and decision-making process.
- Patient will engage in social interaction with others.
- Patient will demonstrate verbal and behavioral decrease in negative self-evaluation.
- Patient will voice acceptance of positive and negative feedback without exaggeration.

Suggested NOC Outcomes

Body Image; Depression Level; Mood Equilibrium; Motivation; Personal Autonomy; Quality of Life; Self-Esteem

INTERVENTIONS AND RATIONALES

PCC — Provide for a specific amount of uninterrupted time each day to engage patient in conversation. *This time will allow the patient time for self-exploration.*

S — When appropriate, institute suicide precaution according to protocol. *Patient needs supervision until patient demonstrates adequate self-control to ensure own safety.*

PCC — Provide patient with a simple structured daily routine. *Structured activity limits the patient's anxious behavior.*

PCC — Spend time alone with patient listening to patient's problems that are important to him or her at this time. Have patient make a list of the three most critical issues currently in focus. *Spending this time can allow the opportunity to help patient identify strengths and begin setting some realistic goals to build self-confidence.*

PCC ■ Encourage bathing, grooming, and other hygiene functions for patient every day as needed. Encourage patient to do as much as possible independently. *Greater independence will help strengthen self-esteem.*

EBP ■ Teach self-healing techniques to both patient and family, such as meditation, guided imagery, yoga, and prayer, *to prevent anxiety and aid in keeping patient in a frame of mind to make positive decisions.*

EBP ■ Teach patient how to incorporate the use of self-healing techniques in carrying out usual daily activities.

EBP ■ Provide patient with concise information about decision-making skills. *This will produce benefits that can reinforce health-seeking behaviors.*

PCC ■ Encourage patient to express feelings about self (past and present). *Self-exploration encourages patient to consider future change.*

PCC ■ Provide patient with positive feedback for verbal reports or behaviors that indicate a return to positive self-appraisal. *This gives patient feelings of significance, approval, and competence, which can help cope effectively with stressful situations.*

PCC ■ Encourage social interaction between patient and others. Disturbed interpersonal relationships are a direct expression of self-hate.

PCC ■ Facilitate opportunities for spiritual nourishment and growth *to address patient's holistic needs for maximal therapeutic environment.*

PCC ■ Encourage patient's cooperation as you continue with healing techniques, such as therapeutic touch.

PCC ■ Provide emotional support to family by being available to answer questions. *Accurate information will help family to cope with current situation.*

T&C ■ Assist patient in mobilizing resources for assistance when discharged in order *to help the patient replace maladaptive coping behaviors with more adaptive ones.*

PCC ■ Schedule time to meet with family and patient to listen to ways in which they plan to enhance their coping skills in the present situation. *Helping patient and/or family develop a realistic plan will better ensure success in meeting established goals.*

T&C ■ Refer family to community resources and support groups available *to assist in managing patient's illness and providing emotional and financial assistance to caregivers.*

Suggested NIC Interventions

Active Listening; Body Image Enhancement; Coping Enhancement; Decision-Making Support; Hope Instillation; Self-Esteem Enhancement; Spiritual Support; Support Group

EVALUATIONS FOR EXPECTED OUTCOMES

■ Patient expresses feelings about self-esteem.
■ Patient participates in at least one aspect of self-care daily.
■ Patient converses with others on daily basis.
■ Patient states at least two positive aspects about self.
■ Patient accepts positive feedback and constructive criticism.

DOCUMENTATION

■ Patient's verbal expressions and behaviors that indicate low self-esteem
■ Mental status examination (baseline and ongoing)
■ Suicide assessment, interventions, and patient's response
■ Nursing interventions implemented to promote self-esteem
■ Patient's response to interventions
■ Evaluations for expected outcomes

REFERENCES

Evans, L., & Allez, K. (2018). Cognitive behaviour therapy for low self-esteem in a person with a learning disability: A case study. *Advances in Mental Health & Intellectual Disabilities, 12*(2), 67–76. doi:10.1108/AMHID-06-2017-0023

Junker, A., Nordahl, H. M., Bjørngaard, J. H., & Bjerkeset, O. (2019). Adolescent personality traits, low self-esteem and self-harm hospitalisation: A 15-year follow-up of the Norwegian Young-HUNT1 cohort. *European Child & Adolescent Psychiatry, 28*(3), 329–339. doi:10.1007/s00787-018-1197-x

van Geel, M., Goemans, A., Zwaanswijk, W., Gini, G., & Vedder, P. (2018). Does peer victimization predict low self-esteem, or does low self-esteem predict peer victimization? Meta-analyses on longitudinal studies. *Developmental Review, 49*, 31–40. doi:10.1016/j.dr.2018.07.001

Risk for Chronic Low Self-Esteem

DEFINITION

Susceptible to long-standing negative perception of self-worth, self-acceptance, self-respect, competence, and attitude toward self, which may compromise health

RISK FACTORS

- Decreased mindful acceptance
- Difficulty managing finances
- Disturbed body image
- Fatigue
- Fear of rejection
- Impaired religiosity
- Inadequate affection received
- Inadequate attachment behavior
- Inadequate family cohesiveness
- Inadequate group membership
- Inadequate respect from others
- Inadequate sense of belonging
- Inadequate social support
- Ineffective communication skills
- Insufficient approval from others
- Low self-efficacy
- Maladaptive grieving
- Negative resignation
- Repeated negative reinforcement
- Spiritual incongruence
- Stigmatization
- Stressors
- Values incongruent with cultural norms

ASSOCIATED CONDITION

Depression
Functional impairment
Mental disorders
Physical illness

ASSESSMENT

- Reason for hospitalization or outpatient treatment
- Age

- Gender
- Developmental stage
- Family system, including marital status, role in family, and sibling position
- Perception of health problem
- Past experience with health care system
- Mental status, including abstract thinking, affect, communication, general appearance, judgment or insight, memory, mood, orientation, perception, and thinking process
- Belief system, including norms, religion, and values
- Social interaction pattern
- Social and occupational history
- Perception of self (past and present), including body image, coping mechanisms, problem-solving ability, and self-worth
- Past experience with crisis
- Past history of treatment for psychosocial disturbance, including hospitalization, medication, psychotherapy, and suicidal ideation, plans, and attempts
- Neurovegetative signs, including ability to experience pleasure, appetite, energy level, and sleep

EXPECTED OUTCOMES

- Patient will attend milieu therapies and interact with peers.
- Patient will use cognitive therapies to modify negative thoughts about self.
- Patient will report decrease in feelings of anger, fear, guilt, and self-doubt.
- Patient will verbalize positive self-characteristics and accomplishments.

Suggested NOC Outcomes

Anxiety Control; Body Image; Coping; Depression Level; Mood Equilibrium; Risk Control; Self-Esteem; Social Interaction Skills

INTERVENTIONS AND RATIONALES

- **PCC** Assess patient's mental status per unit protocols. *Recurring assessments will aid in identifying interventions, expected outcomes, and allow for modifications based on patient's progress.*
- **PCC** Obtain thorough history upon admission *in order to determine if patient past history has additional risk factors for low self-esteem.*
- **PCC** Assist patient in applying cognitive therapies and positive self-talk *in order to identify and modify negative actions and thoughts that lead to feelings of anger, fear, guilt, and self-doubt.*
- **PCC** Work with patient to set a daily schedule that promotes self-care and attendance at milieu therapies and give sincere praise when patient follows through. *Independence and positive feedback from peers and staff will aid in developing self-confidence and increasing self-esteem.*
- **EBP** Educate patient on the importance of being assertive and reinforce by having patient state particular needs or preferences for the day *as this will help build independence, self-confidence, and decrease fear of rejection.*
- **EBP** Educate patient regarding the importance of setting realistic treatment goals *in order to continue to build self-confidence and self-esteem.*
- **EBP** Educate patient regarding resources available in the community, such as support groups, and *their positive impact on building self-esteem.*

PCC ▪ Dedicate quality time to patient in a therapeutic and consistent manner *in order to help patient feel safe, allow time for open expression of feelings, and allow for the development of a trusting relationship.*

PCC ▪ Work together with patient to develop a treatment plan and schedule appointments. *This will help to build patient's independence, confidence, social skills, and self-esteem.*

Suggested NIC Interventions

Anxiety Reduction; Body Image Enhancement; Cognitive Restructuring; Coping Enhancement; Self-Esteem Enhancement; Support Group

EVALUATIONS FOR EXPECTED OUTCOMES

▪ Patient attends milieu therapy.
▪ Patient interacts with peers.
▪ Patient uses cognitive therapies.
▪ Patient expresses reduction in anger, fear, self-doubt, and guilt.
▪ Patient expresses positive thoughts about self.

DOCUMENTATION

▪ Mental status assessment
▪ Cognitive therapies used
▪ Treatment goals set and results achieved
▪ Responses to interventions
▪ External agencies suggested
▪ Changes occurring as a result of using outside resources
▪ Evaluations for expected outcomes

REFERENCES

Park, A., & Kim, Y. (2018). The longitudinal influence of child maltreatment on child obesity in South Korea: The mediating effects of low self-esteem and depressive symptoms. *Children & Youth Services Review, 87,* 34–40. doi:10.1016/j.childyouth.2018.02.012

Pelletier Brochu, J., Meilleur, D., DiMeglio, G., Taddeo, D., Lavoie, E., Erdstein, J., … Frappier, J.-Y. (2018). Adolescents' perceptions of the quality of interpersonal relationships and eating disorder symptom severity: The mediating role of low self-esteem and negative mood. *Eating Disorders, 26*(4), 388–406. doi:10.1080/10640266.2018.1454806

Raykos, B. C., McEvoy, P. M., & Fursland, A. (2017). Socializing problems and low self-esteem enhance interpersonal models of eating disorders: Evidence from a clinical sample. *International Journal of Eating Disorders, 50*(9), 1075–1083. doi:10.1002/eat.22740

Situational Low Self-Esteem

DEFINITION

Change from positive to negative perception of self-worth, self-acceptance, self-respect, competence, and attitude toward self in response to a current situation

RELATED FACTORS (R/T)

▪ Behavior incongruent with values
▪ Decrease in environmental control
▪ Decreased mindful acceptance

- Difficulty accepting alteration in social role
- Difficulty managing finances
- Disturbed body image
- Fatigue
- Fear of rejection
- Impaired religiosity
- Inadequate attachment behavior
- Inadequate family cohesiveness
- Inadequate respect from others
- Inadequate social support
- Ineffective communication skills
- Low self-efficacy
- Maladaptive perfectionism
- Negative resignation
- Powerlessness
- Stigmatization
- Stressors
- Unrealistic self-expectations
- Values incongruent with cultural norms

ASSOCIATED CONDITIONS

- Depression
- Functional impairment
- Mental disorders
- Physical illness

ASSESSMENT

- Age
- Gender
- Developmental stage
- Level of education
- Family history, including marital status of parents, financial status, family rules, ability of family to modify rules, consequences when rules are broken, how family members communicate, quality of communication, methods of conflict resolution, family alliances, family stability, ability of family to meet patient's physical and emotional needs, and disparities between patient's needs and family's ability to meet them
- Goals and values, including extent to which family permits patient to pursue individual goals and values
- Reason for health care visit
- Mental status, including affect, general appearance, and mood
- Cognitive ability
- Behavior
- Perception of self (past and present), including body image, coping mechanisms, and self-worth

DEFINING CHARACTERISTICS

- Depressive symptoms
- Expresses loneliness

- Helplessness
- Indecisive behavior
- Insomnia
- Loneliness
- Nonassertive behavior
- Purposelessness
- Rumination
- Self-negating verbalizations
- Underestimates ability to deal with situation

EXPECTED OUTCOMES

- Patient will describe positive qualities about self.
- Patient will voice feelings related to current situation and its effect on self-esteem.
- Patient will verbally appraise self before and during current health problem.
- Patient will participate in decisions related to care and therapies.
- Patient will report sense of control over life events.
- Patient will articulate return to previous positive feelings about self.

Suggested NOC Outcomes

Decision-Making; Grief Resolution; Psychosocial Adjustment: Life Change; Self-Esteem

INTERVENTIONS AND RATIONALES

S ▪ Assess patient for suicidal ideations or thoughts of violence to self or others. *It is necessary to determine this so early intervention can be taken to prevent injury to patient and those around.*

EBP ▪ Provide a secure, structured environment for patient *to foster open discussion of conflicts.*

PCC ▪ Encourage patient to express feelings about self (past and present). *Self-exploration encourages patient to consider future change.*

PCC ▪ Provide a specific amount of uninterrupted noncare-related time to engage patient in conversation. *Such discussions help patient assume ultimate responsibility for coping responses.*

PCC ▪ Explore patient's usual coping mechanisms in times of stress. Suggest additional positive methods of coping. Role-play with patient in *order to help patient see what healthy coping mechanisms look like.*

PCC ▪ Assess patient's mental status through interview and observation at least once per day. *If anxiety resulting from self-rejection becomes severe, patient may experience disorientation and psychotic symptoms.*

PCC ▪ Involve patient in the decision-making process. *Making such decisions can help combat ambivalence and procrastination associated with low self-esteem.*

PCC ▪ Provide patient with positive feedback for verbal reports or behaviors that indicate a return to positive self-appraisal. *This gives patient feelings of significance, approval, and competence, which can help in coping effectively with stressful situations.*

T&C ▪ Provide information about appropriate support groups and encourage interacting with individuals who have successfully adapted to illness or limitations *to increase patient's coping skills.*

Suggested NIC Interventions

Anticipatory Guidance; Decision-Making Support; Grief Work Facilitation; Self-Esteem Enhancement

EVALUATIONS FOR EXPECTED OUTCOMES

- Patient uses positive statements about self.
- Patient expresses feelings about self in relation to recent stressful events.
- Patient makes decisions related to care daily.
- Patient reports feeling more self-confident and in control of current situation.
- Patient states at least two positive feelings about self.

DOCUMENTATION

- Patient's expressions of lowered self-esteem
- Mental status assessment (baseline and ongoing)
- Nursing interventions directed toward return to previous positive self-esteem
- Patient's response to interventions
- Evaluations for expected outcomes

REFERENCES

Cengiz, M., Demirbag, B. C., & Yıldizlar, O. (2018). The effect of mobbing in workplace on professional self-esteem of nurses. *International Journal of Caring Sciences, 11*(2), 1241–1246.

Kim, H. S., & Shin, S. R. (2017). The Influence of social support among community dwelling elderly and their attitude towards the withdrawal of life-sustaining treatment: A mediating effect of self-esteem. *Korean Journal of Adult Nursing, 29*(4), 373–381. doi:10.7475/kjan.2017.29.4.373

Sharma, G., Prakash, K., & Narayan, P. J. (2018). Effectiveness of teaching regarding individualized coping strategy on self-esteem of cancer patients undergoing radiation therapy in selected cancer research institute, Dehradun, Uttarakhand. *International Journal of Nursing Education, 10*(4), 38–43. doi:10.5958/0974-9357.2018.00098.3

Risk for Situational Low Self-Esteem

DEFINITION

Susceptible to change from positive to negative perception of self-worth, self-acceptance, self-respect, competence, and attitude toward self in response to a current situation, which may compromise health

RISK FACTORS

- Behavior incongruent with values
- Decrease in environmental control
- Decreased mindful acceptance
- Difficulty accepting alteration in social role
- Difficulty managing finances
- Disturbed body image
- Fatigue
- Fear of rejection
- Impaired religiosity
- Inadequate attachment behavior
- Inadequate family cohesiveness
- Inadequate respect from others
- Inadequate social support
- Individuals experiencing repeated failure
- Ineffective communication skills

- Low self-efficacy
- Maladaptive perfectionism
- Negative resignation
- Powerlessness
- Stigmatization
- Stressors
- Unrealistic self-expectations
- Values incongruent with cultural norms

ASSOCIATED CONDITIONS

- Depression
- Functional impairment
- Mental disorders
- Physical illness

ASSESSMENT

- Age
- Gender
- Developmental stage
- Family system, including marital status, role in family, and sibling position
- Reason for health care visit
- Mental status, including affect, general appearance, and mood
- Cognitive ability
- Behavior
- Perception of self (past and present), including body image, coping mechanisms, and self-worth

EXPECTED OUTCOMES

- Patient will participate in decisions related to care and therapy.
- Patient will maintain eye contact and initiate conversation.
- Patient will verbally assess feelings about current situation and health problems and impact on lifestyle.
- Patient will express positive feelings about self (verbally or through behaviors), indicating acceptance of changes caused by health problems or situation.
- Patient will express interest in talking to others who have successfully overcome the problem of low self-esteem.

Suggested NOC Outcomes

Self-Esteem; Life Changes; Decision-Making; Perceived Control; Psychosocial Adjustment

INTERVENTIONS AND RATIONALES

PCC ▪ Assess developmental stage; family system; role in family; sibling position; health history; mental status, including affect, general appearance, mood; cognitive ability; support systems; patient's ability to identify choices; readiness for change to occur; and level of knowledge for positive decision-making, coping mechanisms, and environmental factors. *Information from assessment will assist the nurse in identifying appropriate interventions.*

`PCC` ▦ Encourage bathing, grooming, and other hygiene functions for the patient every day as needed. Encourage patient to do as much as possible for self. *Greater independence will help strengthen self-esteem.*

`PCC` ▦ Keep patient informed about what to expect and when to expect it. *Accurate information reduces anxiety.*

`EBP` ▦ Teach self-healing techniques to both patient and family such as meditation, guided imagery, yoga, and prayer. Teach patient how to incorporate the use of self-healing techniques in carrying out usual daily activities. *These techniques help calm the mind and promote ability to cooperate with the difficulties associated with low self-esteem.*

`PCC` ▦ Encourage patient to talk about personal assets and accomplishments and about improvements in condition no matter how small these may seem. Give positive feedback. *Conversation assists you to evaluate the patient's self-concept and adaptive abilities.*

`PCC` ▦ Provide ongoing, positive feedback about patient's behavior *to clear up misconceptions and increase feelings of self-esteem.*

`PCC` ▦ Direct patient's focus beyond the present state. *Focusing on the present state alone will make it difficult for patient to plan activities that will move patient forward.*

`T&C` ▦ Help patient involve the family, community, clergy, and friends with changes to the care plan *to increase the potential of patient's control over self-care outcomes.*

`T&C` ▦ Refer patient and family to other professional caregivers, for example, dietitian, social worker, clergy, and mental health professional. *Support groups such as ostomy clubs, I Can Cope, and Reach for Recovery can provide physical, material, financial, and emotional resources to patient and the family during the recovery period.*

`T&C` ▦ Assist patient in utilizing appropriate resources by contacting family and scheduling follow-up appointments. *This helps give patient a sense of direction and control over future care.*

Suggested NIC Interventions

Assertiveness Training; Coping Enhancement; Self-Modification Assistance; Self-Responsibility Facilitation

EVALUATIONS FOR EXPECTED OUTCOMES

▦ Patient expresses feelings about self in relation to recent stressful events.
▦ Patient makes decisions related to care daily.
▦ Patient reports feeling more self-confident and in control of current situation.
▦ Patient states at least two positive feelings about self.

DOCUMENTATION

▦ Patient's expressions of lowered self-esteem
▦ Mental status assessment (baseline and ongoing)
▦ Nursing interventions directed toward return to previous positive self-esteem
▦ Patient's response to interventions
▦ Evaluations for expected outcomes

REFERENCES

Keshtkar, Z., Nabavi, M., Bolghan-Abadi, M. (2018). The effectiveness of the integrated group therapy on increasing the prisoners' self-esteem. *International Archives of Health Sciences, 5*(4), 131–134. doi:10.4103/iahs.iahs_19_18

Li, C., & Wu, Y. (2019). Improving Special Olympics volunteers' self-esteem and attitudes towards individuals with intellectual disability. *Journal of Intellectual & Developmental Disability, 44*(1), 35–41. doi:10.3109/13668250.2017.1310815

Mohammadzadeh, M., Awang, H., Kadir Shahar, H., & Ismail, S. (2018). Emotional health and self-esteem among adolescents in Malaysian orphanages. *Community Mental Health Journal, 54*(1), 117–125. doi:10.1007/s10597-017-0128-5

Self-Mutilation

DEFINITION

Deliberate self-injurious behavior causing tissue damage with the intent of causing nonfatal injury to attain relief of tension

RELATED FACTORS (R/T)

- Absence of family confidant
- Alteration in body image
- Dissociation
- Disturbance in interpersonal relationships
- Eating disorder
- Emotional disturbance
- Feeling threatened with loss of significant relationship
- Impaired self-esteem
- Impulsiveness
- Inability to express tension verbally
- Ineffective communication between parent and adolescent
- Ineffective coping strategies
- Irresistible urge for self-directed violence
- Irresistible urge to cut self
- Isolation from peers
- Labile behavior
- Loss of control over problem-solving situation
- Low self-esteem
- Mounting tension that is intolerable
- Negative feeling
- Pattern of inability to plan solutions
- Pattern of inability to see long-term consequences
- Perfectionism
- Requires rapid stress reduction
- Substance misuse
- Use of manipulation to obtain nurturing relationship with others

ASSOCIATED CONDITIONS

- Autism
- Borderline personality disorder
- Character disorder
- Depersonalization
- Psychotic disorder

ASSESSMENT

- Age
- Gender
- Developmental history
- Current stress level and coping behaviors
- Mental status, including judgment, thought content, and mood
- Family history, including abusive behavior
- Previous episodes of self-mutilation or suicide attempts
- Substance abuse history
- Social history, including sexual activity and aggression within peer group

DEFINING CHARACTERISTICS

- Abrading
- Biting
- Constricting a body part
- Cuts on body
- Hitting
- Ingestion of harmful substances
- Inhalation of harmful substance
- Insertion of object into body orifice
- Picking at wound
- Scratches on body
- Self-inflicted burn
- Severing of a body part

EXPECTED OUTCOMES

- Patient will refrain from harming self.
- Patient will express an increased sense of security.
- Patient will report being able to cope better with disorganization, aggressive impulses, anxiety, and hallucinations.
- Patient will verbalize absence of or fewer dissociative states.
- Patient will participate in therapeutic milieu.
- Patient will describe community resources that can provide assistance when the patient feels out of control.

Suggested NOC Outcomes

Impulse Self-Control; Risk Control; Self-Mutilation Restraint

INTERVENTIONS AND RATIONALES

- **PCC** Assess behavioral responses, coping strategies, number and types of stressors, social factors, and spiritual beliefs. *Assessment information will assist in identifying appropriate goal and interventions.*
- **PCC** Move patient to a quiet room *to reduce stimuli if the patient is in a dissociative state.*
- **S** Remove all dangerous objects from patient's room *to prevent injury.* Place patient under observation *to provide protection and increase patient's sense of security.*
- **EBP** Administer psychotropic medications as prescribed *to reduce tension, impulse behavior, hallucinations, and panic.*

EBP ▪ Teach patient's coping strategies to family members. *Family members and friends can help patient practice adaptive methods of coping with self-destructive feelings.*

▪ Have patient and family members practice role-playing *to increase the confidence in the patient's ability to handle difficult situations.*

EBP ▪ Teach self-healing techniques to both patient and family such as meditation, guided imagery, yoga, and prayer. Teach patient how to incorporate the use of self-healing techniques in carrying out usual daily activities. *These techniques can reduce the anxiety that comes from attempting to cope with disease.*

EBP ▪ Teach additional skills that enhance coping and relaxation strategies for the patient and family (i.e., meditation, guided imagery, yoga, exercise). *Self-healing gives patient a better sense of control over regaining independence.*

EBP ▪ Limit the number of staff who interact with patient *to provide continuity of care and enhance a sense of security.*

PCC ▪ If patient is participating in a therapeutic milieu, discuss patient's risk of self-harm with community members *to provide patient with enhanced protection and psychological support.*

PCC ▪ If patient causes harm to self, provide care in a calm, nonjudgmental manner. Encourage discussion of feelings that caused self-mutilation *to help patient connect self-destructive behavior to feelings that preceded it and provide an opportunity to explore alternative ways of dealing with negative feelings.*

PCC ▪ Accept patient's feelings of powerlessness as normal. *This indicates respect for patient and enhances feelings of self-respect.*

PCC ▪ Encourage patient to take an active role in self-care *to promote a sense of control.*

T&C ▪ Organize frequent staff meetings *to ensure patient care is consistent with current behavior.*

T&C ▪ Organize family conferences to allow opportunities for the family to discuss their particular frustrations and hopes in relation to patient's current situation. *Family conferences can help the patient and family members ventilate true feelings in a safe environment.*

Suggested NIC Interventions

Area Restriction; Behavior Management; Self-Harm; Environmental Management; Impulse Control; Coping Behaviors; Guided Imagery; Meditation Facilitation

EVALUATIONS FOR EXPECTED OUTCOMES

▪ Patient keeps terms of verbal contract that the patient won't harm self.
▪ Patient expresses increased sense of security.
▪ Patient describes coping skills that help in dealing better with disorganization, aggressive impulses, anxiety, and hallucinations.
▪ Patient experiences fewer or no dissociative states.
▪ Patient participates in therapeutic milieu.
▪ Patient tells staff member about suicidal thoughts.

DOCUMENTATION

▪ Nursing interventions performed and patient's response to them
▪ Verbal contracts between patient and nurse
▪ Patient's responses to medication and behavior modification program
▪ Revisions to treatment plan
▪ Drawing of self-inflicted injuries
▪ Evidence of suicidal ideation
▪ Evaluations for expected outcomes

REFERENCES

Conde, E., Santos, T., Leite, R., Vicente, C., & Figueiredo, A. M. (2017). A case of genital self-mutilation in a female-symptom choice and meaning. *Journal of Sex & Marital Therapy, 43*(6), 560–566. doi:10.1080/0092623X.2016.1208699

Harner, A., & Young, L. (2019). Nonoperative management of intra-abdominal foreign bodies: Selected cases involving recurrent self-harm. *American Surgeon, 85*(1), e18–e20.

Hosie, L., & Dickens, G. L. (2018). Harm-reduction approaches for self-cutting in inpatient mental health settings: Development and preliminary validation of the Attitudes to Self-cutting Management (ASc-Me) Scale. *Journal of Psychiatric & Mental Health Nursing, 25*(9/10), 531–545. doi:10.1111/jpm.12498

Sullivan, P. J. (2019). Risk and responding to self-injury: Is harm minimisation a step too far? *Journal of Mental Health Training, Education & Practice, 14*(1), 1–11. doi:10.1108/JMHTEP-05-2018-0031

Risk for Self-Mutilation

DEFINITION

Susceptible to deliberate self-injurious behavior causing tissue damage with the intent of causing nonfatal injury to attain relief of tension

RISK FACTORS

- Absence of family confidant
- Alteration in body image
- Dissociation
- Disturbance in interpersonal relationships
- Eating disorder
- Emotional disturbance
- Feeling threatened with loss of significant relationship
- Impaired self-esteem
- Impulsiveness
- Inability to express tension verbally
- Ineffective communication between parent and adolescent
- Ineffective coping strategies
- Irresistible urge for self-directed violence
- Irresistible urge to cut self
- Isolation from peers
- Labile behavior
- Loss of control over problem-solving situation
- Low self-esteem
- Mounting tension that is intolerable
- Negative feeling
- Pattern of inability to plan solutions
- Pattern of inability to see long-term consequences
- Perfectionism
- Requires rapid stress reduction
- Substance misuse
- Use of manipulation to obtain nurturing relationship with others

ASSOCIATED CONDITIONS

- Autism
- Borderline personality disorder

- Character disorder
- Depersonalization
- Psychotic disorder

ASSESSMENT

- Age
- Gender
- Developmental history
- Current stress level and coping behaviors
- Mental status, including judgment, thought content, and mood
- Family history, including abusive behavior
- Previous episodes of self-mutilation or suicide attempts
- Substance abuse history
- Social history, including sexual activity and aggression within peer group

EXPECTED OUTCOMES

- Patient won't harm self.
- Patient will express increased sense of security.
- Patient will report being able to cope better with disorganization, aggressive impulses, anxiety, and hallucinations.
- Patient will experience fewer or no dissociative states.
- Patient will participate in therapeutic milieu.
- Patient will report suicidal thoughts to staff members.

Suggested NOC Outcomes

Abuse Recovery Status; Anxiety Level; Impulse Self-Control; Risk Control; Self-Mutilation Restraint

INTERVENTIONS AND RATIONALES

EBP - Limit the number of staff members interacting with patient *to provide continuity of care and increase patient's sense of security.*

EBP - Have staff members make frequent, short contacts with patient *to reassure patient without stifling independence.*

S - Remove all dangerous objects from patient's environment *to promote safety.*

PCC - Make short-term verbal contracts with patient on not harming self *to make patient aware about being ultimately responsible for own safety and that patient can guarantee it.*

EBP - Administer psychotropic medications as ordered *to reduce tension, impulsive behavior, hallucinations, and panic.*

- If patient enters a dissociative state or hallucinates, move patient to a quiet room with reduced stimuli. If restraint is needed, remain with patient and provide reassurance *to calm and orient patient to reality.*

EBP - As ordered, place patient under observation *to provide protection and increase patient's sense of security.* If hospitalized, patient can be "zoned" or asked to remain in areas within sight of staff members.

PCC - If patient is participating in a therapeutic milieu, discuss patient's risk of self-harm with community members *to provide enhanced protection and psychological support.*

- If patient harms self, care for injuries in a calm, nonjudgmental manner. Encourage patient to talk about the feelings that prompted self-mutilation. *Discussion may help patient connect self-destructive behavior to the feelings that preceded it and allow exploration of alternative ways of dealing with negative thoughts and feelings.*

PCC - If self-destructive acts persist, consider developing a behavior modification program in which patient is rewarded with benefits (personal attention, material items) for demonstrating self-control *to reinforce self-control.*

PCC - Ask patient directly whether patient is thinking of suicide and if so, what the plan is. *A self-destructive patient may become suicidal and may require additional precautions.*

T&C - Hold frequent treatment team meetings *to ensure consistent care that's appropriate to patient's current behavior.*

Suggested NIC Interventions

Area Restriction; Behavior Management: Self-Harm; Environmental Management: Violence Prevention; Impulse Control Training; Limit Setting

EVALUATIONS FOR EXPECTED OUTCOMES

- Patient keeps terms of verbal contract on not harming self.
- Patient expresses increased sense of security.
- Patient describes coping skills that help in dealing better with disorganization, aggressive impulses, anxiety, and hallucinations.
- Patient experiences fewer or no dissociative states.
- Patient participates in therapeutic milieu.
- Patient tells staff member about suicidal thoughts.

DOCUMENTATION

- Nursing interventions performed and patient's response to them
- Verbal contracts between patient and nurse
- Patient's responses to medication and behavior modification program
- Revisions to treatment plan
- Drawing of self-inflicted injuries
- Evidence of suicidal ideation
- Evaluations for expected outcomes

REFERENCES

Cully, G., Corcoran, P., Leahy, D., Griffin, E., Dillon, C., Cassidy, E., … Arensman, E. (2019). Method of self-harm and risk of self-harm repetition: Findings from a national self-harm registry. *Journal of Affective Disorders, 246*, 843–850. doi:10.1016/j.jad.2018.10.372

Dickens, G. L., & Hosie, L. (2018). Self-cutting and harm reduction: Evidence trumps values but both point forward. *Journal of Psychiatric & Mental Health Nursing, 25*(9/10), 529–530. doi:10.1111/jpm.12508

Gholamzadeh, S., Zahmatkeshan, M., Zarenezhad, M., Ghaffari, E., & Hoseni, S. (2017). The pattern of self-harm in Fars Province in South Iran: A population-based study. *Journal of Forensic & Legal Medicine, 51*, 34–38. doi:10.1016/j.jflm.2017.07.003

Gillies, D., Christou, M. A., Dixon, A. C., Featherston, O. J., Rapti, I., Garcia-Anguita, A., … Christou, P. A. (2018). Prevalence and characteristics of self-harm in adolescents: Meta-analyses of community-based studies 1990-2015. *Journal of the American Academy of Child & Adolescent Psychiatry, 57*(10), 733–741. doi:10.1016/j.jaac.2018.06.018

Self-Neglect

DEFINITION

A constellation of culturally framed behaviors involving one or more self-care activities in which there is a failure to maintain a socially accepted standard of health and well-being (Gibbons, Lauder, & Ludwick, 2006)

RELATED FACTORS (R/T)

- Deficient executive function
- Fear of institutionalization
- Inability to maintain control
- Lifestyle choice
- Stressors
- Substance misuse

ASSOCIATED CONDITIONS

- Alteration in cognitive functioning
- Capgras syndrome
- Frontal lobe dysfunction
- Functional impairment
- Learning disability
- Malingering
- Psychiatric disorder
- Psychotic disorder

ASSESSMENT

- Age
- Gender
- Self-care status including bathing, hygiene, grooming, feeding, and toileting
- Cultural status including cultural norms
- Patient's understanding of problem, coping mechanisms, problem-solving ability, and family system

DEFINING CHARACTERISTICS

- Insufficient environmental hygiene
- Insufficient personal hygiene
- Nonadherence to health activity

EXPECTED OUTCOMES

- Patient will demonstrate adequate personal hygiene.
- Patient will adhere to prescribed health activities.
- Patient will demonstrate improved ability to maintain complex health circumstances, including environmental hygiene, nutrition, and fitness.

Suggested NOC Outcomes

Adherence Behavior; Compliance Behavior; Decision-Making; Health Orientation; Motivation; Personal Well-Being; Risk Control; Self-Care Status

PCC ▪ Assess patient with complex health issues for adequate coping abilities. *Poor coping skills may lead to unintentional self-neglect.*

PCC ▪ Assess patient with failing self-care for changes in cognitive function. *Neglected self-care may be the first noticeable sign of diminishing cognitive function.*

PCC ▪ Involve patient's family in care activities as appropriate *to improve the chance that the patient will incorporate recommended regimens into lifestyle as long-term choice.*

EBP ▪ Teach strategies to enhance adherence to medication and other health regimens. *Some instances of self-neglect occur because patient has not been able to incorporate recommended regimens into lifestyle.*

PCC ▪ Encourage patient to identify internally motivating factors for adhering to health regimens. *Persons who intentionally neglect self-care as a lifestyle choice (i.e., fail to comply with medication and treatment regimens) will fare better if the decision to improve self-care is their decision.*

T&C ▪ Refer patient demonstrating a significant decline in self-care abilities (i.e., posing a threat to self and/or community) for competency evaluation. *Unintentional self-neglect may indicate diminished competency.*

Suggested NIC Interventions

Behavior Management; Counseling; Exercise Promotion; Limit Setting; Mutual Goal Setting; Self-Care Assistance; Self-Responsibility Facilitation; Weight Management

EVALUATIONS FOR EXPECTED OUTCOMES

▪ Patient performs adequate personal hygiene.
▪ Patient adheres to prescribed health activities.
▪ Patient demonstrates ability to maintain complex health circumstances, including environmental hygiene, nutrition, and fitness.
▪ Patient is able to cope with complex health situation in a positive way.

DOCUMENTATION

▪ Patient's cognitive, functional, and mental health status
▪ Patient's method of coping with circumstances
▪ Evaluations for expected outcomes

REFERENCES

Gibbons, S., Lauder, W., & Ludwick, R. (2006). Self-neglect: A proposed new NANDA diagnosis. *International Journal of Nursing Terminologies and Classifications*, 17, 10–18. doi:10.1111/j.1744-618X.2006.00018.

Li, J., Zhao, D., Dong, B., Yu, D., Ren, Q., Chen, J., … Sun, Y. (2018). Frailty index and its associations with self-neglect, social support and sociodemographic characteristics among older adults in rural China. *Geriatrics & Gerontology International*, 18(7), 987–996. doi:10.1111/ggi.13280

Preston-Shoot, M. (2019). Self-neglect and hoarding: A guide to safeguarding and support. *Journal of Adult Protection*, 21(1), 65–68. doi:10.1108/JAP-02-2019-052

Storey, J. E., & Prashad, A. A. (2018). Recognizing, reporting, and responding to abuse, neglect, and self-neglect of vulnerable adults: An evaluation of the re:act adult protection worker basic curriculum. *Journal of Elder Abuse & Neglect*, 30(1), 42–63. doi:10.1080/08946566.2017 .1371092

Sexual Dysfunction

DEFINITION

A state in which an individual experiences a change in sexual function during the sexual response phases of desire, arousal, and/or orgasm, which is viewed as unsatisfying, unrewarding, or inadequate

RELATED FACTORS (R/T)

- Absence of privacy
- Inadequate role model
- Insufficient knowledge about sexual function
- Misinformation about sexual function
- Presence of abuse
- Psychosocial abuse
- Value conflict
- Vulnerability

ASSOCIATED CONDITIONS

- Alteration in body function
- Alteration in body structure

ASSESSMENT

- Age
- History of problem that caused change in structure or function
- Patient's perception of change's effect
- Marital status and attitude of spouse or significant other
- Living arrangement
- Usual sexual patterns
- Sexual problems before current health problem
- Patient's attitude toward modifying sexual patterns
- Psychological variables, including patient's perception of sexual performance, relationships, desire for erection, guilt, shame, relationship with parents, and family or social pressures
- Physiologic status, including medication history (response, effectiveness, and adverse reactions) and history of substance abuse (type and effect on mental status)
- Sociocultural factors, including educational level, socioeconomic status, ethnic group, and religious beliefs and practices
- Sexual history, including sexual drive, sexual preference, frequency of impotence, premature ejaculation, spontaneous morning erections, positive coital experiences, types of erotic stimulation used, past professional counseling or sex therapy, homosexual experiences, affairs (other partners or prostitutes), and feelings of anger, hostility, or disgust toward partner
- Patient's present knowledge about appropriate options available

DEFINING CHARACTERISTICS

- Alteration in sexual activity
- Alteration in sexual excitation

- Alteration in sexual satisfaction
- Change in interest toward others
- Change in self-interest
- Change in sexual role
- Decrease in sexual desire
- Perceived sexual limitation
- Seeking confirmation of desirability
- Undesired change in sexual function

EXPECTED OUTCOMES

- Patient will acknowledge problem or potential problem in sexual function.
- Patient will voice feelings about changes in sexual identity.
- Patient will explain reason for sexual dysfunction.
- Patient will reestablish sexual activity at preillness level.
- Patient will learn methods to enhance sexual pleasure for self and partner and incorporate them into sexual activities.
- Patient will continue to communicate with partner about sexual issues and needs.
- Patient will agree to obtain sexual evaluation and therapy, if needed.
- Patient will develop and maintain positive attitude toward own sexuality and sexual performance.

Suggested NOC Outcomes

Adaptation to Physical Disability; Body Image; Fear Level; Physical Aging; Role Performance; Sexual Functioning; Sexual Identity; Stress Level

INTERVENTIONS AND RATIONALES

PCC ▪ Provide a nonthreatening atmosphere and encourage patient to ask questions about personal sexuality. *A nonthreatening atmosphere encourages patient to ask questions specifically related to the current situation.*

PCC ▪ Establish a therapeutic relationship with patient *to provide a safe, comfortable atmosphere for discussing sexual concerns.*

PCC ▪ Encourage patient to discuss feelings and perceptions about sexual dysfunction *to help patient validate perceptions and reduce emotional distress through catharsis.*

PCC ▪ Encourage patient and partner to discuss feelings and perceptions *to help the couple clarify issues about their relationship and improve communication.*

EBP ▪ Educate patient and partner about alternative methods of lovemaking and expressing affection. *Alternative expressions of love and intimacy can raise patient's self-esteem until impotence is evaluated and treated.*

EBP ▪ Encourage use of sexual fantasies and erotica to promote sexual stimulation and erection. *This helps patient and partner achieve sexual satisfaction and decreases "spectatoring" (watching oneself during sexual activity with partner), which can inhibit performance.*

PCC ▪ Allow patient to express feelings openly in a nonjudgmental atmosphere *to enhance communication and understanding between patient and caregiver.*

EBP ▪ Provide answers to specific questions *to help patient focus on specific issues, clarify misconceptions, and build trust in the caregiver.*

PCC ▪ Help patient recognize potentially harmful sexual behavior. Set limits on high-risk sexual behavior. *Indiscriminate, impulsive sexual behavior can lead to unwanted pregnancy, sexually transmitted diseases, and physical and emotional trauma.*

`PCC` ▣ Encourage patient to express sexual urges in socially acceptable ways (including masturbation in a private setting) *to help patient discover positive methods of relieving sexual tension.*

`PCC` ▣ Discuss with patient hypersexual behaviors and feelings associated with hypersexuality *to promote insight into behavior.*

`PCC` ▣ Provide time for privacy *to demonstrate respect for patient, allow time for introspection, and give patient control over time spent interacting with others.*

`PCC` ▣ Suggest that patient discuss concerns with partner. *Open discussion fosters sharing of concerns and strengthens relationships.*

`PCC` ▣ Provide support for the partner. *Supportive interventions such as active listening communicate concern, interest, and acceptance.*

`EBP` ▣ Educate patient and partner about limitations imposed by patient's current physical condition. *Education about limitations imposed on sexual activity by illness helps patient avoid complications or injury.*

`T&C` ▣ Suggest referral to a sex counselor or other appropriate professional for future guidance *to provide patient with a resource for postdischarge support.*

Suggested NIC Interventions

Anxiety Reduction; Emotional Support; Mutual Goal Setting; Role Enhancement; Self-Awareness Enhancement; Self-Esteem Enhancement; Sexual Counseling; Teaching: Individual; Values Clarification

EVALUATIONS FOR EXPECTED OUTCOMES

▣ Patient reports feeling comfortable discussing sexual concerns.
▣ Patient and partner communicate with each other about their sexual relationship.
▣ Patient states specific ways of enhancing sexual pleasure with partner.
▣ Patient continues to communicate with partner about sexual issues and needs.
▣ Patient acknowledges existence of problem or potential problem in sexual function.
▣ Patient expresses anxiety, anger, depression, or frustration over changes in sexual function.
▣ Patient explains relationship between illness or treatment and sexual dysfunction.
▣ Patient expresses willingness to obtain counseling.
▣ Patient resumes usual level of sexual activity.

DOCUMENTATION

▣ Patient's perception of problem
▣ Subtle comments made by patient about inability to cope with change in structure or function
▣ Observations of patient's behavior
▣ Interventions performed to assist patient and spouse or significant other; response to interventions
▣ Evaluations for expected outcomes

REFERENCES

Dahlen, H. (2019). Female sexual dysfunction: Assessment and treatment. *Urologic Nursing, 39*(1), 39–46. doi:10.7257/1053-816X.2019.39.1.39

Dusenbury, W., Palm Johansen, P., Mosack, V., & Steinke, E. E. (2017). Determinants of sexual function and dysfunction in men and women with stroke: A systematic review. *International Journal of Clinical Practice, 71*(7). doi:10.1111/ijcp.12969

İrer, B., Çelikhisar, A., Çelikhisar, H., Bozkurt, O., & Demir, Ö. (2018). Evaluation of sexual dysfunction, lower urinary tract symptoms and quality of life in men with obstructive sleep apnea syndrome and the efficacy of continuous positive airway pressure therapy. *Urology, 121*, 86–92. doi:10.1016/j.urology.2018.08.001

Thakurdesai, A., & Sawant, N. A prospective study on sexual dysfunctions in depressed males and the response to treatment. (2018). *Indian Journal of Psychiatry, 60*(4), 472–477. doi:10.4103/psychiatry. IndianJPsychiatry_386_17

Ineffective Sexuality Pattern

DEFINITION

Expressions of concern regarding own sexuality

RELATED FACTORS (R/T)

- Conflict about sexual orientation
- Conflict about variant preference
- Fear of pregnancy
- Fear of sexually transmitted infection
- Impaired relationship with a significant other
- Inadequate role model
- Insufficient knowledge about alternatives related to sexuality
- Skill deficit about alternatives related to sexuality
- Absence of privacy

ASSESSMENT

- History of current illness
- Current treatment regimen (medications and therapies)
- Patient's perception of changes in sexual activity resulting from illness or treatment
- Changes in female reproductive organs related to aging
- History of hormone replacement therapy (postmenopause or postoophorectomy), including estrogen, progesterone, or both
- Marital status and family members
- Living arrangement
- Patient's perception of sexual identity and role
- Usual sexual activity pattern
- Significance of sexual relationship to patient and partner
- Emotional reactions (affect and mood)
- Behavioral reactions (specify)

DEFINING CHARACTERISTICS

- Alteration in relationship with significant other
- Alteration in sexual activity
- Alteration in sexual behavior
- Change in sexual role
- Difficulty with sexual activity
- Difficulty with sexual behavior
- Value conflict

EXPECTED OUTCOMES

- Patient will voice feelings about changes in usual sexual activity and/or behavior.
- Patient and partner will discuss possible realistic alternatives for intimacy.
- Patient and partner will use available counseling referrals.

Suggested NOC Outcomes

Anxiety Level; Body Image; Role Performance; Self-Esteem; Sexual Identity; Stress Level

INTERVENTIONS AND RATIONALES

PCC • Allow a specific amount of uninterrupted, noncare-related time *to talk with patient to demonstrate your comfort with sexuality issues and reassure patient that personal concerns are acceptable for discussion.*

PCC • Display an accepting, nonjudgmental manner *to encourage patient to discuss concerns about sexuality.* Approach the partner in the same manner and include the partner in discussions with patient, if agreeable to both. *A nonjudgmental approach demonstrates unconditional positive regard for both patient and partner.*

PCC • Include patient in a plan for setting limits on inappropriate behavior, if indicated by behavioral assessment.
  - Explain aspects of patient's behavior that are inappropriate.
  - Share the proposed care plan with patient, including expectations, goals, and approaches for reducing bothersome behavior.
  - Request patient's cooperation, but be willing to compromise if patient offers acceptable alternatives.
  - Working together to set limits allows patient to take part in planning to reduce undesirable behaviors.

PCC • Discuss with patient and partner realistic, acceptable alternatives for intimacy needs. *Discussion encourages open communication between them as sexual partners.*

PCC • Explain to patient and partner the limitations related to illness and facility environment *to establish a standard for realistic and acceptable behavior.*

PCC • Encourage social interaction and communication between patient and partner *to foster sharing of concerns and strengthen relationship.*

PCC • Provide time for privacy to allow patient and partner *to discuss feelings about sexuality and to engage in alternatives for intimacy while patient is hospitalized.*

EBP • Provide information about menopause. *After menopause or hysterectomy, older women may need reassurance that sexual activity can still be enjoyable.*

EBP • Teach patient about the impact of normal physiologic changes caused by aging on sexuality. For example, the vagina becomes smaller and less elastic, vaginal walls become thin and smooth, and external genitalia may become softer. Also, vaginal lubrication may take longer. Patient may also have abdominal pain or bladder irritability during intercourse. *Explaining how aging affects sexuality may help patient accept these physiologic changes.*

EBP • Provide information about alternative techniques and adaptations that can assist sexual satisfaction *to encourage patient to explore and accept her sexuality.* Topics may include the use of lubricants, Kegel exercises (for vaginal muscle tone), self-stimulation, and alternative sexual positions and activities.

T&C • Offer referral for counseling, such as a mental health professional and sex counselor, if indicated. *Referrals provide opportunities for additional ongoing therapy during hospitalization and after discharge.*

Suggested NIC Interventions

Anticipatory Guidance; Anxiety Reduction; Coping Enhancement; Role Enhancement; Self-Esteem Enhancement; Sexual Counseling; Teaching: Sexuality

EVALUATIONS FOR EXPECTED OUTCOMES

- Patient describes usual sexual activity pattern and expresses feelings resulting from changes in pattern.
- Patient and partner request privacy and seek permission to use acceptable alternatives for intimacy, such as holding and kissing.
- Patient and partner seek counseling.

DOCUMENTATION

- Patient's verbal and nonverbal behaviors
- Patient's and partner's perception of current situation
- Specific nursing interventions to reduce emotional and behavioral reactions, such as active listening, limit setting, and counseling referrals
- Patient's and partner's response to nursing interventions
- Evaluations for expected outcomes

REFERENCES

Lyttle, D., Montgomery, A. J., Davis, B. L., Burns, D., McGee, Z. T., & Fogel, J. (2018). An exploration using the Neuman systems model of risky sexual behaviors among African American college students: A brief report. *Journal of Cultural Diversity, 25*(4), 142–147.

Marchese, K. (2017). An overview of erectile dysfunction in the elderly population. *Urologic Nursing, 37*(3), 157–170. doi:10.7257/1053-816X.2017.37.3.157

Vieira Pereira, E., Moreira Belém, J., Henrique Alves, M. J., Rodrigues Maia, E., Alves Firmino, P. R., & da Silva Quirino, G. (2018). Function, practices and sexual positions of pregnant women. *Journal of Nursing UFPE/Revista de Enfermagem UFPE, 12*(3), 772–780. doi:10.5205/1981-8963-v12i3a231225p772-780-2018

Risk for Shock

DEFINITION

Susceptible to an inadequate blood flow to tissues that may lead to cellular dysfunction, which may compromise health

RISK FACTORS

Bleeding
Deficient fluid volume
Factors identified by standardized, validated screening tool
Hyperthermia
Hypothermia
Hypoxemia
Hypoxia
Inadequate knowledge of bleeding management strategies
Inadequate knowledge of infection management strategies
Inadequate knowledge of modifiable factors

Ineffective medication self-management
Nonhemorrhagic fluid losses
Smoking
Unstable blood pressure

ASSOCIATED CONDITIONS

- Artificial respiration
- Burns
- Chemotherapy
- Diabetes mellitus
- Embolism
- Heart diseases
- Hypersensitivity
- Immunosuppression
- Infections
- Lactate levels ≥2 mmol/L
- Liver diseases
- Medical devices
- Neoplasms
- Nervous system diseases
- Pancreatitis
- Radiotherapy
- Sepsis
- Sequential Organ Failure Assessment (SOFA) Score ≥3
- Simplified Acute Physiology Score (SAPS) III gt; 70
- Spinal cord injuries
- Surgical procedures
- Systemic inflammatory response syndrome (SIRS)
- Trauma

ASSESSMENT

- Cardiovascular status including heart rate and rhythm, blood pressure, peripheral pulses
- Signs of dehydration, inflammation, or allergic responses
- Respiratory status including respiratory rate and depth, pulse oximetry
- Renal status, intake and output, urine specific gravity
- Mental status including orientation, level of consciousness

EXPECTED OUTCOMES

- Patient will maintain adequate blood pressure to maintain tissue perfusion.
- Patient will not experience hemodynamic complications from underlying medical condition.
- Patient will understand the need for aggressive management of underlying medical condition in an effort to prevent shock.
- Patient will verbalize signs and symptoms of possible hypotension and hypoperfusion.

Suggested NOC Outcomes

Tissue Perfusion: Cerebral; Hydration; Fluid Balance; Vital Signs

S ▪ Monitor hemodynamic status frequently, including blood pressure, heart rate, oxygen saturation. *Trending of vital signs will provide database for early intervention and treatment.*

S ▪ Assess level of consciousness with each vital sign check. *Change in level of consciousness is an early indicator of cerebral hypoperfusion.*

EBP ▪ Administer intravenous fluids, oxygen, and medications as prescribed *to maintain fluid volume and organ perfusion.*

EBP ▪ Collect and evaluate serum laboratory specimens *to provide data to effectively treat underlying medical condition and avoid complication of shock.*

EBP ▪ Educate patient and family of reportable signs and symptoms of inadequate tissue perfusion, for example, dizziness, confusion, restlessness, and dyspnea. *Early intervention and treatment is essential in preventing permanent organ damage.*

PCC ▪ Encourage patient and family to express concerns and *fears to reduce anxiety.*

T&C ▪ Collaborate with other members of the health care team *to effectively manage underlying medical condition and prevent complications.*

Suggested NIC Interventions

Acid–Base Monitoring; Fluid/Electrolyte Management; Hypovolemia Management; Shock Management

EVALUATIONS FOR EXPECTED OUTCOMES

▪ Patient's blood pressure was adequate to maintain tissue perfusion.
▪ Patient did not experience any complications related to hypoperfusion.
▪ Patient understood the need for aggressive management of underlying medical condition to prevent hypoperfusion.
▪ Patient was able to verbalize reportable signs and symptoms of possible hypoperfusion and shock.

DOCUMENTATION

▪ Patient's vital signs, intake and output, and laboratory results
▪ Patient's response to medical interventions to treat underlying condition
▪ Ability of patient to identify reportable signs and symptoms of hypoperfusion
▪ Evaluations for expected outcomes

REFERENCES

Enslow, M. S., Preece, S. R., Wildman-Tobriner, B., Enslow, R. A., Mazurowski, M., & Nelson, R. C. (2018). Splenic contraction: A new member of the hypovolemic shock complex. *Abdominal Radiology, 43*(9), 2375–2383. doi:10.1007/s00261-018-1478-3

Standl, T., Annecke, T., Cascorbi, I., Heller, A. R., Sabashnikov, A., & Teske, W. (2018). The nomenclature, definition and distinction of types of shock. *Deutsches Aerzteblatt International, 115*(45), 757–767. doi:10.3238/arztebl.2018.0757

Xie, Z., Zhang, Z., Xu, Y., Zhou, H., Wu, S., & Wang, Z. (2018). Effects of arm elevation on radial artery pressure: A new method to distinguish hypovolemic shock and septic shock from hypotension. *Blood Pressure Monitoring, 23*(3), 127–133. doi:10.1097/MBP.0000000000000318

Impaired Sitting

DEFINITION

Limitation of ability to independently and purposefully attain and/or maintain a rest position that is supported by the buttocks and thighs, in which the torso is upright

- Insufficient endurance
- Insufficient energy
- Insufficient muscle strength
- Malnutrition
- Pain
- Self-imposed relief posture

ASSOCIATED CONDITIONS

- Alteration in cognitive functioning
- Impaired metabolic functioning
- Neurological disorder
- Orthopedic surgery
- Prescribed posture
- Psychological disorder
- Sarcopenia

ASSESSMENT

- History of neuromuscular disorder or dysfunction
- Neurologic status, including level of consciousness, motor ability, and sensory ability
- Musculoskeletal status, including coordination, balance, muscle size and strength, muscle tone, range of motion (ROM), and functional mobility scale:

  0 = completely independent
  1 = requires use of equipment or device
  2 = requires help, supervision, or teaching from another person
  3 = requires help from another person and equipment or device
  4 = dependent; doesn't participate in activity

DEFINING CHARACTERISTICS

- Impaired ability to adjust position of one or both lower limbs on uneven surface
- Impaired ability to attain a balanced position of the torso
- Impaired ability to flex or move both hips
- Impaired ability to flex or move both knees
- Impaired ability to maintain the torso in balanced position
- Impaired ability to stress torso with body weight

EXPECTED OUTCOMES

- Patient will achieve highest level of independence possible when sitting.
- Patient will achieve highest level of joint ROM when sitting.
- Patient will show no evidence of complications.
- Patient will achieve balance while sitting.
- Patient will maintain muscle strength.

Suggested NOC Outcomes

Activity Tolerance; Endurance; Joint Movement: Hip; Joint Movement: Spine; Neurological Status: Central Motor Control; Neurological Status: Spinal Sensory/Motor Function; Physical Fitness; Skeletal Function

EBP ▪ Perform ROM exercises to joints, unless contraindicated, at least once every shift. Progress from passive to active, as tolerated. *This prevents joint contractures and muscular atrophy.*

EBP ▪ Place joints in functional position. *Maintain joints in a functional position and prevent musculoskeletal deformities.*

EBP ▪ Identify the level of functioning using a functional mobility scale (see "Assessment"). Communicate patient's skill level to all staff members *to provide continuity and preserve identified level of independence.*

PCC ▪ Encourage independence by helping patient use assistive devices. *This increases muscle tone and patient's self-esteem.*

PCC ▪ Monitor and record daily any evidence of immobility complications (such as contractures, venous stasis, thrombus, pneumonia, and urinary tract infection). *Patients with histories of neuromuscular disorders or dysfunction may be more prone to developing complications.*

S ▪ Instruct patient to call before attempting to stand without assistance. *Ensure patient safety from falls.*

EBP ▪ Carry out a medical regimen to manage or prevent complications; for example, administer prophylactic heparin as ordered for venous thrombosis. *This promotes patient's health and well-being.*

S ▪ Use a transfer belt if necessary *to support patient and prevent staff injury.*

S ▪ Use assistive devices as necessary *to support patient and prevent staff injury.*

T&C ▪ Refer patient to a physical therapist for development of sitting regimen *to help rehabilitate musculoskeletal deficits.*

PCC ▪ Demonstrate the sitting regimen and note date. Have patient and family members return sitting regimen demonstration and note date. *This ensures continuity of care and use of proper technique.*

Suggested NIC Interventions

Body Mechanics Promotion; Exercise Therapy: Balance; Exercise Therapy: Muscle Control; Positioning; Self-Care Assistance

▪ Patient achievement of highest level of independence possible when sitting.
▪ Patient achievement of highest level of joint ROM when sitting.
▪ Patient has no evidence of complications.
▪ Patient achievement of balance while sitting.
▪ Patient maintains muscle strength.

▪ Patient's current status of functional abilities and goals set for self
▪ Observations of patient's mobility status, presence of complications, and response to sitting regimen
▪ Instruction and demonstration of skills in carrying out sitting regimen
▪ Patient's response to nursing interventions
▪ Evaluations for expected outcomes

REFERENCES

Cabanas-Valdés, R., Bagur-Calafat, C., Girabent-Farrés, M., Caballero-Gómez, F. M., du Port de Pontcharra-Serra, H., German-Romero, A., & Urrútia, G. (2017). Long-term follow-up of a randomized controlled trial on additional core stability exercises training for improving dynamic sitting balance and trunk control in stroke patients. *Clinical Rehabilitation, 31*(11), 1492–1499. doi:10.1177/0269215517701804

Kim, D.-H., An, D.-H., & Yoo, W.-G. (2018). Changes in trunk sway and impairment during sitting and standing in children with cerebral palsy. *Technology & Health Care, 26*(5), 761–768. doi:10.3233/THC-181301

Kurita, S., Doi, T., Tsutsumimoto, K., Hotta, R., Nakakubo, S., Kim, M., & Shimada, H. (2019). Cognitive activity in a sitting position is protectively associated with cognitive impairment among older adults. *Geriatrics & Gerontology International, 19*(2), 98–102. doi:10.1111/ggi.13532

Tse, C. M., Chisholm, A. E., Lam, T., Eng, J. J., & the SCIRE Research Team. (2018). A systematic review of the effectiveness of task-specific rehabilitation interventions for improving independent sitting and standing function in spinal cord injury. *Journal of Spinal Cord Medicine, 41*(3), 254–266. doi:10.1080/10790268.2017.1350340

Impaired Skin Integrity

DEFINITION

Altered epidermis and/or dermis

RELATED FACTORS (R/T)

External

- Excessive moisture
- Excretions
- Humidity
- Hyperthermia
- Hypothermia
- Inadequate caregiver knowledge about maintaining tissue integrity
- Inadequate caregiver knowledge about protecting tissue integrity
- Inadequate use of chemical agent
- Pressure over bony prominence
- Psychomotor agitation
- Secretions
- Shearing forces
- Surface friction
- Use of linen with insufficient moisture wicking property

Internal

- Body mass index above normal range for age and gender
- Body mass index below normal range for age and gender
- Decreased physical activity
- Decreased physical mobility
- Edema
- Inadequate adherence to incontinence treatment regimen
- Inadequate knowledge about maintaining tissue integrity
- Inadequate knowledge about protecting tissue integrity
- Malnutrition

- Psychogenic factor
- Self-mutilation
- Smoking
- Substance misuse
- Water–electrolyte imbalance

ASSOCIATED CONDITIONS

- Altered pigmentation
- Anemia
- Cardiovascular diseases
- Decreased level of consciousness
- Decreased tissue oxygenation
- Decreased tissue perfusion
- Diabetes mellitus
- Hormonal change
- Immobilization
- Immunodeficiency
- Impaired metabolism
- Infections
- Medical devices
- Neoplasms
- Peripheral neuropathy
- Pharmaceutical preparations
- Punctures
- Sensation disorders

ASSESSMENT

- Age
- Presence of medical condition that may interfere with healing
- History of skin problems, trauma, chronic debilitating disease, or immobility
- Integumentary status, including color, elasticity, hygiene, lesions, moisture, texture, turgor, sensation, temperature, and quantity and distribution of hair
- Musculoskeletal status, including joint mobility, muscle strength and mass, paralysis, and range of motion
- Nutritional status, including appetite, dietary intake, hydration, current weight, and change from normal weight
- Hemoglobin and serum albumin levels and hematocrit
- Psychosocial status, including coping patterns, family members, mental status, occupation, self-concept, and body image
- Knowledge level, including patient's current understanding of physical condition and physical, mental, and emotional readiness to learn

DEFINING CHARACTERISTICS

- Abscess
- Acute pain
- Altered skin color
- Altered turgor
- Bleeding
- Blister

- Desquamation
- Disrupted skin surface
- Dry skin
- Excoriation
- Foreign matter piercing skin
- Hematoma
- Localized area hot to touch
- Macerated skin
- Peeling
- Pruritus

EXPECTED OUTCOMES

- Patient will not exhibit skin breakdown.
- Patient will exhibit improved or healed lesions or wounds.
- Patient will have few, if any, complications.
- Patient will correlate precipitating factors with appropriate skin care regimen.
- Patient will explain skin care regimen.
- Patient and family members will demonstrate skin care regimen.

Suggested NOC Outcomes

Immobility Consequences: Physiological; Tissue Integrity: Skin & Mucous Membranes; Wound Healing: Secondary Intention

INTERVENTIONS AND RATIONALES

S ▪ Inspect patient's skin every 8 hours, describe and document skin condition, and report changes *to provide evidence of the effectiveness of skin care regimen.*

EBP ▪ Perform prescribed treatment regimen for the skin condition involved; monitor progress. Report favorable and adverse responses to treatment regimen *to maintain or modify current therapies, as needed.*

S ▪ Maintain infection control standards *to help minimize the risk of nosocomial infections.*

EBP ▪ Provide supportive measures, as indicated:
  - Assist with general hygiene and comfort measures *to promote comfort and general sense of well-being.*
  - Administer pain medications and monitor effectiveness. *Patient needs pain relief to maintain health.*
  - Maintain proper environmental conditions, including room temperature and ventilation. *Providing a comfortable environment promotes sense of well-being.*
  - Apply a bed cradle *to protect lesions from bed covers.*
  - Remind patient not to scratch *to avoid skin injury.*
  - Administer and monitor effectiveness of antipruritic medications. *Antipruritics reduce itching sensation.*
  - Explain dietary restrictions; for example, explain that certain foods may cause a skin allergy. *Avoiding foods that cause skin allergy helps prevent skin breakdown.*

PCC ▪ Encourage patient to express feelings about skin condition *to enhance coping.*

EBP ▪ Position patient for comfort and minimal pressure on bony prominences. Change patient's position at least every 2 hours. Monitor frequency of turning and skin condition. *These measures reduce pressure, promote circulation, and minimize skin breakdown.*

EBP ▦ Discuss precipitating factors, if known, and long-term effects of skin integrity interruption. *Knowledge of precipitating factors helps patient reduce their occurrence and severity.*

EBP ▦ Follow facility protocol for treatment of pressure ulcer or surgical wound care *to ensure provision of appropriate care.*

EBP ▦ Instruct patient and family in the skin care regimen *to ensure compliance.*

PCC ▦ Supervise patient and family in the skin care regimen. Provide feedback. *Practice helps improve skill in managing patient's skin care regimen.*

PCC ▦ Encourage adherence to other aspects of health care management *to control or minimize effects on skin.*

T&C ▦ Refer patient to a psychiatric liaison nurse, social service, or support group, as appropriate. *These resources provide additional support for patient and family.*

Suggested NIC Interventions

Infection Control; Nutrition Therapy; Positioning; Pressure Ulcer Prevention; Skin Surveillance

EVALUATIONS FOR EXPECTED OUTCOMES

▦ Patient's skin remains intact.
▦ Patient's wounds or lesions heal.
▦ Patient doesn't experience further skin breakdown or other complications.
▦ Patient lists factors precipitating skin breakdown.
▦ Patient explains skin care regimen.
▦ Patient and family members demonstrate skin care regimen.

DOCUMENTATION

▦ Patient's concerns about skin disorder and its impact on body image and lifestyle
▦ Patient's willingness to participate in care
▦ Observations of skin condition, healing, and response to treatment regimen
▦ Interventions to provide supportive care
▦ Instructions about treatment regimen
▦ Patient's or family members' understanding of and skill in carrying out instructions
▦ Patient's response to nursing interventions
▦ Evaluations for expected outcomes

REFERENCES

Bonifant, H., & Holloway, S. (2019). A review of the effects of ageing on skin integrity and wound healing. *British Journal of Community Nursing, 24*, S28–S33. doi:10.12968/bjcn.2019.24.Sup3.S28

Edwards, H. E., Chang, A. M., Gibb, M., Finlayson, K. J., Parker, C., O'Reilly, M., … Shuter, P. (2017). Reduced prevalence and severity of wounds following implementation of the Champions for Skin Integrity model to facilitate uptake of evidence-based practice in aged care. *Journal of Clinical Nursing, 26*(23–24), 4276–4285. doi:10.1111/jocn.13752

Lee, Y. J., Kim, J. Y., & Shin, W. Y. (2019). Use of prophylactic silicone adhesive dressings for maintaining skin integrity in intensive care unit patients: A randomised controlled trial. *International Wound Journal, 16*, 36–42. doi:10.1111/iwj.13028

Messer, L. H., Berget, C., Beatson, C., Polsky, S., & Forlenza, G. P. (2018). Preserving skin integrity with chronic device use in diabetes. *Diabetes Technology & Therapeutics, 20*, S254–S264. doi:10.1089/dia.2018.0080

Risk for Impaired Skin Integrity

DEFINITION

Susceptible to alteration in epidermis and/or dermis, which may compromise health

RISK FACTORS

External

- Excessive moisture
- Excretions
- Humidity
- Hyperthermia
- Hypothermia
- Inadequate caregiver knowledge about maintaining tissue integrity
- Inadequate caregiver knowledge about protecting tissue integrity
- Inadequate use of chemical agent
- Pressure over bony prominence
- Psychomotor agitation
- Secretions
- Shearing forces
- Surface friction
- Use of linen with insufficient moisture wicking property

Internal

- Body mass index above normal range for age and gender
- Body mass index below normal range for age and gender
- Decreased physical activity
- Decreased physical mobility
- Edema
- Inadequate adherence to incontinence treatment regimen
- Inadequate knowledge about maintaining skin integrity
- Inadequate knowledge about protecting skin integrity
- Malnutrition
- Psychogenic factor
- Self-mutilation
- Smoking
- Substance misuse
- Water–electrolyte imbalance

ASSOCIATED CONDITIONS

- Altered pigmentation
- Anemia
- Cardiovascular diseases
- Decreased level of consciousness
- Decreased tissue oxygenation
- Decreased tissue perfusion
- Diabetes mellitus
- Hormonal change
- Immobilization

- Immunodeficiency
- Impaired metabolism
- Infections
- Medical devices
- Neoplasms
- Peripheral neuropathy
- Pharmaceutical preparations
- Punctures
- Sensation disorders

ASSESSMENT

- Age
- History of skin problems, trauma, chronic debilitating disease, or immobility
- Mental status
- Ability to perform skin care regimen
- Evidence of incontinence
- Recent changes in medication regimen
- Integumentary status, including color, elasticity, hygiene, lesions, moisture, sensation, temperature, texture, turgor, and quantity and distribution of hair
- Musculoskeletal status, including muscle strength and mass, joint mobility, paralysis, and range of motion (ROM)
- Nutritional status, including appetite, dietary intake, hydration, current weight, and change from normal weight
- Hemoglobin and serum albumin levels and hematocrit
- Psychosocial status, including activities of daily living, mental status, occupation (sun exposure), and recreational activities

EXPECTED OUTCOMES

- Patient will not exhibit skin breakdown.
- Patient's mucous membranes will remain intact.
- Patient will maintain adequate skin circulation.
- Patient will communicate understanding of preventive skin care measures.
- Patient and family members will demonstrate preventive skin care measures.
- Patient and family members will correlate risk factors and preventive measures.

Suggested NOC Outcomes

Immobility Consequences: Physiological; Nutritional Status; Physical Aging; Risk Control; Risk Detection; Tissue Integrity: Skin & Mucous Membranes

INTERVENTIONS AND RATIONALES

- **S** Inspect patient's skin every shift; document skin condition and report status changes. *Early detection of changes prevents or minimizes skin breakdown.*
- **S** Change patient's position at least every 2 hours; follow turning schedule posted at bedside. Monitor frequency of turning. *These measures reduce pressure on tissues, promote circulation, and help prevent skin breakdown.*
- **S** Encourage ambulation or perform or assist with active ROM exercises at least every 4 hours while patient is awake. *Exercises prevent muscle atrophy and contracture; ambulation promotes circulation and relieves pressure.*

S ▪ Use preventive skin care devices, as needed, such as a foam mattress, alternating pressure mattress, sheepskin, pillows, and padding, *to avoid discomfort and skin breakdown.*

EBP ▪ Keep patient's skin clean and dry; lubricate, as needed. Don't use irritating soap, and rinse skin well. *These measures alleviate skin dryness, promote comfort, and reduce the risk of irritation and skin breakdown.*

S ▪ Protect bony prominences with foam padding. *Prominences have little subcutaneous fat and are prone to breakdown; using foam padding may help promote skin integrity.*

S ▪ Lift patient's body when moving the patient, using a lifting sheet, if needed. Avoid shearing force. *Shearing force results when tissues slide against each other; a lifting sheet reduces sliding.*

EBP ▪ Keep linen dry, clean, and free from wrinkles or crumbs. Change wet bed linens and incontinence pads immediately. *Dry, smooth linens help prevent excoriation and skin breakdown.*

EBP ▪ Monitor nutritional intake; maintain adequate hydration. *Anemia (<10 mg hemoglobin) and low serum albumin concentrations (<2 mg) are associated with the development of pressure ulcers. Hydration helps maintain skin integrity.*

EBP ▪ Teach patient about the need for good nutrition, including the importance of meeting caloric requirements and benefits of adequate vitamin and protein intake. *Good nutrition helps maintain adequate tissue nourishment, perfusion, and oxygenation.*

EBP ▪ Educate patient and family in preventive skin care. Teach them how to maintain good personal hygiene; use nonirritating (nonalkaline) soap; pat rather than rub skin dry; inspect skin regularly; avoid prolonged exposure to water, sun, cold, and wind; avoid rubber rings; recognize the beginning of skin breakdown (redness, blisters, and discoloration); and report signs and symptoms. *These measures encourage compliance with patient's skin care regimen.*

EBP ▪ Indicate the risk factor potential on patient's chart and care plan, and reevaluate weekly, using an accepted form such as the Braden Scale. *The risk factor score helps evaluate treatment progress.*

PCC ▪ Explain the importance of practicing preventive skin care measures *to encourage compliance with skin care regimen.*

PCC ▪ Supervise patient and family in preventive skin care measures. Give constructive feedback. *Practice helps improve skill in managing the skin care regimen.*

Suggested NIC Interventions

Circulatory Precautions; Infection Prevention; Positioning; Pressure Management; Pressure Ulcer Prevention; Skin Surveillance; Splinting

EVALUATIONS FOR EXPECTED OUTCOMES

▪ Patient's skin remains intact.
▪ Patient's mucous membranes remain intact.
▪ Patient maintains adequate skin circulation.
▪ Patient lists preventive skin care measures.
▪ Patient and family members demonstrate skin care measures.
▪ Patient and family members understand need to avoid prolonged pressure, obtain adequate nutrition, prevent incontinence, and consistently perform skin care measures.

DOCUMENTATION

▪ Patient's and family members' expressions of concern about potential skin breakdown
▪ Observations of risk factors and skin condition

- Use of preventive skin care devices and their effectiveness
- Instructions about preventive skin care; patient's and family members' understanding of instructions
- Patient's and family members' demonstrated skill in carrying out preventive skin care measures
- Results of Braden Scale
- Patient's response to nursing interventions
- Evaluations for expected outcomes

REFERENCES

Ahtiala, M., Soppi, E., & Tallgren, M. (2018). Specific risk factors for pressure ulcer development in adult critical care patients—A retrospective cohort study. *EWMA Journal*, 19(1), 35–42.

Conklin, M. J., Hopson, B., Arynchyna, A., Atchley, T., Trapp, C., Rocque, B. G., & Castillo, J. (2018). Skin breakdown of the feet in patients with spina bifida: Analysis of risk factors. *Journal of Pediatric Rehabilitation Medicine*, 11(4), 237–241. doi:10.3233/PRM-170520

García, M. S., Morilla, H. J. C., Lupiáñez, P. I., Kaknani Uttumchandani, S., León Campos, Á., Aranda, G. M., ... Morales, A. J. M. (2018). Peripheral perfusion and oxygenation in areas of risk of skin integrity impairment exposed to pressure patterns. A phase I trial (POTER Study). *Journal of Advanced Nursing*, 74(2), 465–471. doi:10.1111/jan.13414

Patton, D., Moore, Z., O'Connor, T., Shanley, E., De Oliveira, A. L., Vitoriano, A., ... Nugent, L. E. (2018). Using technology to advance pressure ulcer risk assessment and self-care: Challenges and potential benefits. *EWMA Journal*, 19(2), 23–27.

Readiness for Enhanced Sleep

DEFINITION

A pattern of natural, periodic suspension of relative consciousness to provide rest and sustain a desired lifestyle, which can be strengthened

ASSESSMENT

- Age
- Daytime activity and work patterns
- Cognitive status
- Possible precipitating factors
- Daytime consequences of sleeplessness
- Underlying conditions or medications
- Situational daily stressors
- Overall quality and duration of sleep
- Sleep environment
- Exposure to bright lights, exercise, and social interaction
- Recent changes in health status or lifestyle
- Dietary and drug history, including ingestion of caffeine or other stimulants, nicotine, alcohol, sedatives, hypnotics, and fluid intake

DEFINING CHARACTERISTIC

Expresses desire to enhance sleep

EXPECTED OUTCOMES

- Patient will identify factors that enhance readiness for sleep.
- Patient will demonstrate readiness for enhanced sleep through the use of appropriate sleep hygiene measures.

- Patient's amount of sleep and rapid eye movement (REM) sleep will be congruent with developmental needs.
- Patient will express feeling rested after sleep.
- Institutional policies and staff behaviors will reflect measures to enhance readiness for sleep.

Suggested NOC Outcomes

Anxiety Level; Rest; Sleep

INTERVENTIONS AND RATIONALES

PCC ▪ Ask patient to keep a log of sleep and wake times, number of awakenings, total time asleep, quality of sleep, and any precipitating factors that may influence sleep *to determine sleep efficiency.*

EBP ▪ Educate patient about normal age-related changes to sleep and strategies to improve sleep that are specific to patient's health status, lifestyle, and environment *to decrease anxiety about sleeplessness.*

PCC ▪ Make a behavioral modification plan based on the assessment of condition, patient history, and precipitating factors *to enhance compliance.*

EBP ▪ Provide education about sleep *to dispel myths about sleep requirements and faulty strategies.*

EBP ▪ Increase exposure to light, exercise, and social interaction as synchronizers *to help rematch the circadian rhythms with normal day and night cycles.*

PCC ▪ Provide an environment conducive to relaxation, including low level of stimuli, dimmed lights, silence, and comfortable furniture, *to maximize sleep response.*

PCC ▪ Develop interventions within the facility that address quality sleep; for example, scheduling procedures and care activities *to avoid unnecessary awakenings;* modifying environmental factors *to promote a quiet, warm, relaxed sleep setting;* addressing lifestyle changes, such as having a roommate and the unfamiliarity of relocation; and orienting older adults to facility's setting *to enhance the ability to sleep.*

PCC ▪ Implement environmental strategies that cause people to lower their voices and thereby reduce noise; for example, closing the patient's door, placing phones on low volume, speaking at lower volumes, and dimming lights *to reduce extraneous sounds.*

EBP ▪ Instruct patient to avoid dietary substances and drugs that may influence sleep, including ingestion of caffeine or other stimulants, nicotine, alcohol, sedatives, hypnotics, and fluid intake *to enhance the ability to sleep.*

EBP ▪ Provide warm, light snacks containing protein at bedtime and small amounts of liquids *to promote a sense of comfort.*

EBP ▪ Provide a cup of water close to the bed *to avoid a dry mouth and facilitate returning to sleep after awakening.*

EBP ▪ Advise patient to avoid strenuous exercise at least 2 hours before bedtime *to enhance the ability to sleep.*

▪ Teach patient to relax before going to bed with reading, music, meditation, or other comforting and soothing activity *to enhance the ability to sleep.*

EBP ▪ Educate patient about sleep hygiene measures: to use the bedroom and bed only for sleep or sexual activity and to avoid other activities in the bedroom, such as watching television, reading, and eating, *to enhance the ability to sleep.*

Suggested NIC Interventions

Energy Management; Environmental Management; Environmental Management: Comfort; Progressive Muscle Relaxation; Sleep Enhancement

- Patient identifies factors that enhance readiness for sleep.
- Patient demonstrates readiness for enhanced sleep through the use of appropriate sleep hygiene measures.
- Patient's amount of sleep and REM sleep is congruent with developmental needs.
- Patient expresses feeling rested after sleep.
- Institutional policies and staff behaviors reflect measures to enhance readiness for sleep.

DOCUMENTATION

- Patient's sleep history
- Patient's plan for behavioral modification
- Observations of sleep hygiene behaviors
- Nursing interventions to enhance sleep readiness
- Patient's response to nursing interventions
- Evaluations for expected outcomes

REFERENCES

Bartel, K., Scheeren, R., & Gradisar, M. (2019). Altering adolescents' pre-bedtime phone use to achieve better sleep health. *Health Communication, 34*(4), 456–462. doi:10.1080/10410236.2017.1422099

Jaiswal, S. J., Topol, E. J., & Steinhubl, S. R. (2019). Digitising the way to better sleep health. *Lancet, 393*(10172), 639. doi:10.1016/S0140-6736(19)30240-5

Yackobovitch, G. M., Machtei, A., Lazar, L., Shamir, R., Phillip, M., Lebenthal, Y., & Yackobovitch-Gavan, M. (2018). Randomised study found that improved nutritional intake was associated with better sleep patterns in prepubertal children who were both short and lean. *Acta Paediatrica, 107*(4), 666–671. doi:10.1111/apa.14205

Sleep Deprivation

DEFINITION

Prolonged periods of time without sleep (sustained natural, periodic suspension of relative consciousness)

RELATED FACTORS (R/T)

- Age related sleep stage shifts
- Average daily physical activity is less than recommended for gender and age
- Environmental barrier
- Late day confusion
- Nonrestorative sleep pattern
- Prolonged discomfort
- Sleep terror
- Sleep walking
- Sustained circadian asynchrony
- Sustained inadequate sleep hygiene

ASSOCIATED CONDITIONS

- Conditions with periodic limb movement
- Dementia
- Idiopathic central nervous system hypersomnolence
- Narcolepsy

- Nightmares
- Sleep apnea
- Sleep-related enuresis
- Sleep-related painful erections
- Treatment regimen

ASSESSMENT

- Number of hours of sleep patient usually needs to feel rested
- Premorbid sleep patterns and current sleep patterns
- Daytime activity and work patterns
- Recent changes in health status or lifestyle
- Sleep environment, including recent changes to environment
- Activities that promote sleep
- Quality of sleep, as described by patient
- Dietary and drug history, including ingestion of caffeine or other stimulants, nicotine, alcohol, and sedative-hypnotics

DEFINING CHARACTERISTICS

- Agitation
- Alteration in concentration
- Anxiety
- Apathy
- Combativeness
- Confusion
- Decrease in functional ability
- Decrease in reaction time
- Drowsiness
- Fatigue
- Fleeting nystagmus
- Hallucinations
- Hand tremors
- Heightened sensitivity to pain
- Irritability
- Lethargy
- Malaise
- Perceptual disorders
- Restlessness
- Transient paranoia

EXPECTED OUTCOMES

- Patient will identify factors that prevent or disrupt sleep.
- Patient will sleep _____ (specify) hours without interruption.
- Patient will express feeling well rested.
- Patient will show no physical signs of sleep deprivation.
- Patient will not exhibit complications associated with sleep deprivation, such as sleep apnea and nocturnal hypoxic episodes.
- Patient will alter diet and habits to promote sleep—for example, by reducing caffeine intake and limiting alcohol intake.

- Patient will not exhibit such sleep-related behavioral symptoms as irritability, lethargy, listlessness, restlessness, anxiety, worry, or depression.
- Patient will perform relaxation exercises at bedtime.
- Health care providers will schedule nighttime treatments to allow for maximum restful sleep.

Suggested NOC Outcomes

Concentration; Endurance; Energy Conservation; Mood Equilibrium; Rest; Sleep; Stress Level; Symptom Severity

INTERVENTIONS AND RATIONALES

PCC ▪ Encourage patient to identify factors in the environment that make sleeping difficult. *A strange or new environment may affect rapid eye movement and non–rapid eye movement sleep.*

PCC ▪ Ask patient what changes would help promote sleep *to encourage patient to play an active role in care.*

EBP ▪ Advise patient to avoid daytime naps *to promote restful nocturnal sleep.*

EBP ▪ Tell patient to avoid spending long periods in bed without sleep. *Activity produces healthy fatigue, which promotes restful sleep.*

PCC ▪ Make immediate changes to accommodate patient—for example, reduce noise; change catheterization, medication, or treatment schedule; change lighting; and close door. *These measures promote rest and sleep.*

PCC ▪ Develop a plan to allow patient to have _____ hours of uninterrupted sleep if possible. *This provides consistent nursing care and provides patient with maximum hours of uninterrupted sleep.*

PCC ▪ Perform interventions to promote sleep, such as giving patient a bath or back rub, ensuring patient is positioned properly, or providing pillows, food, or drink. *Personal hygiene routine precedes sleep for many individuals. Milk and some high-protein snacks, such as cheese or nuts, contain L-tryptophan, a sleep promoter.*

PCC ▪ Assess patient each morning to determine quality of sleep the night before *to help detect sleep-related behavioral symptoms.*

EBP ▪ Teach patient relaxation techniques, such as guided imagery, meditation, and progressive muscle relaxation. Practice them with patient at bedtime. *Purposeful relaxation efforts commonly promote sleep.*

EBP ▪ Instruct patient to limit alcohol and caffeine intake and avoid foods that interfere with sleep (such as spicy foods). Foods and beverages with caffeine should be avoided for 4 to 5 hours before bedtime. *Dietary changes may help to promote restful sleep.*

PCC ▪ Avoid quick, unanticipated movements when turning and positioning patients with neuromuscular dysfunction *to prevent spasticity, which may interrupt sleep.*

EBP ▪ In stroke patients with muscle tone problems, plan to position patient on the affected side during the last turn of the night *to promote restful sleep and help normalize patient's muscle tone for morning activities.*

T&C ▪ Refer patient experiencing sleep deprivation to a sleep disorder center, especially if activities of daily living are affected or sleep apnea occurs. *A specialist may be required to assist in treatment.*

PCC ▪ Assess the daytime schedule to ensure adequate time for rest. *Excessive fatigue can result in insomnia.*

T&C ▪ Help patient with chronic illness or disability find resources for addressing psychosocial issues. *Fears and concerns about future prevent restful sleep.*

Suggested NIC Interventions

Anxiety Reduction; Coping Enhancement; Energy Management; Environmental Management: Comfort; Progressive Muscle Relaxation; Sleep Enhancement

EVALUATIONS FOR EXPECTED OUTCOMES

- Patient identifies factors that prevent or disrupt sleep.
- Patient sleeps ____ (specify) hours without interruption.
- Patient expresses feeling of being well rested.
- Patient shows no physical signs of sleep deprivation.
- Patient doesn't exhibit complications associated with sleep deprivation, such as sleep apnea and nocturnal hypoxic episodes.
- Patient alters diet and habits to promote sleep—for example, by reducing caffeine intake and limiting alcohol intake.
- Patient doesn't exhibit sleep-related behavioral symptoms, such as irritability, lethargy, listlessness, restlessness, anxiety, worry, or depression.
- Patient performs relaxation exercises at bedtime.
- Health care providers schedule nighttime treatments to allow for maximum restful sleep.

DOCUMENTATION

- Patient's reports of sleep disturbances
- Patient's expressions of feelings related to sleep deprivation
- Observations of behaviors that indicate sleep deprivation
- Nursing interventions to alleviate sleep deprivation
- Patient's response to nursing interventions
- Evaluations for expected outcomes

REFERENCES

Cerolini, S., Rodgers, R. F., & Lombardo, C. (2018). Partial sleep deprivation and food intake in participants reporting binge eating symptoms and emotional eating: Preliminary results of a quasi-experimental study. *Eating & Weight Disorders, 23*(5), 561–570. doi:10.1007/s40519-018-0547-5

McLaughlin, D. C., Hartjes, T. M., & Freeman, W. D. (2018). Sleep deprivation in neurointensive care unit patients from serial neurological checks: How much is too much? *Journal of Neuroscience Nursing, 50*(4), 205–210. doi:10.1097/JNN.0000000000000378

Pallesen, S., Olsen, O. K., Eide, E. M., Nortvedt, B., Grønli, J., Larøi, F., ... Glomlien, F. E. (2018). Sleep deprivation and hallucinations. A qualitative study of military personnel. *Military Psychology (American Psychological Association), 30*(5), 430–436. doi:10.1080/08995605.2018.1478561

Disturbed Sleep Pattern

DEFINITION

Time-limited awakenings due to external factors

RELATED FACTORS (R/T)

- Disruption caused by sleep partner
- Environmental barrier

- Immobilization
- Insufficient privacy
- Nonrestorative sleep pattern

ASSESSMENT

- Number of hours of sleep patient usually needs to feel rested
- Premorbid sleep patterns and current sleep patterns
- Daytime activity and work patterns
- Recent changes in health status or lifestyle
- Sleep environment, including recent changes to environment
- Activities that promote sleep
- Quality of sleep, as described by patient
- Dietary and drug history, including ingestion of caffeine or other stimulants, nicotine, alcohol, and sedative-hypnotics

DEFINING CHARACTERISTICS

- Difficulty in daily functioning
- Difficulty initiating sleep
- Difficulty maintaining sleep state
- Dissatisfaction with sleep
- Feeling unrested
- Unintentional awakening

EXPECTED OUTCOMES

- Patient will identify factors that changed usual sleep pattern.
- Patient will sleep _____ (specify) hours without interruption.
- Patient will express feeling well rested.
- Patient will alter diet and habits to promote sleep—for example, by reducing caffeine intake and limiting alcohol intake.
- Patient will incorporate sleep preparation measures into evening routine.
- Patient will carry out relaxation exercises that promote sleep.
- Patient will express satisfaction with sleep.

Suggested NOC Outcomes

Rest; Sleep; Symptom Control; Well-Being

INTERVENTIONS AND RATIONALES

- **PCC** Complete a sleep history and help patient identify factors that may impair sleep. *Review of patterns may elicit insights that can be used to correct the problem.*
- **PCC** Assist patient in identifying environmental factors that make sleeping difficult. Suggest the use of "white noise" machines to mask unwanted noise. *A strange or new environment may affect rapid eye movement and non–rapid eye movement sleep.*
- Ask patient what changes would help promote sleep *to encourage patient to play an active role in care.*
- **EBP** Encourage regular evening routines that promote sleep, such as taking a warm bath or eating a small snack. *Personal hygiene routine precedes sleep for many individuals. Milk*

and some high-protein snacks, such as cheese or nuts, contain L-tryptophan, a sleep promoter.

▦ Ask patient to evaluate the quality of sleep the night before *to help detect sleep-related behavioral symptoms.*

EBP ▦ Teach patient relaxation techniques, such as guided imagery, meditation, and progressive muscle relaxation. *Purposeful relaxation efforts commonly promote sleep.*

EBP ▦ Instruct patient to limit alcohol and caffeine intake and avoid foods that interfere with sleep (such as spicy foods). Foods and beverages with caffeine should be avoided for 4 to 5 hours before bedtime. *Dietary changes may help to promote restful sleep.*

T&C ▦ Refer the patient experiencing extended sleep changes to a sleep disorder center, especially if activities of daily living are affected or sleep apnea occurs. *A specialist may be required to assist in treatment.*

PCC ▦ Assess the daytime schedule to ensure adequate time for rest. *Excessive fatigue can result in insomnia.*

T&C ▦ Help patient with chronic illness or disability find resources for addressing psychosocial issues. *Fears and concerns about future prevent restful sleep.*

Suggested NIC Interventions

Anxiety Reduction; Simple Guided Imagery; Energy Management; Environmental Management: Comfort; Progressive Muscle Relaxation; Sleep Enhancement; Anticipatory Guidance; Calming Technique; Simple Relaxation Therapy

EVALUATIONS FOR EXPECTED OUTCOMES

▦ Patient identifies factors that prevent or disrupt sleep.
▦ Patient sleeps _____ (specify) hours without interruption.
▦ Patient expresses feeling of being well rested.
▦ Patient alters diet and habits to promote sleep—for example, by reducing caffeine intake and limiting alcohol intake.
▦ Patient performs relaxation exercises at bedtime.
▦ Patient incorporates sleep techniques into bedtime regimen.

DOCUMENTATION

▦ Patient's reports of sleep disturbances
▦ Patient's responses to sleep routine changes
▦ Observations of behaviors that indicate sleep deprivation
▦ Patient's response to guided imagery or relaxation techniques
▦ Patient's response to nursing interventions
▦ Evaluations for expected outcomes

REFERENCES

Biani Manzoli, J. P., Lopes Correia, M. D., & Marocco Duran, E. C. (2018). Conceptual and operational definitions of the defining characteristics of the nursing diagnosis Disturbed Sleep Pattern. *Revista Latino-Americana de Enfermagem (RLAE), 26*, 1–10. doi:10.1590/1518-8345.2582.3105

Reynolds, M. E., & Cone, P. H. (2018). Managing adult insomnia confidently. *Journal for Nurse Practitioners, 14*(10), 718–724. doi:10.1016/j.nurpra.2018.08.019

Rhéaume, A., & Mullen, J. (2018). The impact of long work hours and shift work on cognitive errors in nurses. *Journal of Nursing Management, 26*(1), 26–32. doi:10.1111/jonm.12513

Wang, X., Li, P., Pan, C., Dai, L., Wu, Y., & Deng, Y. (2019). The effect of mind-body therapies on insomnia: A systematic review and meta-analysis. *Evidence-Based Complementary & Alternative Medicine (ECAM)*, 1–17. doi:10.1155/2019/9359807

Impaired Social Interaction

DEFINITION

Insufficient or excessive quantity or ineffective quality of social exchange

RELATED FACTORS (R/T)

- Altered self-concept
- Cognitive dysfunction
- Depressive symptoms
- Disturbed thought processes
- Environmental constraints
- Impaired physical mobility
- Inadequate communication skills
- Inadequate knowledge about how to enhance mutuality
- Inadequate personal hygiene
- Inadequate social skills
- Inadequate social support
- Maladaptive grieving
- Neurobehavioral manifestations
- Sociocultural dissonance

ASSOCIATED CONDITION

- Halitosis
- Mental diseases
- Neurodevelopmental disorders
- Therapeutic isolation

ASSESSMENT

- Reason for hospitalization (physiologic or psychiatric)
- Usual pattern of social interaction (nonverbal behaviors and verbal communication)
- Neurologic functioning, including level of consciousness, orientation, and sensory and motor ability
- Mental status, including abstract ability, affect, concentration ability, insight and judgment, memory, mood, and thought content
- History of substance abuse
- Education and intelligence level
- Sociocultural background, including beliefs, norms, religion, and values
- Support systems, including clergy, family members, and friends

DEFINING CHARACTERISTICS

- Anxiety during social interaction
- Dysfunctional interaction with others
- Expresses difficulty establishing satisfactory reciprocal interpersonal relations
- Expresses difficulty functioning socially
- Expresses difficulty performing social roles
- Expresses discomfort in social situations
- Expresses dissatisfaction with social connection
- Family reports altered interaction

- Inadequate psychosocial support system
- Inadequate use of social status toward others
- Low levels of social activities
- Minimal interaction with others
- Reports unsatisfactory social engagement
- Unhealthy competitive focus
- Unwillingness to cooperate with others

EXPECTED OUTCOMES

- Patient will have comfortable social interactions.
- Patient's perceptions will be reality based.
- Patient and family members will participate in care and prescribed therapies.
- Patient will verbalize perceptions of difficulty in interaction with others.
- Patient will express needs and will communicate whether needs are met.
- Patient will demonstrate effective social interaction skills in one-on-one and group settings.
- Patient and family members will identify and mobilize resources for rehabilitation and discharge planning, as necessary.

Suggested NOC Outcomes

Family Social Climate; Immobility Consequences: Psycho-Cognitive; Self-Esteem; Social Interaction Skills; Social Involvement

INTERVENTIONS AND RATIONALES

PCC ■ Assign a primary nurse to patient if possible. *Primary nursing provides consistency, enhances trust, and decreases the potential for fragmented care.*

PCC ■ Provide a specific time (e.g., 10 minutes each shift) to talk with patient and family members. *In many cultural groups, trust develops slowly and may be hampered by lengthy interviews.*

PCC ■ Provide specific, noncare-related time with patient each shift *to encourage social interaction.* Begin with one-on-one interaction and increase to group interaction as patient's skills indicate. *Gradually increasing social interaction reduces patient's feeling of being overwhelmed and eliminates sensory input that may renew a cognitive or perceptual disturbance.*

EBP ■ Follow the medical regimen to treat the underlying condition. *The nurse is responsible for following the medical regimen and working with the physician to plan appropriate care.*

S ■ Assess neurologic function and mental status every shift *to monitor changes in patient's status;* reorient patient as often as necessary: *Reorienting patient and involving family members enhance patient's reality-testing ability and overall mental status. Scheduling a daily routine narrows patient's frame of reference, thereby decreasing the potential for increased confusion.*

- Call patient by name and say your name during each interaction.
- Tell patient the correct day, date, time, and place at least once per shift.
- Teach family members how to reorient patient and help them do so.
- Ask family members to bring patient familiar objects from home, such as clock, radio, and photographs.
- Post a structured schedule of daily activities in patient's room within visual range.
- Explain the schedule to family members and other caregivers to provide consistency and continuity.

PCC ▦ If delusions and hallucinations occur, don't focus on them; provide patient with reality-based information and reassure patient of safety *to increase patient's ability to grasp reality and reduce fears associated with these disturbances.*

PCC ▦ Help patient identify and use effective social interaction behaviors, such as increased eye contact, calling people by name, and asking questions. *Teaching patient effective interpersonal communication helps in functioning more effectively in a social environment.*

PCC ▦ Demonstrate respect for patient's privacy, personal belongings, cultural norms, and religious beliefs and practices *to provide sensitive care to patients from varied cultural backgrounds.*

PCC ▦ Give positive reinforcement for appropriate and effective interaction behaviors (verbal and nonverbal) *to help patient recognize progress and enhance feelings of self-worth.*

PCC ▦ Assist patient and family members in progressive participation in care and therapies *to reduce feelings of helplessness and enhance patient's feeling of control and independence.*

T&C ▦ Initiate or participate in multidisciplinary patient-centered conferences to evaluate progress and plan discharge. In addition to patient and family members, conferences may include physical, occupational, and speech therapists; a social worker; the attending physician; and other consultants, as necessary. *These conferences involve patient and family members in a cooperative effort to develop strategies for altering the care plan, as necessary.*

Suggested NIC Interventions

Behavior Modification: Social Skills; Complex Relationship Building; Family Integrity Promotion; Family Therapy; Normalization Promotion; Support System Enhancement

EVALUATIONS FOR EXPECTED OUTCOMES

▦ Patient expresses comfort in social interactions.
▦ Patient's verbal responses and behavior don't indicate delusions or hallucinations.
▦ Patient and family members perform care-related procedures to extent possible.
▦ Patient uses words, gestures, or writing to communicate needs and whether needs are met.
▦ Patient maintains appropriate cognitive and perceptual functioning to extent possible.
▦ Patient communicates effectively in one-on-one and group settings.
▦ Patient and family members identify and contact available support resources, as needed.

DOCUMENTATION

▦ Patient's verbal and nonverbal behaviors
▦ Neurologic and mental status assessment
▦ Observations of patient's social interaction skills
▦ Interventions to facilitate appropriate and effective social interaction
▦ Patient's responses to nursing interventions
▦ Evaluations for expected outcomes

REFERENCES

Bundock, K. E., & Hewitt, O. (2017). A review of social skills interventions for adults with autism and intellectual disability. *Tizard Learning Disability Review, 22*(3), 148–158. doi:10.1108/TLDR-05-2016-0015

Kent, C., Cordier, R., Joosten, A., Wilkes, G. S., & Bundy, A. (2018). Peer-mediated intervention to improve play skills in children with autism spectrum disorder: A feasibility study. *Australian Occupational Therapy Journal, 65*(3), 176–186. doi:10.1111/1440-1630.12459

Zhao, M., & Chen, S. (2018). The effects of structured physical activity program on social interaction and communication for children with autism. *BioMed Research International, 2018,* 1–13. doi:10.1155/2018/1825046

Social Isolation

DEFINITION

A state in which the individual lacks a sense of relatedness connected to positive, lasting, and significant interpersonal relationships

RELATED FACTORS (R/T)

- Cognitive dysfunction
- Difficulty establishing satisfactory reciprocal interpersonal relations
- Difficulty performing activities of daily living
- Difficulty sharing personal life expectations
- Fear of crime
- Fear of traffic
- Impaired physical mobility
- Inadequate psychosocial support system
- Inadequate social skills
- Inadequate social support
- Inadequate transportation
- Low self-esteem
- Negative perception of support system
- Neurobehavioral manifestations
- Values incongruent with cultural norms

ASSOCIATED CONDITIONS

- Chronic disease
- Cognitive disorders

ASSESSMENT

- Age
- Gender
- Developmental stage
- Level of education
- Reason for hospitalization (physiologic or psychiatric)
- Attitudes of family, friends, teachers, and other important individuals toward adolescent
- Available support systems
- Factors contributing to social isolation, including delayed physical development, immaturity, altered mental status, changes in behavior or cognition, illness, and history of trauma
- Self-esteem
- Coping and problem-solving ability
- Evidence of substance abuse
- Current and past stressors
- Health status, including vision or hearing deficits, chronic illness, incontinence, and pain
- Self-care abilities, including knowledge and use of adaptive equipment and supplies, and technical and mechanical skills
- Living conditions, including home environment, site of activities and resources, and transportation
- Mental status, including behavior, mood, and affect

- Musculoskeletal status, including coordination, functional ability, gait, range of motion, presence of tremor or paralysis, and muscle tone, size, and strength
- Sociocultural factors, including ethnic and religious background

DEFINING CHARACTERISTICS

- Altered physical appearance
- Expresses dissatisfaction with respect from others
- Expresses dissatisfaction with social connection
- Expresses dissatisfaction with social support
- Expresses loneliness
- Flat affect
- Hostility
- Impaired ability to meet expectations of others
- Low levels of social activities
- Minimal interaction with others
- Preoccupation with own thoughts
- Purposelessness
- Reduced eye contact
- Reports feeling different from others
- Reports feeling insecure in public
- Sad affect
- Seclusion imposed by others
- Sense of alienation
- Social behavior incongruent with cultural norms
- Social withdrawal

EXPECTED OUTCOMES

- Patient will express feelings associated with social isolation.
- Patient will identify causes of social isolation.
- Patient will participate in planning social activities.
- Patient will identify personal behaviors that are considered socially unacceptable and will acknowledge the need for change.
- Patient will demonstrate more socially acceptable behaviors.
- Patient will make use of community resources.
- Patient will describe increased number of social contacts.
- Patient will express satisfaction with level of social contacts.
- Patient will exhibit effective interpersonal communication skills.
- Patient will report feeling less isolated as social interaction improves and will report improved sense of self-esteem.

Suggested NOC Outcomes

Family Social Climate; Personal Well-Being: Leisure Participation; Loneliness Severity; Social Interaction Skills; Social Involvement; Social Support

INTERVENTIONS AND RATIONALES

`PCC` - Assign a primary nurse to patient *to enhance continuity of care, establish a trusting relationship, and provide an opportunity to practice developing a one-on-one relationship.*

`PCC` ▪ Arrange uninterrupted time to talk with patient during each visit. Listen to patient's concerns and feelings. Provide honest feedback (positive and negative) about patient's behavior *to encourage appropriate behaviors and reinforce awareness of inappropriate ones. Feedback is essential to behavior modification.*

`PCC` ▪ Provide guidance as patient explores possible causes for feelings of social isolation. Help patient identify inappropriate behaviors and provide education about ways to improve communication and interpersonal skills *to foster socially acceptable behavior. Patient may be more willing to learn new skills and behaviors after becoming aware of the connection between unacceptable behavior patterns and feelings of isolation.*

`PCC` ▪ Discuss with patient causes and contributing factors of social isolation. Find out what factors patient believes interfere most with the ability to develop relationships with others *to determine patient's wants and needs.*

`PCC` ▪ Make a contract with patient that requires demonstration of one new behavior within a specific period. Reward successful changes in behavior. *Contracts can enhance self-esteem by giving patient responsibility for making constructive changes and allowing enough time to practice new behavior and communication skills without fear of criticism. Successful completion of the contract provides positive reinforcement.*

`PCC` ▪ Demonstrate appropriate communication skills and behaviors in all interactions with patient *to provide an example of appropriate behavior and reinforce teaching concepts.*

`PCC` ▪ If appropriate, address physical limitations that interfere with patient's ability to form social relationships. For example, if patient has a hearing deficit, make a referral to an audiologist for a hearing aid; if patient has a mobility impairment, make a referral to a physical therapist for an exercise program or for recommendations for assistive devices. *Patient may need physical limitations addressed before patient can overcome social isolation.*

`PCC` ▪ Assess the influence of the home environment on patient's social life. For example, is patient afraid to go outside because of a high crime rate in the neighborhood? If so, consider investigating options, such as a retirement community or residential care facility, which might offer better social opportunities. *Patient may not be aware of alternative living options.*

`PCC` ▪ Engage patient in role-playing activities that simulate social situations. Provide encouragement and positive reinforcement, and avoid criticism *to provide an opportunity to rehearse new skills in a safe environment, which reduces anxiety and boosts self-confidence.*

`T&C` ▪ Encourage patient to participate in group activities and one-on-one interactions with staff members. *Gradual increases in social interaction help reduce patient's feelings of social isolation and instill confidence in newly developed communication and interpersonal skills.*

`PCC` ▪ Encourage patient to increase level of social contact gradually *to avoid becoming overwhelmed.*

`T&C` ▪ Refer patient to social services for follow-up, if necessary, *to ensure a comprehensive approach to care.*

`T&C` ▪ Talk to patient about community resources, such as social services or support groups that can provide ongoing support. Provide names, addresses, and phone numbers whenever possible. *This provides patient with ongoing opportunities for social interaction in a supportive environment.*

Suggested NIC Interventions

Behavior Modification: Social Skills; Coping Enhancement; Counseling; Emotional Support; Socialization Enhancement; Support Group; Support System Enhancement; Therapy Group

EVALUATIONS FOR EXPECTED OUTCOMES

- Patient expresses feelings of social isolation and desire for help.
- Patient identifies causes of social isolation.
- Patient takes part in planning social activities.
- Patient identifies socially unacceptable personal behaviors and acknowledges the need for change.
- Patient demonstrates more socially appropriate behaviors.
- Patient exhibits effective communication skills.
- Patient reports increased social interaction, decreased feelings of isolation, and improved self-esteem.

DOCUMENTATION

- Observations of patient's behavior and communication skills
- Patient's description of causes for impaired social interaction
- Nursing interventions to promote behavior modification and improved socialization
- Patient's response to interventions
- Resources and referrals provided to patient or family members
- Evaluations for expected outcomes

REFERENCES

Bower, M., Conroy, E., & Perz, J. (2018). Australian homeless persons' experiences of social connectedness, isolation and loneliness. *Health & Social Care in the Community, 26*(2), e241–e248. doi:10.1111/hsc.12505

Gardiner, C., Geldenhuys, G., & Gott, M. (2018). Interventions to reduce social isolation and loneliness among older people: An integrative review. *Health & Social Care in the Community, 26*(2), 147–157. doi:10.1111/hsc.12367

Moola, F. (2018). The complexities of contagion: The experience of social isolation among children and youth living with cystic fibrosis in Canada. *Journal of Child Health Care, 22*(4), 631–645. doi:10.1177/1367493518767784

Chronic Sorrow

DEFINITION

Cyclical, recurring, and potentially progressive pattern of pervasive sadness experienced (by a parent, caregiver individual with chronic illness or disability) in response to continual loss, throughout the trajectory of an illness or disability

RELATED FACTORS (R/T)

- Crisis in disability management
- Crisis in illness management
- Missed milestones
- Missed opportunities

ASSOCIATED CONDITIONS

- Chronic disability
- Chronic illness

- Age and sex
- History of recent loss
- Patient's usual pattern of coping with loss, including cultural, intellectual, and emotional responses
- Expressed feelings of loss of control over current situation
- Behavioral manifestations of grieving, including their intensity
- Somatic problems associated with grieving, including changes in appetite, sleep patterns, activity level, and libido
- Lifestyle changes related to illness (mobility restrictions, risk of complications, and medication regimen)
- Psychosocial status, including religious beliefs and practices, personal philosophy, educational background, and effect of altered health status on social life
- Physical and social environment
- Sources of support, including family members, friends, and clergy

- Feeling that interferes with well-being
- Overwhelming negative feelings
- Sadness

- Patient will identify losses associated with changes in health status.
- Patient will express feelings about changes in health status.
- Patient will seek assistance in dealing with emotions related to loss.
- Patient will begin to develop healthy coping mechanisms such as open expression of grief.
- Patient will seek out support from family, friends, clergy, or others when necessary.
- Patient will begin to plan for discharge and for future.
- Patient will express realistic expectations with regard to health status.

Suggested NOC Outcomes

Acceptance: Health Status; Depression Self-Control; Hope; Mood Equilibrium

- **PCC** Spend at least 15 minutes each shift with patient to focus on expression of feelings. Encourage patient to express thoughts and feelings openly. *Dysfunctional grieving may result from the inability to freely express feelings.*
- **PCC** Communicate to patient that feelings of anger are acceptable, but place limits on destructive behavior. *Inability to identify anger as normal response to loss may cause patient to express aggression inappropriately.*
- Help patient focus realistically on changes in health status because of loss *to help patient plan for the future.*
- **T&C** Encourage patient to reach out to people who can offer support, such as family, friends, and clergy, *to increase emotional strength.*
- **PCC** Encourage patient and family members to reminisce. *Engaging in life review promotes a peaceful atmosphere and helps in understanding the meaning of loss in relation to health and life.*
- **T&C** Inform patient and family members about additional sources of support within the facility or community *to facilitate adaptive responses to loss and encourage community integration.*

`PCC` ▦ Encourage patient to take an active part in setting goals for health care *to facilitate independence and enhance self-esteem.*

`PCC` ▦ Help patient and family set realistic goals for discharge and the future *to help patient place the loss in perspective and move on to new opportunities and relationships.*

`PCC` ▦ Encourage patient to be as independent as possible in self-care activities *to enhance self-esteem and promote optimal functioning.*

`T&C` ▦ Refer the patient to a psychologist, psychiatrist, or social worker as appropriate. *Restoring emotional health may require assistance from a mental health professional.*

Suggested NIC Interventions

Coping Enhancement; Decision-Making Support; Emotional Support; Hope Instillation; Mood Management; Spiritual Support; Support Group

EVALUATIONS FOR EXPECTED OUTCOMES

▦ Patient identifies losses associated with changes in health status.
▦ Patient expresses feelings about changes in health status.
▦ Patient seeks assistance in dealing with emotions related to loss.
▦ Patient begins to develop healthy coping mechanisms such as open expression of grief.
▦ Patient seeks out support from family, friends, clergy, or others when necessary.
▦ Patient begins to plan for discharge and for future.
▦ Patient expresses realistic expectations with regard to health status.

DOCUMENTATION

▦ Patient's statements regarding loss
▦ Patient's behavioral response to loss, including interactions with family members and staff
▦ Nursing interventions to help patient overcome chronic sorrow
▦ Patient's response to nursing interventions
▦ Patient's statements indicating understanding that grief is normal
▦ Patient's statements regarding goals for discharge and future
▦ Referrals to a mental health professional
▦ Evaluations for expected outcomes

REFERENCES

Carroll, K. (2019). Bringing joy-sorrow to light: Informing practice utilizing theoretical and research perspectives. *Nursing Science Quarterly, 32*(1), 29–32. doi:10.1177/0894318418807941

Chang, K., Huang, X., Cheng, J., & Chien, C. (2018). The chronic sorrow experiences of caregivers of clients with schizophrenia in Taiwan: A phenomenological study. *Perspectives in Psychiatric Care, 54*(2), 281–286. doi:10.1111/ppc.12235

Coughlin, M. B., & Sethares, K. A. (2017). Chronic sorrow in parents of children with a chronic illness or disability: An integrative literature review. *Journal of Pediatric Nursing, 37*, 108–116. doi:10.1016/j.pedn.2017.06.011

Spiritual Distress

DEFINITION

A state of suffering related to the impaired ability to integrate meaning and purpose in life through connections with self, others, the world, and/or a power greater than oneself

- Altered religious ritual
- Altered spiritual practice
- Anxiety
- Barrier to experiencing love
- Cultural conflict
- Depressive symptoms
- Difficulty accepting the aging process
- Inadequate environmental control
- Inadequate interpersonal relations
- Loneliness
- Loss of independence
- Low self-esteem
- Pain
- Perception of having unfinished business
- Self-alienation
- Separation from support system
- Social alienation
- Sociocultural deprivation
- Stressors
- Substance misuse

- Chronic disease
- Depression
- Loss of a body part
- Loss of function of a body part
- Treatment regimen

- General spiritual beliefs
- Personal spiritual beliefs
- Spiritual support systems
- Religious affiliation
- Impact of illness on spiritual beliefs

- Anger behaviors
- Crying
- Decreased expression of creativity
- Disinterested in nature
- Dysomnias
- Excessive guilt
- Expresses alienation
- Expresses anger
- Expresses anger toward power greater than self
- Expresses concern about beliefs
- Expresses concern about the future
- Expresses concern about values system

- Expresses concerns about family
- Expresses feeling abandoned by power greater than self
- Expresses feeling of emptiness
- Expresses feeling unloved
- Expresses feeling worthless
- Expresses insufficient courage
- Expresses loss of confidence
- Expresses loss of control
- Expresses loss of hope
- Expresses loss of serenity
- Expresses need for forgiveness
- Expresses regret
- Expresses suffering
- Fatigue
- Fear
- Impaired ability for introspection
- Inability to experience transcendence
- Maladaptive grieving
- Perceived loss of meaning in life
- Questions identity
- Questions meaning of life
- Questions meaning of suffering
- Questions own dignity
- Refuses to interact with others

EXPECTED OUTCOMES

- Patient will express feelings of spiritual comfort.
- Patient will express feelings about usual and current spiritual beliefs.
- Patient will identify areas of ambivalence and conflict about beliefs.
- Patient will state an understanding of grief process and its stages.
- Patient will use effective coping strategies to ease spiritual discomfort.
- Patient will seek appropriate support persons (family members, priest, minister, imam, or rabbi) for assistance.

Suggested NOC Outcomes

Hope; Personal Autonomy; Quality of Life; Spiritual Health; Suffering Severity; Will to Live

INTERVENTIONS AND RATIONALES

- **PCC** Approach patient in an accepting, nonjudgmental manner *to demonstrate unconditional positive regard for patient.*
- **PCC** Listen for cues about patient's feelings. ("Why did God do this to me?" or "God is punishing me.") *Active listening demonstrates involvement with patient and allows you to hear important messages indicating spiritual distress.*
- **PCC** Acknowledge patient's spiritual concerns and encourage expression of feelings *to help build a therapeutic relationship.*
- **PCC** Help patient concretely define the problem causing inner conflict. *This is the first step in developing strategies for resolving conflicts.*

PCC ▪ Encourage patient to provide information about personal spiritual or religious beliefs and practices. *Acquiring this initial database is the first step in the nursing process.*

EBP ▪ Instruct patient on stages of grieving and on emotions and behaviors common to each stage *to promote understanding and encourage feelings of normalcy.*

PCC ▪ Arrange for patient to have bedside objects that provide spiritual comfort (such as a Bible, prayer shawl, pictures, statues, and rosary beads). *Items of spiritual significance may influence patient's ability to reduce conflict.*

PCC ▪ Encourage interests in art, music, nature, and so on or wherever patient finds spiritual peace. Offer to help find books, CDs, art supplies, and so on. *Patients differ markedly in what gives them peace and promotes spiritual well-being. For many it is not religion.*

PCC ▪ Provide for the continuation of patient's spiritual or religious practices (allow for specific religious materials or clothing; respect dietary restrictions, if possible). *These measures demonstrate support and convey caring and acceptance to patient.*

T&C ▪ Facilitate visits from clergy and provide privacy during visits *to demonstrate respect for patient's relationship with clergy.*

PCC ▪ Encourage patient to discuss concerns with clergy, *thereby using expert spiritual care resources to help patient.*

Suggested NIC Interventions

Active Listening; Anxiety Reduction; Coping Enhancement; Hope Instillation; Referral; Spiritual Growth Facilitation; Spiritual Support

EVALUATIONS FOR EXPECTED OUTCOMES

▪ Patient discusses feelings about personal spiritual or religious beliefs.
▪ Patient specifies areas of spiritual conflict, such as anger toward God, questioning of own usual beliefs about an afterlife, and guilt related to loss of faith.
▪ Patient communicates understanding of grief process and its stages.
▪ Patient continues religious practices that ease spiritual distress.
▪ Patient makes use of available resources for spiritual assistance.

DOCUMENTATION

▪ Patient's verbal and nonverbal communication of spiritual discomfort
▪ Stage of anticipatory grief, as indicated by behavior
▪ Interventions to promote spiritual comfort
▪ Patient's response to interventions
▪ Evaluations for expected outcomes
▪ Observations about patient's spiritual distress or well-being

REFERENCES

Bhatnagar, S., Gielen, J., Satija, A., Singh, S. P., Noble, S., & Chaturvedi, S. K. (2017). Signs of spiritual distress and its implications for practice in Indian palliative care. *Indian Journal of Palliative Care, 23*(3), 306–312. doi:10.4103/IJPC.IJPC_24_17

King, S., Fitchett, G., Murphy, P., Pargament, K., Harrison, D., Loggers, E., ... Loggers, E. T. (2017). Determining best methods to screen for religious/spiritual distress. *Supportive Care in Cancer, 25*(2), 471–479. doi:10.1007/s00520-016-3425-6

Roze des Ordons, A. L., Sinuff, T., Stelfox, H. T., Kondejewski, J., & Sinclair, S. (2018). Spiritual distress within inpatient settings-A scoping review of patients' and families' experiences. *Journal of Pain & Symptom Management, 56*(1), 122–145. doi:10.1016/j.jpainsymman.2018.03.009

Risk for Spiritual Distress

DEFINITION

Susceptible to a state of suffering related to the impaired ability to integrate meaning and purpose in life through connections with self, others, the world, and/or a power greater than oneself, which may compromise health

RISK FACTORS

- Altered religious ritual
- Altered spiritual practice
- Anxiety
- Barrier to experiencing love
- Cultural conflict
- Depressive symptoms
- Difficulty accepting the aging process
- Inadequate environmental control
- Inadequate interpersonal relations
- Loneliness
- Loss of independence
- Low self-esteem
- Pain
- Perception of having unfinished business
- Self-alienation
- Separation from support system
- Social alienation
- Sociocultural deprivation
- Stressors
- Substance misuse

ASSOCIATED CONDITIONS

- Chronic disease
- Depression
- Loss of a body part
- Loss of function of a body part
- Treatment regimen

ASSESSMENT

- Health history, including debilitating disease (e.g., rheumatoid arthritis); terminal illness; recurrent cancer; conditions that alter body image (e.g., burns and scars); relapse or exacerbation of neurologic disease (e.g., multiple sclerosis); alcoholism, depression, and drug abuse; and major traumatic injury
- Impact of current illness, injury, or disability on lifestyle
- Spiritual status, religious affiliation, beliefs, and practices; relationship with spiritual authority (e.g., priest, rabbi); beliefs about life, death, and suffering
- Psychological status, including perception of self, body image, problem-solving ability, and coping mechanisms; sources of support (family, partner, friends, caregivers); perception of medical diagnosis or health problem (progression, severity,

prognosis, treatment options); reaction to illness, injury, or disability; self-image, mood, behavior, motivation, and energy level; stressors (finances, job, marital or partner discord, losses through death or separation); expressions of grief; and changes in sleep pattern

■ Family status, including socioeconomic status; quality of relationships; communication patterns; methods of conflict resolution; ability of family members to meet patient's physical, emotional, and social needs; and family goals

EXPECTED OUTCOMES

■ Patient will discuss current spiritual beliefs and concerns.
■ Patient will discuss effects of illness, injury, or disability on personal beliefs and spiritual practices.
■ Patient will use healthy coping techniques to maintain spiritual well-being.
■ Patient will express feelings of spiritual well-being.
■ Patient will be supported in efforts to pursue spirituality in coping with illness, injury, or disability.
■ Patient will reach out to family members, partner, priest, minister, imam, rabbi, or others for assistance.

Suggested NOC Outcomes

Coping; Grief Resolution; Hope; Spiritual Health

INTERVENTIONS AND RATIONALES

PCC ■ Assess the importance of spirituality in patient's life and in coping with illness. Note patient's participation in religious rituals and practices and personal desire to discuss spiritual beliefs. Assess the impact of the illness, injury, or disability on patient's spiritual outlook. *Accurate assessment of the meaning of spirituality for patient is necessary before intervening.*

PCC ■ Assess patient's desire for help in coping with spiritual concerns *to determine the extent to which patient is motivated to address spiritual concerns and open to help from others.*

PCC ■ Express your willingness to discuss spirituality if patient desires *to reduce isolation and to bring spiritual issues into the open.*

PCC ■ Encourage patient to talk about spiritual or religious beliefs and practices. Listen actively to patient's discussion of spiritual concerns *to foster open discussion.*

PCC ■ Encourage patient to express feelings related to recent life-threatening experience *to help patient clarify and cope with personal feelings.*

PCC ■ Communicate acceptance of patient's expression of spiritual concerns, even if patient's feelings are angry and negative *to reassure patient that feelings are valid.*

PCC ■ Show willingness to pray with patient, if the patient wishes, *to provide spiritual support.*

PCC ■ Maintain a nonjudgmental manner. Keep conversation focused on patient's spiritual values *to maintain the therapeutic value of your interaction with patient.*

PCC ■ Provide for continuation of patient's religious practices (e.g., help to obtain ritual items and respect dietary restrictions, if possible) *to demonstrate support and convey caring and acceptance to patient.*

T&C ■ Arrange for visits by clergy, as appropriate, *to provide patient with expert spiritual support.* Provide privacy during visits.

T&C ■ Collaborate with patient's clergyman or hospital chaplain to develop a plan to integrate spiritual interventions into patient's care *to ensure continuity of care.*

Suggested NIC Interventions

Active Listening; Anticipatory Guidance; Anxiety Reduction; Caregiver Support; Emotional Support; Hope Instillation; Spiritual Growth Facilitation; Spiritual Support

EVALUATIONS FOR EXPECTED OUTCOMES

- Patient discusses current spiritual or religious beliefs.
- Patient discusses effects of illness, injury, or disability on beliefs and spiritual practices.
- Patient uses healthy coping techniques to maintain spiritual well-being.
- Patient expresses feelings of spiritual well-being.
- Patient is supported in efforts to pursue spirituality in coping with illness, injury, or disability.
- Patient reaches out to family members, partner, priest, minister, rabbi, imam, or others for assistance.

DOCUMENTATION

- Patient's statements regarding religious beliefs and practices
- Patient's statements indicating effect of current crisis on spiritual outlook
- Patient's statements indicating which rituals and practices help maintain spiritual well-being
- Patient's statements indicating effectiveness of interventions to promote spiritual well-being
- Visits with selected spiritual authority
- Additional referrals to clergy or chaplain
- Evaluations for expected outcomes

REFERENCES

Ghotbabadi, S. S., & Alizadeh, K. H. (2018). The effectiveness of spiritual-religion psychotherapy on mental distress (depression, anxiety and stress) in the elderly living in nursing homes. *Health, Spirituality & Medical Ethics Journal, 5*(1), 20–25.

Harris, J. I., Usset, T., Krause, L., Schill, D., Reuer, B., Donahue, R., & Park, C. L. (2018). Spiritual/religious distress is associated with pain catastrophizing and interference in veterans with chronic pain. *Pain Medicine, 19*(4), 757–763. doi:10.1093/pm/pnx225

Schultz, M., Meged-Book, T., Mashiach, T., & Bar-Sela, G. (2017). Distinguishing between spiritual distress, general distress, spiritual well-being, and spiritual pain among cancer patients during oncology treatment. *Journal of Pain & Symptom Management, 54*(1), 66–73. doi:10.1016/j.jpainsymman.2017.03.018

Readiness for Enhanced Spiritual Well-Being

DEFINITION

A pattern of integrating meaning and purpose in life through connections with self, others, the world, and/or a power greater than oneself, which can be strengthened

ASSESSMENT

- Spiritual status, including personal religious habit; religious or church affiliation; perceptions of faith, life, death, and suffering; support network; embarrassment at practicing religious rituals; beliefs opposed by family members, peers, and health care providers; conflicts with belief system
- Health history, including medical conditions that change body image, chronic or terminal illness, debilitating disease

▦ Psychological status, including reactions to illness and disability; change in appetite, energy level, motivation, personal hygiene, self-image, sleep, and sex drive; alcohol or drug abuse; moodiness; recent divorce, job loss, losses through separation or death; personality traits, maladaptive behaviors; relationships with peers, group involvement, life events in childhood, family pressure; recreational activities; quality of authority relationships, peer relationships; situational crisis; occupation changes; dating and marital history
▦ Brief Psychiatric Rating Scale, Hamilton Depression Rating Scale, and others as needed
▦ Self-care status, including neurologic, musculoskeletal, sensory or psychological impairment, ability to carry out activities and adapt
▦ Family status, including marital status; communication, methods of conflict resolution; ability of family to meet physical, social, and emotional needs of its members; socioeconomic factors; family health history; evidence of abuse
▦ Nutritional status, including height, weight, and any special dietary habits
▦ Sleep pattern status, including hours of sleep, energy level before and after sleep, rest and relaxation patterns; difficulty falling asleep, nocturnal awakening, early morning awakening, hypersomnia, insomnia, sleep pattern reversal; sleep EEG; dyssomnia, parasomnia, unipolar depression, bipolar disorder, sleep apnea

DEFINING CHARACTERISTICS

▦ Expresses desire to enhance acceptance
▦ Expresses desire to enhance capacity to self-comfort
▦ Expresses desire to enhance comfort in one's faith
▦ Expresses desire to enhance connection with nature
▦ Expresses desire to enhance connection with power greater than self
▦ Expresses desire to enhance coping
▦ Expresses desire to enhance courage
▦ Expresses desire to enhance creative energy
▦ Expresses desire to enhance forgiveness from others
▦ Expresses desire to enhance harmony in the environment
▦ Expresses desire to enhance hope
▦ Expresses desire to enhance inner peace
▦ Expresses desire to enhance interaction with significant other
▦ Expresses desire to enhance joy
▦ Expresses desire to enhance love
▦ Expresses desire to enhance love of others
▦ Expresses desire to enhance meditative practice
▦ Expresses desire to enhance mystical experiences
▦ Expresses desire to enhance oneness with nature
▦ Expresses desire to enhance oneness with power greater than self
▦ Expresses desire to enhance participation in religious practices
▦ Expresses desire to enhance peace with power greater than self
▦ Expresses desire to enhance prayerfulness
▦ Expresses desire to enhance reverence
▦ Expresses desire to enhance satisfaction with life
▦ Expresses desire to enhance self-awareness
▦ Expresses desire to enhance self-forgiveness
▦ Expresses desire to enhance sense of awe
▦ Expresses desire to enhance sense of harmony within oneself
▦ Expresses desire to enhance sense of identity
▦ Expresses desire to enhance sense of magic in the environment
▦ Expresses desire to enhance serenity

- Expresses desire to enhance service to others
- Expresses desire to enhance strength in one's faith
- Expresses desire to enhance surrender

EXPECTED OUTCOMES

- Patient will discuss spiritual conflicts and concerns.
- Patient will be provided with opportunity to meet with chosen religious authority.
- Patient will be supported in the efforts to pursue enhanced spiritual well-being.
- Patient will pursue religious or spiritual practices to the extent that the patient feels comfortable.
- Patient will describe plan to continue to enhance spiritual well-being.
- Patient will receive referrals for continued support.

Suggested NOC Outcomes

Hope; Quality of Life; Spiritual Health

INTERVENTIONS AND RATIONALES

PCC ▪ Monitor patient for potential signs of spiritual distress that might harm patient's well-being (altered self-care, sleep pattern disturbance, and change in exercise and eating habits) *to plan appropriate interventions.*

PCC ▪ Assess the significance of spirituality in patient's life and in coping with illness. Note whether patient participates in religious rituals, observes religious practices (such as prayer, meditation, or dietary restrictions), or wishes to discuss spiritual beliefs. Keep an open view of what constitutes spirituality. *Before the nurse can intervene in spiritual matters, he or she must determine if spirituality is significant for patient.*

▪ Ask patient if illness has affected the spiritual outlook and tell patient you're willing to help in addressing spiritual issues, if patient wishes, *to reduce isolation and help bring issues related to spiritual distress out into the open.*

PCC ▪ Ask if patient wishes to discuss spiritual concerns with a chosen religious authority *to allow access to expert spiritual care resources.*

PCC ▪ Encourage patient to pursue spiritual questions. Reassure patient that spiritual concerns are valid and that by strengthening spirituality, patient can enhance overall well-being *to demonstrate acceptance.*

EBP ▪ Provide patient with resources for coping with spiritual distress (such as referrals to religious or spiritual organizations or books on prayer and meditation) *to enhance the opportunity to attend to spiritual needs.* Make sure the resources selected are appropriate with regard to patient's religious affiliation and spiritual beliefs *to demonstrate respect for own beliefs and values.* If you lack knowledge about patient's beliefs and practices, consult patient's chosen religious authority *to best meet patient's needs.*

PCC ▪ Help patient arrange travel to a place selected for prayer, reflection, or contemplation. Use resources such as church-affiliated vans or volunteer escorts *to enhance patient's contact with outside sources of support.*

PCC ▪ Demonstrate to patient that you're willing to discuss issues related to spirituality, such as patient's view of God or a higher power, how illness has affected patient's religious beliefs, or how hospital stays affect patient's spiritual practices, *to bring spiritual issues into the open.* Keep an open mind when listening. Keep the conversation focused on patient's spiritual values and the role they play in recovering from illness and coping with changes in body image *to ensure that interaction between the nurse and patient remains therapeutic.*

EBP ▪ Discuss with patient the importance of maintaining a healthy diet, getting regular exercise and sleep, and maintaining healthy interaction with family members and friends. *A patient in spiritual distress may neglect day-to-day well-being.*

PCC ▪ Praise patient for taking time to attend to spiritual needs and encourage patient to continue to develop spirituality after leaving the health care setting *to provide continued encouragement.*

T&C ▪ Provide patient with referrals to appropriate religious groups, spiritually centered organizations, and social service organizations *to help provide additional support and to ensure continuity of care.*

T&C ▪ Consider resources such as parish nurses, home-visiting services, and computer networks *to help provide continued opportunity for spiritual development and to ensure continuity of care.*

Suggested NIC Interventions

Active Listening; Emotional Support; Hope Instillation; Presence; Spiritual Growth Facilitation; Spiritual Support

EVALUATIONS FOR EXPECTED OUTCOMES

▪ Patient becomes comfortable discussing spiritual conflicts.
▪ Patient is visited by a religious representative of choice.
▪ Patient is supported in efforts to pursue enhanced spiritual well-being.
▪ Patient takes the initiative to pursue desire for active religious participation.
▪ Patient openly discusses effects of illness on own beliefs and other spiritual issues.
▪ Patient develops a plan for continued involvement in religious activity.
▪ Patient accepts referrals for continued religious growth.

DOCUMENTATION

▪ Statements about spiritual conflicts
▪ Visits with chosen religious authority
▪ Engagement in religious or spiritual practices
▪ Suggested religious resources outside of hospital
▪ Statements about ability to cope with changes in body image as a result of illness, to maintain spiritual values in face of long-term or chronic illness, and to pursue spiritual practices during hospital stays
▪ Eating patterns, exercise schedules, and sleep patterns
▪ Stated plans to continue to enhance spiritual well-being
▪ Evaluations for expected outcomes

REFERENCES

Chen, Y., Lin, L., Chuang, L., & Chen, M. (2017). The relationship of physiopsychosocial factors and spiritual well-being in elderly residents: Implications for evidence-based practice. *Worldviews on Evidence-Based Nursing, 14*(6), 484–491. doi.org/10.1111/wvn.12243

Jugjali, R., Yodchai, K., & Thaniwattananon, P. (2018). Factors influencing spiritual well-being in patients receiving haemodialysis: A literature review. *Renal Society of Australasia Journal, 14*(3), 90–95.

Liu, M. L., & Hsiao, Y. C. (2019). The impact of demoralization on spiritual well-being in terminally ill patients. *Journal of Nursing, 66*(1), 48–59. doi:10.6224/JN.201902_66(1).07

Impaired Spontaneous Ventilation

DEFINITION

Inability to initiate and/or maintain independent breathing that is adequate to support life

RELATED FACTOR (R/T)

Respiratory muscle fatigue

ASSOCIATED CONDITION

Alteration in metabolism

ASSESSMENT

- Age
- Health history, including previous respiratory problems
- Respiratory status, including rate, rhythm, and depth of respirations; chest excursion and symmetry; presence of cyanosis; and use of accessory muscles
- Effectiveness of cough in clearing secretions
- Suctioning demands, including frequency and tolerance
- Sputum characteristics, including appearance, consistency, color, and odor
- Neuromuscular strength and endurance
- Mental and emotional status, including cognitive state and ability to follow directions
- Laboratory values, including arterial blood gas (ABG) levels (baseline and ongoing), complete blood count, serum electrolyte levels, coagulation studies, serum and sputum cultures, and sensitivity tests
- Vital signs
- Functional status, including ability to perform activities of daily living (ADLs)
- Related or concurrent events that may contribute to respiratory distress, such as bleeding, hypervolemia, hypovolemia, and sepsis

DEFINING CHARACTERISTICS

- Apprehensiveness
- Decrease in arterial oxygen saturation (SaO_2)
- Decrease in cooperation
- Decrease in partial pressure of oxygen (PO_2)
- Decrease in tidal volume
- Dyspnea
- Increase in accessory muscle use
- Increase in heart rate
- Increase in metabolic rate
- Increase in partial pressure of carbon dioxide (PCO_2)
- Restlessness

EXPECTED OUTCOMES

- Patient's respiratory rate will remain within 5 breaths/minute of baseline.
- Patient's ABG levels will be normal.
- Patient will indicate feeling comfortable and won't report pain, dyspnea, or fatigue.

- Patient will carry out ADLs with minimal supplemental oxygen.
- Patient's breathing pattern will return to baseline.
- Patient's PaO_2 will remain within normal limits as activity level increases.
- Patient will breathe spontaneously after ventilator support is withdrawn.

Suggested NOC Outcomes

Anxiety Level; Endurance; Energy Conservation; Respiratory Status: Gas Exchange; Respiratory Status: Ventilation; Vital Signs

INTERVENTIONS AND RATIONALES

- **S** Monitor patient's vital signs every 15 minutes to 1 hour *to detect tachypnea and tachycardia, early indicators of respiratory distress.*
- **S** Monitor patient for nasal flaring, change in depth and pattern of breathing, use of accessory muscles, and cyanosis *to detect signs of severe respiratory distress.*
- **S** Monitor ABG levels and report deviations promptly *to determine the need for changes to the therapeutic regimen.*
- **S** Monitor hemoglobin (Hb) level and hematocrit (HCT). *Low Hb level and HCT indicate decreased oxygen-carrying capacity of the blood.*
- **EBP** Begin oxygen support using the smallest concentration needed to make patient comfortable. Monitor closely *to avoid oxygen toxicity.*
- **EBP** Elevate the head of the bed *to increase comfort and to promote adequate chest expansion and diaphragmatic excursion, thereby decreasing work of breathing.*
- **EBP** Explain the meanings of ventilator alarms and what will happen if alarms sound *to help reduce anxiety and minimize complications.*
- **PCC** Help patient progress gradually from bed rest to increased activity *to improve patient's sense of well-being.* Monitor vital signs and ABG levels closely. If respiratory status is compromised, return patient to bed rest *to decrease basal metabolic rate and lower oxygen demands.*
- **PCC** Explain procedures to patient. Describe specific sensations patient may experience during each procedure *to decrease anxiety.*
- **S** Anticipate possible complications. Keep in mind that if patient decompensates while on 100% fraction of inspired oxygen non-rebreather mask, endotracheal intubation may be required. *Anticipating complications facilitates prompt intervention.*
- **S** If patient requires intubation, monitor for spontaneous breathing and gradually wean the patient from the ventilator. *Progressive weaning helps patient adjust physiologically and emotionally to increased work of breathing.*
- **EBP** Avoid respiratory depressants, such as opioids, sedatives, and paralytics, *to facilitate patient's recovery.*
- **PCC** Provide explanations to the family. Spend time with them at the bedside, demonstrating ways in which to approach and support patient without causing undue anxiety. *Watching someone who is having difficulty breathing makes others anxious, compounding the reaction of the patient to shortness of breath.*

Suggested NIC Interventions

Acid–Base Management; Airway Suctioning; Artificial Airway Management; Aspiration Precautions; Coping Enhancement; Mechanical Ventilation; Oxygen Therapy; Positioning; Respiratory Monitoring; Self-Care Assistance

EVALUATIONS FOR EXPECTED OUTCOMES

- Patient's respiratory rate is within 5 breaths/minute of baseline.
- Patient's ABG levels are normal.
- Patient indicates feeling comfortable and doesn't report pain, dyspnea, or fatigue.
- Patient carries out ADLs with minimal supplemental oxygen.
- Patient's breathing pattern returns to baseline.
- Patient's PaO_2 remains within normal limits when activity level increases.
- Patient breathes spontaneously after ventilator support is withdrawn.

DOCUMENTATION

- Patient's reports of malaise, dyspnea, restlessness, chest pain, dizziness, or light-headedness
- Patient's response to nursing interventions
- Patient's response to initiation of oxygen therapy and progressive changes in therapy
- Laboratory data, including ABG levels
- Respiratory status (baseline and ongoing)
- Subtle personality changes
- Changes in breath sounds revealed by auscultation
- Evaluations for expected outcomes

REFERENCES

Ebrahimabadi, S., Moghadam, A. B., Vakili, M., Modanloo, M., & Khoddam, H. (2017). Studying the power of the integrative weaning index in predicting the success rate of the spontaneous breathing trial in patients under mechanical ventilation. *Indian Journal of Critical Care Medicine, 21*(8), 488–493. doi:10.4103/ijccm.IJCCM_10_17

Liang, G., Liu, T., Zeng, Y., Shi, Y., Yang, W., Yang, Y., & Kang, Y. (2018). Characteristics of subjects who failed a 120-minute spontaneous breathing trial. *Respiratory Care, 63*(4), 388–394. doi:10.4187/respcare.05820

Munshi, L., & Ferguson, N. D. (2018). Weaning from mechanical ventilation: What should be done when a patient's spontaneous breathing trial fails? *JAMA: Journal of the American Medical Association, 320*(18), 1865–1867. doi:10.1001/jama.2018.13762

Impaired Standing

DEFINITION

Limitation of ability to independently and purposefully attain and/or maintain the body in an upright position from feet to head

RELATED FACTORS (R/T)

- Emotional disturbance
- Insufficient endurance
- Insufficient energy
- Insufficient strength
- Malnutrition
- Obesity
- Pain
- Self-imposed relief posture

ASSOCIATED CONDITIONS

- Circulatory perfusion disorder
- Impaired metabolic functioning

- Injury to lower extremity
- Neurological disorder
- Prescribed posture
- Sarcopenia
- Surgical procedure

ASSESSMENT

- History of neuromuscular disorder or dysfunction
- Neurologic status, including level of consciousness, motor ability, and sensory ability
- Musculoskeletal status, including coordination, balance, muscle size and strength, muscle tone, range of motion, and functional mobility scale:

  0 = completely independent
  1 = requires use of equipment or device
  2 = requires help, supervision, or teaching from another person
  3 = requires help from another person and equipment or device
  4 = dependent; doesn't participate in activity

DEFINING CHARACTERISTICS

- Impaired ability to adjust position of one or both lower limbs on uneven surface
- Impaired ability to attain a balanced position of the torso
- Impaired ability to extend one or both hips
- Impaired ability to extend one or both knees
- Impaired ability to flex one or both hips
- Impaired ability to flex one or both knees
- Impaired ability to maintain the torso in balanced position
- Impaired ability to stress torso with body weight

EXPECTED OUTCOMES

- Patient will achieve highest level of independence possible when standing.
- Patient will show no evidence of complications.
- Patient will achieve balance while standing.
- Patient will maintain muscle strength.

Suggested NOC Outcomes

Activity Tolerance; Endurance; Joint Movement: Hip; Joint Movement: Spine; Neurological Status: Central Motor Control; Neurological Status: Spinal Sensory/Motor Function; Physical Fitness; Skeletal Function

INTERVENTIONS AND RATIONALES

- **S** Use a transfer belt if necessary *to support patient and prevent staff injury.*
- **S** Use assistive devices as necessary *to support patient and prevent staff injury.*
- **PCC** Identify the level of functioning using a functional mobility scale (see "Assessment"). Communicate patient's skill level to all staff members *to provide continuity and preserve identified level of independence.*
- **PCC** Encourage independence by helping patient use assistive devices. *This increases muscle tone and patient's self-esteem.*

`PCC`   ▓ Monitor and record daily any evidence of immobility complications (such as contractures, venous stasis, thrombus, pneumonia, and urinary tract infection). *Patients with a history of neuromuscular disorders or dysfunction may be more prone to developing complications.*

`S`   ▓ Instruct patient to call before attempting to stand without assistance. *Ensure patient safety from falls.*

`EBP`   ▓ Carry out a medical regimen to manage or prevent complications; for example, administer prophylactic heparin as ordered for venous thrombosis. *This promotes patient's health and well-being.*

`T&C`   ▓ Refer patient to a physical therapist *to help rehabilitate musculoskeletal deficits.*

`PCC`   ▓ Demonstrate the standing procedure and note date. Have patient and family members return standing procedure demonstration and note date. *This ensures continuity of care and use of proper technique.*

Suggested NIC Interventions

Body Mechanics Promotion; Exercise Therapy: Balance; Exercise Therapy: Muscle Control; Positioning; Self-Care Assistance

EVALUATIONS FOR EXPECTED OUTCOMES

▓ Patient achievement of highest level of independence possible when standing.
▓ Patient has no evidence of complications.
▓ Patient achievement of balance while standing.
▓ Patient maintains muscle strength.

DOCUMENTATION

▓ Patient's current status of functional abilities and goals set for self
▓ Observations of patient's mobility status, presence of complications, and response to standing
▓ Instruction and demonstration of skills in standing
▓ Patient's response to nursing interventions
▓ Evaluations for expected outcomes

REFERENCES

Ota, T., Hashidate, H., Shimizu, N., & Yatsunami, M. (2019). Early effects of a knee-ankle-foot orthosis on static standing balance in people with subacute stroke. *Journal of Physical Therapy Science, 31*(2), 127–131.

Sremakaew, M., Sungkarat, S., Treleaven, J., & Uthaikhup, S. (2018). Impaired standing balance in individuals with cervicogenic headache and migraine. *Journal of Oral & Facial Pain & Headache, 32*(3), 321–328. doi:10.11607/ofph.2029

Walowska, J., Bolach, B., & Bolach, E. (2018). The influence of Pilates exercises on body balance in the standing position of hearing impaired people. *Disability & Rehabilitation, 40*(25), 3061–3069. doi:10.1080/09638288.2017.1370731

Stress Overload

DEFINITION

Excessive amounts and types of demands that require action

- Insufficient resources
- Repeated stressors
- Stressors

- History or current presence of stress reactions in response to internal or external forces expressed by such physical findings as choking sensation, hyperventilation, dizziness, increased heart rate and/or blood pressure, perspiration, pupillary dilation, polyuria, and elevated blood glucose, cholesterol, and free fatty acid levels
- History or current presence of stress reactions expressed by such behavioral cues as insomnia, restlessness, "scattered" thoughts, disorganized speech, restlessness, irritability, and altered concentration
- Physical stressors, including extreme heat or cold, malnutrition, disease, infection, and pain
- Psychological stressors, including fear, sense of failure, change in company or home location, success, holiday, vacation, or promotion
- Level of stress, positive coping mechanisms, realistic thought patterns, behaviors, or energy level
- Medication history, including use of drugs, caffeine, tobacco, or alcohol that stimulates the sympathetic nervous system
- Sleep patterns or changes in daily activities that could be perceived as stressful, including too many or too few activities
- Sociologic factors, including job satisfaction, presence of support systems, family coping mechanisms, or hobbies

- Excessive stress
- Feeling of pressure
- Impaired decision-making
- Impaired functioning
- Increase in anger
- Increase in anger behavior
- Increase in impatience
- Negative impact from stress
- Tension

- Patient will experience reduced signs of stress overload as evidenced by subjective report and observations of reduced stress, such as less facial tension and less restlessness.
- Patient will connect environmental stressors with manifestations of stress such as insomnia, tearful outbursts, irritability, or headache.
- Patients will set limits on activities assumed by saying "No" without expressions of guilt.
- Patient will develop more effective coping strategies to manage stress, such as guided imagery, exercise, healthy diet, and recreation and leisure activities.
- Patient will develop strategies to reframe distorted thinking patterns relating to internal and environmental demands, such as talking about feelings and asking for help.

Suggested NOC Outcomes

Abusive Behavior; Aggression Self-Control; Anxiety Self-Control; Coping; Self-Restraint; Stress Level

INTERVENTIONS AND RATIONALES

- **PCC** ▪ Establish and promote a trusting relationship before asking patient to make any changes. *A trusting relationship can facilitate patient's attempts to make changes, while too many demands early in relationship can foster resistance.*
- **EBP** ▪ Teach prioritization of responsibilities and deadlines to facilitate patient's sense of control over stressors. *Stressors may seem overwhelming, and nurse can promote increased self-esteem when a plan is made cooperatively with nurse and patient as partners.*
- **EBP** ▪ Teach patient about positive self-talk. *Positive self-talk helps change and ultimately reverse negative emotions of guilt, fear, and worry.*
- **EBP** ▪ Teach coping strategies, such as reframing thoughts or using music, guided imagery, yoga, deep breathing exercises, progressive neuromuscular relaxation, or pet therapy. *Strategies that reduce tense muscles and feelings can promote deeper relaxation and reduce heart rate, respirations, and blood pressure by promoting the parasympathetic response.*
- **EBP** ▪ Teach assertiveness training techniques with role-play exercises. *Assertiveness training can provide a concrete way to manage stressors and enhance feeling of being empowered, such as in communicating with demanding individuals.*
- **PCC** ▪ Explore support systems with patient, support groups, or hobbies and outings with partner or family and friends. *Often patient is a caretaker who perceives there is little time for self and is at risk for caregiver burden. Promoting verbalization of feelings with support persons can reduce feeling of stress overload.*
- **EBP** ▪ Explore role of lack of exercise and excessive intake of caffeine, alcohol, nicotine, and carbohydrates during periods of stress overload and adoption of healthier alternatives. *Inappropriate food choices, inactivity, and substance abuse can occur when patient feels stress overload.*
- **PCC** ▪ Provide opportunities for patient to ventilate feelings about stressors. *Promoting a time to talk can help patient share feelings of mounting stress before irritability and tension worsen.*

Suggested NIC Interventions

Anger Control Assistance; Assertiveness Training; Behavior Management; Behavior Modification; Calming Techniques; Cognitive Restructuring; Coping Enhancement; Impulse Control Training; Stress Management Assistance

EVALUATIONS FOR EXPECTED OUTCOMES

- ▪ Patient experiences reduced signs of stress overload as evidenced by subjective report and observations of reduced stress, such as less facial tension and less restlessness.
- ▪ Patient connects environmental stressors with manifestations of stress, such as insomnia, tearful outbursts, irritability, or headache.
- ▪ Patient sets limits on activities assumed by saying "No" without expressions of guilt.
- ▪ Patient addresses usual coping mechanisms for dealing with stress overload, such as increased use of alcohol, caffeine, tobacco, or carbohydrates and adopts more effective coping strategies, such as guided imagery, exercise, healthy diet, and recreation and leisure activities.
- ▪ Patient develops strategies to reframe distorted thinking patterns relating to internal and environmental demands, such as talking about feelings and asking for help.

DOCUMENTATION

▦ Observations of subjective and objective data
▦ Documentation of interventions such as yoga, guided imagery, deep breathing exercises, talking about feelings
▦ Patient's response to interventions
▦ Evaluations for expected outcomes

REFERENCES

Amirkhan, J. H. (2018). A brief stress diagnostic tool: The short stress overload scale. *Assessment, 25*(8), 1001–1013. doi:10.1177/1073191116673173
Amirkhan, J. H., Landa, I., & Huff, S. (2018). Seeking signs of stress overload: Symptoms and behaviors. *International Journal of Stress Management, 25*(3), 301–311. doi:10.1037/str0000066
Duxbury, L., Stevenson, M., & Higgins, C. (2018). Too much to do, too little time: Role overload and stress in a multi-role environment. *International Journal of Stress Management, 25*(3), 250–266. doi:10.1037/str0000062

Ineffective Infant Suck–Swallow Response

DEFINITION

Impaired ability of an infant to suck or to coordinate the suck–swallow response.

RELATED FACTORS (R/T)

▦ Hypoglycemia
▦ Hypothermia
▦ Hypotonia
▦ Inappropriate positioning
▦ Unsatisfactory sucking behavior

ASSOCIATED CONDITIONS

▦ Convulsive episodes
▦ Gastroesophageal reflux
▦ High-flow oxygen by nasal cannula
▦ Lacerations during delivery
▦ Low Appearance, Pulse, Grimace, Activity, & Respiration (APGAR) scores
▦ Neurological delay
▦ Neurological impairment
▦ Oral hypersensitivity
▦ Oropharyngeal deformity
▦ Prolonged enteral nutrition

ASSESSMENT

▦ Perinatal history, including gestational age and Apgar score
▦ Suck and swallow reflex, including condition of lip and palate
▦ Nutritional status, including intake (type, amount, and frequency of feedings), output (frequency, amount, and characteristics of urine), current weight, weight change since birth, skin turgor, and signs of dehydration

- Laboratory studies, including glucose and bilirubin levels
- Parental status, including age, maturity level, and previous experience with infant feeding

DEFINING CHARACTERISTICS

- Arrhythmia
- Bradycardic events
- Choking
- Circumoral cyanosis
- Excessive coughing
- Finger splaying
- Flaccidity
- Gagging
- Hiccups
- Hyperextension of extremities
- Impaired ability to initiate an effective suck
- Impaired ability to sustain an effective suck
- Impaired motor tone
- Inability to coordinate sucking, swallowing, and breathing
- Irritability
- Nasal flaring
- Oxygen desaturation
- Pallor
- Subcostal retraction
- Time-out signals
- Uses accessory muscles to breathe

EXPECTED OUTCOMES

- Neonate won't lose more than 10% of birth weight within first week of life.
- Neonate will gain 4 to 7 oz (113.5 to 198.5 g)/week after first week of life.
- Parents or caregivers will identify factors that interfere with neonate establishing effective feeding pattern.
- Parents will express increased confidence in their ability to perform appropriate feeding techniques.
- Neonate won't become dehydrated.
- Neonate will receive adequate supplemental nutrition until able to suckle sufficiently.
- Neonate will establish effective suck and swallow reflexes that allow for adequate intake of nutrients.

Suggested NOC Outcomes

Breastfeeding Establishment: Infant; Breastfeeding Maintenance; Nutritional Status: Food & Fluid Intake

INTERVENTIONS AND RATIONALES

PCC   Weigh the neonate at the same time each day on the same scale *to detect excessive weight loss early.*

PCC   Assess the neonate's sucking pattern *to monitor for ineffective patterns.*

PCC ■ Assess the parents' knowledge of feeding techniques *to help identify and clear up misconceptions.*

PCC ■ Assess the parents' level of anxiety about the neonate's feeding difficulty. *Anxiety may interfere with the parents' ability to learn new techniques.*

PCC ■ Remain with the parents and neonate during the feeding *to identify problem areas and direct interventions.*

EBP ■ Teach the parents to place the neonate in the upright position during feeding *to prevent aspiration.*

EBP ■ Teach the parents to unwrap and position a sleepy neonate before feeding *to ensure that the neonate is awake and alert enough to suckle sufficiently.*

PCC ■ Provide positive reinforcement for the parents' efforts to improve their feeding technique *to decrease anxiety and enhance feelings of success.*

EBP ■ For bottle-feeding, record the amount ingested at each feeding; for breastfeeding, record the number of minutes the neonate nurses at each breast and the amount of any supplement ingested *to monitor for inadequate caloric and fluid intake.*

EBP ■ Provide an alternative nipple, such as a preemie nipple. *A preemie nipple has a larger hole and softer texture, which makes it easier for the neonate to obtain formula.*

EBP ■ For breastfeeding, ensure the neonate's tongue is properly positioned under the mother's nipple *to promote adequate sucking.*

S ■ Monitor the neonate for poor skin turgor, dry mucous membranes, decreased or concentrated urine, and sunken fontanels and eyeballs *to detect possible dehydration and allow for immediate intervention.*

EBP ■ Record the number of stools and amount of urine voided each shift. *An altered bowel elimination pattern may indicate decreased food intake; decreased amounts of concentrated urine may indicate dehydration.*

EBP ■ Assess the need for gavage feeding. *The neonate may temporarily require alternative means of obtaining adequate fluids and calories.*

EBP ■ Alternate oral and gavage feeding *to conserve the neonate's energy.*

EBP ■ If the neonate requires IV nourishment, assess the insertion site, amount infused, and infusion rate every hour *to monitor fluid intake and identify possible complications, such as infiltration and phlebitis.*

EBP ■ Assess the neonate for neurological deficits or other pathophysiological causes of ineffective sucking *to identify the need for more extensive evaluation.*

Suggested NIC Interventions

Attachment Promotion; Breastfeeding Assistance; Lactation Counseling; Nonnutritive Sucking

EVALUATIONS FOR EXPECTED OUTCOMES

■ Neonate doesn't lose more than 10% of birth weight within first week of life.

■ Neonate gains 4 to 7 oz/week after first week of life.

■ Parents identify factors that interfere with effective feeding.

■ Parents express increased confidence in their ability to perform appropriate feeding techniques.

■ Neonate maintains urine output of 1 mL/kg/day, urine specific gravity of 1.003 to 1.013, good skin turgor, moist mucous membranes, and soft, flat fontanels.

■ Neonate receives adequate nutrition.

■ Neonate establishes effective sucking reflex and coordinated suck and swallow response.

DOCUMENTATION

- Frequency, amount, and type of fluid ingested by neonate
- Effectiveness of suck reflex
- Neonate's daily weight
- Parents' knowledge of feeding techniques, involvement with caregiving, and bonding with neonate
- Frequency of neonate's bowel elimination and urination
- Signs of dehydration
- Nursing interventions
- Use of special feeding techniques and equipment
- Parents' and neonate's responses to nursing interventions
- Evidence of neurological or other physical impairment in neonate
- Evaluations for expected outcomes

REFERENCES

Giannì, M. L., Sannino, P., Bezze, E., Plevani, L., Esposito, C., Muscolo, S., Roggero, P., & Mosca, F. (2017). Usefulness of the infant driven scale in the early identification of preterm infants at risk for delayed oral feeding independency. *Early Human Development, 115*, 18–22.

Mckean, E. B., Kasparian, N. A., Batra, S., Sholler, G. F., Winlaw, D. S., & Dalby-Payne, J. (2017). Feeding difficulties in neonates following cardiac surgery: Determinants of prolonged feeding-tube use. *Cardiology in the Young, 27*(6), 1203–1211.

Roess, A. A., Jacquier, E. F., Catellier, D. J., Carvalho, R., Lutes, A. C., Anater, A. S., & Dietz, W. H. (2018). Food consumption patterns of infants and toddlers: Findings from the feeding infants and toddlers study (FITS) 2016. *Journal of Nutrition, 148*, 1525S–1535S.

Zimmerman, E., & Rosner, A. (2018). Feeding swallowing difficulties in the first three years of life: A preterm and full-term infant comparison. *Journal of Neonatal Nursing, 24*(6), 331–335.

Risk for Sudden Infant Death

DEFINITION

Susceptible to unpredicted death of an infant

RISK FACTORS

- Delay in prenatal care
- Exposure to second hand smoke
- Infant overheating
- Infant overwrapping
- Infant placed in prone position to sleep
- Infant placed in side-lying position to sleep
- Insufficient prenatal care
- Soft sleep surface
- Soft, loose objects placed near infant
- Infant less than 4 months placed in sitting devices for routine sleep

ASSOCIATED CONDITION

Cold weather

ASSESSMENT

- Age, sex, weight, ethnic background
- Perinatal history (gestational age, Apgar score, birth weight, birth order)

- Maternal history (age, socioeconomic status, level of education, parenting experience; smoking, alcohol, and drug history)
- Cardiovascular status (pulse, blood pressure, heart sounds)
- Respiratory status (respiratory rate, quality, depth, breath sounds)
- Neurologic status (alertness, reflexes—especially gag, suck, swallow, response to touch)
- Sleep routines (position, mattress, sleepwear, room temperature, cobedding)
- Feeding routines (breast- or bottle-fed, ease of feeding, spitting up)

EXPECTED OUTCOMES

- Parents will be receptive to teaching and guidance.
- Parents will verbalize understanding of risk factors and provide all precautions possible to prevent disorder.
- Infant will be placed in proper position on back with head of crib slightly elevated.
- Infant will be able to move extremities and head freely without restriction or without becoming tangled in loose bedding or articles.
- Infant will sleep alone in appropriate crib on firm sleep surface.
- Infant's body temperature will remain within normal limits.
- Infant will be monitored with apnea monitor during sleep.
- Parents state that they feel prepared and have the ability to handle emergencies utilizing CPR techniques and 911 services.
- Parents will handle the stress of knowing they have a high-risk infant with appropriate coping skills.

Suggested NOC Outcomes

Risk Control; Risk Detection

INTERVENTIONS AND RATIONALES

- **EBP** Educate family about the risk factors of sudden infant death syndrome (SIDS) *so that they'll be aware of the current practices to reduce risk and prevent its occurrence.*
- **S** Position infant on the back when placed in the crib. *Incidence of SIDS is higher among infants placed prone.*
- **S** Make sure infant's head is slightly elevated *to decrease abdominal pressure on the diaphragm and allow better expansion of the lungs.*
- **EBP** Teach parents to avoid having loose blankets, toys, or other articles in the crib *to decrease the risk of accidental suffocation.*
- **S** Make sure infant lies on a firm surface so that infant doesn't sink into the mattress, mattress cover, or blanket *to decrease the risk of suffocation.*
- **S** Avoid overheating the room and wrapping infant's body in heavy blankets. *Overheating infant increases the body's demand for oxygen.*
- **PCC** Encourage mother to breastfeed infant *because this is associated with a lower incidence of SIDS.*
- **S** When an apnea monitor is ordered for high-risk infant, teach parents how to correctly apply the apparatus and leads and ensure that alarms are set correctly. The machine will sound an alarm if the respiratory rate or heart rate falls below a predetermined level (typically specified by the physician). *The benefit of the monitor can only be achieved if it is utilized appropriately.*
- **EBP** Instruct parents in the correct application of CPR *to reduce anxiety and promote confidence in technique.*

▓ Assess the level of anxiety in parents and family members routinely and provide suggestions for coping mechanisms *to assist family in dealing with the period of vulnerability for infant.*

 ▓ Make appropriate referrals for community health nursing and home visits *to allow an opportunity to assess the home situation, care provided, and coping level of the family.*

Suggested NIC Interventions

Anticipatory Guidance; Anxiety Reduction; Caregiver Support; Coping-Enhancement; Emotional Support; Environmental Management: Safety; Family Integrity Promotion: Childbearing Family; Infant Care; Learning Facilitation; Parent Education: Childrearing Family; Positioning; Risk Identification: Childbearing Family; Teaching: Infant Safety

EVALUATIONS FOR EXPECTED OUTCOMES

▓ Parents listen and cooperate with patient teaching.
▓ Parents readily participate in education regarding SIDS risk factors and management.
▓ Parents utilize appropriate positioning of infant in crib.
▓ Infant moves freely without entanglement or suffocation in crib during sleep.
▓ Parents allow infant to sleep alone on firm surface.
▓ Infant's temperature remains within normal limits.
▓ Apnea monitor is utilized correctly.
▓ Parents utilize CPR and activate emergency services appropriately.
▓ Family members recognize need for heightened coping skills to deal with stress of high-risk infant.

DOCUMENTATION

▓ Information given to parents regarding SIDS, positioning the infant, and sleeping arrangements
▓ Infant's temperature
▓ Demonstration of apnea monitor
▓ Attendance at CPR class
▓ Evaluations for expected outcomes

REFERENCES

Bartick, M., & Tomori, C. (2019). Sudden infant death and social justice: A syndemics approach. *Maternal & Child Nutrition, 15*(1), e12652. doi:10.1111/mcn.12652

Dufer, H., & Godfrey, K. (2017). Integration of safe sleep and sudden infant death syndrome (SIDS) education among parents of preterm infants in the Neonatal Intensive Care Unit (NICU). *Journal of Neonatal Nursing, 23*(2), 103–108. doi:10.1016/j.jnn.2016.09.001

Friedmann, I., Dahdouh, E. M., Kugler, P., Mimran, G., & Balayla, J. (2017). Maternal and obstetrical predictors of sudden infant death syndrome (SIDS). *Journal of Maternal-Fetal & Neonatal Medicine, 30*(19), 2315–2323. doi:10.1080/14767058.2016.1247265

Risk for Suffocation

DEFINITION

Susceptible to inadequate air availability for inhalation, which may compromise health

RISK FACTORS

▓ Access to empty refrigerator/freezer
▓ Eating large mouthfuls of food

- Emotional disturbance
- Gas leak
- Insufficient knowledge of safety precautions
- Low-strung clothesline
- Pacifier around infant's neck
- Playing with plastic bag
- Propped bottle in infant's crib
- Small object in airway
- Smoking in bed
- Soft underlayment
- Unattended in water
- Unvented fuel-burning heater
- Vehicle running in closed garage

ASSOCIATED CONDITIONS

- Alteration in cognitive functioning
- Alteration in olfactory function
- Face/neck disease
- Face/neck injury
- Impaired motor functioning

ASSESSMENT

- Health history, including accidents, allergies, exposure to pollutants, falls, hyperthermia, hypothermia, poisoning, seizures, sensory or perceptual changes (auditory, gustatory, kinesthetic, olfactory, tactile, or visual), and trauma
- Circumstances of current situation that might lead to injury
- Neurological status, including level of consciousness, mental status, and orientation
- Laboratory studies, including clotting factors, hemoglobin level, hematocrit, platelet count, and white blood cell count

EXPECTED OUTCOMES

- Patient will avoid accidental suffocation.
- Patient's airway will remain patent at all times.
- Patient's vital signs will remain within normal parameters.
- Patient and family members will demonstrate knowledge of safety measures to prevent suffocation.

Suggested NOC Outcomes

Aspiration Prevention; Personal Safety Behavior; Respiratory Status: Ventilation; Risk Control; Risk Detection

INTERVENTIONS AND RATIONALES

- **S** Monitor and record patient's respiratory status. *Changes in parameters (such as respiratory rate, cough, sputum production, and skin color) may indicate airway obstruction.*
- **S** Monitor and record patient's neurologic status. *Headache, depression, apathy, memory loss, poor muscle coordination, fatigue, stupor, and loss of consciousness may indicate hypoxia.*

S ▪ Monitor patient's vital signs and report changes. *Tachycardia and a slight rise in blood pressure may indicate hypoxia. Reduced heart rate and loss of consciousness indicate advanced hypoxia.*

S ▪ Position patient on the side or adjust position of head and neck to prevent relaxed neck muscles from obstructing airway *to allow maximal chest expansion and prevent aspiration and airway obstruction.*

S ▪ Check all ventilator connections every 30 minutes if patient is on mechanical ventilation *to ensure patient receives proper amount of oxygen at appropriate volume and rate.*

S ▪ Check ventilator alarms every 30 minutes and after suctioning *to ensure proper alarm function.*

S ▪ Obtain suction equipment, assemble, and keep at bedside *to assure equipment readiness in case of need.*

S ▪ Suction airway, as needed, *to prevent secretion accumulation. Do this only as needed to prevent tracheal irritation.*

S ▪ Make sure patient lies on a firm surface and doesn't sink into the mattress, mattress cover, or blanket *to decrease the risk of suffocation.*

EBP ▪ Teach parents to maintain child's bed with sheets that fit snugly on the mattress *to keep it from coming off and getting wrapped around child's head.*

EBP ▪ Teach parents of infants and small children to avoid having loose blankets, toys, or other articles in the crib and bed *to decrease the risk of accidental suffocation.*

EBP ▪ Teach parents of infants and small children to promptly dispose of plastic shopping bags and plastic dry-cleaning bags and to keep all plastic bags, including garbage bags and sandwich-style plastic bags, out of the reach of young children *to avoid playing with plastic bags and to decrease the risk of accidental suffocation.*

EBP ▪ Provide patient and family members with information about safety practices including appliance (refrigerator/freezer) disposal, home environment, swimming pool safety, and use of space heating equipment *to enable them to take an active role in patient's care and ensure performance of safety measures.*

Suggested NIC Interventions

Airway Management; Aspiration Precautions; Energy Management; Respiratory Monitoring; Security Enhancement; Surveillance; Vital Signs Monitoring

EVALUATIONS FOR EXPECTED OUTCOMES

▪ Patient's airway remains free from obstruction.
▪ Patient's vital signs remain within normal parameters.
▪ Patient and family members demonstrate safety measures to prevent suffocation.

DOCUMENTATION

▪ Patient's statements that indicate potential for injury
▪ Physical findings
▪ Observations or knowledge of unsafe practices
▪ Interventions performed to prevent injury
▪ Patient's response to nursing interventions
▪ Evaluations for expected outcomes

REFERENCES

Carlin, R. F., Abrams, A., Mathews, A., Joyner, B. L., Oden, R., Mccarter, R., & Moon, R. Y. (2018). The impact of health messages on maternal decisions about infant sleep position: A randomized controlled trial. *Journal of Community Health, 43*(5), 977–985. doi:10.1007/s10900-018-0514-0

Gaw, C. E., Chounthirath, T., Midgett, J., Quinlan, K., & Smith, G. A. (2017). Types of objects in the sleep environment associated with infant suffocation and strangulation. *Academic Pediatrics, 17*(8), 893–901. doi:10.1016/j.acap.2017.07.002

Sasso, R., Bachir, R., & El Sayed, M. (2018). Suffocation injuries in the United States: Patient characteristics and factors associated with mortality. *Western Journal of Emergency Medicine: Integrating Emergency Care with Population Health, 19*(4), 707–714. doi:10.5811/westjem.2018.4.37198

Simonit, F., Bassan, F., Scorretti, C., & Desinan, L. (2018). Complex suicides: A review of the literature with considerations on a single case of abdominal self stabbing and plastic bag suffocation. *Forensic Science International, 290,* 297–302. doi:10.1016/j.forsciint.2018.07.027

Risk for Suicidal Behavior

DEFINITION

Susceptible to self-injurious acts associated with some intent to die

RISK FACTORS

Behavioral

- Apathy
- Difficulty asking for help
- Difficulty coping with unsatisfactory performance
- Difficulty expressing feelings
- Ineffective chronic pain self-management
- Ineffective impulse control
- Self-injurious behavior
- Self-negligence
- Stockpiling of medication
- Substance misuse

Psychological

- Anxiety
- Depressive symptoms
- Hostility
- Expresses deep sadness
- Expresses frustration
- Expresses loneliness
- Low self-esteem
- Maladaptive grieving
- Perceived dishonor
- Perceived failure
- Reports excessive guilt
- Reports helplessness
- Reports hopelessness
- Reports unhappiness
- Suicidal ideation

Situational

- Easy access to weapon
- Loss of independence
- Loss of personal autonomy

Social

- Dysfunctional family processes
- Inadequate social support
- Inappropriate peer pressure
- Legal difficulty
- Social deprivation
- Social devaluation
- Social isolation
- Unaddressed violence by others

Verbal

- Reports desire to die
- Threat of killing self

Other

Chronic pain

ASSOCIATED CONDITIONS

- Depression
- Mental disorders
- Physical illness
- Terminal illness

ASSESSMENT

- Age
- Gender
- Medical history
- Patient's life situation
- Recent stressors and coping behaviors
- Available support systems
- History of suicide attempts, including aggressiveness of suicide attempts, lethality of suicide attempts, and number of prior suicide attempts
- History of substance abuse (type and effects on mental status)
- Reaction of family members
- Safety hazards
- Mental status, including abstract thinking, affect, content of thought, general information, insight, judgment, mood, orientation, recent and remote memory, and thought processes

EXPECTED OUTCOMES

- Patient will not attempt suicide.
- Patient's environment will be free from potential suicide weapons.
- Patient will recover from suicidal episode.
- Patient will discuss feelings that precipitated suicide attempt.
- Patient will consult mental health professional.
- Patient will describe available resources for crisis prevention and management.
- Patient will voice improvement in self-worth.

Suggested NOC Outcomes

Impulse Self-Control; Self-Mutilation Restraint; Suicide Self-Restraint

INTERVENTIONS AND RATIONALES

- **PCC** ▪ Ask patient directly, "Have you thought about killing yourself?" If so, ask, "What do you plan to do?" *Suicide risk increases if patient has a definite plan.*
- **S** ▪ Initiate appropriate safety protocols by removing from patient's environment anything that could be used to inflict further self-injury (razor blades, belts, glass objects, pills) *to help ensure patient's safety.*
- **PCC** ▪ Make a short-term contract with patient on not harming self during a specific period. Continue negotiating until no evidence of suicidal ideation exists. *A contract gets the subject of suicide out in the open, places some responsibility for safety on patient, and conveys acceptance of patient as a worthwhile person.*
- **S** ▪ Supervise the administration of prescribed medications. *Medications may be appropriate alternative to verbal interventions.* Be aware of drug actions and adverse effects. Make sure that patient doesn't hoard medications.
- **S** ▪ Provide supervision (one-on-one observation when possible) for patient based on facility policy *to ensure compliance with legal requirements to protect patient and to reassure patient of staff concern.*
- **PCC** ▪ Use a warm, caring, nonjudgmental manner *to show unconditional positive regard.*
- **PCC** ▪ Listen carefully to patient and don't challenge patient *to communicate care and support.*
- **PCC** ▪ Demonstrate understanding, but don't reinforce denial of the current situation *because denial can mask the roots of suicidal feelings.*
- **T&C** ▪ Make appropriate referrals to mental health professionals *to help patient work through suicidal feelings and develop healthier alternatives.*
- **PCC** ▪ Help patient set a goal for obtaining long-term psychiatric care. *Ambivalence about psychiatric care or refusal to consult with a therapist marks the suicidal patient's lack of insight and use of denial.*
- **T&C** ▪ Provide patient with telephone numbers and other information about crisis centers, hot lines, and counselors. *Alternatives may ease anxiety about the perceived threat of long-term psychotherapy.*

Suggested NIC Interventions

Behavior Management: Self-Harm; Environmental Management: Violence Prevention; Impulse Control Training; Suicide Prevention

EVALUATIONS FOR EXPECTED OUTCOMES

- ▪ Patient won't harm self.
- ▪ In the aftermath of initial suicide attempt, patient makes commitment not to act on suicidal thoughts.
- ▪ Patient states reasons for suicide attempt.
- ▪ Patient contacts mental health professional.

- Patient identifies crisis prevention resources, such as hotline phone number, local crisis center, and name of therapist.
- Patient expresses positive feelings about self.

DOCUMENTATION

- Patient's comments about suicide attempt and current feelings about it
- Observations of patient's behavior
- Interventions to reduce or prevent self-destructive behavior
- Patient's observable response to interventions
- Evaluations for expected outcomes

REFERENCES

di Giacomo, E., Krausz, M., Colmegna, F., Aspesi, F., & Clerici, M. (2018). Estimating the risk of attempted suicide among sexual minority youths: A systematic review and meta-analysis. *JAMA Pediatrics, 172*(12), 1145–1152. doi:10.1001/jamapediatrics.2018.2731

La Guardia, A. C., Cramer, R. J., Brubaker, M., & Long, M. M. (2019). Community mental health provider responses to a competency-based training in suicide risk assessment and prevention. *Community Mental Health Journal, 55*(2), 257–266. doi:10.1007/s10597-018-0314-0

Miller, S. N., Bozzay, M. L., Ben-Porath, Y. S., & Arbisi, P. A. (2019). Distinguishing levels of suicide risk in depressed male veterans: The role of internalizing and externalizing psychopathology as measured by the MMPI-2-RF. *Assessment, 26*(1), 85–98. doi:10.1177/1073191117743787

Struszczyk, S., Galdas, P. M., & Tiffin, P. A. (2019). Men and suicide prevention: A scoping review. *Journal of Mental Health, 28*(1), 80–88. doi:10.1080/09638237.2017.1370638

Delayed Surgical Recovery

DEFINITION

Extension of the number of postoperative days required to initiate and perform activities that maintain life, health, and well-being

RELATED FACTORS (R/T)

- Delirium
- Impaired physical mobility
- Increased blood glucose level
- Malnutrition
- Negative emotional response to surgical outcome
- Obesity
- Persistent nausea
- Persistent pain
- Persistent vomiting
- Smoking

ASSOCIATED CONDITIONS

- Anemia
- Diabetes mellitus
- Extensive surgical procedures
- Pharmaceutical preparations

- Prolonged duration of perioperative surgical wound infection
- Psychological disorder in postoperative period
- Surgical wound infection

ASSESSMENT

- Age
- Gender
- Reason for surgery
- Type and length of surgical procedure
- Current health status, including weight, vital signs, temperature, nutritional status, integumentary status, neurologic status, cardiovascular status, musculoskeletal status, and pain status
- Laboratory studies, including complete blood count, electrolyte studies, urinalysis, blood cultures, blood coagulation studies, immunologic and serologic tests, liver function tests, cardiac enzyme studies, and arterial blood gas levels
- Health history, including past surgical procedures, food or drug allergies, substance abuse, mental illness, and chronic metabolic or systemic disease (diabetes mellitus; cardiovascular, hepatic, renal, or immunologic disease; coagulation disorders; and splenic or bone marrow disorders)
- Mobility status
- Complications during surgical procedure, such as hemorrhage, drop in blood pressure, and cardiac arrhythmias
- Current medical treatments, including radiation therapy, chemotherapy, antibiotic or antifungal therapy, steroid treatment, anticoagulant or thrombolytic therapy, and immunosuppressive therapy
- Social support, including family status and presence of caregiver and health care provider

DEFINING CHARACTERISTICS

- Anorexia
- Difficulty in moving about
- Difficulty resuming employment
- Excessive time required for recuperation
- Expresses discomfort
- Fatigue
- Interrupted surgical area healing
- Perceives need for more time to recover
- Postpones resumption of work
- Requires assistance for self-care

EXPECTED OUTCOMES

- Patient's vital signs and laboratory values will return to normal limits.
- Patient's wound will begin to heal; incision site will appear free from signs and symptoms of infection.
- Patient will exhibit improved nutritional status.
- Patient's postoperative complications will be resolved.
- Patient will resume normal mobility status.
- Patient will seek and obtain emotional support from family and friends.
- Patient will resume normal eating, bowel, and bladder habits.
- Patient and family members will use community resources that are available to assist after discharge.

Suggested NOC Outcomes

Ambulation; Endurance; Health Beliefs; Immobility Consequences: Physiological; Nutritional Status; Pain Level; Wound Healing: Primary Intention

INTERVENTIONS AND RATIONALES

S ▪ Assess for factors that may be related to a delay in recovery, such as respiratory complications and infection. Document and report assessment findings *to facilitate the development of an individualized care plan.*

S ▪ Monitor wound healing. Assess the surgical site for signs of infection, such as erythema, edema, pain, drainage, odor, incision approximation, and intact sutures. *Infection may delay surgical recovery.*

EBP ▪ Monitor nutritional status by evaluating intake, output, and integumentary status. Consult a dietitian regarding changes to diet *to promote optimal nutritional status. Optimal nutritional status promotes wound healing and provides energy for recovery.*

EBP ▪ Assess all body systems *to detect signs and symptoms of postoperative complications that can delay surgical recovery.*

EBP ▪ Follow the prescribed pulmonary regimen *to facilitate resolution of respiratory complications if present. Respiratory complications can lead to decreased oxygen levels, which can slow wound healing and delay mobility.*

S ▪ Following postoperative bleeding, monitor hemoglobin level and hematocrit. *Bleeding can lead to a low hemoglobin level and hematocrit, reducing the ability of red blood cells to carry oxygen, which can hinder wound healing and diminish patient's energy level.*

PCC ▪ If patient is suffering from psychosis, continue to reorient him or her during the postoperative recovery period. Report any psychological reaction, such as development of depression-like symptoms. *Psychosis or depression may delay recovery.*

EBP ▪ Administer pain medication as prescribed. *A patient in pain may not move, cough, and deep-breathe as needed for timely recovery from surgery.*

S ▪ As appropriate, make sure someone is available to walk with patient or that such devices as walkers or canes are available. Don't allow patient to ambulate alone until steady. *Assistance (from staff or with devices) enhances safety and encourages patient to improve mobility without fear of falling. Mobility will facilitate improved strength, help prevent such complications as deep vein thrombosis, and ultimately enhance recovery.*

S ▪ Make sure patient wears support stockings or a sequential compression device as prescribed *to facilitate venous return and prevent deep vein thrombosis.*

EBP ▪ Monitor bowel and bladder activity. Report urine retention and absent or decreased bowel sounds. *Abnormal bowel and bladder patterns slow surgical recovery. Continual assessment ensures prompt treatment and enhances recovery.*

T&C ▪ Initiate a multidisciplinary care conference for patient with care providers from all disciplines as well as the patient and family. Facilitating this type of communication will help *to develop a plan that will put the patient on a faster track to recovery.*

T&C ▪ Make sure patient and family members have access to community resources to assist with recovery when patient returns home *to ensure ongoing recovery.*

EBP ▪ Educate patient and family members regarding appropriate care after discharge *to help them carry out medication and treatment regimens.*

Suggested NIC Interventions

Bed Rest Care; Case Management; Discharge Planning; Energy Management; Exercise Therapy: Ambulation; Incision Site Care; Multidisciplinary Care Conference; Nutrition Management; Pain Management; Sleep Enhancement

EVALUATIONS FOR EXPECTED OUTCOMES

- Patient's vital signs and laboratory values return to normal limits.
- Patient's wound begins to heal; incision site appears free from signs and symptoms of infection.
- Patient exhibits improved nutritional status.
- Patient's postoperative complications are resolved.
- Patient resumes normal mobility status.
- Patient seeks and obtains emotional support from family and friends.
- Patient resumes normal eating, bowel, and bladder habits.
- Patient and family members use community resources that are available to assist after discharge.

DOCUMENTATION

- Assessment findings
- Type and length of operation
- Type of anesthesia
- Intraoperative complications
- Postoperative complications (as they occur)
- Results of ongoing multisystem assessment
- Treatment regimen (for normal recovery and complications)
- Patient's and family members' progress in following treatment regimen
- Teaching provided to patient and family members
- Discharge plans
- Evaluations for expected outcomes

REFERENCES

dos Santos Cardozo, A., Ferreira Santana, R., Moraes da Rocha, I. da C., Cassiano, K. M., Delphino Mello, T., & Garcia Melo, U. (2017). Phone follow-ups as a nursing intervention in the surgical recovery of prostatectomized elderly. *Journal of Nursing UFPE/Revista de Enfermagem UFPE, 11*(8), 3005–3012. doi:10.5205/reuol.11064-98681-4-ED.1108201703

Kang, E., Gillespie, B. M., Tobiano, G., & Chaboyer, W. (2018). Discharge education delivered to general surgical patients in their management of recovery post discharge: A systematic mixed studies review. *International Journal of Nursing Studies, 87,* 1–13. doi:10.1016/j.ijnurstu.2018.07.004

Lee, J., Seo, E., Choi, J., & Min, J. (2018). Effects of patient participation in the management of daily nursing goals on function recovery and resilience in surgical patients. *Journal of Clinical Nursing, 27*(13–14), 2795–2803. doi:10.1111/jocn.14302

Rembold, S. M., Santana, R. F., de Souza, P. A., & Schwartz, S. M. de O. X. (2018). Nursing diagnosis risk for delayed surgical recovery (00246): Concept clarification and definition of empirical referents. *International Journal of Nursing Knowledge, 29*(4), 263–268. doi:10.1111/2047-3095.12176

Risk for Delayed Surgical Recovery

DEFINITION

Susceptible to an extension of the number of postoperative days required to initiate and perform activities that maintain life, health, and well-being, which may compromise health

RISK FACTORS

- Delirium
- Impaired physical mobility
- Increased blood glucose level
- Malnutrition

- Negative emotional response to surgical outcome
- Obesity
- Persistent nausea
- Persistent pain
- Persistent vomiting
- Smoking

ASSOCIATED CONDITIONS

- Anemia
- Diabetes mellitus
- Extensive surgical procedures
- Pharmaceutical preparations
- Prolonged duration of perioperative surgical wound infection
- Psychological disorder in postoperative period
- Surgical wound infection

ASSESSMENT

- Age
- Gender
- Reason for surgery
- Type and length of surgical procedure
- Current health status, including weight, vital signs, temperature, nutritional status, integumentary status, neurologic status, cardiovascular status, musculoskeletal status, and pain status
- Laboratory studies, including complete blood count, electrolyte studies, urinalysis, blood cultures, blood coagulation studies, immunologic and serologic tests, liver function tests, cardiac enzyme studies, and arterial blood gas levels
- Health history, including past surgical procedures, food or drug allergies, substance abuse, mental illness, and chronic metabolic or systemic disease (diabetes mellitus; cardiovascular, hepatic, renal, or immunologic disease; coagulation disorders; and splenic or bone marrow disorders)
- Mobility status
- Complications during surgical procedure, such as hemorrhage, drop in blood pressure, and cardiac arrhythmias
- Current medical treatments, including radiation therapy, chemotherapy, antibiotic or antifungal therapy, steroid treatment, anticoagulant or thrombolytic therapy, and immunosuppressive therapy
- Social support, including family status and presence of caregiver and health care provider

EXPECTED OUTCOMES

- Patient's vital signs and laboratory values will be within normal limits.
- Patient's incision site will be free from signs and symptoms of infection.
- Patient will exhibit optimal nutritional status.
- Patient will not experience postoperative complications.
- Patient will resume normal mobility status.
- Patient will seek and obtain emotional support from family and friends.
- Patient will resume normal eating, bowel, and bladder habits.
- Patient and family members will use community resources that are available to assist after discharge.

Suggested NOC Outcomes

Ambulation; Mobility; Self-Care: Activities of Daily Living (ADLs); Knowledge: Treatment Regimen

INTERVENTIONS AND RATIONALES

EBP ▪ Assess for factors that may be related to a delay in recovery, such as respiratory complications and infection. Document and report assessment findings *to facilitate the development of an individualized care plan.*

EBP ▪ Assess preoperative nutritional status by evaluating intake, output, and integumentary status. *Optimal nutritional status promotes wound healing and provides energy for recovery.*

S ▪ Assess all body systems *to detect signs and symptoms of postoperative complications that can delay surgical recovery.*

EBP ▪ Preprocedure, teach patient use of incentive spirometer and encourage use. *Respiratory complications can lead to decreased oxygen levels, which can slow wound healing and delay mobility.*

S ▪ Monitor hemoglobin level and hematocrit. *Bleeding can lead to a low hemoglobin level and hematocrit, reducing the ability of red blood cells to carry oxygen, which can hinder wound healing and diminish patient's energy level.*

EBP ▪ Assess pain level. Administer as prescribed. *A patient in pain may not move, cough, and deep-breathe as needed for timely recovery from surgery.*

S ▪ Make sure patient wears support stockings or a sequential compression device as prescribed *to facilitate venous return and prevent deep vein thrombosis.*

T&C ▪ Initiate a multidisciplinary care conference for patient with care providers from all disciplines as well as patient and family. Facilitating this type of communication will help *to develop a plan that will put patient on a faster track to recovery.*

T&C ▪ Make sure patient and family members have access to community resources to assist with recovery when patient returns home *to ensure ongoing recovery.*

EBP ▪ Educate patient and family members regarding appropriate care after discharge *to help them carry out medication and treatment regimens.*

Suggested NIC Interventions

Embolus Precautions; Exercise Therapy: Ambulation; Medication Management; Pain Management; Self-Care Assistance; Vital Signs Monitoring

EVALUATIONS FOR EXPECTED OUTCOMES

▪ Patient's vital signs and laboratory values return to normal limits.
▪ Patient's wound begins to heal; incision site appears free from signs and symptoms of infection.
▪ Patient exhibits improved nutritional status.
▪ Patient resumes normal mobility status.
▪ Patient seeks and obtains emotional support from family and friends.
▪ Patient resumes normal eating, bowel, and bladder habits.
▪ Patient and family members use community resources that are available to assist after discharge.

DOCUMENTATION

▪ Assessment findings
▪ Type and length of operation
▪ Type of anesthesia
▪ Intraoperative complications
▪ Postoperative complications (as they occur)
▪ Results of ongoing multisystem assessment

▦ Treatment regimen (for normal recovery and complications)
▦ Teaching provided to patient and family members
▦ Evaluations for expected outcomes

REFERENCES

Barker, K. L., Hannink, E., Pemberton, S., & Jenkins, C. (2018). Knee arthroplasty patients predicted versus actual recovery: What are their expectations about time of recovery after surgery and how long before they can do the tasks they want to do? *Archives of Physical Medicine & Rehabilitation, 99*(11), 2230–2237. doi:10.1016/j.apmr.2018.03.022

Lirosi, M. C., Tirelli, F., Biondi, A., Mele, M. C., Larotonda, C., Lorenzon, L., … Persiani, R. (2019). Enhanced recovery program for colorectal surgery: A focus on elderly patients over 75 years old. *Journal of Gastrointestinal Surgery, 23*(3), 587–594. doi:10.1007/s11605-018-3943-2

Nwaezeapu, K. (2018). Enhanced recovery after surgery and opioid-sparing techniques. *International Student Journal of Nurse Anesthesia, 17*(2), 31–34.

Risk for Surgical Site Infection

DEFINITION

Susceptible to invasion of pathogenic organisms at surgical site, which may compromise health

RISK FACTORS

▦ Alcoholism
▦ Obesity
▦ Smoking

ASSOCIATED CONDITIONS

▦ Comorbidity
▦ Diabetes mellitus
▦ Duration of surgery
▦ Hypertension
▦ Immunosuppression
▦ Inadequate antibiotic prophylaxis
▦ Ineffective antibiotic prophylaxis
▦ Infections at other surgical sites
▦ Invasive procedure
▦ Post-traumatic osteoarthritis
▦ Rheumatoid arthritis
▦ Type of anesthesia
▦ Type of surgical procedure
▦ Use of implants and/or prostheses

ASSESSMENT

▦ Age, gender, weight, vital signs
▦ Current health status, including vital signs, nutritional status, and integumentary status
▦ Type and duration of procedure
▦ Location of incision
▦ Blood transfusion

- Current infection
- Health history, presence of medical conditions such as diabetes mellitus that may increase incidence of infection, history of smoking
- Presence of invasive devices, including indwelling urinary catheter, endotracheal tube, tracheostomy tube, IV lines, central venous and arterial lines, drains, and gastric feeding tubes

EXPECTED OUTCOMES

- Patient's incision site will remain free of signs and symptoms of infection.
- Patient's incision will appear clean, pink, and free from purulent drainage.
- Patient's vital signs will remain within normal range.
- Patient's WBC count and differential will stay within normal range.
- Patient's cultures won't show evidence of pathogens.
- Patient will identify signs and symptoms of infection.

Suggested NOC Outcomes

> Immune Status; Infection Status; Knowledge: Infection Control; Knowledge: Treatment Procedure(s); Nutritional Status; Risk Control; Risk Detection; Wound Healing: Primary Intention; Wound Healing: Secondary Intention

INTERVENTIONS AND RATIONALES

Preprocedure

EBP
- If indicated, bathe patient with antimicrobial soap or antiseptic agent soap the night before surgery. *Antimicrobial baths decrease the number of pathogens on the skin surface.*

EBP
- Administer antibiotic prophylaxis as ordered by provider. *Prophylactic antibiotic administration helps reduce the pathogenic organisms.*

EBP
- Follow skin preparation guidelines unless contraindicated. *Skin preparation decreases the number of pathogens on the skin surface.*

Postprocedure

S
- Minimize patient's risk of infection by:
  - washing hands before and after providing care. *Hand washing is the single best way to avoid spreading pathogens.*
  - wearing gloves to maintain asepsis when providing direct care. *Gloves offer protection when handling wound dressings or carrying out various treatments.*

S
- Identify risk factors predisposing patient to infection. *A complete nursing assessment allows development of an individualized care plan.*

S
- Monitor blood glucose levels and maintain under 200 mg/dL. *High blood glucose levels increase the risk of infection.*

S
- Follow the facility's infection control policy *to minimize the risk of nosocomial infection.*

EBP
- Maintain standard precautions. Wear gloves if you might come into contact with patient's blood and body secretions. *Standard precautions protect you and patient from the transfer of microorganisms.*

S
- Monitor temperature at least every 4 hours and record on graph paper. Report elevations immediately. *Sustained temperature elevation after surgery may signal onset of wound infection or dehiscence.*

S
- Monitor white blood cell (WBC) count, as ordered. Report elevations or depressions. *Elevated total WBC count indicates infection. Markedly decreased WBC count may indicate*

decreased production resulting from extreme debilitation or severe lack of vitamins and amino acids. Any damage to bone marrow may suppress WBC formation.

PCC ■ Help patient wash hands before and after meals and after using bathroom, bedpan, or urinal. *Hand washing prevents spread of pathogens to other objects and food.*

EBP ■ Ensure adequate nutritional intake. Offer high-protein supplements, unless contraindicated. *This helps stabilize weight, improves muscle tone and mass, and aids wound healing.*

EBP ■ Administer topical, oral, and parenteral antibiotics as ordered *to eradicate pathogenic organisms.*

EBP ■ Teach patient about:
  ▪ good hand washing technique;
  ▪ factors that increase infection risk;
  ▪ signs and symptoms of infection.
  These measures allow patient to participate in care and help patient modify lifestyle to maintain optimum health.

Suggested NIC Interventions

Incision Site Care; Infection Control; Infection Protection; Teaching: Nutrition Therapy; Procedure/Treatment; Wound Care

EVALUATIONS FOR EXPECTED OUTCOMES

▪ Patient's incisions or wounds remain clear, pink, and free from purulent drainage.
▪ Patient's vital signs remain within normal limits.
▪ Patient's WBC count and differential remain within normal range.
▪ Patient's cultures don't exhibit pathogen growth.
▪ Patient does not experience signs and symptoms of infection.

DOCUMENTATION

▪ Patient's activity level
▪ Temperature
▪ Dates, times, and sites of all cultures
▪ Appearance of all invasive catheter sites, tube sites, and wounds
▪ Interventions performed to reduce infection risk
▪ Patient's response to nursing interventions
▪ Evaluations for expected outcomes

REFERENCES

Burden, M., & Thornton, M. (2018). Reducing the risks of surgical site infection: The importance of the multidisciplinary team. *British Journal of Nursing, 27*(17), 976–979. doi:10.12968/bjon.2018.27.17.976

de Castro Franco, L. M., Fernandes Cota, G., Ignacio de Almeida, A. G., Marques Horta Duarte, G., Lamounier, L., Ferreira Souza Pereira, P., & Falci Ercole, F. (2018). Hip arthroplasty: Incidence and risk factors for surgical site infection. *Canadian Journal of Infection Control, 33*(1), 14–19.

Hijas-Gómez, A. I., Lucas, W. C., Checa-García, A., Martínez-Martín, J., Fahandezh-Saddi, H., Gil-de-Miguel, Á., … Rodríguez-Caravaca, G. (2018). Surgical site infection incidence and risk factors in knee arthroplasty: A 9-year prospective cohort study at a university teaching hospital in Spain. *American Journal of Infection Control, 46*(12), 1335–1340. doi:10.1016/j.ajic.2018.06.010

Saeed, K. B., Corcoran, P., O'Riordan, M., & Greene, R. A. (2019). Risk factors for surgical site infection after cesarean delivery: A case-control study. *American Journal of Infection Control, 47*(2), 164–169. doi:10.1016/j.ajic.2018.07.023

Impaired Swallowing

DEFINITION

Abnormal functioning of the swallowing mechanism associated with deficits in oral, pharyngeal, or esophageal structure or function

RELATED FACTORS (R/T)

- Altered attention
- Behavioral feeding problem
- Protein-energy malnutrition
- Self-injurious behavior

ASSOCIATED CONDITIONS

- Acquired anatomic defects
- Brain injuries
- Cerebral palsy
- Conditions with significant muscle hypotonia
- Congenital heart disease
- Cranial nerve involvement
- Developmental disabilities
- Esophageal achalasia
- Gastroesophageal reflux disease
- Laryngeal diseases
- Mechanical obstruction
- Nasal defect
- Nasopharyngeal cavity defect
- Neurological problems
- Neuromuscular diseases
- Oropharynx abnormality
- Pharmaceutical preparations
- Prolonged intubation
- Respiratory condition
- Tracheal defect
- Trauma
- Upper airway anomaly
- Vocal cord dysfunction

ASSESSMENT

- History of neuromuscular, cerebral, or respiratory disease
- Age
- Gender
- Nutritional status, including appetite, dietary intake, hydration, current weight, and change from normal weight
- Neurologic status, including barium swallow; chest X-ray; cognition; esophageal video fluoroscopy; gag reflex; level of consciousness; memory; motor ability; orientation; symmetry of face, mouth, and neck; sensory function; and tongue movement

First Stage: Oral

- Abnormal oral phase of swallow study
- Bruxism
- Choking prior to swallowing
- Choking when swallowing cold water
- Coughing prior to swallowing
- Drooling
- Food falls from mouth
- Food pushed out of mouth
- Gagging prior to swallowing
- Impaired ability to clear oral cavity
- Inadequate consumption during prolonged meal time
- Inadequate lip closure
- Inadequate mastication
- Incidence of wet hoarseness twice within 30 seconds
- Inefficient nippling
- Inefficient suck
- Nasal reflux
- Piecemeal deglutition
- Pooling of bolus in lateral sulci
- Premature entry of bolus
- Prolonged bolus formation
- Tongue action ineffective in forming bolus

Second Stage: Pharyngeal

- Abnormal pharyngeal phase of swallow study
- Altered head position
- Choking
- Coughing
- Delayed swallowing
- Fevers of unknown etiology
- Food refusal
- Gagging sensation
- Gurgly voice quality
- Inadequate laryngeal elevation
- Nasal reflux
- Recurrent pulmonary infection
- Repetitive swallowing

Third Stage: Esophageal

- Abnormal esophageal phase of swallow study
- Acidic-smelling breath
- Difficulty swallowing
- Epigastric pain
- Food refusal
- Heartburn
- Hematemesis

- Hyperextension of head
- Nighttime awakening
- Nighttime coughing
- Odynophagia
- Regurgitation
- Repetitive swallowing
- Reports "something stuck"
- Unexplained irritability surrounding mealtimes
- Volume limiting
- Vomiting
- Vomitus on pillow

EXPECTED OUTCOMES

- Patient won't show evidence of aspiration pneumonia.
- Patient will achieve adequate nutritional intake.
- Patient will maintain weight.
- Patient will maintain oral hygiene.
- Patient and caregiver will demonstrate correct feeding techniques to maximize swallowing.
- Patient and caregiver will list strategies to prevent aspiration.

Suggested NOC Outcomes

Appetite; Aspiration Prevention; Cognition; Nutritional Status: Food & Fluid Intake; Swallowing Status; Swallowing Status: Esophageal Phase; Swallowing Status: Oral Phase; Swallowing Status: Pharyngeal Phase

INTERVENTIONS AND RATIONALES

- **S** Elevate the head of the bed 90 degrees during mealtimes and for 30 minutes after the completion of a meal *to decrease the risk of aspiration.*
- **S** Position patient on the side when recumbent *to decrease the risk of aspiration.*
- **S** Keep suction apparatus at the bedside; observe and report instances of cyanosis, dyspnea, or choking. *Symptoms indicate the presence of material in the lungs.*
- **EBP** Monitor intake and output and weight daily until stabilized. Establish an intake goal—for example, "Patient consumes ____mL of fluid and ____ % of solid food." Record and report any deviation from this. *Evaluating calorie and protein intake daily allows any necessary modifications to begin quickly.*
- **T&C** Consult with a dietitian to modify patient's diet and conduct a calorie count as needed *to establish nutritional requirements.*
- **T&C** Consult with a dysphagia rehabilitation team, if available, *to obtain expert advice.*
- **EBP** Provide mouth care three times daily *to promote comfort and enhance appetite.*
- **EBP** Keep the oral mucous membrane moist by frequent rinses; use a bulb syringe or suction if necessary *to promote comfort.*
- **PCC** Lubricate patient's lips *to prevent cracking and blisters.*
- **PCC** Encourage patient to wear properly fitted dentures *to enhance chewing ability.*
- **PCC** Serve food in attractive surroundings; encourage patient to smell and look at food. Remove soiled equipment, control smells, and provide a quiet atmosphere for eating. *A pleasant atmosphere stimulates appetite; food aroma stimulates salivation.*

EBP   ■ Teach patient and family members about positioning, dietary requirements, and specific feeding techniques, including facial exercises (such as whistling), using a short straw to provide sensory stimulation to patient's lips, tipping the head forward to decrease aspiration, applying pressure above the lip to stimulate mouth closure and the swallowing reflex, and checking the oral cavity frequently for food particles (remove if present). *These measures allow patient to take an active role in maintaining health.*

Suggested NIC Interventions

Airway Suctioning; Aspiration Precautions; Feeding; Positioning; Referral; Risk Identification; Swallowing Therapy

EVALUATIONS FOR EXPECTED OUTCOMES

■ Patient shows no evidence of aspiration pneumonia. Breath sounds remain bilaterally clear; fever, chills, purulent sputum, and rapid shallow respirations are absent.
■ Patient's fluid and dietary intake remains within established daily limits.
■ Patient's weight remains stable.
■ Patient demonstrates appropriate oral hygiene practices.
■ Patient and caregiver demonstrate feeding techniques to maximize swallowing and minimize risk of complications.
■ Patient and caregiver list strategies to prevent aspiration.

DOCUMENTATION

■ Patient's expressions of feelings about current situation
■ Observations of weight, swallowing ability, intake and output, and oral hygiene
■ Patient's response to nursing interventions
■ Instructions about diet monitoring and feeding techniques
■ Evaluations for expected outcomes

REFERENCES

Govender, R., Smith, C. H., Taylor, S. A., Barratt, H., & Gardner, B. (2017). Swallowing interventions for the treatment of dysphagia after head and neck cancer: A systematic review of behavioural strategies used to promote patient adherence to swallowing exercises. *BMC Cancer, 17*, 1–15. doi:10.1186/s12885-016-2990-x

Martin-Harris, B., Garand, K. L. (Focht), & McFarland, D. (2017). Optimizing respiratory-swallowing coordination in patients with oropharyngeal head and neck cancer. *Perspectives of the ASHA Special Interest Groups, 2*(13), 103–110. doi:10.1044/persp2.SIG13.103

Masilamoney, M., & Dowse, R. (2018). Knowledge and practice of healthcare professionals relating to oral medicine use in swallowing-impaired patients: A scoping review. *International Journal of Pharmacy Practice, 26*(3), 199–209. doi:10.1111/ijpp.12447

Wakasugi, Y., Yamamoto, T., Oda, C., Murata, M., Tohara, H., & Minakuchi, S. (2017). Effect of an impaired oral stage on swallowing in patients with Parkinson's disease. *Journal of Oral Rehabilitation, 44*(10), 756–762. doi:10.1111/joor.12536

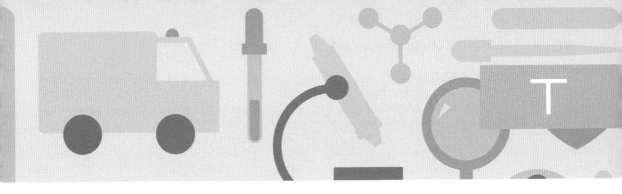

Ineffective Thermoregulation

DEFINITION

Temperature fluctuation between hypothermia and hyperthermia

RELATED FACTORS (R/T)

- Dehydration
- Fluctuating environmental temperature
- Inactivity
- Inappropriate clothing for environmental temperature
- Increase in oxygen demand
- Vigorous activity

ASSOCIATED CONDITIONS

- Alteration in metabolic rate
- Brain injury
- Condition affecting temperature regulation
- Decrease in sweat response
- Illness
- Inefficient nonshivering thermogenesis
- Pharmaceutical agent
- Sedation
- Sepsis
- Trauma

ASSESSMENT

- Age
- Vital signs
- History of current illness
- Medication history
- Neurologic status, including level of consciousness (LOC), mental status, motor status, and sensory status
- Cardiovascular status, including blood pressure, capillary refill time, electrocardiogram, heart rate and rhythm, pulses (apical and peripheral), and temperature
- Respiratory status, including arterial blood gas measurements; breath sounds; and rate, depth, and character of respirations
- Integumentary status, including color, temperature, and turgor

- Fluid and electrolyte status, including blood urea nitrogen level, intake and output, serum electrolyte levels, and urine specific gravity
- Laboratory studies, including clotting factors, hemoglobin level, hematocrit, platelet count, and white blood cell count

DEFINING CHARACTERISTICS

- Cyanotic nail beds
- Flushed skin
- Hypertension
- Increase in body temperature above normal range
- Increase in respiratory rate
- Mild shivering
- Moderate pallor
- Piloerection
- Reduction in body temperature below normal range
- Seizures
- Skin cool to touch
- Skin warm to touch
- Slow capillary refill
- Tachycardia

EXPECTED OUTCOMES

- Patient will maintain body temperature at normothermic levels.
- Patient won't shiver.
- Patient will express feelings of comfort.
- Patient will have warm, dry skin.
- Patient will maintain heart rate, respiratory rate, and blood pressure within normal range.
- Patient won't exhibit signs of compromised neurologic status.
- Patient and family members will voice an understanding of health problem.

Suggested NOC Outcomes

Hydration; Thermoregulation; Vital Signs

INTERVENTIONS AND RATIONALES

S ▪ Monitor patient's body temperature every 4 hours or more often if indicated. Record the temperature and route (keep in mind that the baseline depends on the route). *Monitoring determines the effectiveness of therapy or whether intervention is required and allows accurate comparison of data.*

S ▪ Monitor and record patient's neurologic status every 8 hours. Report any changes to the physician. *Changes in LOC can result from tissue hypoxia related to altered tissue perfusion. Hyperthermia increases cerebral edema and thus intracranial pressure (ICP); hypothermia depresses metabolic rate.*

▪ Monitor and record patient's heart rate and rhythm, blood pressure, and respiratory rate every 4 hours. *Hyperthermia may create hypoxia by increasing oxygen demand, which results from increased tissue metabolism (metabolism increases 7% with each increase of 1° F [0.6° C]). This in turn results in faster breathing and a rising pulse rate.*

EBP ▪ Administer analgesics, antipyretics, and medications that prevent shivering, as prescribed. Monitor and record their effectiveness. *Antipyretics help reduce fever. Shivering tends to retard the lowering of body temperature.*

EBP ▪ If patient develops excessive fever, take the following steps following institutional protocol:
  ▪ Remove blankets; place a loincloth over patient.
  ▪ Apply ice bags to the axilla and groin.
  ▪ Initiate a tepid water sponge bath.
  ▪ Use a hypothermia blanket if temperature rises above ____. Cool patient to ____.
  These measures help reduce excessive fever.

EBP ▪ Maintain hydration.
  ▪ Monitor intake and output.
  ▪ Administer parenteral fluids, as ordered.
  ▪ Determine patient's fluid preference. Keep oral fluids at the bedside and encourage patient to drink.
  These measures help maintain fluid balance. Keeping preferred fluids at the bedside allows patient to actively participate in the prescribed treatment.

EBP ▪ Maintain the environmental temperature at a comfortable setting.
  ▪ Ensure that all metal and plastic surfaces that come into contact with patient's body are covered.
  ▪ Use or remove blankets as necessary for comfort.
  ▪ Make sure that linens and clothing are clean and dry.
  The temperature of the external environment affects ease of body temperature regulation.

EBP ▪ Instruct patient and family members about:
  ▪ signs and symptoms of altered body temperature;
  ▪ precautionary measures to avoid hypothermia or hyperthermia;
  ▪ adherence to other aspects of health care management to help normalize patient's temperature (such as dietary habits and measures to prevent increased ICP);
  ▪ rationale for treatment.
  These measures allow patient to take an active role in health maintenance.

Suggested NIC Interventions

Bathing; Environmental Management; Fever Treatment; Fluid Management; Fluid Monitoring; Temperature Regulation; Vital Signs Monitoring

EVALUATIONS FOR EXPECTED OUTCOMES

▪ Patient's temperature remains within normal parameters.
▪ Patient doesn't shiver.
▪ Patient indicates feelings of comfort, either verbally or through behavior.
▪ Patient's skin remains warm and dry.
▪ Patient's heart rate and blood pressure remain within normal range.
▪ Patient and family state understanding of health problem.

DOCUMENTATION

▪ Patient's needs and perceptions of current problem
▪ Physical findings
▪ Intake and output
▪ Patient's response to nursing interventions
▪ Evaluations for expected outcomes

REFERENCES

Davis, J. K., Stolworthy, N. I., Laurent, C. M., Allen, K. E., Zhang, Y., Welch, T. R., & Nevett, M. E. (2017). Influence of clothing on thermoregulation and comfort during exercise in the heat. *Journal of Strength & Conditioning Research (Lippincott Williams & Wilkins), 31*(12), 3435–3443. doi:10.1519/JSC.0000000000001754

Iyoho, A. E., Ng, L. J., & MacFadden, L. (2017). Modeling of gender differences in thermoregulation. *Military Medicine, 182*, 295–303. doi:10.7205/MILMED-D-16-00213

Saqe-Rockoff, A., Schubert, F. D., Ciardiello, A., & Douglas, E. (2018). Improving thermoregulation for trauma patients in the emergency department : An evidence-based practice project. *Journal of Trauma Nursing, 25*(1), 14–20. doi:10.1097/JTN.0000000000000336

Risk for Ineffective Thermoregulation

DEFINITION

Susceptible to temperature fluctuation between hypothermia and hyperthermia, which may compromise health

RISK FACTORS

- Dehydration
- Fluctuating environmental temperature
- Inactivity
- Inappropriate clothing for environmental temperature
- Increase in oxygen demand
- Vigorous activity

ASSOCIATED CONDITIONS

- Alteration in metabolic rate
- Brain injury
- Condition affecting temperature regulation
- Decrease in sweat response illness
- Inefficient nonshivering thermogenesis
- Pharmaceutical agent
- Sedation
- Sepsis
- Trauma

ASSESSMENT

- Age
- Vital signs
- History of current illness
- Medication history
- Neurologic status, including level of consciousness (LOC), mental status, motor status, and sensory status
- Cardiovascular status, including blood pressure, capillary refill time, electrocardiogram, heart rate and rhythm, pulses (apical and peripheral), and temperature
- Respiratory status, including arterial blood gas measurements; breath sounds; and rate, depth, and character of respirations

- Integumentary status, including color, temperature, and turgor
- Fluid and electrolyte status, including blood urea nitrogen level, intake and output, serum electrolyte levels, and urine specific gravity
- Laboratory studies, including clotting factors, hemoglobin level, hematocrit, platelet count, and white blood cell count

EXPECTED OUTCOMES

- Patient will maintain body temperature at normothermic levels.
- Patient will express feelings of comfort.
- Patient will have warm, dry skin.
- Patient will maintain heart rate, respiratory rate, and blood pressure within normal range.
- Patient won't exhibit signs of compromised neurologic status.

Suggested NOC Outcomes

Hydration; Thermoregulation; Tissue Perfusion: Peripheral; Vital Signs

INTERVENTIONS AND RATIONALES

S ▪ Monitor patient's body temperature every 4 hours or more often if indicated. Record the temperature and route (keep in mind that the baseline depends on the route). *Regular monitoring will identify when an intervention is required and allows accurate comparison of data.*

S ▪ Monitor and record patient's neurologic status every 8 hours. Report any changes to the physician. *Changes in LOC can result from tissue hypoxia related to altered tissue perfusion. Hyperthermia increases cerebral edema and thus intracranial pressure (ICP); hypothermia depresses metabolic rate.*

S ▪ Monitor and record patient's heart rate and rhythm, blood pressure, and respiratory rate every 4 hours. *Hyperthermia may create hypoxia by increasing oxygen demand, which results from increased tissue metabolism (metabolism increases 7% with each increase of 1° F [0.6° C]). This in turn results in faster breathing and a rising pulse rate.*

EBP ▪ Maintain hydration.
  - Monitor intake and output.
  - Administer parenteral fluids, as ordered.
  - Determine patient's fluid preference. Keep oral fluids at the bedside and encourage patient to drink.
  These measures help maintain fluid balance. Keeping preferred fluids at the bedside allows patient to actively participate in the prescribed treatment.

EBP ▪ Maintain the environmental temperature at a comfortable setting.
  - Ensure that all metal and plastic surfaces that come into contact with patient's body are covered.
  - Use or remove blankets as necessary for comfort.
  - Make sure that linens and clothing are clean and dry.
  The temperature of the external environment affects ease of body temperature regulation.

EBP ▪ Instruct patient and family members about:
  - signs and symptoms of altered body temperature;
  - precautionary measures to avoid hypothermia or hyperthermia;
  - adherence to other aspects of health care management to help normalize patient's temperature (such as dietary habits and measures to prevent increased ICP);
  - rationale for treatment.
  These measures allow patient to take an active role in health maintenance.

Suggested NIC Interventions

Environmental Management; Fever Treatment; Fluid Management; Fluid Monitoring; Temperature Regulation; Vital Signs Monitoring

EVALUATIONS FOR EXPECTED OUTCOMES

- Patient's temperature remains within normal parameters.
- Patient indicates feelings of comfort, either verbally or through behavior.
- Patient's skin remains warm and dry.
- Patient's heart rate and blood pressure remain within normal range.

DOCUMENTATION

- Patient's vital signs
- Patient's needs and perceptions of current problem
- Physical findings
- Intake and output
- Patient's response to nursing interventions
- Evaluations for expected outcomes

REFERENCES

Balmain, B. N., Sabapathy, S., Louis, M., & Morris, N. R. (2018). Aging and thermoregulatory control: The clinical implications of exercising under heat stress in older individuals. *BioMed Research International, 2018*, 1–12. doi:10.1155/2018/8306154

Iyoho, A. E., Ng, L. J., & MacFadden, L. (2017). Modeling of gender differences in thermoregulation. *Military Medicine, 182*, 295–303. doi:10.7205/MILMED-D-16-00213

Saqe-Rockoff, A., Schubert, F. D., Ciardiello, A., & Douglas, E. (2018). Improving thermoregulation for trauma patients in the emergency department: An evidence-based practice project. *Journal of Trauma Nursing, 25*(1), 14–20. doi:10.1097/JTN.0000000000000336

Zawadzka, M., Szmuda, M., & Mazurkiewicz-Bełdzińska, M. (2017). Thermoregulation disorders of central origin—How to diagnose and treat. *Anaesthesiology Intensive Therapy, 49*(3), 227–234. doi:10.5603/AIT.2017.0042

Disturbed Thought Process

DEFINITION

Disruption in cognitive functioning that affects the mental processes involved in developing concepts and categories, reasoning, and problem solving

RELATED FACTORS (R/T)

- Acute confusion
- Anxiety
- Disorientation
- Fear
- Grieving
- Nonpsychotic depressive symptoms
- Pain
- Stressors

- Substance misuse
- Unaddressed trauma

ASSOCIATED CONDITIONS

- Brain injuries
- Critical illness
- Hallucinations
- Mental disorders
- Neurodegenerative disorders
- Pharmaceutical preparations

ASSESSMENT

- Age, gender, level of education, and occupation
- Health history, including use of medications, recent surgery, allergies, history of alcoholism, drug abuse, and depression
- Neurologic status, including level of consciousness (LOC); orientation; thought and speech; mood; affect; memory; visual and spatial ability; judgment and insight; psychomotor activity; perceptions; delusions, illusions, and hallucinations; pain level; recent behavioral changes; and history of transient ischemic attacks, head injury, early dementia, AIDS, or schizophrenia
- Cardiovascular status, including vital signs, skin color, auscultation of carotid artery and heart sounds, and history of coronary artery disease or hypertension
- Respiratory status, including rate, depth, and pattern of respirations; auscultation for breath sounds; smoking history; shortness of breath; and history of chronic obstructive pulmonary disease, cancer, or tuberculosis
- Sensory status, including results of vision and hearing examination, use of corrective lenses or hearing aid, and history of eye or ear disorders
- Ability to make decisions and/or problem solve
- Nutritional status, including typical daily food intake and weight loss
- Laboratory values for abnormalities (e.g., metabolic alkalosis, hypokalemia, anemia, elevated ammonia levels, and signs of infection)
- Sleep status, including recent change in sleep pattern or environment (recent hospitalization)

DEFINING CHARACTERISTICS

- Difficulty communicating verbally
- Difficulty performing instrumental activities of daily living
- Disorganized thought sequence
- Expresses unreal thoughts
- Impaired interpretation of events
- Impaired judgment
- Inadequate emotional response to situations
- Limited ability to find solutions to everyday situations
- Limited ability to make decisions
- Limited ability to perform expected social roles
- Limited ability to plan activities
- Limited impulse control ability
- Obsessions

■ Phobic disorders
■ Suspicions

■ Patient will effectively communicate verbally.
■ Patient expresses thoughts and feelings.
■ Patient will perform instrumental activities of daily living.
■ Patient will have organized thought sequence.
■ Patient will express realistic thoughts.
■ Patient will interpret events appropriately.
■ Patient will exhibit reasonable judgment.
■ Patient will find solutions to everyday situations, make decisions, and plan activities.
■ Patient will perform expected social roles.
■ Patient will exhibit impulse control.
■ Patient will use appropriate coping strategies.

Suggested NOC Outcomes

Cognition; Cognition Orientation; Concentration; Decision-Making; Information Processing; Memory

PCC ■ Assess for underlying problems (brain injury, critical illness, mental disorders, neurodegenerative disorders, or substance misuse). *The thought process may improve with treatment of medical problems.*

PCC ■ Assess and reorient to patient to person/place/time as needed. *Inability to maintain orientation indicates thought deterioration.*

PCC ■ Provide clear communication and do not challenge illogical thinking. *Challenging can lead to distrust or reinforce delusions.*

PCC ■ Use therapeutic touch cautiously. *May be perceived as aggression or create anxiety.*

S ■ Implement safety measures as needed (e.g., use of side rails, padding, supervision). *Disoriented thinking may lead to unsafe behaviors.*

PCC ■ Encourage patient to verbalize thoughts and feelings. *Verbalizing feelings in a nonthreatening environment helps patient come identify issues and formulate solutions.*

PCC ■ Encourage patient to participate in social/groups activities. *To maximize functioning and thought processes.*

EBP ■ Maintain quiet environment and avoid loud noise and sudden movements. *Prevents overstimulation and anxiety.*

EBP ■ Educate patient and family about options for long-term plans. *To provide home care, transportation, assistance with care, support, and respite for caregivers.*

T&C ■ Refer to community resources (e.g., support groups, substance rehabilitation, mental health treatment programs). *To promote wellness.*

Suggested NIC Interventions

Anxiety Reduction; Behavior Management; Calming Technique; Cognitive Restructuring; Cognitive Stimulation; Memory Training; Planning Assistance; Sequence Guidance

EVALUATIONS FOR EXPECTED OUTCOMES

▦ Patient effectively communicates and verbally expresses thoughts and feelings.
▦ Patient performs instrumental activities of daily living.
▦ Patient has organized thought sequence.
▦ Patient expresses realistic thoughts.
▦ Patient interprets events appropriately.
▦ Patient exhibits appropriate judgment and decision-making.
▦ Patient plans activities.
▦ Patient performs expected social roles.
▦ Patient exhibits impulse control.
▦ Patient uses appropriate coping strategies.

DOCUMENTATION

▦ Description of episodes of disturbed thought process
▦ Assessment of patient's cognitive abilities, behavior, and self-care status
▦ Changes in patient's mental status as they occur
▦ Patient's statements of improved thought processes
▦ Patient's stated goals for activity planning and execution
▦ Teaching sessions and referrals
▦ Evaluations for expected outcomes

REFERENCES

Blanke, E. S., Schmidt, M. J., Riediger, M., & Brose, A. (2020). Thinking mindfully: How mindfulness relates to rumination and reflection in daily life. *Emotion, 20*(8), 1369–1381. http://dx.doi.org/10.1037/emo0000659

Gehrt, T. B., Frostholm, L., Pallesen, K. J., Obermann, M., & Berntsen, D. (2020). Conscious thought during the resting state in patients with severe health anxiety and patients with obsessive–compulsive disorder. *Psychology of Consciousness: Theory, Research, and Practice, 7*(3), 207–217. http://dx.doi.org/10.1037/cns0000256

Larsen, S. E., Fleming, C. J. E., & Resick, P. A. (2019). Residual symptoms following empirically supported treatment for PTSD. *Psychological Trauma: Theory, Research, Practice, and Policy, 11*(2), 207–215. http://dx.doi.org/10.1037/tra0000384

Or, G., Levi-Belz, Y., & Aisenberg, D. (2021). Death anxiety and intrusive thinking during the COVID-19 pandemic. *GeroPsych: The Journal of Gerontopsychology and Geriatric Psychiatry, 34*(4), 201–212. http://dx.doi.org/10.1024/1662-9647/a000268

Risk for Thrombosis

DEFINITION

Susceptible to obstruction of a blood vessel by a thrombus that can break off and lodge in another vessel, which may compromise health

RISK FACTORS

▦ Atherogenic diet
▦ Dehydration
▦ Excessive stress
▦ Impaired physical mobility
▦ Inadequate knowledge of modifiable factors
▦ Ineffective management of preventive measures

- Ineffective medication self-management
- Obesity
- Sedentary lifestyle
- Smoking

ASSOCIATED CONDITIONS

- Atherosclerosis
- Autoimmune diseases
- Blood coagulation disorders
- Chronic inflammation
- Critical illness
- Diabetes mellitus
- Dyslipidemias
- Endovascular procedures
- Heart diseases
- Hematologic diseases
- High-acuity illness
- Hormonal therapy
- Hyperhomocysteinemia
- Infections
- Kidney diseases
- Medical devices
- Metabolic syndrome
- Neoplasms
- Surgical procedures
- Trauma
- Vascular diseases

ASSESSMENT

- Age
- Weight
- Vital signs
- Fluid volume status, intake and output
- Mobility patterns, sedentary lifestyle
- Cardiovascular status, including blood pressure, cardiac output, patient and family history of cardiovascular disease, peripheral pulses, and smoking history
- Neurologic status, including level of consciousness (LOC), mental status, motor function, and sensory pattern
- Respiratory status, including breath sounds, respiratory rate, and pattern
- Presence of health condition that may interfere with blood clotting, such as coagulopathies
- Laboratory studies, including complete blood count, liver profile, serum electrolyte levels, platelet count, D-Dimer, and blood coagulation studies

EXPECTED OUTCOMES

- Patient will be free of thromboembolism.
- Patient will not experience complications from thromboembolism.
- Patient will demonstrate adequate peripheral perfusion and oxygenation.
- Patient will identify risk factors for thrombus formation.

- Patient will identify signs and symptoms of thrombus formation or embolus.
- Patient will maintain prothrombin time (PT), international normalized ratio (INR), and partial thromboplastin time (PTT) within desired range.

Suggested NOC Outcomes

Knowledge: Thrombus Prevention; Medication Response; Risk Control: Thrombus

INTERVENTIONS AND RATIONALES

S - Observe patient for new onset wheezing or difficulty breathing. *Emboli that travels to the pulmonary system can be life threatening.*

S - Perform comprehensive assessment of peripheral circulation and pulses *to identify the signs and symptoms of thromboembolism—weak pulses, swelling, or elevated skin temperature.*

S - Apply and maintain elastic compression stockings, remove for 15 to 20 minutes every 8 hours *to avoid development of deep vein thrombosis.*

S - Apply intermittent pneumatic compression device *to aid in venous blood return.*

EBP - Encourage flexion and extension of feet and legs at least 10 times every hour *to stimulate adequate circulation and blood return.*

S - Alert provider immediately of any redness, swelling, and heat in the calf *for further evaluation.*

EBP - Administer prophylactic low-dose anticoagulant medications as prescribed by provider *to maintain serum levels of anticoagulant therapy.*

EBP - Monitor patient's prothrombin time (PT) and partial thromboplastin time (PTT) *to maintain serum levels of anticoagulant therapy.*

EBP - Instruct patient not to cross legs and to avoid sitting for long periods with legs dependent. *Crossing legs and sitting for long periods of time inhibits blood flow and perfusion.*

EBP - Instruct patient if traveling for long periods of time to take breaks and walk *to stimulate blood flow and return.*

Suggested NIC Interventions

Bleeding Precautions; Embolus Care: Peripheral; Embolus Precautions; Risk Identification; Thrombolytic Therapy Management

EVALUATIONS FOR EXPECTED OUTCOMES

- Patient remains free from developing a venous thromboembolism.
- Patient does not experience complications from venous thromboembolism.
- Patient demonstrates adequate peripheral perfusion and oxygenation.
- Patient seeks information about embolus prevention.
- Patient identifies risk factors for thrombus formation.
- Patient identifies signs and symptoms of thrombus formation or embolus.
- Patient maintains prothrombin time (PT), international normalized ratio (INR), and partial thromboplastin time (PTT) within desired range.

DOCUMENTATION

- Recording of assessments
- Lab values and vital signs
- Signs and symptoms of thrombus formation

- Intake and output
- Nursing interventions
- Patient's response to nursing interventions
- Patient's concern about the risk for thrombus formation
- Patient's understanding of practical ways in which to avoid risk

REFERENCES

Geraldini, F., De Cassai, A., Correale, C., Andreatta, G., Grandis, M., Navalesi, P., & Munari, M. (2020). Predictors of deep-vein thrombosis in subarachnoid hemorrhage: A retrospective analysis. *Acta Neurochirurgica, 162*(9), 2295–2301. http://dx.doi.org/10.1007/s00701-020-04455-x

Wei, L., Li-li, W., Hai-yan, L., & Rui, F. (2021). Analysis of risk factors for asymptomatic deep venous thrombosis in patients with acute ischemic stroke. *Chinese Journal of Contemporary Neurology & Neurosurgery, 21*(7), 592–597.

Ren, Z., Yuan, Y., Qi, W., Li, Y., & Wang, P. (2021). The incidence and risk factors of deep venous thrombosis in lower extremities following surgically treated femoral shaft fracture: A retrospective case-control study. *Journal of Orthopaedic Surgery & Research, 16*(1), 1–9.

Timp, J. F., Braekkan, S. K., Lijfering, W. M., van Hylckama Vlieg, A., Hansen, J.-B., Rosendaal, F. R., le Cessie, S., & Cannegieter, S. C. (2019). Prediction of recurrent venous thrombosis in all patients with a first venous thrombotic event: The Leiden Thrombosis Recurrence Risk Prediction Model (L-TRRiP). *PLoS Medicine, 16*(10). http://dx.doi.org/10.1371/journal.pmed.1002883

Impaired Tissue Integrity

DEFINITION

Damage to the mucous membranes, cornea, integumentary system, muscular fascia, muscle, tendon, bone, cartilage, joint capsule, and/or ligament

RELATED FACTORS (R/T)

External Factors

- Excretions
- Humidity
- Hyperthermia
- Hypothermia
- Inadequate caregiver knowledge about maintaining tissue integrity
- Inadequate caregiver knowledge about protecting tissue integrity
- Inadequate use of chemical agent
- Pressure over bony prominence
- Psychomotor agitation
- Secretions
- Shearing forces
- Surface friction
- Use of linen with insufficient moisture wicking property

Internal Factors

- Body mass index above normal range for age and gender
- Body mass index below normal range for age and gender
- Decreased blinking frequency

- Decreased physical activity
- Fluid imbalance
- Impaired physical mobility
- Impaired postural balance
- Inadequate adherence to incontinence treatment regimen
- Inadequate blood glucose level management
- Inadequate knowledge about maintaining tissue integrity
- Inadequate knowledge about restoring tissue integrity
- Inadequate ostomy care
- Malnutrition
- Psychogenic factor
- Self-mutilation
- Smoking
- Substance misuse

ASSOCIATED CONDITIONS

- Anemia
- Autism spectrum disorder
- Cardiovascular diseases
- Chronic neurological conditions
- Critical illness
- Decreased level of consciousness
- Decreased serum albumin level
- Decreased tissue oxygenation
- Decreased tissue perfusion
- Hemodynamic instability
- Immobilization
- Intellectual disability
- Medical devices
- Metabolic diseases
- Peripheral neuropathy
- Pharmaceutical preparations
- Sensation disorders
- Surgical procedures

ASSESSMENT

- History of peripheral vascular disease or surgery
- Age
- Gender
- Mobility status, including range of motion
- Integumentary status, including color, skin care practices, temperature, tenderness, texture, turgor, and edema
- Cardiovascular status, including blood pressure, cardiac output, patient and family history of cardiovascular disease, peripheral pulses, and smoking history
- Nutritional status, including dietary patterns, laboratory tests, serum lipid level, serum protein level, and change from normal weight
- Neurologic status, including motor function and sensory pattern

DEFINING CHARACTERISTICS

- Abscess
- Acute pain
- Bleeding
- Decreased muscle strength
- Decreased range of motion
- Difficulty bearing weight
- Dry eye
- Hematoma
- Impaired skin integrity
- Localized area hot to touch
- Localized deformity
- Localized loss of hair
- Localized numbness
- Localized swelling
- Muscle spasm
- Reports lack of balance
- Reports tingling sensation
- Stiffness
- Tissue exposure below the epidermis

EXPECTED OUTCOMES

- Patient will attain relief from immediate signs and symptoms (pain, ulcers, color changes, and edema).
- Patient will maintain collateral circulation.
- Patient will voice intent to stop smoking.
- Patient will voice intent to follow specific management routines after discharge.

Suggested NOC Outcomes

Knowledge: Treatment Regimen; Self-Care Hygiene; Tissue Integrity: Skin & Mucous Membranes; Tissue Perfusion: Peripheral; Wound Healing: Secondary Intention

INTERVENTIONS AND RATIONALES

EBP ▪ Provide scrupulous foot care. Administer and monitor treatments according to institutional protocols. *Foot care prevents fungal infections and ingrown toenails, stimulates circulation, and allows detection of signs and symptoms you should immediately report to the physician.*

EBP ▪ Use padding, special mattresses, and support devices if needed. *These measures reduce undue pressure and decrease the risk of impaired tissue integrity.*

EBP ▪ Instruct patient to avoid pressure on popliteal space. For example, say "Don't cross your legs or wear constrictive clothing" *to avoid reducing arterial blood supply and increasing venous congestion.*

PCC ▪ Encourage adherence to an exercise regimen as tolerated. *Exercise improves arterial circulation and venous return by promoting muscle contraction and relaxation.*

EBP ▪ Educate patient about risk factors and prevention of injury. Refer patient to a smoking cessation program. *Teaching about factors influencing peripheral vascular disease and prevention of tissue damage helps prevent complications.*

EBP ▪ Maintain adequate hydration. Monitor intake and output and record daily weight. *Adequate hydration reduces blood viscosity and decreases the risk of clot formation.*

EBP ▪ If patient has venous insufficiency, apply antiembolism stockings or intermittent pneumatic compression stockings as prescribed, removing them for 1 hour every 8 hours or according to institutional protocol. Elevate patient's feet when sitting and elevate foot of bed 6 to 9 inches (15 to 20.5 cm) when lying down. *These measures promote venous return and decrease venous congestion in lower extremities.*

EBP ▪ If patient has arterial insufficiency, elevate the head of the bed 6 to 9 in (15 to 20.5 cm) when lying down *to increase arterial blood supply to extremities.*

Suggested NIC Interventions

Circulatory Care: Arterial Insufficiency; Circulatory Precautions; Nutrition Management; Oral Health Maintenance; Positioning; Pressure Management; Pressure Ulcer Prevention; Skin Surveillance; Teaching: Foot Care

EVALUATIONS FOR EXPECTED OUTCOMES

▪ Patient attains relief from immediate symptoms.
  ▪ Patient's feet show no signs of infection, ingrown toenails, or impaired circulation.
  ▪ Patient maintains normal skin turgor.
  ▪ Patient's mucous membranes remain moist.
  ▪ Patient maintains balanced intake and output.
  ▪ Patient's weight remains stable.
▪ Patient's vital signs remain within normal parameters.
▪ Patient uses interventions (antiembolism stockings or intermittent pneumatic compression stockings, elevation of feet, and elevation of head of bed) to promote arterial and venous circulation.
▪ Patient states rationale for quitting smoking and begins smoking cessation program.
▪ Patient describes plan to incorporate prescribed treatment program into postdischarge routine, including avoiding risk factors and activities that contribute to vascular compression (such as popliteal compression, leg crossing, and wearing constrictive clothing), following exercise program, and practicing foot care.

DOCUMENTATION

▪ Patient's expressions of feelings about current situation
▪ Observations of skin color, turgor, temperature, and ulcer size
▪ Patient's response to nursing interventions
▪ Evaluations for expected outcomes

REFERENCES

Avşar, P., & Karadağ, A. (2018). Efficacy and cost-effectiveness analysis of evidence-based nursing interventions to maintain tissue integrity to prevent pressure ulcers and incontinence-associated dermatitis. *Worldviews on Evidence-Based Nursing, 15*(1), 54–61. doi:10.1111/wvn.12264

Chantal Magalhães da Silva, N., de Souza Oliveira, K. A. R., Moorhead, S., Pace, A. E., & Carvalho, E. (2017). Clinical validation of the indicators and definitions of the nursing outcome "Tissue integrity: Skin and mucous membranes" in people with diabetes mellitus. *International Journal of Nursing Knowledge, 28*(4), 165–170. doi:10.1111/2047-3095.12150

Kottner, J., Sigaudo-Roussel, D., & Cuddigan, J. (2019). From bed sores to skin failure: Linguistic and conceptual confusion in the field of skin and tissue integrity. *International Journal of Nursing Studies, 92*, 58–59. doi:10.1016/j.ijnurstu.2019.01.007

Risk for Impaired Tissue Integrity

DEFINITION

Susceptible to damage to the mucous membrane, cornea, integumentary system, muscular fascia, muscle, tendon, bone, cartilage, joint capsule, and/or ligament, which may compromise health

RISK FACTORS

External Factors

- Excretions
- Humidity
- Hyperthermia
- Hypothermia
- Inadequate caregiver knowledge about maintaining tissue integrity
- Inadequate caregiver knowledge about protecting tissue integrity
- Inadequate use of chemical agent
- Pressure over bony prominence
- Psychomotor agitation
- Secretions
- Shearing forces
- Surface friction
- Use of linen with insufficient moisture wicking property

Internal Factors

- Body mass index above normal range for age and gender
- Body mass index below normal range for age and gender
- Decreased blinking frequency
- Decreased physical activity
- Fluid imbalance
- Impaired physical mobility
- Impaired postural balance
- Inadequate adherence to incontinence treatment regimen
- Inadequate blood glucose level management
- Inadequate knowledge about maintaining tissue integrity
- Inadequate knowledge about restoring tissue integrity
- Inadequate ostomy care
- Malnutrition
- Psychogenic factor
- Self-mutilation
- Smoking
- Substance misuse

ASSOCIATED CONDITIONS

- Anemia
- Autism spectrum disorder
- Cardiovascular diseases
- Chronic neurological conditions

- Critical illness
- Decreased level of consciousness
- Decreased serum albumin level
- Decreased tissue oxygenation
- Decreased tissue perfusion
- Hemodynamic instability
- Immobilization
- Intellectual disability
- Medical devices
- Metabolic diseases
- Peripheral neuropathy
- Pharmaceutical preparations
- Sensation disorders
- Surgical procedures

ASSESSMENT

- History of peripheral vascular disease or surgery
- Age
- Gender
- Integumentary status, including color, skin care practices, temperature, tenderness, texture, turgor, and edema
- Cardiovascular status, including blood pressure, cardiac output, patient and family history of cardiovascular disease, peripheral pulses, and smoking history
- Mobility status, including range of motion
- Nutritional status, including dietary patterns, laboratory tests, serum lipid level, serum protein level, and change from normal weight
- Neurologic status, including motor function and sensory pattern
- Current medical treatments, including surgery, chemotherapy and radiation, steroid, immunosuppressive, anticoagulant, thrombolytic, and antibiotic therapy

EXPECTED OUTCOMES

- Patient will not experience tissue impairment.
- Patient will maintain collateral circulation.
- Patient will describe measures to protect tissue.
- Patient will have adequate hydration.

Suggested NOC Outcomes

Body Positioning: Self-Initiated; Circulation Status; Hydration; Mobility; Nutritional Status; Tissue Perfusion: Peripheral

INTERVENTIONS AND RATIONALES

- **S** Inspect patient's skin every shift; document skin condition and report status changes. *Early detection of changes prevents or minimizes skin breakdown.*
- **S** Monitor any wounds and surrounding tissue. *Allows for individualized care.*
- **S** Monitor placement of tubing and devices. *Correct placement and frequent inspection of devices prevent skin breakdown.*

S   ▪ Evaluate need for specialty pressure redirecting devices. *Pressure redirecting devices help to eliminate pressure points on skin and tissue.*

S   ▪ Provide scrupulous foot care. Administer and monitor treatments according to institutional protocols. *Foot care prevents fungal infections and ingrown toenails, stimulates circulation, and allows detection of signs and symptoms you should immediately report to the physician.*

EBP   ▪ Instruct patient to avoid pressure on popliteal space. For example, say "Don't cross your legs or wear constrictive clothing" *to avoid reducing arterial blood supply and increasing venous congestion.*

EBP   ▪ Encourage exercise as tolerated. *Exercise improves arterial circulation and venous return by promoting muscle contraction and relaxation.*

EBP   ▪ Educate patient about risk factors and prevention of injury. Refer patient to a smoking cessation program. *Teaching about factors influencing peripheral vascular disease and prevention of tissue damage help prevent complications.*

EBP   ▪ Maintain adequate hydration. Monitor intake and output and record daily weight. *Adequate hydration reduces blood viscosity and decreases the risk of clot formation.*

PCC   ▪ Identify and document factors that predispose patient to impaired tissue integrity. *A complete nursing assessment allows the development of an individualized care plan.*

Suggested NIC Interventions

Electrolyte Monitoring; Fluid Monitoring; Nutrition Management; Positioning; Pressure Ulcer Prevention; Skin Surveillance

EVALUATIONS FOR EXPECTED OUTCOMES

▪ Patient's tissue remains intact.
▪ Patient's mucous membranes remain moist.
▪ Patient's weight remains stable.
▪ Patient's vital signs remain within normal parameters.
▪ Patient uses interventions (antiembolism stockings or intermittent pneumatic compression stockings, elevation of feet, and elevation of head of bed) to promote arterial and venous circulation.
▪ Patient states rationale for quitting smoking and begins smoking cessation program.
▪ Patient doesn't develop rash, edema, bruises, discoloration, redness, skin breakdown, or other signs of altered tissue integrity related to physical hazards.
▪ Patient maintains adequate circulation to tissue.

DOCUMENTATION

▪ Observations of skin color, turgor, and temperature
▪ Preexisting conditions that increase risk of tissue injury
▪ Nursing interventions performed to protect tissue integrity
▪ Medications administered
▪ Presence of lines, tubes, catheters, and drains
▪ Evaluations for expected outcomes

REFERENCES

Bonifant, H., & Holloway, S. (2019). A review of the effects of ageing on skin integrity and wound healing. *British Journal of Community Nursing, 24,* S28–S33. doi:10.12968/bjcn.2019.24.Sup3.S28

Grap, M. J., Munro, C. L., Schubert, C. M., Wetzel, P. A., Burk, R. S., Pepperl, A., & Lucas, V. (2018). Lack of association of high backrest with sacral tissue changes in adults receiving mechanical ventilation. *American Journal of Critical Care, 27*(2), 104–113. doi:10.4037/ajcc2018419

Grap, M. J., Munro, C. L., Wetzel, P. A., Schubert, C. M., Pepperl, A., Burk, R. S., & Lucas, V. (2017). Tissue interface pressure and skin integrity in critically ill, mechanically ventilated patients. *Intensive & Critical Care Nursing, 38*, 1–9. doi:10.1016/j.iccn.2016.07.004

Ineffective Peripheral Tissue Perfusion

DEFINITION

Decrease in blood circulation to the periphery, which may compromise health

RELATED FACTORS (R/T)

- Excessive sodium intake
- Insufficient knowledge of disease process
- Insufficient knowledge of modifiable factors
- Sedentary lifestyle
- Smoking

ASSOCIATED CONDITIONS

- Diabetes mellitus
- Endovascular procedure
- Hypertension
- Trauma

ASSESSMENT

- Cardiovascular status including blood pressure, heart rate, and rhythm
- Peripheral vascular assessment, peripheral pulses, temperature and color of extremities, skin integrity
- Activity status
- Pain assessment

DEFINING CHARACTERISTICS

- Absence of peripheral pulses
- Alteration in motor functioning
- Alteration in skin characteristic
- Ankle-brachial index <0.90
- Capillary refill time >3 seconds
- Color does not return to lowered limb after 1-minute leg elevation
- Decrease in blood pressure in extremities
- Decrease in pain-free distances achieved in the 6-minute walk test
- Decrease in peripheral pulses
- Delay in peripheral wound healing
- Distance in the 6-minute walk test below normal range
- Edema
- Extremity pain
- Femoral bruit
- Intermittent claudication
- Paresthesia
- Skin color pales with limb elevation

EXPECTED OUTCOMES

- Patient will understand the need to maintain moderate activity level to promote circulation.
- Patient will articulate the need and rationale for smoking cessation.
- Patient will not experience ischemic damage to involved extremity.
- Patient will experience adequate perfusion to promote wound healing.
- Patient will acknowledge the importance of protecting involved extremity from injury.
- Patient will recognize reportable changes in skin characteristics to the involved extremity that indicate decreased perfusion.

Suggested NOC Outcomes

Activity Tolerance; Tissue Integrity: Skin and Mucous Membranes; Tissue Perfusion: Peripheral

INTERVENTIONS AND RATIONALES

- **EBP** Evaluate involved extremity for clinical signs (pain, decreased temperature, pallor, delayed capillary refill, weak or absent pulse, decreased sensation, and decreased pulse oximetry), *which are indicators of ineffective peripheral perfusion.*
- **S** Protect the extremity from injury using sheepskin or bed cradle and position extremity at or lower than level of heart *to promote collateral blood flow.*
- **EBP** Instruct patient to increase walking activity *to promote collateral circulation and improve blood supply to the extremity.*
- **S** Encourage patient to protect extremity from injury or extreme hot or cold temperatures. *Infection or ulcer formation may develop more easily due to decreased blood supply.*
- **T&C** Refer patients who smoke to smoking cessation program *since continued smoking will significantly increase risks for further damage.*

Suggested NIC Interventions

Circulatory Care: Arterial Insufficiency; Exercise Promotion; Positioning; Skin Surveillance

EVALUATIONS FOR EXPECTED OUTCOMES

- Patient understands the need to maintain moderate activity to promote blood flow to extremity.
- Patient states the need for smoking cessation.
- Patient's involved extremity is free of injury or ischemic damage.
- Patient recognizes reportable changes to involved extremity that indicate decreased perfusion.

DOCUMENTATION

- Patient's understanding of need for moderate activity and implementation plan
- Patient's plan for smoking cessation
- Assessment of involved extremity
- Assessment of peripheral pain
- Evaluations for expected outcomes

REFERENCES

Heringlake, M., & Maurer, H. (2017). Taking two steps at a time does not necessarily bring you forward! Monitoring peripheral tissue perfusion with near-infrared spectroscopy. *BJA: The British Journal of Anaesthesia, 118*(4), 485–486. doi:10.1093/bja/aex032

Hotfiel, T., Swoboda, B., Krinner, S., Grim, C., Engelhardt, M., Uder, M., & Heiss, R. U. (2017). Acute effects of lateral thigh foam rolling on arterial tissue perfusion determined by spectral Doppler and power Doppler ultrasound. *Journal of Strength & Conditioning Research (Lippincott Williams & Wilkins), 31*(4), 893–900. doi:10.1519/JSC.0000000000001641

Kilgas, M. A., McDaniel, J., Stavres, J., Pollock, B. S., Singer, T. J., & Elmer, S. J. (2019). Limb blood flow and tissue perfusion during exercise with blood flow restriction. *European Journal of Applied Physiology, 119*(2), 377–387. doi:10.1007/s00421-018-4029-2

Risk for Ineffective Peripheral Tissue Perfusion

DEFINITION

Susceptible to a decrease in blood circulation to the periphery, which may compromise health

RISK FACTORS

- Excessive sodium intake
- Insufficient knowledge of disease process
- Insufficient knowledge of modifiable factors
- Sedentary lifestyle
- Smoking

ASSOCIATED CONDITIONS

- Diabetes mellitus
- Endovascular procedure
- Hypertension
- Trauma

ASSESSMENT

- Pain sensation, including characteristics (sharp, dull, constant, or intermittent); precipitating factors
- Psychosocial status, including age, learning ability, decision-making ability, developmental stage, financial resources, health beliefs, knowledge and skill regarding current health problem, usual coping patterns
- Cardiovascular status including heart rate and rhythm, blood pressure, and peripheral pulses
- Neurologic status including level of consciousness, orientation, motor activity, and strength of all extremities
- Behavioral status, understanding of health problem and treatment plan, past history with health care providers, participation in health care planning and decision-making; recognition and realization of potential growth, health, autonomy

EXPECTED OUTCOMES

- Patient will be free from tissue injury due to decreased peripheral perfusion.
- Patient will understand the need for smoking cessation.
- Patient will understand the need for moderate activity to promote circulation.
- Patient will state reportable changes that indicate decreased peripheral perfusion.

Suggested NOC Outcomes

Activity Tolerance; Tissue Integrity: Skin and Mucous Membranes; Tissue Perfusion: Peripheral

INTERVENTIONS AND RATIONALES

S ▪ Assess lower extremities for early signs of ineffective peripheral perfusion. *Early identification and intervention will improve patient outcomes.*

S ▪ Assess patient's history for presence of heart disease, hyperlipidemia, diabetes, and smoking, *which are significant risk factors for impaired peripheral tissue perfusion.*

PCC ▪ Evaluate patient's understanding of lifestyle modifications *to enable patient participation in risk factor reduction.*

EBP ▪ Administer and evaluate effectiveness of medications to treat underlying medical conditions that place patient at risk for decreased peripheral perfusion. *Control of risk factors will prevent or delay onset of tissue hypoperfusion.*

EBP ▪ Position extremity at or lower than level of the heart *to promote peripheral perfusion.*

EBP ▪ Instruct patient to initiate a regular walking program *to promote collateral circulation* and improve perfusion.

EBP ▪ Teach patient to avoid crossing of the legs *to avoid constriction.*

PCC ▪ Encourage patient to carefully follow treatment regimens for existing medical conditions *that are risk factors for decreased peripheral tissue perfusion.*

T&C ▪ Refer patients who smoke to smoking cessation program *because continued smoking will significantly increase risks for development of peripheral tissue damage.*

Suggested NIC Interventions

Circulatory Care: Arterial Insufficiency; Exercise Promotion; Positioning; Skin Surveillance

EVALUATIONS FOR EXPECTED OUTCOMES

▪ Patient has no tissue injury due to decreased peripheral perfusion.
▪ Patient understands need for smoking cessation.
▪ Patient understands need for moderate activity.
▪ Patient states changes that may indicate poor peripheral perfusion.

DOCUMENTATION

▪ Observations of lower extremity status
▪ Interventions performed to manage decreased peripheral perfusion
▪ Patient's response to interventions
▪ Evaluations for expected outcomes

REFERENCES

García-Mayor, S., Morilla-Herrera, J. C., Lupiáñez-Pérez, I., Kaknani Uttumchandani, S., León Campos, Á., Aranda-Gallardo, M., . . . Morales-Asencio, J. M. (2018). Peripheral perfusion and oxygenation in areas of risk of skin integrity impairment exposed to pressure patterns. A phase I trial (POTER Study). *Journal of Advanced Nursing, 74*(2), 465–471. doi:10.1111/jan.13414

Gobbo, M., Gaffurini, P., Vacchi, L., Lazzarini, S., Villafane, J., Orizio, C., . . . Bissolotti, L. (2017). Hand passive mobilization performed with robotic assistance: Acute effects on upper limb perfusion and spasticity in stroke survivors. *BioMed Research International, 2017*, 1–6. doi:10.1155/2017/2796815

Urbina, T., Bigé, N., Nguyen, Y., Boelle, P.-Y., Dubée, V., Joffre, J., . . . Ait-Oufella, H. (2018). Tissue perfusion alterations correlate with mortality in patients admitted to the intensive care unit for acute pulmonary embolism: An observational study. *Medicine, 97*(42), 1–5. doi:10.1097/MD.0000000000011993

Risk for Decreased Cardiac Tissue Perfusion

DEFINITION

Susceptible to a decrease in cardiac (coronary) circulation, which may compromise health

RISK FACTORS

- Insufficient knowledge about modifiable risk factors
- Substance misuse

ASSOCIATED CONDITIONS

- Cardiac tamponade
- Cardiovascular surgery
- Coronary artery spasm
- Diabetes mellitus
- Hyperlipidemia
- Hypertension
- Hypovolemia
- Hypoxemia
- Hypoxia
- Increase in C-reactive protein
- Pharmaceutical agent

ASSESSMENT

- Cardiovascular status including blood pressure, heart rate and rhythm, skin color, temperature, and peripheral pulses
- Results of echocardiogram and other diagnostic tests
- Medical history including family history, history of cardiovascular disease, and medication history

EXPECTED OUTCOMES

- Patient will remain hemodynamically stable.
- Patient will not experience any signs or symptoms of decreased cardiac tissue perfusion.
- Patient will verbalize modifiable risk factors for decreased cardiac perfusion.
- Patient will identify reportable symptoms of possible decreased cardiac perfusion.

Suggested NOC Outcomes

Knowledge: Cardiac Disease Management; Cardiac Pump Effectiveness; Circulation Status; Tissue Perfusion: Cardiac

INTERVENTIONS AND RATIONALES

S - Assess hemodynamic status, including blood pressure, heart rate, oxygen saturation, and respiratory rate for any abnormalities *that may be early indicators of altered perfusion.*

S - Monitor cardiac rhythm for any irregularities *that may indicate cardiac irritability.*

EBP - Assist with preparation and completion of diagnostic tests and the postprocedural care. *Safe completion of diagnostic tests will result in improved patient outcomes.*

S ■ Treat episodes of tachycardia promptly. *Cardiac tissue is perfused during diastole and perfusion is decreased if tachycardia is not treated.*

EBP ■ Provide patient with information regarding modifiable risk factors. *Knowledge of risk factors will contribute to informed decisions about lifestyle changes.*

PCC ■ Encourage patient and family to share concerns regarding outcomes of tests *to reduce anxiety.*

T&C ■ Collaborate with other members of the health care team to ensure that all underlying medical conditions are being managed effectively. *This will minimize the possibility of cardiac perfusion complications.*

Suggested NIC Interventions

Risk Identification; Teaching: Disease Process; Cardiac Care; Hemodynamic Regulation

EVALUATIONS FOR EXPECTED OUTCOMES

■ Patient remained hemodynamically stable.
■ Patient did not experience any signs or symptoms of decreased cardiac tissue perfusion.
■ Patient verbalized modifiable risk factors for decreased cardiac perfusion.
■ Patient identified reportable symptoms of possible decreased cardiac perfusion.

DOCUMENTATION

■ Hemodynamic status including vital signs and physical assessment findings
■ Patient's report of any symptoms related to decreased cardiac tissue perfusion
■ Patient's understanding of risk reduction interventions
■ Evaluation of expected outcomes

REFERENCES

Kim, H.-L., Kim, M.-A., Oh, S., Kim, M., Yoon, H. J., Park, S. M., … Shim, W.-J. (2019). Sex differences in traditional and nontraditional risk factors for obstructive coronary artery disease in stable symptomatic patients. *Journal of Women's Health (15409996), 28*(2), 212–219. doi:10.1089/jwh.2017.6834

Smith, R. (2018). Myocardial perfusion study to detect coronary artery disease. *Radiologic Technology, 90*(2), 131–146.

Song, I., Yi, J. G., Park, J. H., Kim, M. Y., Shin, J. K., & Ko, S. M. (2018). Diagnostic performance of static single-scan stress perfusion cardiac computed tomography in detecting hemodynamically significant coronary artery stenosis: A comparison with combined invasive coronary angiography and cardiovascular magnetic resonance-myocardial perfusion imaging. *Acta Radiologica, 59*(10), 1184–1193. doi:10.1177/0284185117752553

Risk for Ineffective Cerebral Tissue Perfusion

DEFINITION

Susceptible to a decrease in cerebral tissue circulation, which may compromise health

RISK FACTOR

Substance misuse

ASSOCIATED CONDITIONS

- Abnormal partial thromboplastin time (PTT)
- Abnormal prothrombin time (PT)
- Akinetic left ventricular wall segment
- Aortic atherosclerosis
- Arterial dissection
- Atrial fibrillation
- Atrial myxoma
- Brain injury
- Brain neoplasm
- Carotid stenosis
- Cerebral aneurysm
- Coagulopathy
- Dilated cardiomyopathy
- Disseminated intravascular coagulopathy
- Embolism
- Hypercholesterolemia
- Hypertension
- Infective endocarditis
- Mechanical prosthetic valve
- Mitral stenosis
- Pharmaceutical agent
- Sick sinus syndrome
- Treatment regimen

ASSESSMENT

- Cardiovascular status including heart rate and rhythm, blood pressure, and peripheral pulses
- Neurologic status including level of consciousness, orientation, motor activity, and strength of all extremities
- History of recent trauma, injury
- Results of diagnostic and laboratory tests

EXPECTED OUTCOMES

- Patient will understand the need for frequent neurologic assessments to evaluate for any changes.
- Patient will experience adequate cerebral perfusion evidenced by normal neurologic checks.
- Patient will remain hemodynamically stable.
- Patient will participate in diagnostic testing when necessary.
- Patient will verbalize strategies to minimize or decrease modifiable risk factors.

Suggested NOC Outcomes

Tissue Perfusion: Cerebral; Neurological Status; Circulation Status

S ▪ Assess patient for positive risk factors for decrease in cerebral perfusion, including carotid stenosis, hypertension, coagulopathies, atrial fibrillation, and smoking. *Risk factor reduction will result in positive patient outcomes.*

EBP ▪ Facilitate completion of diagnostic tests and provide postprocedural care to prevent complications *to ensure accurate, safe, and timely diagnosis and treatment.*

S ▪ Maintain adequate oxygenation *to ensure cerebral perfusion.*

EBP ▪ Educate at-risk patients of the signs of decreased cerebral perfusion and the importance of timely medical intervention for positive symptoms. *Change in mental status is a sensitive indicator for decreased cerebral perfusion.*

PCC ▪ Encourage at-risk patient and family to ask questions and share concerns *to increase their confidence and ability to recognize and respond to warning signs of decreased cerebral perfusion.*

T&C ▪ Collaborate with community organizations to educate public on risk factors for and symptoms of decreased cerebral perfusion and the appropriate response. *Increased community awareness may result in a more timely intervention for decreased cerebral perfusion conditions.*

Suggested NIC Interventions

Cerebral Perfusion Promotion; Neurologic Monitoring

▪ Patient accepts the need for frequent neurologic assessments to evaluate changes in condition.

▪ Patient condition reflects normal cerebral perfusion.

▪ Patient's hemodynamic status supports adequate cerebral perfusion.

▪ Patient participates in diagnostic testing.

▪ Patient identifies modifiable risk factors for decreased cerebral perfusion.

▪ Trending of neurologic assessments

▪ Vital sign results, including blood pressure, heart rate, and oxygenation status

▪ Patient tolerance and results of diagnostic tests

▪ Evaluations for expected outcomes

REFERENCES

He, M., Cui, B., Wu, C., Meng, P., Wu, T., Wang, M., … Sun, Y. (2018). Blood pressures immediately following ischemic strokes are associated with cerebral perfusion and neurologic function. *Journal of Clinical Hypertension, 20*(6), 1008–1015. doi:10.1111/jch.13310

Kramer, A. H., Couillard, P. L., Zygun, D. A., Aries, M. J., & Gallagher, C. N. (2019). Continuous assessment of "optimal" cerebral perfusion pressure in traumatic brain injury: A cohort study of feasibility, reliability, and relation to outcome. *Neurocritical Care, 30*(1), 51–61. doi:10.1007/s12028-018-0570-4

McNett, M., Livesay, S., Yeager, S., Moran, C., Supan, E., Ortega, S., & Olson, D. M. (2018). The impact of head-of-bed positioning and transducer location on cerebral perfusion pressure measurement. *Journal of Neuroscience Nursing, 50*(6), 322–326. doi:10.1097/JNN.0000000000000398

Sharma, V. K., Tan, B. Y. Q., Sim, M. Y., Kulkarni, A., Seow, P. A., Hong, C. S., … Butcher, K. (2018). Rationale and design of a randomized trial of early intensive blood pressure lowering on cerebral perfusion parameters in thrombolysed acute ischemic stroke patients. *Medicine, 97*(40), 1–6. doi:10.1097/MD.0000000000012721

Impaired Transfer Ability

DEFINITION

Limitation of independent movement between two nearby surfaces

RELATED FACTORS (R/T)

- Environmental barrier
- Impaired balance
- Insufficient knowledge of transfer techniques
- Insufficient muscle strength
- Obesity
- Physical deconditioning
- Pain

ASSOCIATED CONDITIONS

- Alteration in cognitive functioning
- Impaired vision
- Musculoskeletal impairment
- Neuromuscular impairment

ASSESSMENT

- Age
- Gender
- Vital signs
- Drug history
- History of neuromuscular disorder or dysfunction
- Musculoskeletal status, including coordination, muscle size and strength, muscle tone, range of motion (ROM), functional mobility as follows:
  0 = completely independent
  1 = requires use of equipment or device
  2 = requires help, supervision, or teaching from another person
  3 = requires help from another person and equipment or device
  4 = dependent; doesn't participate in activity
- Neurologic status, including level of consciousness, motor ability, and sensory ability
- Endurance, for example, how long patient can remain sitting in wheelchair before becoming fatigued
- Knowledge of wheelchair transfer techniques

DEFINING CHARACTERISTICS

- Impaired ability to transfer between bed and chair
- Impaired ability to transfer between bed and standing position
- Impaired ability to transfer between car and chair
- Impaired ability to transfer between chair and floor
- Impaired ability to transfer between chair and standing position
- Impaired ability to transfer between floor and standing position
- Impaired ability to transfer between uneven levels
- Impaired ability to transfer in or out of bath tub

- Impaired ability to transfer in or out of shower
- Impaired ability to transfer on or off a commode
- Impaired ability to transfer on or off a toilet

EXPECTED OUTCOMES

- Patient won't exhibit complications associated with impaired wheelchair transfer mobility, such as depression, altered health maintenance, and falls.
- Patient will maintain or improve muscle strength and joint ROM.
- Patient will achieve highest level of mobility possible (independence with regard to wheelchair transfer, ability to transfer to wheelchair with assistance, verbalization of needs regarding wheelchair transfer).
- Patient will maintain safety during wheelchair transfer.
- Patient will adapt to alteration in ability to perform wheelchair transfer.
- Patient will demonstrate understanding of wheelchair transfer techniques.
- Patient will participate in social and occupational activities to the greatest extent possible.

Suggested NOC Outcomes

Balance; Body Positioning: Self-Initiated; Transfer Performance; Coordinated Movement; Mobility

INTERVENTIONS AND RATIONALES

EBP ▪ Perform ROM exercises to the joints of affected limbs, unless contraindicated, at least once every 8 hours. Progress from passive to active ROM as tolerated *to prevent joint contractures and muscle atrophy.*

EBP ▪ Identify patient's level of independence using the functional mobility scale. Report the findings to the staff *to provide continuity and preserve or improve the documented level of independence.*

PCC ▪ Monitor and record daily evidence of complications related to altered mobility or decreased ability to perform wheelchair transfer (contractures, venous stasis, skin breakdown, thrombus formation, depression, altered health maintenance, or self-care deficit). *Patients with neuromuscular dysfunction are at risk for complications.*

EBP ▪ Teach patient wheelchair transfer techniques, such as performing a standing or sitting transfer, *to maintain muscle tone, prevent complications of immobility, and promote independence.* Adapt teaching to the limits imposed by patient's condition *to prevent injury.*

T&C ▪ Refer patient to a physical therapist for the development of a wheelchair mobility program *to assist with rehabilitation of musculoskeletal deficits.*

PCC ▪ Encourage patient to attend physical therapy. Request a written copy of wheelchair transfer instructions to use as a reference *to maintain continuity of care and foster safety.*

S ▪ Assess patient's skin upon return to bed and request a wheelchair cushion if necessary *to maintain skin integrity.*

EBP ▪ As part of your teaching plan, demonstrate transfer techniques to family members and note the date. Have them perform a return demonstration *to ensure the use of proper technique and to promote continuity of care.*

T&C ▪ Identify resources (stroke program, sports association for the disabled, National Multiple Sclerosis Society) *to promote patient's reintegration into the community.*

Suggested NIC Interventions

Body Mechanics Promotion; Energy Management; Exercise Promotion: Strength Training; Exercise Therapy: Balance; Fall Prevention; Self-Care Assistance: Transfer

EVALUATIONS FOR EXPECTED OUTCOMES

- Patient doesn't exhibit complications associated with impaired wheelchair transfer mobility, such as depression, altered health maintenance, and falls.
- Patient maintains or improves muscle strength and joint ROM.
- Patient achieves highest level of mobility possible (independence with regard to wheelchair transfer, ability to transfer to wheelchair with assistance, verbalization of needs regarding wheelchair transfer).
- Patient maintains safety during wheelchair transfer.
- Patient adapts to alteration in ability to perform wheelchair transfer.
- Patient demonstrates understanding of wheelchair transfer techniques.
- Patient participates in social and occupational activities to the greatest extent possible.

DOCUMENTATION

- Patient's mobility status
- Presence of complications
- Evidence of alterations in patient's ability to perform wheelchair transfer
- Patient's statements regarding difficulties in wheelchair transfer
- Instruction of transfer techniques
- Patient's and family members' return demonstration of skills
- Patient's response to nursing interventions
- Evaluations for expected outcomes

REFERENCES

Ferreira, M. S., de Melo Franco, F. G., Rodrigues, P. S., da Silva de Poli Correa, V. M., Akopian, S. T. G., Cucato, G. G., ... de Carvalho, J. A. M. (2019). Impaired chair-to-bed transfer ability leads to longer hospital stays among elderly patients. *BMC Geriatrics, 19*(1), 89. doi:10.1186/s12877-019-1104-4

Loomer, L., Downer, B., & Thomas, K. S. (2019). Relationship between functional improvement and cognition in short-stay nursing home residents. *Journal of the American Geriatrics Society, 67*(3), 553–557. doi:10.1111/jgs.15708

Münter, K. H., Clemmesen, C. G., Foss, N. B., Palm, H., & Kristensen, M. T. (2018). Fatigue and pain limit independent mobility and physiotherapy after hip fracture surgery. *Disability & Rehabilitation, 40*(15), 1808–1816. doi:10.1080/09638288.2017.1314556

Risk for Physical Trauma

DEFINITION

Susceptible to physical injury of sudden onset and severity, which requires immediate attention

RISK FACTORS

External

- Absence of call-for-aid device
- Absence of stairway gate
- Absence of window guard
- Access to weapon
- Bathing in very hot water
- Bed in high position
- Children riding in front seat of car

- Defective appliance
- Delay in ignition of gas appliance
- Dysfunctional call-for-aid device
- Electrical hazard
- Exposure to corrosive product
- Exposure to dangerous machinery
- Exposure to radiation
- Exposure to toxic chemical
- Extremes of environmental temperature
- Flammable object
- Grease on stove
- Icicles hanging from roof
- Inadequate stair rails
- Inadequately stored combustible
- Inadequately stored corrosive
- Insufficient anti-slip material in bathroom
- Insufficient lighting
- Insufficient protection from heat source
- Misuse of headgear
- Misuse of seat restraint
- Nonuse of seat restraints
- Obstructed passageway
- Playing with dangerous object
- Playing with explosive
- Pot handle facing front of stove
- Proximity to vehicle pathway
- Slippery floor
- Smoking in bed
- Smoking near oxygen
- Struggling with restraints
- Unanchored electric wires
- Unsafe operation of heavy equipment
- Unsafe road
- Unsafe walkway
- Use of cracked dishware
- Use of throw rugs
- Use of unstable chair
- Use of unstable ladder
- Wearing loose clothing around open flames

Internal

- Emotional disturbance
- Impaired balance
- Insufficient knowledge of safety precautions
- Insufficient vision
- Weakness

ASSOCIATED CONDITIONS

- Alteration in cognitive functioning
- Alteration in sensation

- Decrease in eye–hand coordination
- Decrease in muscle coordination

ASSESSMENT

- Age
- Gender
- Level of education
- Developmental factors, including tendency to test independence and take risks (especially in company of peers), feelings of indestructibility, high level of energy, need for peer approval, and access to potential safety hazards (such as complex machinery or tools, farm equipment, car, motorcycle, jet ski, or snowmobile)
- Health history, including accidents, allergies, exposure to pollutants, falls, hyperthermia, hypothermia, poisoning, sensory or perceptual changes (auditory, gustatory, kinesthetic, olfactory, tactile, and visual), seizures, and trauma
- Social history, including academic performance, sports, hobbies, social activities, and occupation
- Circumstances of current situation that might lead to injury from surgery or from chemical, physical, or human agents
- Neurologic status, including level of consciousness, mental status, and orientation
- Laboratory studies, including clotting factors, hemoglobin level, hematocrit, and platelet and white blood cell counts

EXPECTED OUTCOMES

- Patient will avoid injury.
- Patient will state understanding of safety precautions.
- Patient will use assistive devices correctly (e.g., walker or cane).

Suggested NOC Outcomes

Balance; Coordinated Movement; Fall Prevention Behavior; Knowledge: Fall Prevention; Risk Control; Safe Home Environment

INTERVENTIONS AND RATIONALES

- **[S]** Observe, record, and report falls, seizures, and unsafe practices. *Accurate assessment promotes appropriate interventions; documentation ensures continuity of care.*
- **[S]** Assess and document risk factors and unsafe practices discovered through observation or through discussions with patient *to plan effective interventions.*
- **[S]** Monitor and record patient's respiratory status. *Trauma increases respiratory rate; other respiratory effects depend on the nature of the trauma.*
- **[S]** Monitor and record patient's neurologic status *to detect changes and to report deteriorated status.*
- **[S]** Remain with patient in case of a seizure; loosen restrictive clothing, and protect patient from environmental hazards. Don't restrain patient or pry the mouth open. Keep an oral airway at the bedside and maintain a patent airway. Turn patient to the side after the seizure stops and suction if secretions occlude the airway. Record seizure characteristics, including onset, duration, and body movements. Reorient patient to surroundings and allow a rest period. *Remaining with patient provides safety and information for accurate documentation of the event. Loosening clothing and proper positioning may prevent further harm.*

S ▥ Keep the bed in a low position except when providing direct care *to minimize the effects of a possible fall.*

S ▥ Emphasize the importance of asking for help before getting up. *Illness or injury may have weakened patient.*

S ▥ Help debilitated, weak, or unsteady patient to get out of bed. Ensure that the floor is dry and that furniture and litter don't block patient's way *to help prevent falls.*

EBP ▥ When using soft restraints, don't secure them too tightly *to avoid skin burns.*

EBP ▥ Use leather restraints following facility policy; pad them well before applying. Release each extremity on a rotation basis every hour; check for skin burns. *Such restraints should be used only when other kinds are ineffective.*

EBP ▥ Instruct patient and family members on safety practices such as correct use of a walker, crutches, or cane. *These enable patient and family members to take an active role in health care and maintain a safe environment.*

EBP ▥ Demonstrate the use of appropriate safety equipment, such as protective sports gear, and have patient perform a return demonstration *to reinforce learning.*

EBP ▥ Select teaching topics that will help patient prevent future injuries and promote personal health—for example, automotive and motorcycle safety, proper use of protective equipment in sports, or alcohol and drug awareness. *Teaching patient increases knowledge and reinforces the notion of responsibility for ensuring personal safety.*

Suggested NIC Interventions

Environmental Management: Safety; Fall Prevention; Health Education; Pressure Ulcer Prevention; Seizure Precautions; Surveillance: Safety; Teaching: Disease Process

EVALUATIONS FOR EXPECTED OUTCOMES

▥ Patient remains free from injury.

▥ Patient identifies specific safety precautions.

▥ Patient identifies risks and behaviors that should be avoided.

▥ Patient demonstrates proper use of safety devices and equipment, as appropriate (e.g., using protective sports gear, seat belt, and motorcycle helmet).

▥ Patient demonstrates proper use of assistive devices (specify).

▥ Patient states intention to adopt safety precautions.

DOCUMENTATION

▥ Patient's statements that indicate potential for injury

▥ Physical findings

▥ Observations or knowledge of unsafe practices

▥ Interventions performed to prevent injury

▥ Patient's response to nursing interventions

▥ Evaluations for expected outcomes

REFERENCES

Anderson, S., Stuckey, R., Fortington, L. V., & Oakman, J. (2019). Workplace injuries in the Australian allied health workforce. *Australian Health Review, 43*(1), 49–54. doi:10.1071/AH16173

Duzinski, S. V., Guevara, L. M., Barczyk, A. N., Garcia, N. M., Cassel, J. L., & Lawson, K. A. (2018). Effectiveness of a pediatric abusive head trauma prevention program among Spanish-speaking mothers. *Hispanic Health Care International, 16*(1), 5–10. doi:10.1177/1540415318756859

Eastern Association for the Surgery of Trauma Firearm Injury Prevention Statement. (2019). *Journal of Trauma & Acute Care Surgery, 86*(1), 168–170. doi:10.1097/TA.0000000000002148

Galic, T., Kuncic, D., Pericic, T. P., Galic, I., Mihanovic, G., Bozic, J., ... Herceg, M. (2018). Knowledge and attitudes about sports-related dental injuries and mouthguard use in young athletes in four different contact sports-water polo, karate, taekwondo and handball. *Dental Traumatology, 34*(3), 175–181. doi:10.1111/edt.12394

Risk for Vascular Trauma

DEFINITION

Susceptible to damage to vein and its surrounding tissues related to the presence of a catheter and/or infused solutions, which may compromise health

RISK FACTORS

- Inadequate available insertion site
- Prolonged period of time catheter is in place

ASSOCIATED CONDITIONS

- Irritating solution
- Rapid infusion rate

ASSESSMENT

- Integumentary status including color, turgor, lesions, and wounds
- Fluid and electrolyte and medication therapies
- Mobility status

EXPECTED OUTCOMES

- Patient will not experience vascular trauma as a result of catheter or infused solution.
- Patient will communicate reportable signs and symptoms indicating possible catheter infusion–related problems.
- Patient will maintain recommended position of extremity during treatment.

Suggested NOC Outcomes

Tissue Integrity: Skin & Mucous Membranes; Comfort Status: Physical; Knowledge: Treatment Procedure

INTERVENTIONS AND RATIONALES

- **S** Assess patient for pain at insertion site. *Pain is often the first symptom of vascular trauma.*
- **S** Use transparent dressing over the insertion site. *This will secure the catheter and facilitate frequent assessment of the insertion site.*
- **S** Perform prescribed insertion site checks and progress of the infusion *to ensure early identification of problems and timely interventions to avoid vascular trauma.*

EBP ▪ Educate patient about the purpose of the infusion and reportable symptoms indicative of trauma, for example, burning, swelling, and warmth. *Prompt termination of the infusion and the catheter will minimize damage to the tissue.*

PCC ▪ Support patient throughout intravenous therapy *to decrease anxiety and promote positive patient outcomes.*

T&C ▪ Collaborate with experienced team members in the management of complex intravenous therapy *to ensure all possible steps are taken to minimize complications.*

Suggested NIC Interventions

Intravenous Therapy; Medication Administration: Intravenous (IV); Skin Surveillance; Teaching: Procedure/Treatment

EVALUATIONS FOR EXPECTED OUTCOMES

▪ Patient did not experience vascular trauma as a result of intravenous therapy.
▪ Patient was able to maintain proper position of the extremity during treatment.
▪ Patient was able to identify reportable signs and symptoms of infusion-related problems.

DOCUMENTATION

▪ Intravenous site checks and interventions
▪ Patient reports of possible complications of intravenous therapy
▪ Intake and output including type of intravenous fluid and rate of infusion
▪ Evaluations for expected outcomes

REFERENCES

Braga, L. M., Parreira, P. M., Oliveira, A. S. S., Mónico, L. D. S. M., Arreguy-Sena, C., & Henriques, M. A. (2018). Phlebitis and infiltration: Vascular trauma associated with the peripheral venous catheter. *Revista Latino-Americana de Enfermagem (RLAE), 26,* 1–8. doi:10.1590/1518-8345.2377.3002

Perkins, Z. B., Yet, B., Glasgow, S., Marsh, W. R., Tai, N. R. M., Rasmussen, T. E., ... Marsh, D. W. R. (2018). Long-term, patient-centered outcomes of lower-extremity vascular trauma. *Journal of Trauma & Acute Care Surgery, 85,* S104–S111. doi:10.1097/TA.0000000000001956

Wesslén, C., & Wahlgren, C.-M. (2018). Contemporary management and outcome after lower extremity fasciotomy in non-trauma-related vascular surgery. *Vascular & Endovascular Surgery, 52*(7), 493–497. doi:10.1177/1538574418773503

Wlodarczyk, J. R., Thomas, A. S., Schroll, R., Campion, E. M., Croyle, C., Menaker, J., ... Moore, M. M. (2018). To shunt or not to shunt in combined orthopedic and vascular extremity trauma. *Journal of Trauma & Acute Care Surgery, 85*(6), 1038–1042. doi:10.1097/TA.0000000000002065

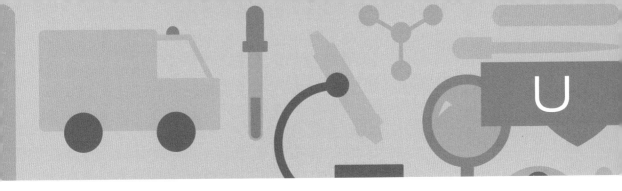

Unilateral Neglect

Impairment in sensory and motor response, mental representation, and spatial attention of the body, and the corresponding environment, characterized by inattention to one side and over-attention to the opposite side. Left-side neglect is more severe and persistent than right-side neglect

To be developed

Brain injury

- History of neurologic impairment
- Age
- Neurologic status, including awareness of body parts, cognition, level of consciousness, mental status, memory, sensory function, orientation, position sense, visual acuity, visual fields, ability to communicate (verbally and nonverbally), and bowel and bladder control
- Musculoskeletal status, including coordination, muscle size and strength, muscle tone, range of motion (ROM), and functional mobility scale:
  - 0 = completely independent
  - 1 = requires use of equipment or device
  - 2 = requires help, supervision, or teaching from another person
  - 3 = requires help from another person and equipment or device
  - 4 = dependent; doesn't participate in activity
- Integumentary status, including color, texture, turgor, temperature, elasticity, sensation, moisture, hygiene, and lesions
- Psychosocial status, including coping mechanisms, support systems (family and others), lifestyle, and understanding of physical condition
- Self-care abilities, including preparation of equipment and supplies, technical or mechanical skills, and use of assistive devices

- Alteration in safety behavior on neglected side
- Disturbance of sound lateralization

- Failure to dress neglected side
- Failure to eat food from portion of plate on neglected side
- Failure to groom neglected side
- Failure to move eyes in the neglected hemisphere
- Failure to move head in the neglected hemisphere
- Failure to move limbs in the neglected hemisphere
- Failure to move trunk in the neglected hemisphere
- Failure to notice people approaching from the neglected side
- Hemianopsia
- Impaired performance on line cancellation, line bisection, and target cancellation tests
- Left hemiplegia from cerebrovascular accident
- Marked deviation of the eyes to stimuli on the non neglected side
- Marked deviation of the trunk to stimuli on the non neglected side
- Omission of drawing on the neglected side
- Perseveration
- Representational neglect
- Substitution of letters to form alternative words when reading
- Transfer of pain sensation to the non neglected limb
- Unaware of positioning of neglected limb
- Unilateral visuospatial neglect
- Use of vertical half of page only when writing

EXPECTED OUTCOMES

- Patient will avoid injury to affected body part.
- Patient will avoid skin breakdown.
- Patient will avoid contractures.
- Patient will recognize neglected body part.
- Patient and family members will demonstrate exercises for affected body part.
- Patient and family members will demonstrate measures for maximum functioning and arrange environment to protect affected body part.
- Patient and family members will express feelings about altered state of health and neurologic deficits.
- Patient and family members will identify community resources and support groups to help cope with the effects of illness.

Suggested NOC Outcomes

Adaptation to Physical Disability; Body Image; Body Mechanics Performance; Body Positioning: Self-Initiated; Self-Care: Activities of Daily Living (ADLs)

INTERVENTIONS AND RATIONALES

S ■ Place a sling on the affected arm *to prevent dangling or injury*. Support the affected leg and foot while in bed, place a foot strap on the wheelchair, and perform other measures as appropriate *to keep patient's limbs in functional position and avoid contractures*. Use a draw sheet to move patient up in bed *to avoid skin abrasions*.

PCC ■ Touch the affected limb. Describe it in conversation with patient *to remind patient of neglected body part*.

PCC ■ Direct patient to perform activities that require the use of the affected limb. *A patient who uses a paretic or paralyzed limb will more easily integrate the affected limb into his or her body image.*

S ▪ Encourage patient to check the position of the affected body part with each repositioning or transfer *to reestablish awareness of the body part.*

S ▪ Establish and follow a regular turning schedule *to maintain skin integrity.*

T&C ▪ Request consultations with occupational and physical therapists about adaptive equipment, exercise program, and other recommendations *to increase patient's awareness of the affected limb.*

S ▪ Use safety belts or protective devices according to facility policy. *Safety devices remind patient of self-limitations and help prevent falls.*

S ▪ Remove splints and other devices at least every 2 hours. Inspect the skin for pressure areas. Reapply the splint. *Proper use of splints and other devices prevents deformities and maintains skin integrity.*

EBP ▪ Perform ROM exercises on the affected side at least once every shift unless medically contraindicated *to maintain joint flexibility and prevent contractures.*

S ▪ Instruct family and nursing personnel to observe the position of the affected body part frequently. Remove food or drainage from the face if unnoticed by patient. Place the arm or leg in the proper position as often as necessary *to prevent injury.*

PCC ▪ When approaching the patient, do so from the non neglected side in order that the patient will see you and not become startled. *Patient will not move the eyes in the neglected hemisphere and so will not see you.*

S ▪ Arrange the environment for maximum functioning; for example, place water, television controls, and the call bell within reach on the non neglected side. *These measures enhance orientation and encourage independence.*

EBP ▪ Assist with ADLs or provide supervision as appropriate *to protect patient's affected side.* Teach the family the reasons for unilateral neglect. Help them to understand how they can work with patient to minimize frustration. *Families not understanding can challenge patient inappropriately by ignoring patient's ability to use the neglected side.*

PCC ▪ Encourage patient and family members to express their feelings regarding patient's condition and level of functioning *to release tension and enhance coping.*

T&C ▪ Refer patient and family members to appropriate support groups and other community resources *to assist patient and family in adjusting to patient's altered state of health.*

Suggested NIC Interventions

Anticipatory Guidance; Body Image Enhancement; Coping Enhancement; Exercise Therapy: Joint Mobility; Mutual Goal Setting; Self-Care Assistance; Unilateral Neglect Management

EVALUATIONS FOR EXPECTED OUTCOMES

▪ Patient doesn't experience injury.

▪ Patient's skin doesn't show signs of breakdown.

▪ Patient doesn't show evidence of contractures.

▪ Patient recognizes and protects neglected body part when carrying out ADLs.

▪ Patient and family members demonstrate exercise routine for affected body part.

▪ Patient and family members demonstrate measures for maximum functioning and arrange environment to protect affected body part.

▪ Patient and family members openly express fear and other feelings associated with patient's neurologic deficits and altered level of functioning.

▪ Patient and family members identify and contact appropriate community resources and support groups.

DOCUMENTATION

- Patient's expressions of feelings about neglected side of body
- Safety measures taken to prevent injury
- Patient's ability to perform ADLs and nursing measures taken to overcome deficits
- Observations of patient's and family's coping skills
- Patient's response to nursing interventions, including verbal expressions or behavior, that indicates increased awareness of affected limb
- Evaluations for expected outcomes

REFERENCES

Cotoi, A., Mirkowski, M., Iruthayarajah, J., Anderson, R., & Teasell, R. (2019). The effect of theta-burst stimulation on unilateral spatial neglect following stroke: A systematic review. *Clinical Rehabilitation, 33*(2), 183–194. doi:10.1177/0269215518804018

Fan, J., Li, Y., Yang, Y., Qu, Y., & Li, S. (2018). Efficacy of noninvasive brain stimulation on unilateral neglect after stroke: A systematic review and meta-analysis. *American Journal of Physical Medicine & Rehabilitation, 97*(4), 261–269. doi:10.1097/PHM.0000000000000834

Yang, N. Y. H., Fong, K. N. K., Li-Tsang, C. W. P., & Zhou, D. (2017). Effects of repetitive transcranial magnetic stimulation combined with sensory cueing on unilateral neglect in subacute patients with right hemispheric stroke: a randomized controlled study. *Clinical Rehabilitation, 31*(9), 1154–1163. doi:10.1177/0269215516679712

Impaired Urinary Elimination

DEFINITION

Dysfunction in urinary elimination

RELATED FACTORS (R/T)

- Alcohol consumption
- Altered environmental factor
- Caffeine consumption
- Environmental constraints
- Fecal impaction
- Improper toileting posture
- Ineffective toileting habits
- Insufficient privacy
- Involuntary sphincter relaxation
- Obesity
- Pelvic organ prolapse
- Smoking
- Use of aspartame
- Weakened bladder muscle
- Weakened supportive pelvic structure

ASSOCIATED CONDITIONS

- Anatomic obstruction
- Diabetes mellitus
- Sensory motor impairment
- Urinary tract infection

- History of sensory or neuromuscular impairment, urinary tract disease, trauma, surgery, or previous urethral infection
- Age
- Gender
- Vital signs
- Genitourinary status, including characteristics of urine, excretory urography, pain or discomfort, palpation of bladder, urinalysis, and voiding patterns
- Fluid and electrolyte status, including blood urea nitrogen and creatinine levels, intake and output, mucous membranes (inspection), serum electrolyte levels, skin turgor, and urine specific gravity
- Nutritional status, including appetite, constipation, dietary intake, elimination habits, current weight and change from normal, and rectal examination
- For females—labor and delivery, including anesthesia (regional or local) and oxytocin induction or augmentation
- Sexuality status, including capability, concerns, habits, and sexual partners
- Neuromuscular status, including ability to perceive bladder fullness
- Psychosocial status, including coping skills, patient's perception of health problem, self-concept (body image), family members, and stressors (such as finances and job)

- Dysuria
- Frequent voiding
- Nocturia
- Urinary hesitancy
- Urinary incontinence
- Urinary retention
- Urinary urgency

- Patient's urinary function will be free from complications.
- Patient will voice understanding of treatment.
- Patient will empty bladder regularly, as confirmed by abdominal palpation or bladder scan.
- Patient will discuss impact of urologic disorder on self.
- Patient will demonstrate skill in managing urinary elimination problem.
- Patient will maintain urinary continence.
- Patient and family members will identify resources to assist with care following discharge.

Suggested NOC Outcomes

Urinary Continence; Urinary Elimination

S ▪ Observe patient's voiding pattern. Document urine color and characteristics, intake and output, and patient's daily weight. Report any changes. *Urine characteristics help to identify potential problems.*

S ▦ Assess for dehydration (poor skin turgor; flushed, dry skin; confusion; dry mucous membranes; fever; and rapid, thready pulse). *Dehydration leads to decreased circulatory blood volume and decreased urine output.*

S ▦ Palpate the abdomen above the symphysis pubis every 2 hours *to detect bladder distention and the degree of fullness.*

EBP ▦ Administer appropriate care for the urologic condition and monitor progress (e.g., strain urine). Report favorable and adverse responses to the treatment regimen. *Appropriate care helps patient recover from the underlying disorder. Reporting responses to treatment allows modification of the treatment, as needed.*

PCC ▦ Explain reasons for therapy and intended effects to patient and family members *to increase patient's understanding and build trust in caregivers.* If urinary diversion is needed, prepare the patient for a change in body appearance (instruct patient and family members how to care for the ostomy site postoperatively). *Preparation and appropriate information helps patient and family members cope with changes.*

EBP ▦ If patient requires surgery, give appropriate preoperative and postoperative instructions and care. *Accurate information allows patient to understand the procedure and builds trust in caregivers.*

EBP ▦ Assist with bladder elimination procedure as indicated.

▦ For bladder training, place patient on the commode or toilet every 2 hours while awake and once during the night. Maintain regular fluid intake while patient is awake. Provide privacy. Teach patient how to perform Kegel exercises to strengthen sphincter control. *These measures aid adaptation to routine physiologic function. Women with good muscle tone can improve levator muscle action significantly if they perform Kegel exercises regularly.*

▦ For intermittent catheterization, catheterize patient using clean or sterile technique every 2 hours. Record amount voided spontaneously and amount obtained with catheterization (e.g., 7 a.m., spontaneous void of 200 mL; catheter void of 150 mL). Record bladder balance daily. *These measures promote normal voiding, prevent infection, and help maintain integrity of ureterovesical function. Catheterization schedule is based on flow sheet data and can provide a baseline chart.*

▦ Monitor bladder balance for amount of residual urine/amount of voided urine.

▦ For external catheterization (in a male patient), monitor patency. Apply a condom catheter according to the established policy. *Applying a foam strip in a spiral fashion increases the adhesive surface and reduces the risk of impairing circulation.* Avoid constriction. Observe the skin condition of the penis, and clean with soap and water at least twice daily. *These measures prevent infection and ensure therapeutic effectiveness.*

▦ For an indwelling urinary catheter, monitor patency. Keep the tubing free from kinks, and keep the drainage bag below the level of the bladder *to avoid urine reflux.* Clean the urinary meatus according to the established policy, and maintain a closed drainage system *to prevent skin irritation and bacteriuria.* Secure the catheter to patient's leg (female) or abdomen (male); avoid tension on the sphincter. *Anchoring the catheter avoids straining the trigone muscle of the bladder and prevents friction leading to inflammation.*

▦ For a suprapubic catheter, monitor patency. Change the dressing, and clean the catheter site according to policy. Keep the tubing free from kinks; keep the drainage bag below bladder level. Maintain a closed drainage system. *Suprapubic drainage allows increased patient mobility and reduces the risk of bladder infection.*

PCC ▦ Provide supportive measures, as indicated:

 ▦ Encourage fluids, as ordered, to moisten mucous membranes and maintain fluid balance.

 ▦ Refer patient to a dietitian for instructions on diet. Dietary changes may decrease urinary infections.

- Assist with general hygiene and comfort measures, as needed. Cleanliness prevents bacterial growth and promotes comfort.
- Maintain the patency of catheters, drainage bags, and other urinary elimination equipment to avoid reflux and risk of infection and ensure the effectiveness of therapy.
- Provide meatal care according to facility policy to promote cleanliness and comfort and reduce the risk of infection.
- Provide privacy during the toileting procedure to avoid inhibiting elimination.
- Respond to patient's call bell quickly, assign patient to the bed next to the bathroom, and have patient wear easily removed clothing (such as a gown rather than pajamas). These measures reduce delay and impediments to the voiding routine.

S - Alert patient and family members to the signs and symptoms of a full bladder: restlessness, abdominal discomfort, sweating, and chills. *Adequate education increases patient's and family members' ability to maintain health level and to prevent patient from harming himself.*

EBP - Instruct patient and family members on catheterization techniques to be used at home; provide time for return demonstrations until they can perform the procedure well. *Knowledge of procedures and rationales reduces anxiety and promotes comfort. Demonstrations may progress through several sessions until patient can perform independently.*

PCC - Encourage patient to ventilate feelings and concerns related to his or her urologic problem. *Active listening conveys respect for patient; ventilation helps pinpoint patient's fears.*

T&C - Refer patient and family members to a psychiatric liaison nurse, sex counselor, or support group, when appropriate. *These resources help patient gain knowledge of self and the situation, reduce anxiety, and promote personal growth. Community resources usually provide support and care not available in other health agencies.*

EBP - Explain the urologic condition to patient and family members, including instructions on preventive measures, if appropriate. Prepare for discharge according to individual needs. *Accurate health knowledge increases patient's ability to maintain health. Involving family members assures patient of continued care.*

Suggested NIC Interventions

Anxiety Reduction; Fluid Management; Urinary Elimination Management; Urinary Retention Care; Weight Management; Urinary Bladder Training; Urinary Catheterization

EVALUATIONS FOR EXPECTED OUTCOMES

- Patient maintains urinary continence.
- Patient empties bladder adequately at least every 2 hours.
- Patient's urinary function remains free from complications.
- Patient voices understanding of treatment, including urinary diversion therapy, if appropriate.
- Patient discusses disease, signs and symptoms, complications, treatments, and adjustments to lifestyle caused by altered urinary pattern.
- Patient and family members demonstrate skill in managing urinary elimination problem, including catheterization techniques to be used at home.
- Patient demonstrates proficiency in steps necessary to manage urinary elimination problems.
- Patient and family members identify and contact home health care agency, support group, or other resources, as needed.

DOCUMENTATION

- Results of bladder assessment
- Observations of urologic condition and response to treatment regimen
- Interventions to provide supportive care and patient's response

- Nursing interventions performed to promote voiding
- Patient's response to nursing interventions
- Instructions given to patient and family members on urologic problem, response to instructions, and demonstrated ability to manage patient's urinary elimination needs
- Patient's expression of concern about urologic problem and its impact on body image and lifestyle; patient's motivation to participate in self-care
- Evaluations for expected outcomes

REFERENCES

Bitencourt, G. R., Alves Lde, A., Santana, R. F., & Lopes, M. V. (2016). Agreement between experts regarding assessment of postoperative urinary elimination nursing outcomes in elderly patients. *International Journal of Nursing Knowledge, 27*(3), 143–148.

Fowler, S., Urban, T., & Taggart, H. (2018). Factors affecting urinary retention in critically ill trauma patients. *Journal of Trauma Nursing, 25*(6), 356–359.

Lynser, D., Marbaniang, E., & Khongsni, P. (2016). Lower urinary tract obstruction in male children—A report of three cases. *Medical Ultrasonography, 18*(3), 400–402.

Shaid, E. C. (2017). Meeting the needs of the complex older adult patient with urinary retention: A case study. *Urologic Nursing, 37*(2), 75–100.

Urinary Retention

DEFINITION

Incomplete emptying of the bladder

RELATED FACTORS (R/T)

- Environmental constraints
- Fecal impaction
- Improper toileting posture
- Inadequate relaxation of pelvic floor muscles
- Insufficient privacy
- Pelvic organ prolapse
- Weakened bladder muscle

ASSOCIATED CONDITIONS

- Benign prostatic hyperplasia
- Diabetes mellitus
- Nervous system diseases
- Pharmaceutical preparations
- Urinary tract obstruction

ASSESSMENT

- Age
- Gender
- Vital signs
- History of sensory or neuromuscular impairment, prostate enlargement, surgery, urethral trauma or tumor, or urinary tract disease
- Genitourinary status, including pain or discomfort, palpation of bladder, residual urine volume after voiding, urethral obstruction (prostate hyperplasia or masses, fecal impaction, masses, and swelling), urinalysis, urine characteristics, and voiding patterns

- Fluid and electrolyte status, including inspection of mucous membranes, intake and output, skin turgor, urine specific gravity, and serum electrolyte, blood urea nitrogen, and creatinine levels
- Medication history
- Neuromuscular status, including anal sphincter tone, motor ability to start and stop stream, neuromuscular function, and sensory ability to perceive bladder fullness and voiding
- Sexuality status, including capability and concerns or partner's concerns
- Psychosocial status, including coping skills, patient's or family members' perception of problem, self-concept, and stressors (such as finances and job)

DEFINING CHARACTERISTICS

- Absence of urinary output
- Bladder distention
- Dysuria
- Increased daytime urinary frequency
- Minimal void volume
- Overflow incontinence
- Reports sensation of bladder fullness
- Reports sensation of residual urine
- Weak urine stream

EXPECTED OUTCOMES

- Patient will empty bladder.
- Patient will voice understanding of treatment.
- Patient will have few, if any, complications.
- Patient will avoid bladder distention.
- Patient and family members will demonstrate skill in managing urine retention.
- Patient will discuss impact of urologic disorder on self and family members.
- Patient and family members will identify resources to assist with care following discharge.

Suggested NOC Outcomes

Knowledge: Treatment Regimen; Symptom Control; Symptom Severity; Urinary Continence; Urinary Elimination

INTERVENTIONS AND RATIONALES

S - Monitor intake and output. Report if intake exceeds output. *Accurate intake and output measurements are essential for correct fluid replacement therapy.*

S - Monitor voiding pattern. *Data on time, place, amount, and patient's awareness of micturition are needed to establish a pattern of incontinence.*

EBP - Assist with the ordered bladder elimination procedure as follows:
  - Voiding techniques. Perform Credé or Valsalva maneuver every 2 to 3 hours *to increase bladder pressure to pass urine.* Repeat until empty.
  - Intermittent catheterization. Catheterize using clean or sterile technique every 2 hours. Record amount voided spontaneously and amount obtained with catheterization. *These measures promote normal voiding, prevent infection, and help maintain the integrity of ureterovesical function.*
  - Use of an indwelling urinary catheter. Monitor patency and avoid kinks in tubing. Keep the drainage bag below bladder level *to avoid urine reflux.* Perform catheter

care according to established policy and maintain a closed drainage system *to prevent skin irritation and bacteriuria.* Secure the catheter to patient's leg (female) or abdomen (male), avoiding tension on the sphincter. *Anchoring the catheter prevents straining of the bladder's trigone muscle and prevents friction leading to inflammation.*

▨ Use of a suprapubic catheter. Change dressings according to facility policy. Monitor patency and avoid kinks in the tubing. Keep drainage bag below bladder level. Maintain closed drainage system. *Suprapubic drainage allows for increased mobility and reduces the risk of bladder infection.*

▨ Administer pain medication, as ordered, and monitor patient *to reduce pain and assess the medication's effects.*

EBP ▨ For fecal impaction, disimpact and institute a bowel regimen *to promote comfort and prevent the loss of rectal muscle tone from prolonged distention.*

EBP ▨ Encourage a high fluid intake of 2 L/day, unless contraindicated, *to moisten mucous membranes and dilute chemical materials within the body.* Limit fluid intake after 7 p.m. *to prevent nocturia.*

▨ Monitor therapeutic and adverse effects of prescribed medications *for early recognition and treatment of drug reactions.*

▨ If patient requires surgery, give appropriate preoperative and postoperative instructions and care *to increase patient's understanding.* If urinary diversions are being considered, prepare patient for a change in body image. *Preparation and appropriate information help patient and family members cope with changes.*

EBP ▨ Instruct patient and family members on voiding techniques to be used at home. Provide for return demonstrations until they can perform the procedure well. *Knowledge of procedures and rationales reduces anxiety and promotes comfort. Demonstrations may progress through several sessions until patient can perform independently.*

PCC ▨ Encourage patient and family members to share feelings and concerns related to urologic problems. *Ventilation helps pinpoint patient's fears and establishes an environment of trust in which patient and family members can begin to deal with the situation.*

T&C ▨ Refer patient and family members to a psychiatric liaison nurse, enterostomal therapist, sex counselor, support group, or home health care agency, when appropriate. *These resources help patient gain knowledge of self and situation, reduce anxiety, and help promote personal growth. Community resources usually provide services not available at other health agencies.*

Suggested NIC Interventions

Distraction; Perineal Care; Urinary Bladder Training; Urinary Catheterization: Intermittent; Urinary Elimination Management

EVALUATIONS FOR EXPECTED OUTCOMES

▨ Patient empties bladder.

▨ Patient expresses understanding of treatment, including ordered bladder elimination procedure and surgery, if appropriate.

▨ Patient's urinalysis remains normal.

▨ Patient avoids bladder distention.

▨ Patient and family members demonstrate skill in managing urine retention, including voiding techniques to be used at home.

▨ Patient or family contacts home health care agency, support group, or other resources, as needed.

- Observations of urologic condition and response to treatment regimen
- Interventions to provide supportive care and patient's response
- Instructions given to patient and family members on urologic problem and their returned response and demonstrated ability to manage patient's urinary elimination
- Patient's concerns about urologic problem and its impact on body image and lifestyle; motivation to participate in self-care
- Evaluations for expected outcomes

REFERENCES

Downey, J., Kruse, D., & Plonczynski, D. J. (2019). Nurses reduce epidural-related urinary retention and postpartum hemorrhages. *Journal of PeriAnesthesia Nursing, 34*(1), 206–210. doi:10.1016/j.jopan.2018.09.001

Fowler, S., Urban, S., & Taggart, H. (2018). Factors affecting urinary retention in critically ill trauma patients. *Journal of Trauma Nursing, 25*(6), 356–359. doi:10.1097/JTN.0000000000000400

Shaid, E. C. (2017). Meeting the needs of the complex older adult patient with urinary retention: A case study. *Urologic Nursing, 37*(2), 75–100. doi:10.7257/1053-816X.2017.37.2.75

Wehner, S. D. (2018). Acute urinary retention 49 years post-injury: An unusual case study. *Urologic Nursing, 38*(2), 81–84. doi:10.7257/1053-816X.2018.38.2.81

Risk for Urinary Retention

Susceptible to incomplete emptying of the bladder

- Environmental constraints
- Fecal impaction
- Improper toileting posture
- Inadequate relaxation of pelvic floor muscles
- Insufficient privacy
- Pelvic organ prolapse
- Weakened bladder muscle

- Benign prostatic hyperplasia
- Diabetes mellitus
- Nervous system diseases
- Pharmaceutical preparations
- Urinary tract obstruction

- Age
- Gender
- Vital signs
- History of sensory or neuromuscular impairment, prostate enlargement, surgery, urethral trauma or tumor, or urinary tract disease

- Genitourinary status, including pain or discomfort, palpation of bladder, residual urine volume after voiding, urethral obstruction (prostate hyperplasia or masses, fecal impaction, masses, and swelling), urinalysis, urine characteristics, and voiding patterns
- Fluid and electrolyte status, including inspection of mucous membranes, intake and output, skin turgor, urine specific gravity, and serum electrolyte, blood urea nitrogen, and creatinine levels
- Medication history
- Neuromuscular status, including anal sphincter tone, motor ability to start and stop stream, neuromuscular function, and sensory ability to perceive bladder fullness and voiding
- Sexuality status, including capability and concerns or partner's concerns
- Psychosocial status, including coping skills, patient's or family members' perception of problem, self-concept, and stressors (such as finances and job)

EXPECTED OUTCOMES

- Patient will empty bladder.
- Patient will identify risk factors associated with urinary retention.
- Patient will voice understanding of treatment.
- Patient will have few, if any, complications.
- Patient will avoid bladder distention.
- Patient and family members will demonstrate skill in managing urine retention.
- Patient will discuss impact of urologic disorder on self and family members.
- Patient and family members will identify resources to assist with care following discharge.

Suggested NOC Outcomes

Knowledge: Treatment Regimen; Symptom Control; Symptom Severity; Urinary Continence; Urinary Elimination

INTERVENTIONS AND RATIONALES

S — Monitor intake and output. Report if intake exceeds output. *Accurate intake and output measurements are essential for correct fluid replacement therapy.*

S — Monitor voiding pattern. *Data on time, place, amount, and patient's awareness of micturition are needed to establish a pattern of incontinence.*

EBP — Assist with the ordered bladder elimination procedure as follows:
  - Voiding techniques. Perform Credé's or Valsalva's maneuver every 2 to 3 hours *to increase bladder pressure to pass urine.* Repeat until empty.
  - Intermittent catheterization. Catheterize using clean or sterile technique every 2 hours. Record amount voided spontaneously and amount obtained with catheterization. *These measures promote normal voiding, prevent infection, and help maintain the integrity of ureterovesical function.*
  - Use of an indwelling urinary catheter. Monitor patency and avoid kinks in tubing. Keep the drainage bag below bladder level *to avoid urine reflux.* Perform catheter care according to established policy and maintain a closed drainage system *to prevent skin irritation and bacteriuria.* Secure the catheter to patient's leg (female) or abdomen (male), avoiding tension on the sphincter. *Anchoring the catheter prevents straining of the bladder's trigone muscle and prevents friction leading to inflammation.*

- Use of a suprapubic catheter. Change dressings according to facility policy. Monitor patency and avoid kinks in the tubing. Keep drainage bag below bladder level. Maintain closed drainage system. *Suprapubic drainage allows for increased mobility and reduces the risk of bladder infection.*
- Administer pain medication, as ordered, and monitor patient *to reduce pain and assess the medication's effects.*
- **EBP** For fecal impaction, disimpact and institute a bowel regimen *to promote comfort and prevent the loss of rectal muscle tone from prolonged distention.*
- **EBP** Encourage a high fluid intake 2 L/day, unless contraindicated, *to moisten mucous membranes and dilute chemical materials within the body.* Limit fluid intake after 7 p.m. *to prevent nocturia.*
- **EBP** Monitor therapeutic and adverse effects of prescribed medications *for early recognition and treatment of drug reactions.*
- **EBP** Instruct patient and family members on voiding techniques to be used at home. Provide for return demonstrations until they can perform the procedure well. *Knowledge of procedures and rationales reduces anxiety and promotes comfort. Demonstrations may progress through several sessions until patient can perform independently.*
- **PCC** Encourage patient and family members to share feelings and concerns related to urologic problems. *Ventilation helps pinpoint patient's fears and establishes an environment of trust in which patient and family members can begin to deal with the situation.*
- **T&C** Refer patient and family members to a psychiatric liaison nurse, enterostomal therapist, sex counselor, support group, or home health care agency, when appropriate. *These resources help patient gain knowledge of self and situation, reduce anxiety, and help promote personal growth. Community resources usually provide services not available at other health agencies.*

Suggested NIC Interventions

Distraction; Perineal Care; Urinary Bladder Training; Urinary Catheterization: Intermittent; Urinary Elimination Management

EVALUATIONS FOR EXPECTED OUTCOMES

- Patient empties bladder.
- Patient lists risk factors associated with urinary retention.
- Patient expresses understanding of treatment, including ordered bladder elimination procedure and surgery, if appropriate.
- Patient's urinalysis remains normal.
- Patient avoids bladder distention.
- Patient and family members demonstrate skill in managing urine retention, including voiding techniques to be used at home.
- Patient or family contacts home health care agency, support group, or other resources, as needed.

DOCUMENTATION

- Observations of urologic condition and response to treatment regimen
- Interventions to provide supportive care and patient's response
- Instructions given to patient and family members on urologic problem and their returned response and demonstrated ability to manage patient's urinary elimination

▧ Patient's concerns about urologic problem and its impact on body image and lifestyle; motivation to participate in self-care

▧ Evaluations for expected outcomes

REFERENCES

Çakmak, M., Yıldız, M., Akarken, İ., Karaman, Y., & Çakmak, Ö. (2020). Risk factors for postoperative urinary retention in surgical population: A prospective cohort study. *Journal of Urological Surgery, 7*(2), 144–148.

Hall, B. R., Armijo, P. R., Grams, B., Lomelin, D., & Oleynikov, D. (2019). Identifying patients at risk for urinary retention following inguinal herniorrhaphy: A single institution study. *Hernia, 23*(2), 311–315.

Lamblin, G., Chene, G., Aeberli, C., Soare, R., Moret, S., Bouvet, L., & Doret-Dion, M. (2019). Identification of risk factors for postpartum urinary retention following vaginal deliveries: A retrospective case-control study. *European Journal of Obstetrics & Gynecology & Reproductive Biology, 243*, 7–11.

Schettini, D. A., Freitas, F. G., Tomotani, D. Y., Alves, J. C., Bafi, A. T., & Machado, F. R. (2019). Incidence and risk factors for urinary retention in critically ill patients. *Nursing in Critical Care, 24*(6), 355–361.

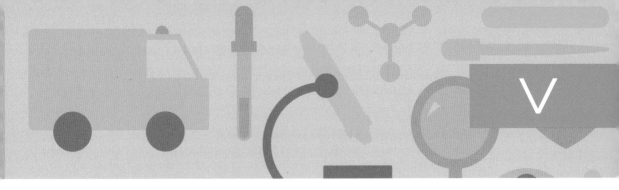

Dysfunctional Adult Ventilatory Weaning Response

Inability of individuals greater than 18 years of age, who have required mechanical ventilation at least 24 hours, to successfully transition to spontaneous ventilation

- Altered sleep–wake cycle
- Excessive airway secretions
- Ineffective cough
- Malnutrition

- Acid–base imbalance
- Anemia
- Cardiogenic shock
- Decreased level of consciousness
- Diaphragm dysfunction acquired in the intensive care unit
- Endocrine system diseases
- Heart diseases
- High acuity illness
- Hyperthermia
- Hypoxemia
- Infections
- Neuromuscular diseases
- Pharmaceutical preparations
- Water–electrolyte imbalance

- Vital signs
- Pulse oximetry readings
- Health history, including previous respiratory problems
- Nutritional status, including caloric intake and type of and tolerance for feeding
- Neurologic status, including mental status and level of consciousness

- Emotional status, including signs of anxiety or stress
- Laboratory values, including arterial blood gas (ABG) levels (baseline and ongoing), serum electrolyte and blood glucose levels, complete blood count, blood and sputum culture, and sensitivity tests
- Weaning parameters and current ventilator settings
- Respiratory status, including respiratory rate, pattern, character, and depth; chest expansion and symmetry; sputum characteristics (color, amount, odor, and consistency); cough effectiveness; presence of cyanosis in mucous membranes and nail beds; and auscultation of breath sounds
- Need for suctioning, including frequency and patient's response
- Musculoskeletal status, including muscle mass, strength, and endurance level
- Cognitive state, including patient's ability to follow directions and readiness to learn
- Recent administration of potential respiratory-depressant medications, such as opioids, sedatives, and neuromuscular blockers

DEFINING CHARACTERISTICS

Early Response (less than 30 minutes)

- Adventitious breath sounds
- Audible airway secretions
- Decreased blood pressure (<90 mm Hg or >20% reduction from baseline)
- Decreased heart rate (>20% reduction from baseline)
- Decreased oxygen saturation (<90% when fraction of inspired oxygen ratio >40%)
- Expresses apprehensiveness
- Expresses distress
- Expresses fear of machine malfunction
- Expresses feeling warm
- Hyperfocused on activities
- Increased blood pressure (systolic pressure >180 mm Hg or >20% from baseline)
- Increased heart rate (>140 bpm or >20% from baseline)
- Increased respiratory rate (>35 rpm or >50% over baseline)
- Nasal flaring
- Panting
- Paradoxical abdominal breathing
- Perceived need for increased oxygen
- Psychomotor agitation
- Shallow breathing
- Uses significant respiratory accessory muscles
- Wide-eyed appearance

Intermediate Response (30–90 minutes)

- Decreased pH (<7.32 or >0.07 reduction from baseline)
- Diaphoresis
- Difficulty cooperating with instructions
- Hypercapnia (>50 mm Hg increase in partial pressure of carbon dioxide or >8 mm Hg increase from baseline)
- Hypoxemia (Partial pressure of oxygen 50% or oxygen >6L/min)

Late Response (>90 minutes)

- Cardiorespiratory arrest
- Cyanosis

■ Fatigue
■ Recent onset arrhythmias

■ Patient will maintain respiratory rate within 5 breaths/minute of baseline during weaning period.
■ Patient's ABG levels will remain within acceptable limits (specify).
■ Patient's mental status and emotional state will remain stable during gradual withdrawal of ventilatory support.
■ Patient will express comfort with progressive ventilator changes.
■ Patient will experience no dyspnea, fatigue, or pain during progressive ventilator changes.
■ Patient will remain within adequate weaning parameters:
  ■ Tidal volume: 4 to 5 cc/kg
  ■ Negative inspiratory force: ≥-20 cm H_2O
  ■ Vital capacity: 10 to 15 cc/kg
  ■ Minute ventilation: 6 to 10 L
■ Patient's cough will effectively clear secretions.

Suggested NOC Outcomes

Anxiety Self-Control; Client Satisfaction: Technical Aspects of Care; Depression Self-Control; Respiratory Status: Gas Exchange; Respiratory Status: Ventilation; Risk Control; Vital Signs

[S] ■ Monitor patient's vital signs every hour when changing ventilator settings. *Fever, tachycardia, tachypnea, and elevated blood pressure may indicate hypoxemia.*

[S] ■ Auscultate for breath sounds every 2 hours and report deviations. *Adventitious sounds may precede respiratory failure.*

[EBP] ■ Place patient in a comfortable position (preferably Fowler's) *to facilitate adequate chest expansion and drainage.*

[PCC] ■ Describe all weaning procedures to patient. Explain that he may experience changes in breathing rate and pattern, increased difficulty breathing, and fatigue *to decrease anxiety.*

[EBP] ■ If patient is receiving intermittent mandatory ventilation (IMV), begin to decrease IMV by increments of 2 breaths/minute. This process may take place over days or weeks. *Lowering IMV encourages patient to take own breaths, thereby exercising respiratory muscles.*

[S] ■ Monitor ABG levels with every ventilator change *to assess for adequate oxygenation and acid–base balance.*

[PCC] ■ Include periods of rest between ventilator changes, especially at night, *to reduce tissue oxygen demand.*

[EBP] ■ If patient tolerates IMV of 2 to 4 breaths/minute, try pressure support ventilation (PSV). *PSV prolongs positive airway pressure during inspiration, allowing patient to regulate own respiratory rate and tidal volume.*

[EBP] ■ When patient is breathing adequately without IMV, place the patient on continuous positive airway pressure (CPAP) of 5 cm H_2O *to prevent alveolar collapse.*

[EBP] ■ When patient tolerates CPAP, place on T-piece (T-bar) of 30% to 50% fraction of inspired oxygen. *This allows patient to breathe independently, continue to receive oxygen, and remain intubated in the event of respiratory compromise.*

PCC ▪ When patient tolerates longer weaning periods, incorporate activities of daily living into patient's daily routine *to increase muscular strength and endurance.*

PCC ▪ When patient has satisfactory respiratory status, weaning parameters, and ABG levels, assist with the removal of the ventilator tubes and keep the oxygen mask on hand *to prevent respiratory compromise.*

S ▪ Assess patient for stridor, respiratory distress, and dysphonia and report these findings to the physician *to monitor the need for renewed ventilatory assistance.*

S ▪ Perform chest physiotherapy and suctioning, as needed, *to maintain a patent airway.*

S ▪ Monitor the respiratory effects of medications closely and evaluate the response to bronchodilators *to detect respiratory status compromise. Avoid respiratory depressants.*

Suggested NIC Interventions

Acid–Base Management; Airway Management; Anxiety Reduction; Aspiration Precautions; Mechanical Ventilatory Weaning; Respiratory Monitoring; Support System Enhancement; Teaching: Procedure/Treatment; Vital Signs Monitoring

EVALUATIONS FOR EXPECTED OUTCOMES

▪ Patient's respiratory rate is within 5 breaths/minute of baseline during weaning period.
▪ Patient's ABG levels are within specified acceptable limits.
▪ Patient maintains stable mental and emotional status during withdrawal of ventilatory support.
▪ Patient expresses comfort with progressive ventilator changes.
▪ Patient doesn't experience dyspnea, fatigue, or pain during progressive ventilator changes.
▪ Patient remains within adequate weaning parameters.
▪ Patient's cough effectively clears secretions.

DOCUMENTATION

▪ Patient's reports of malaise, anxiety, restlessness, breathlessness, and unusual pain
▪ Patient's response to ventilator changes
▪ Subtle changes in patient's mental or emotional status
▪ Laboratory data, including ABG levels
▪ Patient's response to nursing interventions, including positioning, chest physiotherapy, and suctioning
▪ Patient's response to medications, including opioids, bronchodilators, and neuromuscular blockers
▪ Respiratory rate, pattern, and depth, including changes from baseline
▪ Evaluations for expected outcomes

REFERENCES

Ghiani, A., Paderewska, J., Sainis, A., Crispin, A., Walcher, S., & Neurohr, C. (2020). Variables predicting weaning outcome in prolonged mechanically ventilated tracheotomized patients: A retrospective study. *Journal of Intensive Care, 8*, 1–10. doi:10.1186/s40560-020-00437-4

Hadfield, D., Rose, L., Reid, F., Cornelius, V., Hart, N., Finney, C., … Rafferty, G. F. (2020). Factors affecting the use of neurally adjusted ventilatory assist in the adult critical care unit: A clinician survey. *BMJ Open Respiratory Research, 7*(1). doi:10.1136/bmjresp-2020-000783

Rosa da Silva, L. C., Soto Tonelli, I., Costa Oliveira, R. C., Lage Lemos, P., Silqueira de Matos, S., & Machado Chianca, T. C. (2020). Clinical study of dysfunctional ventilatory weaning response in critically ill patients. *Revista Latino-Americana de Enfermagem (RLAE), 28*, 1–13.

Saint Clair Gomes, B. N., Torres-Castro, R., Lima, Í., Resqueti, V. R., & Fregonezi, G. A. F. (2021). Weaning from mechanical ventilation in people with neuromuscular disease: A systematic review. *BMJ Open, 11*(9). doi:10.1136/bmjopen-2020-047449

Dysfunctional Ventilatory Weaning Response

DEFINITION

Inability to adjust to lowered levels of mechanical ventilator support that interrupts and prolongs the weaning process

RELATED FACTORS (R/T)

Physiological

- Alteration in sleep pattern
- Inadequate nutrition
- Ineffective airway clearance
- Pain

Psychological

- Anxiety
- Decrease in motivation
- Fear
- Hopelessness
- Insufficient knowledge of weaning process
- Insufficient trust in health care professional
- Low self-esteem
- Powerlessness
- Uncertainty about ability to wean

Situation

- Environmental barrier
- Inappropriate pace of weaning process
- Insufficient social support
- Uncontrolled episodic energy demands

ASSOCIATED CONDITIONS

- History of unsuccessful weaning attempt
- History of ventilator dependence >4 days

ASSESSMENT

- Health history, including previous respiratory problems
- Nutritional status, including caloric intake and type of and tolerance for feeding
- Neurologic status, including mental status and level of consciousness
- Emotional status, including signs of anxiety or stress
- Laboratory values, including arterial blood gas (ABG) levels (baseline and ongoing), serum electrolyte and blood glucose levels, complete blood count, blood and sputum culture, and sensitivity tests
- Weaning parameters and current ventilator settings
- Respiratory status, including respiratory rate, pattern, character, and depth; chest expansion and symmetry; sputum characteristics (color, amount, odor, and consistency); cough effectiveness; presence of cyanosis in mucous membranes and nail beds; and auscultation of breath sounds

- Need for suctioning, including frequency and patient's response
- Musculoskeletal status, including muscle mass, strength, and endurance level
- Cognitive state, including patient's ability to follow directions and readiness to learn
- Recent administration of potential respiratory-depressant medications, such as opioids, sedatives, and neuromuscular blockers
- Vital signs
- Pulse oximetry readings

DEFINING CHARACTERISTICS

Mild

- Breathing discomfort
- Fatigue
- Fear of machine malfunction
- Feeling warm
- Increase in focus on breathing
- Mild increase of respiratory rate over baseline
- Perceived need for increase in oxygen
- Restlessness

Moderate

- Abnormal skin color
- Apprehensiveness
- Decrease in air entry on auscultation
- Diaphoresis
- Facial expression of fear
- Hyperfocused on activities
- Impaired ability to cooperate
- Impaired ability to respond to coaching
- Increase in blood pressure from baseline (<20 mm Hg)
- Increase in heart rate from baseline (<20 beats/minute)
- Minimal use of respiratory accessory muscles
- Moderate increase in respiratory rate over baseline

Severe

- Abnormal skin color
- Adventitious breath sounds
- Agitation
- Asynchronized breathing with the ventilator
- Decrease in level of consciousness
- Deterioration in arterial blood gases from baseline
- Gasping breaths
- Increase in blood pressure from baseline (≥20 mm Hg)
- Increase in heart rate from baseline (≥20 beats/minute)
- Paradoxical abdominal breathing
- Profuse diaphoresis
- Shallow breathing
- Significant increase in respiratory rate above baseline
- Use of significant respiratory accessory muscles

▧ Patient will maintain respiratory rate within 5 breaths/minute of baseline during weaning period.

▧ Patient's ABG levels will remain within acceptable limits (specify).

▧ Patient's mental status and emotional state will remain stable during gradual withdrawal of ventilatory support.

▧ Patient will express comfort with progressive ventilator changes.

▧ Patient will experience no dyspnea, fatigue, or pain during progressive ventilator changes.

▧ Patient will remain within adequate weaning parameters:

  ▧ Tidal volume: 4 to 5 cc/kg

  ▧ Negative inspiratory force: greater than or equal to -20 cm H_2O

  ▧ Vital capacity: 10 to 15 cc/kg

  ▧ Minute ventilation: 6 to 10 L

▧ Patient's cough will effectively clear secretions.

Suggested NOC Outcomes

Anxiety Self-Control; Client Satisfaction: Technical Aspects of Care; Depression Self-Control; Respiratory Status: Gas Exchange; Respiratory Status: Ventilation; Risk Control; Vital Signs

S ▧ Monitor patient's vital signs every hour when changing ventilator settings. *Fever, tachycardia, tachypnea, and elevated blood pressure may indicate hypoxemia.*

S ▧ Auscultate for breath sounds every 2 hours and report deviations. *Adventitious sounds may precede respiratory failure.*

EBP ▧ Place patient in a comfortable position (preferably Fowler) *to facilitate adequate chest expansion and drainage.*

PCC ▧ Describe all weaning procedures to patient. Explain that he or she may experience changes in breathing rate and pattern, increased difficulty breathing, and fatigue *to decrease anxiety.*

EBP ▧ If patient is receiving intermittent mandatory ventilation (IMV), begin to decrease IMV by increments of 2 breaths/minute. This process may take place over days or weeks. *Lowering IMV encourages patient to take own breaths, thereby exercising respiratory muscles.*

S ▧ Monitor ABG levels with every ventilator change *to assess for adequate oxygenation and acid–base balance.*

PCC ▧ Include periods of rest between ventilator changes, especially at night, *to reduce tissue oxygen demand.*

EBP ▧ If patient tolerates IMV of 2 to 4 breaths/minute, try pressure support ventilation (PSV). *PSV prolongs positive airway pressure during inspiration, allowing patient to regulate own respiratory rate and tidal volume.*

EBP ▧ When patient is breathing adequately without IMV, place patient on continuous positive airway pressure (CPAP) of 5 cm H_2O *to prevent alveolar collapse.*

EBP ▧ When patient tolerates CPAP, place on T-piece (T-bar) of 30% to 50% fraction of inspired oxygen. *This allows patient to breathe independently, continue to receive oxygen, and remain intubated in the event of respiratory compromise.*

PCC ▧ When patient tolerates longer weaning periods, incorporate activities of daily living into patient's daily routine *to increase muscular strength and endurance.*

PCC ▪ When patient has satisfactory respiratory status, weaning parameters, and ABG levels, assist with the removal of the ventilator tubes and keep the oxygen mask on hand *to prevent respiratory compromise*.

S ▪ Assess patient for stridor, respiratory distress, and dysphonia and report these findings to the physician *to monitor the need for renewed ventilatory assistance*.

S ▪ Perform chest physiotherapy and suctioning as needed *to maintain a patent airway*.

S ▪ Monitor the respiratory effects of medications closely and evaluate the response to bronchodilators *to detect respiratory status compromise*. Avoid respiratory depressants.

Suggested NIC Interventions

Acid–Base Management; Airway Management; Anxiety Reduction; Aspiration Precautions; Mechanical Ventilatory Weaning; Respiratory Monitoring; Support System Enhancement; Teaching: Procedure/Treatment; Vital Signs Monitoring

EVALUATIONS FOR EXPECTED OUTCOMES

▪ Patient's respiratory rate is within 5 breaths/minute of baseline during weaning period.
▪ Patient's ABG levels are within specified acceptable limits.
▪ Patient maintains stable mental and emotional status during withdrawal of ventilatory support.
▪ Patient expresses comfort with progressive ventilator changes.
▪ Patient doesn't experience dyspnea, fatigue, or pain during progressive ventilator changes.
▪ Patient remains within adequate weaning parameters.
▪ Patient's cough effectively clears secretions.

DOCUMENTATION

▪ Patient's reports of malaise, anxiety, restlessness, breathlessness, and unusual pain
▪ Patient's response to ventilator changes
▪ Subtle changes in patient's mental or emotional status
▪ Laboratory data, including ABG levels
▪ Patient's response to nursing interventions, including positioning, chest physiotherapy, and suctioning
▪ Patient's response to medications, including opioids, bronchodilators, and neuromuscular blockers
▪ Respiratory rate, pattern, and depth, including changes from baseline
▪ Evaluations for expected outcomes

REFERENCES

Chen, Y. J., Hwang, S. L., Li, C. R., Yang, C. C., Huang, K. L., Lin, C. Y., & Lee, C. Y. (2017). Vagal withdrawal and psychological distress during ventilator weaning and the related outcomes. *Journal of Psychosomatic Research, 101*, 10–16. doi:10.1016/j.jpsychores.2017.07.012

Chuang, Y. C. (2017). A nursing experience of assisting a patient weaning from ventilator. *Tzu Chi Nursing Journal, 16*(4), 87–96.

Füssenich, W., Hirschfeld Araujo, S., Kowald, B., Hosman, A., Auerswald, M., & Thietje, R. (2018). Discontinuous ventilator weaning of patients with acute SCI. *Spinal Cord, 56*(5), 461–468. doi:10.1038/s41393-017-0055-x

Greenberg, J. A., Balk, R. A., & Shah, R. C. (2018). Score for predicting ventilator weaning duration in patients with tracheostomies. *American Journal of Critical Care, 27*(6), 477–485. doi:10.4037/ajcc2018532

Impaired Verbal Communication

DEFINITION

Decreased, delayed, or absent ability to receive, process, transmit, and/or use a system of symbols

RELATED FACTORS (R/T)

- Altered self-concept
- Cognitive dysfunction
- Dyspnea
- Emotional lability
- Environmental constraints
- Inadequate stimulation
- Low self-esteem
- Perceived vulnerability
- Psychological barriers
- Values incongruent with cultural norms

ASSOCIATED CONDITIONS

- Altered perception
- Central nervous system diseases
- Developmental disabilities
- Flaccid facial paralysis
- Hemifacial spasm
- Motor neuron disease
- Neoplasms
- Neurocognitive disorders
- Oropharyngeal defect
- Peripheral nervous system diseases
- Psychotic disorders
- Respiratory muscle weakness
- Sialorrhea
- Speech disorders
- Tongue diseases
- Tracheostomy
- Treatment regimen
- Velopharyngeal insufficiency
- Vocal cord dysfunction

ASSESSMENT

- Age
- Neurologic status, including level of consciousness, orientation, cognition, memory (recent and remote), insight, and judgment
- Speech characteristics, including pattern (garbled, incomprehensible, difficulty forming words), language and vocabulary, level of comprehension and expression, and ability to use other forms of communication (such as eye blinks, gestures, pictures, and nods)
- Motor ability
- Circulatory status, including a history of cardiac and circulatory problems, pulse, blood pressure, arteriogram, electroencephalography, and computed tomography scan
- Respiratory status, including dyspnea and use of accessory muscles

DEFINING CHARACTERISTICS

- Absence of eye contact
- Agraphia
- Alternative communication
- Anarthria
- Aphasia
- Augmentative communication
- Decline of speech productivity
- Decline of speech rate
- Decreased willingness to participate in social interaction
- Difficulty comprehending communication
- Difficulty establishing social interaction
- Difficulty maintaining communication
- Difficulty using body expressions
- Difficulty using facial expressions
- Difficulty with selective attention
- Displays negative emotions
- Dysarthria
- Dysgraphia
- Dyslalia
- Dysphonia
- Fatigued by conversation
- Impaired ability to speak
- Impaired ability to use body expressions
- Impaired ability to use facial expressions
- Inability to speak language of caregiver
- Inappropriate verbalization
- Obstinate refusal to speak
- Slurred speech

EXPECTED OUTCOMES

- Patient will communicate needs and desires without undue frustration.
- Patient will use alternate means of communication.
- Patient will demonstrate correct use of adaptive equipment.
- Patient will express plans to use appropriate resources to maximize communication skills.
- Patient and family members will express satisfaction with level of communication ability.
- Patient will maintain effective level of communication.
- Patient will answer direct questions correctly.

Suggested NOC Outcomes

Cognition; Communication; Communication: Expressive; Communication: Receptive; Information Processing; Sensory Function Status

INTERVENTIONS AND RATIONALES

PCC ■ Observe patient closely for cues to personal needs and desires, such as gestures, pointing to objects, looking at items, and pantomime *to enhance understanding*. Don't continually respond to gestures if the potential exists to improve speech *to avoid discouraging improvement*.

DEFINING CHARACTERISTICS

ASSOCIATED CONDITIONS

ASSOCIATED CONDITIONS

- Deficient knowledge (specify)
- Impaired skin integrity
- Ineffective breastfeeding
- Ineffective coping
- Insufficient breast milk production
- Labor pain
- Readiness for enhanced childbearing
- Risk for bleeding
- Risk for disturbed maternal–fetal dyad
- Risk for dry mouth
- Risk for injury
- Urinary retention

Leukemia
- Acute pain
- Hopelessness
- Imbalanced nutrition: Less than body requirements
- Impaired gas exchange
- Impaired oral mucous membrane integrity
- Impaired tissue integrity
- Ineffective protection
- Ineffective tissue perfusion (cardiopulmonary)
- Ineffective tissue perfusion (renal)
- Risk for bleeding
- Risk for contamination
- Risk for adult falls
- Risk for infection
- Risk for injury

Liver transplantation
- Anxiety
- Compromised family coping
- Defensive coping
- Deficient knowledge (specify)
- Delayed surgical recovery
- Fear
- Ineffective coping
- Ineffective protection
- Ineffective tissue perfusion (cardiopulmonary)
- Ineffective tissue perfusion (GI)
- Ineffective tissue perfusion (renal)
- Moral distress
- Risk for impaired liver function
- Risk for electrolyte imbalance
- Risk for imbalanced fluid volume
- Risk for infection
- Risk for injury

Lung abscess
- Acute pain
- Anxiety
- Impaired gas exchange

- Ineffective airway clearance
- Ineffective breathing pattern
- Ineffective coping
- Ineffective tissue perfusion (cardiopulmonary)

Lung cancer
- Decreased activity tolerance
- Death anxiety
- Fear
- Hopelessness
- Imbalanced nutrition: Less than body requirements
- Impaired gas exchange
- Impaired tissue integrity
- Impaired verbal communication
- Ineffective airway clearance
- Ineffective breathing pattern
- Powerlessness
- Risk for infection

Lupus erythematosus
- Acute pain
- Decreased cardiac output
- Deficient knowledge
- Fatigue
- Hyperthermia
- Imbalanced nutrition: Less than body requirements
- Impaired oral mucous membrane integrity
- Impaired physical mobility
- Impaired skin integrity
- Ineffective coping
- Ineffective tissue perfusion
- Risk for infection
- Risk-prone health behavior

Lyme disease
- Decreased activity tolerance
- Acute pain
- Fatigue
- Hyperthermia
- Impaired skin integrity

Lymphomas
- Death anxiety
- Disturbed sleep pattern
- Hopelessness
- Impaired tissue integrity
- Ineffective protection
- Readiness for enhanced decision-making
- Risk for impaired religiosity
- Risk for infection

Macular degeneration
⬚ Decreased activity tolerance
⬚ Deficient knowledge
⬚ Ineffective denial
⬚ Powerlessness
⬚ Readiness for enhanced hope
⬚ Risk for caregiver role strain
⬚ Risk for low situational self-esteem
⬚ Risk for adult falls
⬚ Risk for physical trauma

Malnutrition
⬚ Imbalanced nutrition: Less than body requirements
⬚ Ineffective adolescent eating dynamics
⬚ Ineffective child eating dynamics
⬚ Ineffective infant feeding dynamics
⬚ Ineffective community coping
⬚ Risk for electrolyte imbalance
⬚ Risk for impaired oral mucous membrane integrity
⬚ Risk for injury

Maternal psychological stress
⬚ Anxiety
⬚ Deficient knowledge
⬚ Ineffective breastfeeding
⬚ Ineffective infant suck-swallow response
⬚ Ineffective role performance
⬚ Interrupted breastfeeding
⬚ Neonatal abstinence syndrome
⬚ Parental role conflict
⬚ Risk for impaired attachment
⬚ Risk for disturbed maternal–fetal dyad
⬚ Risk for ineffective childbearing process
⬚ Risk for sudden infant death
⬚ Powerlessness

Meconium aspiration syndrome
⬚ Ineffective breathing pattern
⬚ Impaired gas exchange
⬚ Impaired spontaneous ventilation
⬚ Risk for aspiration
⬚ Risk for injury

Melanoma
⬚ Death anxiety
⬚ Decisional conflict
⬚ Defensive coping
⬚ Disturbed body image
⬚ Fatigue
⬚ Hopelessness
⬚ Impaired resilience

⬚ Impaired oral mucous membrane integrity
⬚ Impaired skin integrity
⬚ Powerlessness
⬚ Spiritual distress

Ménière's disease
⬚ Impaired physical mobility
⬚ Insomnia
⬚ Nausea
⬚ Risk for adult falls
⬚ Risk for injury
⬚ Risk for physical trauma

Meningitis
⬚ Acute pain
⬚ Impaired bowel continence
⬚ Deficient fluid volume
⬚ Excess fluid volume
⬚ Fatigue
⬚ Fear
⬚ Hyperthermia
⬚ Ineffective airway clearance
⬚ Ineffective breathing pattern
⬚ Risk for imbalanced fluid volume
⬚ Risk for infection
⬚ Risk for injury

Menopause
⬚ Ineffective sexuality patterns
⬚ Insomnia
⬚ Sexual dysfunction
⬚ Situational low self-esteem
⬚ Stress overload

Metabolic acidosis
⬚ Deficient knowledge (specify)
⬚ Impaired airway clearance
⬚ Impaired gas exchange
⬚ Impaired oral mucous membrane integrity
⬚ Ineffective breathing pattern
⬚ Risk for acute confusion
⬚ Risk for electrolyte imbalance
⬚ Risk for injury
⬚ Risk for poisoning
⬚ Risk for shock

Metabolic alkalosis
⬚ Deficient fluid volume
⬚ Disturbed thought processes
⬚ Impaired oral mucous membrane integrity
⬚ Ineffective breathing pattern
⬚ Risk for electrolyte imbalance
⬚ Risk for injury

Mitral insufficiency

- Decreased activity tolerance
- Decreased cardiac output
- Deficient knowledge (specify)
- Fatigue
- Ineffective tissue perfusion (cardiopulmonary)
- Risk for infection

Mitral stenosis

- Decreased activity tolerance
- Decreased cardiac output
- Deficient knowledge (specify)
- Fatigue
- Ineffective tissue perfusion (cardiopulmonary)
- Risk for infection

Mood disorders

- Deficient community health
- Impaired religiosity
- Ineffective adolescent eating dynamics
- Ineffective child eating dynamics
- Ineffective infant feeding dynamics
- Ineffective health self-management
- Labile emotional control
- Powerlessness
- Readiness for enhanced health self-management
- Risk for impaired resilience
- Risk for suicidal behavior
- Self-mutilation
- Social isolation
- Spiritual distress

Multiple births

- Anxiety
- Deficient knowledge (specify)
- Impaired parenting
- Ineffective coping
- Interrupted family processes
- Risk for injury
- Risk for impaired parenting
- Risk for urinary tract injury
- Stress urinary incontinence

Multiple myeloma

- Decreased activity tolerance
- Acute pain
- Excess fluid volume
- Fatigue
- Imbalanced nutrition: Less than body requirements
- Ineffective tissue perfusion (cerebral)
- Risk for infection

Multiple sclerosis

- Acute pain
- Impaired bowel continence
- Caregiver role strain
- Chronic low self-esteem
- Death anxiety
- Deficient knowledge (specify)
- Disturbed sensory perception
- Dressing self-care deficit
- Fatigue
- Imbalanced nutrition: Less than body requirements
- Impaired bed mobility
- Impaired comfort
- Impaired memory
- Impaired physical mobility
- Impaired sitting
- Impaired spontaneous ventilation
- Impaired standing
- Impaired urinary elimination
- Impaired wheelchair mobility
- Ineffective airway clearance
- Ineffective health maintenance
- Ineffective sexuality patterns
- Ineffective health self-management
- Readiness for enhanced family coping
- Readiness for enhanced spiritual well-being
- Risk for decreased activity tolerance
- Risk for caregiver role strain
- Risk for infection
- Risk for spiritual distress
- Risk for urge urinary incontinence
- Risk-prone health behavior

Multisystem trauma

- Anxiety
- Bathing self-care deficit
- Deficient fluid volume
- Dysfunctional ventilatory weaning response
- Ineffective tissue perfusion
- Impaired spontaneous ventilation
- Powerlessness
- Risk for electrolyte imbalance
- Risk for ineffective cardiac tissue perfusion
- Risk for ineffective cerebral tissue perfusion
- Risk for infection
- Risk for suffocation
- Risk for physical trauma
- Risk for unstable blood pressure

Muscular dystrophy

- Caregiver role strain
- Deficient knowledge (specify)
- Disturbed sensory perception (kinesthetic)
- Feeding self-care deficit
- Hopelessness
- Impaired physical mobility
- Impaired sitting
- Impaired standing
- Impaired swallowing
- Impaired transfer ability
- Ineffective health maintenance behaviors
- Readiness for enhanced family coping
- Risk for caregiver role strain
- Risk for adult pressure injury
- Risk for urge urinary incontinence
- Risk-prone health behavior

Myasthenia gravis

- Impaired bowel continence
- Chronic low self-esteem
- Dressing self-care deficit
- Dysfunctional ventilatory weaning response
- Fatigue
- Fear
- Impaired gas exchange
- Impaired physical mobility
- Impaired verbal communication
- Ineffective airway clearance
- Readiness for enhanced self-care
- Risk for urge urinary incontinence

Myocardial infarction

- Decreased activity tolerance
- Acute pain
- Anxiety
- Compromised family coping
- Death anxiety
- Decreased cardiac output
- Health-seeking behaviors
- Ineffective coping
- Ineffective denial
- Ineffective role performance
- Ineffective sexuality patterns
- Ineffective tissue perfusion
- Readiness for enhanced spiritual well-being
- Readiness for enhanced relationships
- Risk for decreased cardiac function
- Risk for ineffective cardiac tissue perfusion
- Risk for metabolic syndrome
- Risk for spiritual distress

- Risk-prone health behavior
- Sedentary lifestyle
- Sexual dysfunction
- Situational low self-esteem
- Sleep deprivation
- Spiritual distress

Neonatal asphyxia

- Compromised family coping
- Hypothermia
- Ineffective breathing pattern
- Risk for aspiration
- Risk for hypothermia
- Risk for injury
- Risk for sudden infant death
- Risk for suffocation

Neonatal hyperbilirubinemia

- Interrupted breastfeeding
- Neonatal hyperbilirubinemia
- Risk for neonatal hyperbilirubinemia

Neurologic impairment (neonatal)

- Compromised family coping
- Disorganized infant behavior
- Ineffective infant suck-swallow response
- Neonatal abstinence syndrome
- Readiness for enhanced organized infant behavior
- Risk for disorganized infant behavior
- Risk for ineffective thermoregulation

Neuromuscular trauma

- Impaired skin integrity
- Impaired swallowing
- Post-trauma syndrome
- Risk for aspiration
- Risk for constipation
- Risk for disuse syndrome
- Unilateral neglect

Nutritional deficiencies

- Imbalanced nutrition: Less than body requirements
- Impaired skin integrity
- Risk for impaired parenting
- Risk for infection

Obesity

- Ineffective adolescent eating dynamics
- Ineffective child eating dynamics
- Ineffective infant feeding dynamics
- Obesity
- Readiness for enhanced nutrition
- Readiness for enhanced self-concept

- Risk for constipation
- Risk for impaired skin integrity
- Risk for impaired tissue integrity
- Risk for metabolic syndrome
- Situational low self-esteem
- Stress urinary incontinence

Obsessive-compulsive disorder
- Anxiety
- Compromised family coping
- Decisional conflict
- Disturbed personal identity
- Ineffective home maintenance behaviors
- Ineffective coping
- Ineffective denial
- Insomnia
- Risk for impaired religiosity
- Risk for injury
- Risk for spiritual distress
- Risk for self-directed violence
- Risk for other-directed violence
- Risk for suicidal behavior
- Self-mutilation
- Sleep deprivation
- Social isolation

Organic brain syndrome
- Frail elderly syndrome
- Impaired verbal communication
- Risk for deficient fluid volume
- Risk for frail elderly syndrome
- Wandering

Osteoarthritis
- Decreased activity tolerance
- Acute pain
- Compromised family coping
- Deficient knowledge (specify)
- Disturbed body image
- Dressing self-care deficit
- Ineffective home maintenance behaviors
- Impaired physical mobility
- Impaired wheelchair ability
- Ineffective health maintenance behaviors
- Ineffective health self-management
- Risk for injury
- Risk for adult falls

Osteomyelitis
- Acute pain
- Disturbed body image
- Impaired coping
- Impaired physical mobility
- Impaired skin integrity

- Impaired tissue integrity
- Ineffective coping
- Ineffective tissue perfusion (specify)
- Risk for infection
- Risk for injury
- Risk for adult falls

Osteoporosis
- Deficient knowledge (specify)
- Disturbed body image
- Fear
- Ineffective denial
- Ineffective health self-management
- Ineffective sexuality patterns
- Loneliness
- Nutrition imbalanced: Less than body requirements
- Powerlessness
- Risk for adult falls
- Risk for injury
- Risk for physical trauma
- Risk-prone health behaviors
- Self-neglect
- Social isolation

Ovarian cancer
- Constipation
- Death anxiety
- Fear
- Imbalanced nutrition: Less than body requirements
- Impaired tissue integrity
- Ineffective coping
- Ineffective protection
- Nausea
- Powerlessness
- Readiness for enhanced hope
- Readiness for enhanced resilience
- Readiness for enhanced spiritual well-being
- Risk for adult falls
- Spiritual distress
- Urinary retention

Panic disorder
- Anxiety
- Chronic low self-esteem
- Deficient knowledge (specify)
- Fear
- Impaired emancipated decision-making
- Impaired resilience
- Impaired mood regulation
- Ineffective coping
- Insomnia

- Powerlessness
- Risk for impaired emancipated decision-making
- Risk for post-trauma syndrome
- Sleep deprivation
- Risk for spiritual distress

Paralysis

- Autonomic dysreflexia
- Impaired bowel continence
- Caregiver role strain
- Compromised family coping
- Disuse syndrome
- Hopelessness
- Impaired bed mobility
- Impaired physical mobility
- Impaired sitting
- Impaired skin integrity
- Impaired standing
- Impaired walking
- Ineffective coping
- Ineffective health maintenance behaviors
- Ineffective role performance
- Ineffective sexuality patterns
- Maladaptive grieving
- Powerlessness
- Risk for caregiver role strain
- Risk for dry mouth
- Risk for impaired skin integrity
- Risk for impaired tissue integrity
- Risk for adult pressure injury

Parkinson's disease

- Decreased activity tolerance
- Impaired bowel continence
- Caregiver role strain
- Chronic low self-esteem
- Compromised family coping
- Death anxiety
- Deficient knowledge (specify)
- Disturbed body image
- Feeding self-care deficit
- Hopelessness
- Imbalanced nutrition: Less than body requirements
- Ineffective home maintenance behaviors
- Impaired resilience
- Impaired physical mobility
- Impaired transfer ability
- Ineffective breathing pattern
- Ineffective coping
- Ineffective health maintenance behaviors

- Ineffective role performance
- Ineffective sexuality patterns
- Loneliness
- Powerlessness
- Readiness for enhanced therapeutic regimen management
- Risk for aspiration
- Risk for caregiver role strain
- Risk for compromised human dignity
- Risk for injury
- Risk for adult falls
- Risk for loneliness
- Risk for urge urinary incontinence
- Social isolation

Pelvic inflammatory disease

- Acute pain
- Deficient fluid volume
- Ineffective sexuality pattern
- Risk for infection
- Risk-prone health behavior
- Sexual dysfunction

Pericarditis

- Decreased activity tolerance
- Acute pain
- Anxiety
- Decreased cardiac output
- Deficient knowledge
- Ineffective tissue perfusion (cardiopulmonary)
- Risk for decreased cardiac output
- Risk for ineffective cardiac tissue perfusion
- Risk for infection
- Risk for shock

Perinatal trauma

- Decisional conflict
- Hypothermia
- Impaired gas exchange
- Impaired spontaneous ventilation
- Risk for hypothermia
- Risk for injury
- Risk for ineffective cardiac tissue perfusion
- Risk for ineffective cerebral tissue perfusion
- Risk for shock
- Risk for vascular trauma

Peripheral vascular disease

- Decreased activity tolerance
- Acute pain
- Decreased diversional activity engagement
- Deficient knowledge (specify)

- Impaired physical mobility
- Impaired skin integrity
- Impaired tissue integrity
- Ineffective health self-management
- Risk for adult falls
- Risk for impaired skin integrity
- Risk for ineffective peripheral tissue perfusion
- Risk for vascular trauma
- Risk for impaired tissue integrity
- Risk for infection
- Risk for injury
- Risk for peripheral neurovascular dysfunction
- Risk-prone health behavior

Peritoneal dialysis
- Caregiver role strain
- Defensive coping
- Deficient fluid volume
- Deficient knowledge (specify)
- Disabled family coping
- Disturbed body image
- Excess fluid volume
- Imbalanced nutrition: Less than body requirements
- Impaired resilience
- Interrupted family processes
- Risk for electrolyte imbalance
- Risk for infection
- Risk for injury

Peritonitis
- Acute pain
- Anxiety
- Decreased cardiac output
- Deficient fluid volume
- Nausea
- Risk for decreased cardiac output
- Risk for electrolyte imbalance
- Risk for ineffective cardiac tissue perfusion
- Risk for imbalanced fluid volume
- Risk for infection
- Risk for shock

Personality disorders
- Decisional conflict
- Deficient knowledge
- Disturbed personal identity
- Impaired resilience
- Interrupted family processes
- Loneliness
- Risk for loneliness
- Risk for self-directed violence
- Risk for suicidal behavior

- Sexual dysfunction
- Social isolation

Phobic disorder
- Anxiety
- Disturbed personal identity
- Fear
- Hopelessness
- Ineffective coping
- Powerlessness
- Risk for impaired resilience
- Risk for loneliness
- Social isolation

Placenta previa
- Anxiety
- Fear
- Ineffective denial
- Risk for disturbed maternal–fetal dyad
- Risk for situational low self-esteem

Pleural effusion
- Acute pain
- Dysfunctional ventilatory weaning response
- Hyperthermia
- Impaired gas exchange
- Ineffective breathing pattern
- Risk for infection

Pleurisy
- Acute pain
- Fatigue
- Impaired gas exchange
- Ineffective breathing pattern

Pneumonia
- Bathing self-care deficit
- Feeding self-care deficit
- Toileting self-care deficit
- Deficient fluid volume
- Imbalanced nutrition: Less than body requirements
- Impaired gas exchange
- Impaired physical mobility
- Impaired spontaneous ventilation
- Impaired verbal communication
- Ineffective airway clearance
- Ineffective breathing pattern
- Ineffective tissue perfusion (cardiopulmonary)
- Readiness for enhanced sleep
- Risk for aspiration
- Risk for electrolyte imbalance
- Risk for imbalanced fluid volume
- Risk for infection

Pneumothorax
- Anxiety
- Ineffective breathing pattern
- Fear
- Impaired gas exchange
- Acute pain
- Ineffective tissue perfusion (cardiopulmonary)
- Impaired spontaneous ventilation

Poisoning
- Contamination
- Ineffective tissue perfusion (renal)
- Nausea
- Risk for aspiration
- Risk for bleeding
- Risk for injury
- Risk for poisoning
- Risk for shock

Polycystic kidney disease
- Acute pain
- Anxiety
- Defensive coping
- Deficient knowledge (specify)
- Fear
- Ineffective tissue perfusion (renal)
- Interrupted family processes
- Moral distress
- Risk for infection
- Risk for urinary tract injury

Polycythemia vera
- Acute pain
- Fatigue
- Impaired gas exchange
- Impaired skin integrity
- Ineffective breathing pattern
- Risk for bleeding
- Risk for injury

Postpartum hemorrhage
- Anxiety
- Deficient fluid volume
- Ineffective tissue perfusion
- Risk for bleeding
- Risk for shock
- Risk for unstable blood pressure

Post-traumatic stress disorder
- Ineffective impulse control
- Ineffective relationships
- Defensive coping
- Disabled family coping
- Disturbed personal identity
- Hopelessness
- Ineffective activity planning
- Interrupted family processes

Post-trauma syndrome
- Powerlessness
- Risk for loneliness
- Risk for post-trauma syndrome
- Risk for other-directed violence
- Risk for self-directed violence
- Risk for self-mutilation
- Risk for suicidal behavior
- Situational low self-esteem
- Sleep deprivation

Pregnancy
- Anxiety
- Deficient knowledge (specify)
- Impaired tissue integrity
- Ineffective coping
- Ineffective tissue perfusion (peripheral)
- Interrupted family processes
- Readiness for enhanced childbearing
- Readiness for enhanced relationship
- Risk for constipation

Premature labor
- Anxiety
- Deficient knowledge (specify)
- Effective breastfeeding
- Impaired parenting
- Ineffective coping
- Risk for disturbed maternal–fetal dyad
- Risk for infection
- Situational low self-esteem

Premature rupture of membranes
- Risk for infection

Prematurity
- Compromised family coping
- Disorganized infant behavior
- Hypothermia
- Imbalanced nutrition: Less than body requirements
- Impaired verbal communication
- Ineffective breastfeeding
- Ineffective breathing pattern
- Ineffective infant feeding dynamics
- Ineffective infant suck-swallow response
- Ineffective thermoregulation
- Interrupted breastfeeding
- Neonatal abstinence syndrome
- Readiness for enhanced parenting

▦ Risk for aspiration
▦ Risk for delayed child development
▦ Risk for disorganized infant behavior
▦ Risk for disturbed maternal–fetal dyad
▦ Risk for hypothermia
▦ Risk for impaired parent–infant–child attachment
▦ Risk for ineffective thermoregulation
▦ Risk for sudden infant death

Pressure ulcers
▦ Imbalanced nutrition: Less than body requirements
▦ Impaired physical mobility
▦ Impaired skin integrity
▦ Impaired tissue integrity
▦ Ineffective protection
▦ Risk for deficient fluid volume
▦ Risk for infection

Prolapsed intervertebral disc
▦ Acute pain
▦ Impaired physical mobility
▦ Powerlessness
▦ Urinary retention

Prostate cancer
▦ Acute pain
▦ Chronic sorrow
▦ Deficient knowledge
▦ Imbalanced energy field
▦ Impaired skin integrity
▦ Impaired tissue integrity
▦ Risk for situational low self-esteem
▦ Risk for urinary tract injury
▦ Sexual dysfunction
▦ Urinary retention

Prostatectomy
▦ Acute pain
▦ Disturbed body image
▦ Ineffective protection
▦ Ineffective role performance
▦ Impaired skin integrity
▦ Risk for infection
▦ Urinary retention

Pseudomembranous colitis
▦ Deficient fluid volume
▦ Diarrhea
▦ Impaired skin integrity
▦ Ineffective tissue perfusion (cardiopulmonary)
▦ Ineffective tissue perfusion (GI)
▦ Ineffective tissue perfusion (renal)

▦ Risk for bleeding
▦ Risk for electrolyte imbalance

Psoriasis
▦ Deficient knowledge
▦ Disturbed body image
▦ Impaired skin integrity
▦ Powerlessness
▦ Social isolation
▦ Risk for infection

Pulmonary edema
▦ Decreased activity tolerance
▦ Bathing self-care deficit
▦ Decreased cardiac output
▦ Dysfunctional ventilatory weaning response
▦ Excess fluid volume
▦ Fear
▦ Impaired gas exchange
▦ Impaired verbal communication
▦ Ineffective airway clearance
▦ Ineffective breathing pattern
▦ Ineffective tissue perfusion (cardiopulmonary)
▦ Risk for decreased cardiac output
▦ Risk for ineffective cardiac tissue perfusion
▦ Risk for ineffective cerebral tissue perfusion

Pulmonary embolus
▦ Acute pain
▦ Anxiety
▦ Decreased activity tolerance
▦ Decreased cardiac output
▦ Deficient fluid volume
▦ Impaired gas exchange
▦ Impaired verbal communication
▦ Ineffective breathing pattern
▦ Ineffective tissue perfusion (cardiopulmonary)
▦ Risk for decreased cardiac output
▦ Risk for ineffective cardiac tissue perfusion

Pyelonephritis
▦ Acute pain
▦ Excess fluid volume
▦ Impaired physical mobility
▦ Risk for infection
▦ Risk for electrolyte balance
▦ Risk for imbalanced fluid volume

Pyloric stenosis
▦ Acute pain
▦ Imbalanced nutrition: Less than body requirements
▦ Risk for aspiration

Radiation therapy
- Acute pain
- Deficient fluid volume
- Diarrhea
- Imbalanced nutrition: Less than body requirements
- Impaired oral mucous membrane integrity
- Impaired physical mobility
- Impaired tissue integrity
- Ineffective protection
- Nausea
- Risk for dry mouth
- Risk for impaired oral mucous membrane integrity
- Risk for impaired tissue integrity
- Sexual dysfunction

Rape
- Anxiety
- Fear
- Maladaptive grieving
- Post-trauma syndrome
- Rape-trauma syndrome
- Risk for compromised human dignity
- Risk for thermal injury
- Situational low self-esteem
- Social isolation

Raynaud's disease
- Deficient knowledge (specify)
- Impaired tissue integrity
- Ineffective tissue perfusion (peripheral)
- Risk for impaired skin integrity
- Risk for ineffective peripheral tissue perfusion

Renal calculi
- Acute pain
- Ineffective denial
- Risk for infection
- Risk for urinary tract injury
- Urinary retention

Renal cancer
- Acute pain
- Deficient fluid volume
- Imbalanced energy field
- Readiness for enhanced health literacy
- Risk for electrolyte balance
- Risk for imbalanced fluid volume

Renal disease: End-stage
- Caregiver role strain
- Chronic low self-esteem
- Decisional conflict

- Defensive coping
- Excess fluid volume
- Hopelessness
- Ineffective coping
- Ineffective denial
- Ineffective role performance
- Ineffective sexuality patterns
- Risk for caregiver role strain
- Risk for disuse syndrome
- Risk for infection
- Risk for poisoning
- Risk for spiritual distress
- Risk for unstable blood pressure
- Spiritual distress

Respiratory distress syndrome
- Dysfunctional ventilatory weaning response
- Impaired gas exchange
- Impaired spontaneous ventilation
- Ineffective airway clearance
- Ineffective breathing pattern
- Ineffective thermoregulation
- Risk for infection

Reye's syndrome
- Hyperthermia
- Impaired physical mobility
- Ineffective thermoregulation
- Risk for ineffective thermoregulation

Rheumatoid arthritis
- Decreased activity tolerance
- Acute pain
- Deficient knowledge (specify)
- Disturbed body image
- Dressing self-care deficit
- Impaired physical mobility
- Impaired skin integrity
- Impaired transfer ability
- Ineffective coping
- Ineffective denial
- Ineffective health maintenance behaviors
- Ineffective protection
- Ineffective health self-management
- Insomnia
- Risk for disuse syndrome
- Risk for adult falls
- Risk for ineffective activity planning
- Risk for injury
- Risk-prone health management
- Sexual dysfunction

Salmonella

- Constipation
- Diarrhea
- Hyperthermia
- Nausea
- Risk for imbalanced fluid volume
- Risk for dysfunctional gastrointestinal motility
- Risk for electrolyte imbalance
- Risk for imbalanced fluid volume
- Risk for infection
- Urinary retention

Sarcoidosis

- Decreased activity tolerance
- Acute pain
- Decreased cardiac output
- Disturbed body image
- Impaired gas exchange
- Ineffective breathing pattern

Schizophrenia

- Anxiety
- Bathing self-care deficit
- Caregiver role strain
- Disturbed personal identity
- Dysfunctional family processes
- Disability-associated urinary incontinence
- Hopelessness
- Impaired emancipated decision-making
- Ineffective home maintenance behaviors
- Impaired mood regulation
- Impaired social interaction
- Interrupted family processes
- Ineffective coping
- Ineffective therapeutic family regimen management
- Ineffective health maintenance behaviors
- Ineffective relationship
- Ineffective role performance
- Interrupted family processes
- Insomnia
- Labile emotional control
- Risk for caregiver role strain
- Risk for impaired emancipated decision-making
- Risk for injury
- Risk for poisoning
- Risk for self-directed violence
- Risk for suicidal behavior
- Sexual dysfunction
- Social isolation

Seizure disorders

- Anxiety
- Chronic low self-esteem
- Impaired memory
- Ineffective airway clearance
- Ineffective breathing pattern
- Ineffective coping
- Ineffective health self-management
- Risk for delayed child development
- Risk for adult falls
- Risk for impaired oral mucous membrane integrity
- Risk for injury
- Risk for spiritual distress
- Risk for physical trauma
- Risk-prone health behavior
- Social isolation
- Self-neglect

Self-destructive behavior

- Anxiety
- Chronic low self-esteem
- Ineffective denial
- Risk for poisoning
- Risk for self-directed violence
- Risk for self-mutilation

Sepsis

- Acute confusion
- Acute pain
- Diarrhea
- Dysfunctional ventilatory weaning response
- Hyperthermia
- Hypothermia
- Nausea
- Imbalanced nutrition: Less than body requirements
- Impaired spontaneous ventilation
- Ineffective thermoregulation
- Risk for hypothermia
- Risk for ineffective cardiac tissue perfusion
- Risk for shock

Sexual assault

- Post-trauma syndrome
- Rape-trauma syndrome
- Risk for self-directed violence
- Risk for suicidal behavior

Shaken baby syndrome

- Disabled family coping
- Impaired parenting

- Interrupted family processes
- Risk for impaired parenting
- Risk for ineffective cerebral tissue perfusion
- Risk for impaired attachment
- Risk for injury
- Risk for other-directed violence

Shock

- Decreased cardiac output
- Deficient fluid volume
- Impaired gas exchange
- Impaired oral mucous membrane integrity
- Impaired spontaneous ventilation
- Ineffective airway clearance
- Ineffective tissue perfusion (cardiopulmonary)
- Ineffective tissue perfusion (cerebral)
- Ineffective tissue perfusion (renal)
- Risk for decreased cardiac output
- Risk for electrolyte imbalance
- Risk for infection
- Risk for unstable blood pressure

Sickle cell anemia

- Acute pain
- Impaired gas exchange
- Impaired physical mobility
- Ineffective protection
- Ineffective tissue perfusion (peripheral)
- Ineffective tissue perfusion (renal)

Sjögren's syndrome

- Acute pain
- Risk for corneal injury
- Risk for dry eye
- Impaired oral mucous membrane integrity

Spina bifida

- Impaired bowel continence
- Impaired skin integrity
- Risk for physical immobility
- Risk for latex allergy reaction
- Urinary incontinence

Spinal cord defects

- Chronic low self-esteem
- Impaired urinary elimination
- Readiness for enhanced family coping
- Risk-prone health behavior
- Total urinary incontinence

Spinal cord injury

- Decreased activity tolerance
- Autonomic dysreflexia

- Bathing self-care deficit
- Impaired bowel continence
- Chronic functional constipation
- Chronic pain
- Chronic sorrow
- Constipation
- Decreased diversional activity engagement
- Deficient knowledge (specify)
- Disturbed body image
- Fear
- Hopelessness
- Impaired physical mobility
- Impaired sitting
- Impaired spontaneous ventilation
- Impaired standing
- Impaired transfer ability
- Impaired urinary elimination
- Ineffective airway clearance
- Ineffective health maintenance behaviors
- Ineffective sexuality patterns
- Ineffective health self-management
- Maladaptive grieving
- Moral distress
- Post-trauma syndrome
- Powerlessness
- Readiness for enhanced communication
- Readiness for enhanced therapeutic regimen management
- Risk for autonomic dysreflexia
- Risk for chronic functional constipation
- Risk for constipation
- Risk for delayed child development
- Risk for disuse syndrome
- Risk for impaired skin integrity
- Risk for impaired tissue integrity
- Risk for infection
- Risk for physical trauma
- Risk for adult pressure injury
- Risk for urge urinary incontinence
- Risk-prone health behavior
- Sleep deprivation
- Social isolation
- Mixed urinary incontinence
- Urinary retention

Spinal tumor

- Autonomic dysreflexia
- Impaired bowel continence
- Chronic low self-esteem
- Dressing self-care deficit
- Imbalanced energy field

- Impaired physical mobility
- Impaired urinary elimination
- Ineffective breathing pattern
- Risk for autonomic dysreflexia
- Risk for impaired skin integrity
- Risk for injury
- Risk for urge urinary incontinence
- Sexual dysfunction
- Situational low self-esteem
- Mixed urinary incontinence

Spouse abuse
- Anxiety
- Defensive coping
- Deficient knowledge (specify)
- Fear
- Hopelessness
- Impaired emancipated decision-making
- Post-trauma syndrome
- Powerlessness
- Rape-trauma syndrome
- Readiness for enhanced hope
- Readiness for enhanced knowledge
- Readiness for enhanced parenting
- Readiness for enhanced power
- Readiness for enhanced self-concept
- Readiness for enhanced health self-management
- Risk for impaired emancipated decision-making
- Risk for other-directed violence
- Risk for suicidal behavior
- Stress overload

Streptococcal throat
- Acute pain
- Hyperthermia
- Impaired oral mucous membrane integrity
- Risk for infection

Stroke
- Acute confusion
- Bathing self-care deficit
- Impaired bowel continence
- Caregiver role strain
- Chronic confusion
- Chronic functional constipation
- Chronic sorrow
- Compromised family coping
- Constipation
- Death anxiety
- Deficient knowledge (specify)

- Disturbed body image
- Fatigue
- Frail elderly syndrome
- Disability-associated urinary incontinence
- Hopelessness
- Imbalanced nutrition: Less than body requirements
- Impaired bed mobility
- Impaired gas exchange
- Ineffective home maintenance behaviors
- Impaired memory
- Impaired physical mobility
- Impaired sitting
- Impaired social interaction
- Impaired standing
- Impaired swallowing
- Impaired urinary elimination
- Impaired verbal communication
- Impaired walking
- Ineffective airway clearance
- Ineffective breathing pattern
- Ineffective health maintenance behaviors
- Ineffective sexuality patterns
- Ineffective thermoregulation
- Ineffective tissue perfusion (cerebral)
- Interrupted family processes
- Powerlessness
- Readiness for enhanced family processes
- Risk for decreased activity tolerance
- Risk for aspiration
- Risk for caregiver role strain
- Risk for chronic functional constipation
- Risk for compromised human dignity
- Risk for disuse syndrome
- Risk for frail elderly syndrome
- Risk for impaired skin integrity
- Risk for ineffective thermoregulation
- Risk for injury
- Risk for poisoning
- Risk for adult pressure injury
- Situational low self-esteem
- Sleep deprivation
- Social isolation
- Stress urinary incontinence
- Mixed urinary incontinence
- Unilateral neglect

Suicidal behavior
- Anxiety
- Chronic low self-esteem
- Disturbed personal identity

- Ineffective denial
- Readiness for enhanced spiritual well-being
- Risk for poisoning
- Risk for self-directed violence
- Risk for self-mutilation

Tendinitis
- Acute pain
- Decreased activity tolerance
- Impaired physical mobility
- Ineffective role performance

Testicular cancer
- Acute pain
- Death anxiety
- Disturbed body image
- Fear
- Hopelessness
- Powerlessness
- Sexual dysfunction
- Risk for situational low self-esteem

Thoracic surgery
- Acute pain
- Deficient fluid volume
- Fatigue
- Fear
- Impaired gas exchange
- Ineffective airway clearance
- Ineffective breathing pattern
- Risk for bleeding
- Risk for delayed surgical recovery
- Risk for infection
- Risk for perioperative position injury
- Risk for surgical site infection
- Risk for unstable blood pressure

Thrombophlebitis
- Acute pain
- Impaired gas exchange
- Impaired skin integrity
- Ineffective tissue perfusion (peripheral)
- Risk for impaired skin integrity
- Risk for infection
- Risk for injury
- Risk for vascular trauma

Tracheoesophageal fistula
- Imbalanced nutrition: Less than body requirements
- Risk for aspiration

Tracheostomy
- Imbalanced nutrition: Less than body requirements
- Impaired skin integrity
- Impaired verbal communication
- Risk for dry mouth

Transient ischemic attacks
- Acute confusion
- Impaired memory
- Ineffective tissue perfusion (cerebral)
- Risk for bleeding
- Risk for ineffective cerebral tissue perfusion

Trauma
- Death anxiety
- Disabled family coping
- Risk for bleeding
- Risk for corneal injury
- Risk for ineffective thermoregulation
- Risk for self-directed violence
- Risk for shock
- Risk for urinary tract injury

Trigeminal neuralgia
- Acute pain
- Anxiety
- Deficient knowledge (specify)
- Imbalanced nutrition: Less than body requirements

Tuberculosis
- Deficient community health
- Deficient knowledge
- Fatigue
- Fear
- Impaired dentition
- Impaired gas exchange
- Ineffective airway clearance
- Ineffective breathing pattern
- Ineffective community coping
- Risk for infection
- Risk for loneliness
- Social isolation

Urinary calculi
- Acute pain
- Anxiety
- Impaired urinary elimination
- Ineffective tissue perfusion (renal)
- Risk for infection
- Risk for urinary tract injury

Urinary diversion
- Acute pain
- Constipation
- Disturbed personal identity
- Impaired skin integrity
- Ineffective breathing pattern
- Ineffective sexuality patterns
- Risk for infection
- Sexual dysfunction

Urinary incontinence
- Anxiety
- Disability-associated urinary incontinence
- Impaired skin integrity
- Social isolation
- Stress urinary incontinence
- Mixed urinary incontinence

Urinary tract infection
- Acute pain
- Impaired urinary elimination
- Risk for infection
- Risk for urge urinary incontinence
- Stress urinary incontinence
- Urge urinary incontinence

Uterine prolapse
- Disturbed body image
- Stress urinary incontinence
- Risk for situational low self-esteem

Uterine rupture
- Acute pain
- Deficient fluid volume
- Ineffective tissue perfusion (cardiopulmonary)
- Ineffective tissue perfusion (cerebral)
- Ineffective tissue perfusion (renal)
- Risk for bleeding
- Risk for electrolyte imbalance
- Risk for shock

Vascular insufficiency
- Impaired tissue integrity
- Risk for peripheral neurovascular dysfunction

Viral hepatitis
- Deficient fluid volume
- Imbalanced nutrition: Less than body requirements
- Impaired skin integrity
- Risk for impaired skin integrity
- Risk for infection
- Social isolation

Select Nursing Diagnoses by Population Focus

Adult Health

A

- Decreased Activity Tolerance
- Risk for Decreased Activity Tolerance
- Ineffective Activity Planning
- Risk for Ineffective Activity Planning
- Ineffective Airway Clearance
- Risk for Allergy Reaction
- Anxiety
- Risk for Aspiration
- Autonomic Dysreflexia
- Risk for Autonomic Dysreflexia

B

- Risk for Bleeding
- Risk for Unstable Blood Glucose Level
- Risk for Unstable Blood Pressure
- Disturbed Body Image
- Impaired Bowel Continence
- Ineffective Breathing Pattern

C

- Decreased Cardiac Output
- Risk for Decreased Cardiac Output
- Impaired Comfort
- Acute Confusion
- Risk for Acute Confusion
- Chronic Confusion
- Constipation
- Risk for Constipation
- Perceived Constipation
- Defensive Coping
- Ineffective Coping

- Compromised Family Coping
- Disabled Family Coping

D

- Death Anxiety
- Decisional Conflict
- Ineffective Denial
- Diarrhea
- Risk for Disuse Syndrome
- Decreased Diversional Activity
- Risk for Dry Eye
- Risk for Peripheral Neurovascular Dysfunction

E

- Risk for Electrolyte Imbalance
- Imbalanced Energy Field

F

- Interrupted Family Processes
- Fatigue
- Fear
- Deficient Fluid Volume
- Risk for Deficient Fluid Volume
- Excess Fluid Volume
- Risk for Imbalanced Fluid Volume

G

- Impaired Gas Exchange
- Dysfunctional Gastrointestinal Motility
- Risk for Dysfunctional Gastrointestinal Motility
- Maladaptive Grieving
- Risk for Maladaptive Grieving

H

- Risk-Prone Health Behavior
- Ineffective Health Maintenance Behaviors

- Ineffective Health Self-Management
- Ineffective Family Health Self-Management
- Ineffective Home Maintenance Behaviors
- Hopelessness
- Risk for Compromised Human Dignity
- Hyperthermia
- Hypothermia

I

- Risk for Complicated Immigration Transition
- Disability-Associated Urinary Incontinence
- Mixed Urinary Incontinence
- Stress Urinary Incontinence
- Urge Urinary Incontinence
- Risk for Infection
- Risk for Injury
- Risk for Urinary Tract Injury
- Insomnia

K

- Deficient Knowledge

L

- Risk for Latex Allergy Reaction
- Sedentary Lifestyle
- Risk for Impaired Liver Function
- Risk for Loneliness

M

- Impaired Memory
- Risk for Metabolic Syndrome
- Impaired Physical Mobility
- Moral Distress
- Impaired Oral Mucous Membrane Integrity

N

- Nausea
- Imbalanced Nutrition: Less Than Body Requirements

O

- Obesity
- Risk for Occupational Injury
- Overweight
- Risk for Overweight

P

- Acute Pain
- Chronic Pain
- Chronic Pain Syndrome
- Risk for Poisoning
- Risk for Perioperative-Positioning Injury
- Post-Trauma Syndrome
- Risk for Post-Trauma Syndrome
- Powerlessness

- Risk for Powerlessness
- Risk for Adult Pressure Injury
- Ineffective Protection

R

- Risk for Adverse Reaction to Iodinated Contrast Media
- Impaired Religiosity
- Readiness for Enhanced Religiosity
- Risk for Impaired Religiosity
- Relocation Stress Syndrome
- Ineffective Role Performance
- Caregiver Role Strain
- Risk for Caregiver Role Strain

S

- Bathing Self-Care Deficit
- Dressing Self-Care Deficit
- Feeding Self-Care Deficit
- Toileting Self-Care Deficit
- Readiness for Enhanced Self-Care
- Chronic Low Self-Esteem
- Situational Low Self-Esteem
- Risk for Situational Low Self-Esteem
- Self-Neglect
- Sexual Dysfunction
- Ineffective Sexuality Pattern
- Risk for Shock
- Impaired Sitting
- Impaired Skin Integrity
- Risk for Impaired Skin Integrity
- Sleep Deprivation
- Disturbed Sleep Pattern
- Impaired Social Interaction
- Spiritual Distress
- Risk for Spiritual Distress
- Impaired Spontaneous Ventilation
- Impaired Standing
- Stress Overload
- Risk for Suffocation
- Delayed Surgical Recovery
- Risk for Surgical Site Infection
- Impaired Swallowing

T

- Risk for Thermal Injury
- Ineffective Thermoregulation
- Impaired Tissue Integrity
- Risk for Impaired Tissue Integrity
- Risk for Decreased Cardiac Tissue Perfusion
- Risk for Ineffective Cerebral Tissue Perfusion
- Risk for Ineffective Peripheral Tissue Perfusion

- Impaired Transfer Ability
- Risk for Physical Trauma
- Risk for Vascular Trauma

U

- Unilateral Neglect
- Impaired Urinary Elimination
- Urinary Retention

V

- Dysfunctional Adult Ventilatory Weaning Response
- Dysfunctional Ventilatory Weaning Response
- Impaired Verbal Communication

W

- Impaired Walking
- Wandering

Adolescent Health

B

- Disturbed Body Image

D

- Decisional Conflict

E

- Ineffective Adolescent Eating Dynamics

F

- Risk for Female Genital Mutilation

H

- Ineffective Health Maintenance Behaviors

P

- Risk for Poisoning

R

- Risk for Caregiver Role Strain

S

- Risk for Self-Directed Violence
- Situational Low Self-Esteem
- Social Isolation

T

- Risk for Physical Trauma

Child Health

A

- Risk for Aspiration
- Risk for Impaired Attachment

B

- Disturbed Body Image
- Ineffective Breathing Pattern

C

- Chronic Functional Constipation
- Disabled Family Coping

D

- Impaired Dentition
- Risk for Delayed Child Development
- Diarrhea
- Decreased Diversional Activity

E

- Ineffective Child Eating Dynamics

F

- Fear
- Deficient Fluid Volume
- Risk for Deficient Fluid Volume

H

- Hyperthermia

I

- Risk for Injury
- Risk for Corneal Injury

K

- Deficient Knowledge

N

- Imbalanced Nutrition: Less Than Body Requirements

O

- Overweight
- Risk for Overweight

P

- Acute Pain
- Impaired Parenting
- Risk for Impaired Parenting

R

- Parental Role Conflict

S

- Bathing Self-Care Deficit
- Dressing Self-Care Deficit
- Feeding Self-Care Deficit
- Toileting Self-Care Deficit

T

- Ineffective Thermoregulation

V

- Impaired Verbal Communication

Maternal–Neonatal Health

A
- Anxiety
- Risk for Aspiration

B
- Disorganized Infant Behavior
- Readiness for Enhanced Organized Infant Behavior
- Risk for Disorganized Infant Behavior
- Insufficient Breast Milk Production
- Ineffective Breastfeeding
- Interrupted Breastfeeding
- Readiness for Enhanced Breastfeeding
- Ineffective Breathing Pattern

C
- Ineffective Childbearing Process
- Risk for Ineffective Childbearing Process
- Ineffective Coping
- Compromised Family Coping

E
- Imbalanced Energy Field

F
- Interrupted Family Processes
- Readiness for Enhanced Family Processes
- Deficient Fluid Volume
- Ineffective Infant Feeding Dynamics

H
- Hypothermia
- Risk for Hypothermia

I
- Risk for Infection
- Risk for Injury

J
- Neonatal Abstinence Syndrome
- Neonatal Hyperbilirubinemia
- Risk for Neonatal Hyperbilirubinemia

K
- Deficient Knowledge

M
- Risk for Disturbed Maternal–Fetal Dyad

N
- Imbalanced Nutrition: Less Than Body Requirements

P
- Acute Pain
- Labor Pain
- Impaired Parenting
- Readiness for Enhanced Parenting

S
- Risk for Situational Low Self-Esteem
- Impaired Skin Integrity
- Ineffective Infant Suck-Swallow Response
- Risk for Sudden Infant Death

T
- Ineffective Thermoregulation
- Risk for Ineffective Thermoregulation

U
- Impaired Urinary Elimination

Geriatric Health

A
- Risk for Decreased Activity Tolerance

B
- Risk for Bleeding
- Risk for Unstable Blood Glucose Level
- Risk for Unstable Blood Pressure
- Disturbed Body Image

C
- Decreased Cardiac Output
- Constipation
- Ineffective Coping
- Compromised Family Coping

D
- Ineffective Denial
- Risk for Dry Mouth

E
- Imbalanced Energy Field

F
- Risk for Adult Falls
- Frail Elderly Syndrome
- Risk for Frail Elderly Syndrome

G
- Impaired Gas Exchange

H

- Ineffective Home Maintenance Behaviors
- Risk for Perioperative Hypothermia

I

- Stress Urinary Incontinence
- Risk for Urge Urinary Incontinence
- Risk for Injury

K

- Deficient Knowledge (Specify)

M

- Risk for Metabolic Syndrome
- Impaired Bed Mobility
- Impaired Wheelchair Mobility
- Risk for Impaired Oral Mucous Membrane Integrity

N

- Readiness for Enhanced
- Nutrition

P

- Risk for Poisoning
- Powerlessness

R

- Risk for Relocation Stress Syndrome
- Ineffective Role Performance

S

- Risk for Self-Directed Violence
- Situational Low Self-Esteem
- Ineffective Sexuality Pattern
- Risk for Impaired Skin Integrity
- Social Isolation
- Readiness for Enhanced Spiritual Well-Being
- Risk for Surgical Site Infection

T

- Risk for Ineffective Thermoregulation

V

- Impaired Verbal Communication

Psychiatric and Mental Health

A

- Acute Substance Withdrawal Syndrome
- Risk for Acute Substance Withdrawal Syndrome
- Anxiety

C

- Ineffective Coping

E

- Impaired Emancipated Decision-Making
- Readiness for Enhanced Emancipated Decision-Making
- Risk for Impaired Emancipated Decision-Making
- Labile Emotional Control

F

- Dysfunctional Family Processes
- Interrupted Family Processes

H

- Hopelessness

I

- Risk for Complicated Immigration Transition
- Ineffective Impulse Control
- Risk for Injury

K

- Deficient Knowledge

M

- Impaired Mood Regulation

O

- Risk for Other-Directed Violence

P

- Disturbed Personal Identity
- Risk for Disturbed Personal Identity
- Post-Trauma Syndrome
- Powerlessness

R

- Rape-Trauma Syndrome
- Ineffective Relationship
- Risk for Ineffective Relationship
- Impaired Resilience
- Risk for Impaired Resilience
- Caregiver Role Strain

S

- Risk for Chronic Low Self-Esteem
- Self-Mutilation
- Risk for Self-Mutilation
- Sexual Dysfunction
- Social Isolation
- Chronic Sorrow
- Risk for Suicidal Behavior

V

- Impaired Verbal Communication

Community-Based Health

C
- Contamination
- Risk for Contamination
- Ineffective Community Coping

F
- Fear

H
- Deficient Community Health
- Ineffective Health Maintenance Behaviors

I
- Risk for Infection

K
- Deficient Knowledge

N
- Imbalanced Nutrition: Less Than Body Requirements

P
- Risk for Poisoning

R
- Risk for Caregiver Role Strain

S
- Readiness for Enhanced Spiritual Well-Being
- Impaired Spontaneous Ventilation

Wellness

C
- Readiness for Enhanced Childbearing Process
- Readiness for Enhanced Comfort
- Readiness for Enhanced Communication
- Readiness for Enhanced Coping
- Readiness for Enhanced Community Coping
- Readiness for Enhanced Family Coping

D
- Readiness for Enhanced Decision-Making

H
- Readiness for Enhanced Health Literacy
- Readiness for Enhanced Hope

K
- Readiness for Enhanced Knowledge

P
- Readiness for Enhanced Power

R
- Readiness for Enhanced Relationship
- Readiness for Enhanced Resilience

S
- Readiness for Enhanced Self-Care
- Readiness for Enhanced Self-Concept
- Readiness for Enhanced Sleep
- Readiness for Enhanced Spiritual Well-Being

Organizing Assessment Data

Organizing assessment data assists the nurse in developing patient-centered plans of care. Creating lists of objective and subjective data gives the nurse an overview of the patient's condition; however, it can sometimes be difficult to identify an appropriate nursing diagnosis without grouping assessment data into categories.

Concept maps and care maps are tools that create a visual representation of assessment data that can be organized to identify patient problems, appropriate nursing diagnoses, and relevant nursing interventions. Grouping information in a concept map fosters critical thinking needed to make connections between the patient problem, the medical condition, and nursing interventions, which provide a more holistic view of planning patient care.

To understand the multidimensional nature of patient problems, concept maps can be arranged in many ways. The following concept maps are examples of possible ways to cluster, sort, and organize your patient assessment data to plan and implement nursing care.

Concept map template 1 organizes patient assessment data into categories that provide an overview of the patient condition. This basic concept map will give you an idea of where actual and potential patient problems may exist.

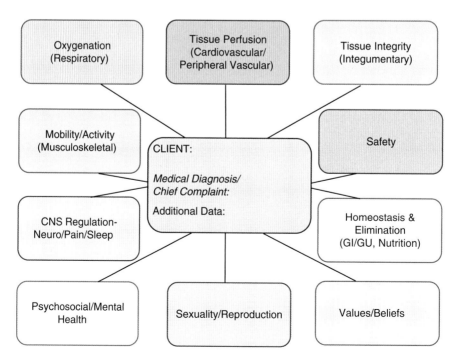

Concept map template 2 follows the nursing process to organize patient data. The problem is identified and stated in NANDA-I terms and the goal and outcomes are established. Nursing interventions can then be identified for the specific patient problem.

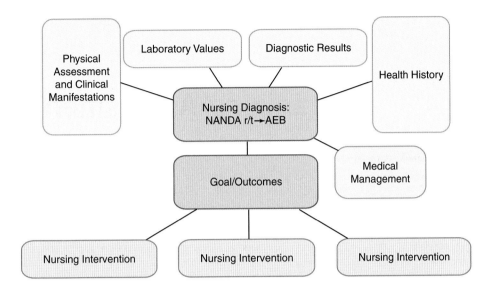

Concept map templates 3 and 4 provide a visual representation of the relationships between the disease process or illness, medical management, and nursing care.

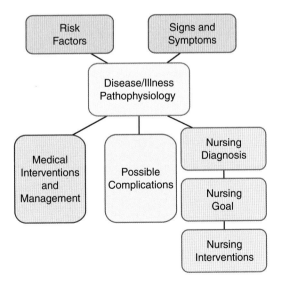

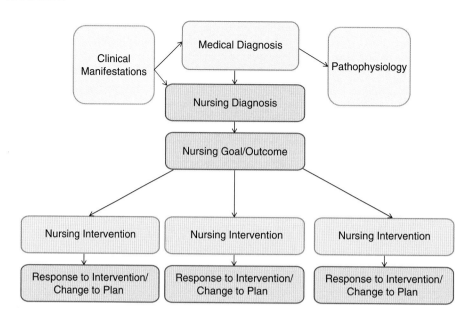

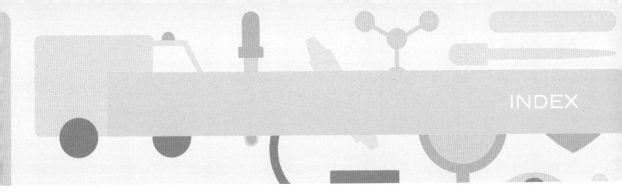

A

Activity Planning, Ineffective, 9
Activity Planning, Risk for Ineffective, 11
Activity Tolerance, Decreased, 2
Activity Tolerance, Risk for Decreased, 5
Acute Substance Withdrawal Syndrome, 12
Acute Substance Withdrawal Syndrome, Risk for, 15
Adolescent Eating Dynamics, Ineffective, 199
Adult Falls, Risk for, 226
Adult Pressure Injury, 510
Adult Pressure Injury, Risk for, 514
Adverse Reaction to Iodinated Contrast Media, Risk for, 17
Airway Clearance, Ineffective, 20
Allergy Reaction, Risk for, 23
Anxiety, 25
Anxiety, Death, 156
Aspiration, Risk for, 30
Attachment, Risk for Impaired, 33
Autonomic Dysreflexia, 36
Autonomic Dysreflexia, Risk for, 40

B

Bathing Self-Care Deficit, 575
Bed Mobility, Impaired, 408
Bleeding, Risk for, 51
Blood Glucose Level, Risk for Unstable, 55
Blood Pressure, Risk for Unstable, 57
Body Image, Disturbed, 60
Bowel Continence, Impaired, 63
Breast Milk Production, Insufficient, 66
Breastfeeding, Ineffective, 69
Breastfeeding, Interrupted, 72
Breastfeeding, Readiness for Enhanced, 74
Breathing Pattern, Ineffective, 77

C

Cardiac Output, Decreased, 81
Cardiac Output, Risk for Decreased, 85
Cardiovascular Function, Risk for Impaired, 87
Caregiver Role Strain, 565
Caregiver Role Strain, Risk for, 571
Child Development, Delayed, 168
Child Development, Risk for Delayed, 171
Child Eating Dynamics, Ineffective, 202
Child Falls, Risk for, 229
Child Pressure Injury, 517
Child Pressure Injury, Risk for, 521
Childbearing Process, Ineffective, 90
Childbearing Process, Readiness for Enhanced, 93
Childbearing Process, Risk for Ineffective, 95
Comfort, Impaired, 98

Comfort, Readiness for Enhanced, 100
Communication, Readiness for Enhanced, 102
Community Health, Deficient, 293
Compromised Human Dignity, Risk for, 324
Confusion, Acute, 104
Confusion, Chronic, 110
Confusion, Risk for Acute, 107
Constipation, 113
Constipation, Chronic Functional, 119
Constipation, Perceived, 126
Constipation, Risk for, 117
Constipation, Risk for Chronic Functional, 123
Contamination, 128
Contamination, Risk for, 131
Coping, Compromised Family, 146
Coping, Defensive, 134
Coping, Disabled Family, 150
Coping, Ineffective, 136
Coping, Ineffective Community, 142
Coping, Readiness for Enhanced, 140
Coping, Readiness for Enhanced Community, 144
Coping, Readiness for Enhanced Family, 153
Corneal Injury, Risk for, 370

D

Decision-Making, Readiness for Enhanced, 159
Decisional Conflict, 161
Denial, Ineffective, 163
Dentition, Impaired, 166
Diarrhea, 180
Disuse Syndrome, Risk for, 183
Diversional Activity Engagement, Decreased, 187
Dressing Self-Care Deficit, 577
Dry Eye, Risk for, 189
Dry Eye Self-Management, Ineffective, 192
Dry Mouth, Risk for, 196

E

Electrolyte Imbalance, Risk for, 206
Elopement Attempt, Risk for, 207
Emancipated Decision-Making, Impaired, 209
Emancipated Decision-Making, Readiness for Enhanced, 215
Emancipated Decision-Making, Risk for Impaired, 212
Energy Field, Imbalanced, 221
Exercise Engagement, Readiness for Enhanced, 223

F

Family Health Self-Management, Ineffective, 308
Family Identity Syndrome, Disturbed, 232
Family Identity Syndrome, Risk for Disturbed, 235

Family Processes, Dysfunctional, 237
Family Processes, Interrupted, 242
Family Processes, Readiness for Enhanced, 245
Fatigue, 248
Fear, 251
Feeding Self-Care Deficit, 580
Female Genital Mutilation, Risk for, 257
Fluid Volume, Deficient, 259
Fluid Volume, Excess, 265
Fluid Volume, Risk for Deficient, 262
Fluid Volume, Risk for Imbalanced, 269
Frail Elderly Syndrome, 271
Frail Elderly Syndrome, Risk for, 274

G

Gas Exchange, Impaired, 277
Gastrointestinal Motility, Dysfunctional, 280
Gastrointestinal Motility, Risk for Dysfunctional, 282
Grieving, Readiness for Enhanced, 289

H

Health Behavior, Risk-Prone, 295
Health Literacy, Readiness for Enhanced, 298
Health Maintenance Behaviors, Ineffective, 300
Health Self-Management, Ineffective, 303
Health Self-Management, Readiness for Enhanced, 306
Home Maintenance Behaviors, Ineffective, 311
Home Maintenance Behaviors, Readiness for Enhanced, 317
Home Maintenance Behaviors, Risk for Ineffective, 315
Hope, Readiness for Enhanced, 319
Hopelessness, 321
Hyperthermia, 331
Hypothermia, 334
Hypothermia, Risk for, 337

I

Immigration Transition, Risk for Complicated, 344
Impulse Control, Ineffective, 346
Infant Behavior, Disorganized, 44
Infant Behavior, Readiness for Enhanced Organized, 47
Infant Behavior, Risk for Disorganized, 49
Infant Feeding Dynamics, Ineffective, 254
Infant Motor Development, Delayed, 174
Infant Motor Development, Risk for Delayed, 177
Infant Suck–Swallow Response, Ineffective, 661
Infection, Risk for, 363
Injury, Risk for, 367
Insomnia, 376

K

Knowledge, Deficient, 380
Knowledge, Readiness for Enhanced, 383

L

Labile Emotional Control, 217
Latex Allergy Reaction, Risk for, 385
Lifestyle, Sedentary, 387
Liver Function, Risk for Impaired, 390
Loneliness, Risk for, 393
Low Self-Esteem, Chronic, 592

Low Self-Esteem, Risk for Chronic, 595
Low Self-Esteem, Risk for Situational, 600
Low Self-Esteem, Situational, 597
Lymphedema Self-Management, Ineffective, 395
Lymphedema Self-Management, Risk for Ineffective, 398

M

Maladaptive Grieving, 285
Maladaptive Grieving, Risk for, 287
Maternal–Fetal Dyad, Risk for Disturbed, 401
Memory, Impaired, 403
Metabolic Syndrome, Risk for, 405
Mobility, Impaired Physical, 412
Mobility, Impaired Wheelchair, 415
Mood Regulation, Impaired, 419
Moral Distress, 422

N

Nausea, 431
Neglect, Unilateral, 719
Neonatal Abstinence Syndrome, 439
Neonatal Hyperbilirubinemia, 326
Neonatal Hyperbilirubinemia, Risk for, 328
Neonatal Hypothermia, 339
Neonatal Hypothermia, Risk for, 341
Neonatal Pressure Injury, 525
Neonatal Pressure Injury, Risk for, 528
Nipple-Areolar Complex Injury, 433
Nipple-Areolar Complex Injury, Risk for, 436
Nutrition, Imbalanced: Less than Body Requirements, 444
Nutrition, Readiness for Enhanced, 448

O

Obesity, 450
Occupational Injury, Risk for, 453
Oral Mucous Membrane Integrity, Impaired, 425
Oral Mucous Membrane Integrity, Risk for Impaired, 428
Other-Directed Violence, Risk for, 455
Overweight, 457
Overweight, Risk for, 460

P

Pain, Acute, 463
Pain, Chronic, 466
Pain, Labor, 471
Pain Syndrome, Chronic, 469
Parental Role Conflict, 559
Parenting, Impaired, 475
Parenting, Readiness for Enhanced, 481
Parenting, Risk for Impaired, 478
Performance, Ineffective Role, 562
Perioperative Hypothermia, Risk for, 484
Perioperative-Positioning Injury, Risk for, 485
Peripheral Neurovascular Dysfunction, Risk for, 441
Personal Identity, Disturbed, 489
Personal Identity, Risk for Disturbed, 492
Poisoning, Risk for, 494
Post-Trauma Syndrome, 497
Post-Trauma Syndrome, Risk for, 501
Power, Readiness for Enhanced, 503
Powerlessness, 504
Powerlessness, Risk for, 508
Protection, Ineffective, 531

R

Rape-Trauma Syndrome, 535
Relationship, Ineffective, 537
Relationship, Readiness for Enhanced, 541
Relationship, Risk for Ineffective, 540
Religiosity, Impaired, 543
Religiosity, Readiness for Enhanced, 545
Religiosity, Risk for Impaired, 547
Relocation Stress Syndrome, 549
Relocation Stress Syndrome, Risk for, 551
Resilience, Impaired, 553
Resilience, Readiness for Enhanced, 557
Resilience, Risk for Impaired, 555

S

Self-Care, Readiness for Enhanced, 585
Self-Concept, Readiness for Enhanced, 587
Self-Directed Violence, Risk for, 589
Self-Mutilation, 603
Self-Mutilation, Risk for, 606
Self-Neglect, 609
Sexual Dysfunction, 611
Sexuality Pattern, Ineffective, 614
Shock Risk for, 616
Sitting, Impaired, 618
Skin Integrity, Impaired, 621
Skin Integrity, Risk for Impaired, 625
Sleep Deprivation, 630
Sleep Pattern, Disturbed, 633
Sleep, Readiness for Enhanced, 628
Social Interaction, Impaired, 636
Social Isolation, 639
Sorrow, Chronic, 642
Spiritual Distress, 644
Spiritual Distress, Risk for, 648
Spiritual Well-Being, Readiness for Enhanced, 650
Spontaneous Ventilation, Impaired, 654
Standing, Impaired, 656
Stress Overload, 658
Stress Urinary Incontinence, 354
Sudden Infant Death, Risk for, 664
Suffocation, Risk for, 666
Suicidal Behavior, Risk for, 669
Surgical Recovery, Delayed, 672

Surgical Recovery, Risk for Delayed, 675
Surgical Site Infection, Risk for, 678
Swallowing, Impaired, 681

T

Thermal Injury, Risk for, 372
Thermoregulation, Ineffective, 685
Thermoregulation, Risk for Ineffective, 688
Thought Process, Disturbed, 690
Thrombosis, Risk for, 693
Tissue Integrity, Impaired, 696
Tissue Integrity, Risk for Impaired, 700
Tissue Perfusion, Ineffective Peripheral, 703
Tissue Perfusion, Risk for Decreased Cardiac, 707
Tissue Perfusion, Risk for Ineffective Cerebral, 708
Tissue Perfusion, Risk for Ineffective Peripheral, 705
Toileting Self-Care Deficit, 583
Transfer Ability, Impaired, 711
Trauma, Risk for Physical, 713

U

Urge Urinary Incontinence, 357
Urge Urinary Incontinence, Risk for, 360
Urinary Elimination, Impaired, 722
Urinary Incontinence, Disability-Associated, 348
Urinary Incontinence, Mixed, 352
Urinary Retention, 726
Urinary Retention, Risk for, 729
Urinary Tract Injury, Risk for, 374

V

Vascular Trauma, Risk for, 717
Ventilatory Weaning Response, Dysfunctional, 737
Ventilatory Weaning Response, Dysfunctional Adult, 733
Verbal Communication, Impaired, 741

W

Walking, Impaired, 745
Wandering, 748